COMMUNITY
NUTRITION

Applying Epidemiology to Contemporary Practice

Gail C. Frank-Spohrer, DrPH, MPH, RD, CHES

Professor of Nutrition
California State University-Long Beach
Long Beach, California

AN ASPEN PUBLICATION®
Aspen Publishers, Inc.
Gaithersburg, Maryland
1996

Library of Congress Cataloging-in-Publication Data

Frank-Spohrer, Gail C.
Community nutrition : applying epidemiology to contemporary
practice / Gail C. Frank-Spohrer.
p.   cm.
Includes bibliographical references and index.
ISBN 0-8342-0784-2
1. Nutritionally induced diseases–Epidemiology. 2. Nutritionally
induced diseases–United States–Epidemiology. I. Title.
RA645.N87F73   1996
614.5'939–dc20
95-48149
CIP

Editorial Resources: Amy Myers-Payne

Library of Congress Catalog Number: 95-48149
ISBN: 0-8342-0784-2

Printed in the United States of America

1 2 3 4 5

*Broad strokes with a population approach
are needed to shift US eating patterns to a
healthier track and to insult the
chronic disease process.*

This book is dedicated with love to my family

my mother, who wanted me to do what she could not,
my father, whose talents were many and whose life was too brief,
my brother Lew and sisters Susan and Deb, who knew I had to do this,
my grandparents, Poppy and Gammy, who helped me find a guiding star
when I was a child,
my sons, Steve and Greg, who intensified the purpose of my life,
my stepdaughter, Heather, who will write her own book someday,
and my husband, Bill, who was always there.

Table of Contents

*For a detailed listing of chapter contents,
please see the first page of each Part.*

Preface

Nutrition is a common word in today's society, but that does not mean that those who say the word understand it. Yet, nutrition science should be translated for all to use and apply to their daily lives for quality living.

The heterogeneity of communities challenges professionals to identify groups at highest risk for nutritional deficiencies, excesses, and chronic disease onset. Community nutrition professionals must know the basic relationship of nutrition to the disease process. This includes the role of nutrition in promoting health and preventing disease and its complications.

Community health, health education, and community nutrition are distinct undergraduate disciplines taught on many US college and university campuses. Graduate programs in nutrition, nursing, and health science, and schools of public health in general, expand the repertoire of health care professionals. A graduate student today may work directly with the public in community-based organizations, clinics, hospitals, and government agencies or plan and implement programs to meet *Healthy People 2000* objectives. Advanced training in community nutrition requires entrance into applied nutritional epidemiology. Professionals must blend the science of nutrition with the principles of epidemiology. This achievement equips the individual with the knowledge and skill to function more effectively and efficiently in the real world.

This book is written to fill the need for an intensive one-semester course in advanced community nutrition or nutritional epidemiology. There are 17 chapters that form three major parts. Each part focuses on a certain level of understanding about disease progression and health care intervention, basically,

- how the health of a community and its members are related to nutrition and eating behavior
- how maintaining a science base and research interest strengthens community nutrition
- how professionals can tackle specific needs of groups based on the age of the group or the disease(s) experienced by the group
- how community nutrition professionals can direct their programs and interventions to either a primary, secondary, or tertiary prevention level

Part I addresses nutrition in US communities and lays the groundwork for primary, secondary, and tertiary prevention. This section contains five chapters, beginning with a discussion of epidemiology and the progression of nutrition care from early activities in public health to today's multicommunity approach to health promotion and disease prevention. Chapter 2 highlights nutrition in the United States today, including a thorough review of allowed health claims on foods, nutraceuticals, and the nutrition education icons such as the Recommended Dietary Allowances and the Food Guide Pyramid. Development of competent community nutrition professionals is presented in Chapter 3, with attention given to developing media savvy and research skills. Chapter 4 addresses groups in the community with special needs such as minority groups and individuals with human immunodeficiency virus (HIV) infection, anorexia, and sustained hunger. Strategic planning for the 21st century concludes Part I by discussing community-based approaches including legislation designed to address community nutrition needs.

Part II focuses on primary prevention of disease by first addressing food-borne illness as a recurrent concern in a community and then stepping across the life cycle with nutritional concerns of each age-specific group. Chapter 6 reinforces the need to maintain the health of a community with a healthy food base, sanitary conditions, and properly trained food service employees. Chapter 7 initiates the discussion on nutrition in the life cycle, with attention to infancy and the preschool years and discussion of the golden window of opportunity to set the foundation for healthy food choices and physically active bodies throughout life. Nutrition issues relevant to school-age children are outlined in a detailed and somewhat urgent manner in Chapter 8. The young-adult and middle-adult years present new challenges to communities as disease morbidity takes form. The needs of adult men and women present challenges in assessment, intervention, and treatment. Chapter 9 discusses issues of concern and strategies for adults. Older adults present a new frontier; more individuals are living longer productive lives, yet many experience extended years of comorbidity with decreasing resources and limited physical abilities. Nutrition issues for older adults are presented in Chapter 10.

Part III broadens the base of understanding of specific chronic diseases and the role of eating behavior in disease development. Both secondary and tertiary prevention are presented. Coronary heart disease and the role of food as an intermediate substrate are presented in Chapter 11. Cancer risk and food components identified in the promotion of the disease are highlighted in Chapter 12. Chapter 13 documents the pivotal role that eating behavior plays in the onset and management of diabetes mellitus. Hypertension and obesity, which are interrelated and respond to similar eating behaviors, are addressed separately in Chapters 14 and 15. With an aging population, nutrition issues related to osteoporosis, arthritis, alcoholism, and renal disease are discussed in Chapter 16. Chapter 17 addresses tertiary prevention and the challenge to avoid complications when clustering of disease occurs (e.g., syndrome X). The development of health education, a framework for diagnosing health problems and programs, and the role of self-management for health and well-being are discussed.

Learning objectives are listed at the beginning of each chapter. The section entitled *High Definition Nutrition* provides key words and definitions within each chapter. "Info Line" presents specific information about professional organizations, educational materials, and resource materials. Relevant *Healthy People 2000* objectives are listed at the end of each chapter beginning in Chapter 3.

Students in various segments of health care—such as health educators, nurses, nutritionists, physical therapists, medical students, sociologists, and behavioral psychologists—often search to understand nutrition and how they can apply nutrition principles to their field. On a daily basis, for example, a health educator may conduct classes for low-income, hypertensive individuals who may depend on the health educator's specific recommendations to alter the health crisis. The health educator may spend one-third of his or her time talking about the role of food and the types of foods to moderate. On the other hand, the health educator may set up a program to monitor the weight and blood pressure of hypertensives and refer them to in-depth classes conducted by a nutritionist. The nutritionist, often a registered dietitian, may deal directly with eating and exercise programs, one-on-one counseling, and specific weight management issues. This professional may review objective data including biochemical and physiological measures, integrate information on food preferences, and then recommend practical eating patterns for individuals. In both of the situations described, the health care professional needs a working knowledge of the hypertensive disease, the role of foods in the disease process, the best approach for managing an eating and exercise change process, and communication skills to convey important nutrition education information to the clients.

This text is written to assist professionals with their many and varied tasks. To contribute to society, health care professionals must know the science, recognize the ills, and apply their skills to everyday events. The author hopes you have a fruitful semester journey through this book. May it serve as your blueprint to build a healthier society.

Acknowledgments

This book was a labor of love and discipline. Without my love for the science of nutrition and the field of epidemiology blended with my passion for merging the two, I do not think I would have accepted the challenge of writing this text. The process was consuming.

Now, surprisingly, the task of writing a book actually seems minor! It is behind me. What else would I have been doing with my extra time? How else could I contribute to both fields and to the newer generations who will be climbing the professional mountain of nutritional epidemiology.

Many individuals have framed my thoughts—and yes, indeed, the writing process has been a scholarly effort. I hope it has been one that even two very important public school teachers might be proud—Mrs. Scott, my 8th grade English teacher who drilled the "helping verbs" into my head in Shamrock, Texas, and Mrs. Malone, my 11th grade English teacher who rejected my use of the word *blueprint* in a report I wrote at Cooper High School in Abilene, Texas.

Maybe even my professors from Texas Tech University, Lubbock, Texas, and Tulane University in New Orleans, would be proud to read and use my work. They were all with me for every page, especially Willa Vaughn Tinsley, Ph.D.; Mina Lamb, Ph.D.; Clara McPherson, Ph.D.; Angela Boren, Ph.D.; and Margaret Harden, Ph.D.; from my Tech years; and Grace Goldsmith, M.D.; Ann Metzinger, Dr.P.H., R.D.; and Bill Bertrand, Ph.D.; at Tulane University. Tucked away on a few pages are motivating memories such as attending the First White House Conference on Food, Nutrition and Health in Washington, DC, in 1969 when I was a college senior at Texas Tech University. At the conference, everyone had a different definition for the word *hunger*. Equally motivating was taking maternal and child health classes from Cecily Williams, M.D., who coined the word *kwashiorkor*, and participating in project meetings with Rose Ann Langham, Dr.P.H., R.D., at the Louisiana State Department of Health.

I have been fortunate to have worked beside many veterans of public health and public health nutrition, such as Margaret Moore, H.Ph.D. We spent many hot, sticky summer days in her French Quarter apartment in New Orleans working on computerization of nutrient data. How blessed I was to have been selected to complete my public health field experience in Florida with Mildred Kaufman, M.S., R.D., and Francis Hoffman, M.S., R.D., in various counties stretching from the Gulf to the Atlantic Ocean in the summer of 1972.

A decade of experience working with the late Antonie Wouter Voors, M.D., Dr.P.H., and the late John Harris, M.D., both in the Bogalusa Heart

Study (BHS), enriched my understanding of risk factors in children. The Community Coordinator for the first decade of the BHS, Imogene Talley, remains a dear friend and a mentor in securing community support for research. My 16-year experience with the BHS will always flavor my thinking and writing. Thanks go to Gerald Berenson, M.D., for selecting me to direct the dietary investigations and to the multidisciplinary BHS staff with whom I worked. Developing and adhering to protocols, publishing dozens of manuscripts, and helping to write several books equipped me with skills to write my own book.

All these past events and people, and numerous other individuals not mentioned herein, motivated me on a daily basis to write yet one more page, to add just one more reference, and to share just one more avenue of thought. The past truly complemented the present. The present is likewise dotted with many friends who have supported the cause.

Pam Harris, M.S., R.D., L.D., and Michael Brown, Aspen Publishers, Inc., had faith in my ability to write a new text for community nutrition. I am extremely grateful for their support and vision.

Shelly Hirabayashi, B.S., was indispensable as my typist. She was dedicated to the effort for two years and may not realize how much a partner she was in seeing this book to completion. Thank you so very much, Shelly! Diana Lamb, B.S., R.D., worked diligently formatting and organizing references. She worked around a pregnancy and the birth of her second child, Kyle. Thanks for the support, Diana! Ranya Atiyeh, M.S., R.D., created many of the illustrations using her computer skills. Thanks, Ranya!

Numerous people assisted with identification of materials and references. Dwayne Reed, M.D., constructively reviewed several chapters. R.J. Kuczmarski, Ph.D., provided reprints of manuscripts and tabular data on height and weight of children. Doris Fredericks located material on preschool children's nutrition. Michelle van Eyken, M.P.H., R.D., provided community nutrition reference material and shared her philosophy and thoughts. Edwina Williams, R.D., M.P.A. compiled information on the Cooperative Extension System. Judith Wylie-Rosett, Ed.D., R.D., and Barbara Paprock, R.D., assisted with diabetes mellitus reference material. Arnell Hinkel, M.S., R.D., supplied several articles on community-based programs. Diane Allensworth, Ph.D., R.N., provided material on comprehensive school health. Mindy Kurzer, Ph.D., Elaine Stone, Ph.D., Winston Craig, Ph.D., and Michael Mudd located important illustrative material. Pat McKinney, M.S., R.D., provided information on US Department of Agriculture programs. Staff at the National Heart, Lung and Blood Institute were generous in providing reports and reference material.

Judy Ogunji, M.S., R.D., and Cindy Baylis, R.D., both of the Long Beach WIC Program, provided historic information about WIC (Special Supplemental Food Program for Women, Infants and Children). Jennifer Gilbertson, B.S., assisted with the tedious task of obtaining permissions to reprint tables and figures. Kim Bailey, B.S., collated materials for chapters. Tracy Lundy, M.S., assisted with a case study illustration.

This community of friends fueled my effort and I am sincerely grateful.

Part I

Nutrition in US Communities

Epidemiology—The Foundation of Community Nutrition

Learning Objectives

- Define epidemiology, the traditional epidemiologic model to explore disease causation, and various types of epidemiologic studies.
- Track the early history of epidemiologic exploration.
- Characterize nutritional epidemiology.
- Identify the characteristics of a chronic disease.
- Discuss the purpose of surveillance and monitoring in epidemiologic exploration.
- Describe various rates used to characterize or monitor health status of samples or populations of people.

High Definition Nutrition

Confidence interval (CI)—the probability that a value would be within a range (e.g., 95% CI).
Nutritional epidemiology—the study of eating behavior and how it influences the etiology, occurrence, prevention, and treatment of disease.
Pathway linking food and health—dietary component → food → food group → eating pattern → health/disease.

Sample size—the number of individuals surveyed.
Standard error—the square root of the variance divided by the sample size.
Variance—the extent of dispersion of individual data points around the mean value for a variable.

The epidemiologic fabric was woven together largely from the numerical (quantitative) method, the development of a vital statistics system, the stimulus of a hygienic or public health movement, and the concept of comparative studies. It has now matured as a scientific discipline so that its study is necessary for a full understanding of the etiology of human and other diseases as well as their prevention and treatment.[1(p43)]

Epidemiology is the study of the occurrence and determinants of health events among people. It is a process to identify and to control health problems.[2] It uses biostatistics, statistical processes and methods applied to the analysis of biological phenomena, to describe and quantitate health events and the factors that place individuals at risk for health events. Epidemiology began as an approach to control communicable disease.

The methods and principles have been applied with equal success to improve our understanding of chronic disease.[3]

Epidemiology is the basic science for public and community health. It characterizes the health status of a community and can influence public health policy. Baseline data are used as the foundation for program planning, which may involve treatment and monitoring an intervention or monitoring the effectiveness of a primary prevention or awareness campaign. The epidemiologic scope ranges from maternal and child health to adolescent school health, on one hand, and from health education in the managed-care setting to well-defined protocols to treat life-threatening disease among older adults, on the other hand. Epidemiology provides a canvas upon which health care paints the story of people in their daily life.

The role of human behavior in health and illness has created a new generation of approaches to explore disease etiology and treatment.[4] Behavioral epidemiology assesses what people do and what they avoid. Nutritional epidemiology focuses on eating behavior and how that behavior influences health status, disease morbidity, and mortality. These approaches are in contrast to clinical medicine, which focuses on diagnosing and treating "sick" people. As the 21st century begins, community nutrition has reached a new level of functioning—one that complements what people choose to eat with programs and guidance about how to make healthy food choices for health promotion and disease prevention.

EPIDEMIOLOGY'S EARLY HISTORY

Twentieth-century epidemiology is built on events that occurred over 200 years ago. In 1662 John Graunt, of England, quantified birth, death, and disease occurrence. He identified differences between men and women, and between urban and rural locations. He also analyzed infant deaths and characterized seasonal variations. William Farr extended Graunt's contribution by collecting and analyzing mortality statistics for Great Britain. He developed the field of vital statistics and disease classifications and identified the effects of marital status and occupation on morbidity and mortality.

Noah Webster (1758–1843), who compiled the first American dictionary, studied epidemics of the New World. In *Epidemic and Pestilential Diseases*, he related specific events in the environment to influenza, yellow fever, and scarlet fever.

John Snow (1813–1858), an anesthesiologist, is called "the father of field epidemiology." In 1854 he studied cholera outbreaks in London; after determining where cases lived and worked, he created a spot map. Snow hypothesized that water was a source of cholera infection and marked where water pumps were located. He linked cases to the water source. He noted that a number of cases occurred around the Broad Street pump. Further, he observed that individuals who did not contract cholera lived near a brewery, where they worked and received their water supply. To thwart the disease, the handle of the Broad Street pump was removed and the source of the cholera was stopped.

Snow studied another cholera outbreak and developed sequential steps to investigate disease outbreaks. He provided the classical process of describing individuals with and without disease, establishing testable hypotheses, and then testing the hypotheses with individuals matched on important characteristics. In effect, Snow used what we now call epidemiologic techniques to identify water as a substrate for transmitting cholera and to evoke public health action.[4]

MODERN EPIDEMIOLOGY

By the 1900s epidemiologic methods were extended to noninfectious diseases. Since World War II, research methods and theoretical frameworks for epidemiologic exploration have flourished. Epidemiology has expanded to include health-related outcomes other than disease.[5] For example, behaviors, knowledge, and attitudes of individuals and groups have been evaluated as predisposing or antecedent to the occurrence of health events. This is demonstrated in studies by Doll and Hill linking smoking to lung cancer.[6] The Framingham Heart Study, spanning over

40 years, has observed the role of men's personal and physiological characteristics on cardiovascular disease morbidity and mortality.[7] The Bogalusa Heart Study (BHS), using an observational, natural history design, focuses on an entire community of school-age children.[8] The Minnesota Heart Health Program, the Stanford Heart Disease Prevention Trials, and the North Karelia Study have multidimensional study designs.[9-11] The Multiple Risk Factor Intervention Trial was a major clinical trial enrolling more than 50,000 men at clinical sites across the United States.[12]

NUTRITIONAL EPIDEMIOLOGY

James Lind conducted one of the first if not the first experimental trial of a nutrition-based disease, scurvy, which was common on all long trips by sea. On May 20, 1747, he set sail on the *Salisbury*. While at sea, 12 sailors developed scurvy. Symptoms were identical among the individuals: all had "putrid" gums and weakness in their limbs. Their breakfast consisted of water and sweetened gruel, and other meals consisted of fresh mutton broth or puddings with a boiled sweet biscuit. Sometimes barley and raisins, rice and currants, or sago and wine were served.

Lind devised a modern intervention trial with five strategies:

1. Once a day, two patients received a quart of cider to gargle and then swallow on an empty stomach.
2. Two patients were given two spoons of vinegar, three times a day on an empty stomach, and had vinegar added to their cereals and other foods. They were also required to gargle with vinegar.
3. Two patients drank a half pint of sea water every day.
4. Two others received two oranges and one lemon every day on an empty stomach.
5. The final pair consumed a mixture consisting of nutmeg tree, garlic, mustard seed, and other herbs. They also drank barley water that was mixed with tamarind, and periodically they had a gentle enema.

The men who consumed oranges and lemons had the most rapid recovery and reported to duty after six days. Their bloody gums disappeared, and they appeared healthy before the ship reached land on June 16.

The result of this experiment was the identification of an effective therapeutic agent for treating a disorder and preventing its occurrence. The experiment resulted in a health policy in 1795 that required that limes or lime juice be included in the meals of all sailors. Thus, sailors were nicknamed "limeys."[1]

In 1923 Joseph Goldberger conducted what is considered a classic epidemiologic investigation that altered the belief that pellagra was an infectious disease. Goldberger observed that health care personnel attending patients with pellagra did not develop the disease. By studying individuals with and without the disease, he hypothesized and proved that diet initiated the disease.[13,14] Nicotinic acid was later determined to be the specific dietary deficiency causing pellagra among the patients.[5]

These classical studies and events laid the groundwork for nutritional epidemiology. Simply defined, nutritional epidemiology is the study of eating behavior and how it influences the etiology, occurrence, prevention, and treatment of disease. Nutritional epidemiology is the great-grandchild and hybrid of epidemiology, nutrition, and public health. The sequence of development might be envisioned as follows:

> Public health → Epidemiology → Public health nutrition → Community nutrition → Nutritional epidemiology

Community nutrition is a contemporary and comprehensive discipline that encompasses, among other disciplines, public health nutrition. The beginning of public health nutrition can be traced to the early efforts of Ellen Richards and Mary Abel in home economics and public health in the late 1800s.[15,16] The US Children's Bureau was formed as a result of the first White House Conference on Children in 1909. Considered the mother of public health nutrition, the Children's Bureau initiated nutrition publications, led children's campaigns, and pioneered community-based programs.[17]

In 1917, the state of Massachusetts employed its first nutritionist and followed in 1922 to employ a second one.[18] Responsibilities involved development and distribution of nutrition pamphlets and professional education. These early efforts complemented the work of Frances Stern and Lucy Gillett, who blended nutrition education into pediatricians' practices and special clinics.[19] A brief chronology of the development of nutrition positions, services, and departments at the state level is outlined in Table 1-1.

Public health nutrition has developed in the United States in response to numerous societal events and changes, including the following:

- infant mortality, access to health care
- epidemics of communicable disease
- poor hygiene and sanitation, malnutrition
- agriculture and food production
- economic depression, wars, civil rights
- aging of the population
- behavior-related problems, chronic diseases
- poverty, immigration
- preschool/after-school child care, and school-based meals

As public health nutrition has evolved, professional practice standards and training qualifications have developed.[20] Assessing, screening, and monitoring individuals, groups, and communities have become more common. Indicators of effectiveness and efficiency have been identified and have set the stage for improved opportunities for research.[21,22]

Public health nutrition has developed in response to federal legislation, but the field has also lead the charge to create new or to change old legislation. The WIC program demonstrates the arduous effort on the part of public health nutritionists to market the program to nonbelievers, to evaluate and enroll eligible women and children, to employ and train staff, and to testify and lobby for increased funding for prenatal and infant care to meet the needs of a growing target population.[17]

Today an environment exists in which chronic disease control has emerged as a priority. Public health nutrition provides a national resource base to address nutritional needs across the life cycle. The emerging field of nutritional epidemiology is enriched by this valuable resource base, yet it has its own identity. Eating behavior (rather than diet) and specific methods to collect data about

---

Table 1-1 Chronology of the Early Development of Nutrition Positions and Services within the United States

Year	Activity
1917	First public health nutritionist employed in Massachusetts.
1922	Second public health nutritionist employed in Massachusetts.
1936	11 nutrition positions established in 4 states.
1936	First nutrition consultant, Marjorie Heseltine, employed at the US Children's Bureau, which initiated a concerted effort to include nutrition services at the state level.
1939	39 nutrition positions existed in 24 states.
1938	First qualifications established for nutritionists in public health.
1945	45 state health departments had nutritionists.
1952	Association of State and Territorial Public Health Nutrition Directors was organized.
1969	More than 300 nutrition positions established in 53 Maternal and Infant Health Programs and 58 Children and Youth Programs.
1973	Nutrition programs for older patients began to establish nutrition staff positions at the state level.
1981	Guidelines for specialized services in prenatal care were developed and revised in 1992.
1995	US Congress appropriated $3.5 billion for the Special Supplemental Food Program for Women, Infant and Children (WIC), which included coverage of positions for nutritionists and nutrition aides.

Source: Data from Egan M.C., Public Health Nutrition: A Historic Perspective, *Journal of the American Dietetic Association*, Vol. 94, No. 3, pp. 298–304, American Dietetic Association, © 1994.

eating behavior and its relation to wellness and disease are the essence of nutritional epidemiology. The process is dynamic. Nutritional epidemiology explores what people eat and how long they follow certain food patterns; how much people eat on the average and how their eating patterns change over time, as they age; why they choose the foods they eat; whether lifestyles, taste, economics, food availability, or some other factor has the greatest impact on health; and who eats what (for example, who avoids certain foods while eating other foods in excess). The methods used to investigate, monitor, or ensure adherence to an intervention not only follow the epidemiologic process and study designs but also address reliability, validity, and standardization. Conducting community nutrition programs to meet *Healthy People 2000* objectives presents the current challenge and the agenda for nutritional epidemiology.

THE TERRITORY OF EPIDEMIOLOGY— PRINCIPLES AND APPLICATION

Epidemiologic methods are tools to explore disease occurrence, treatment, prevention, and cure. A traditional model explores the causes of infectious disease, using three components: an agent, a host, and an environment that is conducive to linking the first two components. This model does not differentiate between the strength of any of the three components. The environment influences agent, host, and the process that links the two. Figure 1-1 illustrates this model.[1,5]

In the infectious disease model, an agent has historically been an infectious microorganism, bacterium, virus, parasite, or other microbe whose presence is required for disease occurrence. The agent alone may cause disease. In a noninfectious disease model, an agent may be a chemical or toxin, or a missing physical or behavioral factor. It might even be multifactorial. An example of a chemical factor is coal tar, which causes lung cancer. An example of a behavioral factor is a sedentary lifestyle, which promotes weight gain.

Host factors are personal characteristics that are influenced by the type, intensity, duration, and response of one's exposure to an etiologic agent. Age, ethnicity, sex, socioeconomic status, eating patterns, exercise behaviors, and lifestyle are examples. Some personal characteristics such as age, sex, and ethnicity are nonmodifiable, but some are modifiable. Characteristics that can be changed include nutritional status, leisure time activity, geographic location, and occupation.

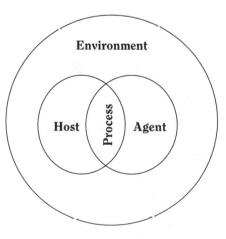

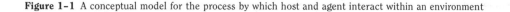

Figure 1-1 A conceptual model for the process by which host and agent interact within an environment

These modifiable host characteristics can be considered environmental factors.

Environmental factors are external factors that encompass an agent and a host. They may be exclusively physical such as geology, climate, or living surroundings (e.g., an urban housing area in the southern United States). An environmental factor may have multiple levels, such as low, middle, and high socioeconomic status (SES). Low SES is often linked to crowding, poor sanitation, and reduced availability of health and social services. High SES may evoke excessive behaviors such as heavy drinking, overeating, and risk taking.

The required trio of agent, host, and environment interact to produce various health outcomes including disease. Exploration of disease etiology demands an awareness of each component and a vigilance using epidemiologic methods.[5]

The *natural history* of a disease is the progression of a disease in an individual or group over time. No interventions occur, other than changes occurring naturally for all people. To document natural history, the individual's or group's exposure to environmental factors that place them at risk of diseases are assessed.

As the individual or group is followed, morbidity and mortality are monitored. Outcomes are compared with host and environmental factors to estimate the effect each has on morbidity or mortality.[23] A model that shows the relationship between understanding of disease progression and level of intervention is presented in Figure 1-2.

Natural history is influenced by the genetic variability of individuals and their response to the environment. With an infectious disease, if a host is exposed to a causal agent frequently and with great intensity, disease will likely occur. For a chronic disease such as breast cancer, the critical factors causing the disease may include an initiating factor (such as not breastfeeding) and a promoter (such as dietary fat and low fiber intake) to cause an effect. Reduced exposure to the promoter at the early stage of development constitutes *primary prevention*.

Because chronic disease progression generally includes an asymptomatic period, individuals and groups are unaware of their exposure and the effect their behavior can have on the disease. This phase is called an incubation period for infectious disease and a latency period for chronic disease. The range of time for this phase varies

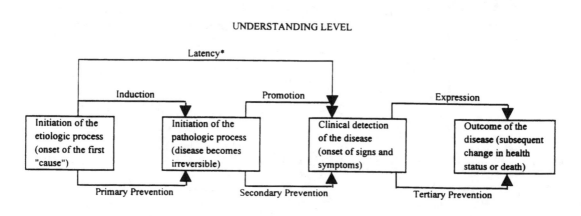

UNDERSTANDING LEVEL

INTERVENTION LEVEL

*Observed duration from the onset of any particular cause to disease detection.

Figure 1-2 Levels of epidemiologic research: a conceptual elaboration. *Source:* Adapted from *Epidemiologic Research: Principles and Quantitative Methods* solution manual by D.G. Kleinbaum and L.L. Kupper, p. 22, with permission of Van Nostrand Reinhold, © 1982.

greatly—from two to four hours for a food-borne illness such as salmonella poisoning, to as many as 20 to 40 years for arteriosclerosis. Even for one specific disease, the incubation period will vary as a result of environmental and host characteristics. For a chronic disease, positive eating or exercise habits may forestall the disease progression by years.

Another example is a nutritionally deprived older person who may demonstrate signs of degenerative diseases earlier than a nutritionally sound individual. Screening programs can identify risk factor levels as the individual ages and can alert health professionals to potential high-risk individuals or groups who require intervention. Early screening for chronic disease risk factors and an intervention focused on those factors may forestall the disease progression.

Once symptoms appear, the individual moves from a subclinical to a clinical disease phase. The clinical diagnosis documents this transition. Intervention at this point is termed *secondary prevention*. The outcome varies, and clinical disease may or may not progress. The disease expression may result in a single diagnosis sustained and treated for 20 years. Such is the case for a single, treatable diagnosis of hypercholesterolemia. On the other hand, comorbidity or multiple illnesses may occur that include the initial diagnosis of hypercholesterolemia but later combine with obesity, diabetes, and hypertension. Intervention to reduce the severity of the comorbidity and death is called *tertiary prevention*.

In primary, secondary, and tertiary prevention, the association of factors or variables is the basis of action. The association between two variables can be explored by statistical means. If the change (increase or decrease) of one variable parallels a change in a second variable, then an association may exist. A *positive association* occurs when two variables increase (e.g., as body weight increases, blood pressure increases). When one variable increases and a second decreases, an *inverse or negative association* occurs (e.g., as insulin level increases, blood sugar level decreases). Significance of association can be tested using a Pearson product moment correlation, for example. The statistical r value

of 1 is perfect agreement; a value of 0 means no agreement.

Rarely are significant correlations of the magnitude of >0.600 found when testing the association between a dietary component and a risk factor variable. In fact, it is more common to see significant correlation analysis at the p <0.05 level of significance, at r = 0.250 to 0.400, depending on the sample size.

Error can occur. Bias, which might be considered an error that occurs in unknown ways, can lead to overestimating or underestimating a characteristic, quality, or variable. An error or bias that can occur in the exploration of a diseases is called *confounding*. A factor is considered a *confounding variable* if it is associated with both the health outcome and the risk factor being studied. Obesity and smoking are considered confounding variables in many studies.

Measurement of confounding variables increases one's precision when evaluating how variables relate and how they influence potential health outcome. When published research studies identify variables that are associated with health outcomes, these variables could then become potential confounders to be assessed in the next research study. The purpose is to explore further their true association or effect on the outcome.

Extreme *outliers* or unusual values can distort the statistical description of the data. To avoid this distortion, researchers often remove these values from the analysis, but the process is complicated by the ambiguity in defining the outliers. They can be unreasonable on the basis of biological fact, or they may represent measurement error from a human or from equipment failure. Outliers can be defined statistically as significant deviations from a measure of central tendency of the distribution.

The easiest way to identify outliers is to examine bivariate scatterplots of the distribution of the data. The values that lie markedly outside the population are suspect. If the outliers are confirmed as errors, they can be removed from subsequent analyses. There are two concerns for nutrition or dietary variables: (1) outliers are often dismissed as errors to "clean" the data and increase the r value, which may be a mistake;

(2) the extreme values may be real, because individuals can make severe behavioral changes (for example, individuals can have fat intake less than 20% or more than 40% of total energy), which dramatically alters a mean value for a group or a correlation coefficient.

Surveillance or monitoring are processes used to assess community health. They allow an individual, agency, or research group to collect, analyze, interpret, and disseminate health data on a continuous basis.[24] Surveillance in public health is called "information for action,"[25] and it profiles a community's health status. Programs can later address the identified community health problems with prevention and control strategies. Sophisticated surveillance systems use computer technology, link data from several communities and states to provide a broader base of data, detect potential problems, and influence programs and policy. Surveillance data can guide policy makers to develop and to reassess interventions. Epidemiologic techniques are used to assess community health and to identify potential solutions to problems. Several types of studies are described below.

Types of Studies

Population or Community Health Assessment

This type of study assesses the health of the population or community. The type, cost, availability, and accessibility of services are studied. Health status—defined as disease risk factor levels, morbidity, and mortality—is measured. Public policy and program planning may stem from these assessments.

The Minnesota Community Prevention Program for Cardiovascular Diseases paired six Minnesota communities: one community provided an intensive educational program for cardiovascular risk factor reduction, and the other served as a comparison. A pair of medium-sized towns were studied initially, then a set of larger towns, and then suburban census tracts. This sequential, comparative design had the scientific advantage of control and repetition, and the practical value of economy and opportunity to improve as the program advanced (Appendix 1–A).

Assessment of Individual Health Choices

Often, individuals unknowingly base decisions on epidemiologic data. For example, when an individual walks a minimum of 20 minutes three times a day, eats five fruits or vegetables a day, or trims the fat from a serving of meat, that person bases his or her knowledge and behavior on epidemiologic data linking these behaviors to health promotion. Today, epidemiologists may explore how leisure activities and eating behaviors influence chronic disease risk factors such as adiposity, serum total cholesterol, and blood pressure. The Stanford Three-Community Heart Disease Prevention Program used mass media campaigns and face-to-face instruction to change knowledge and improve attitudes and behaviors about cardiovascular risk factors. Significant change was noted and sustained for the intervention communities compared to the control community.[26]

Clinical Profile

Epidemiologists collaborate with clinicians to diagnose individuals and to classify them accurately into groups or communities with and without risk factors and with and without disease. The Pawtucket Heart Study demonstrates this type of approach. From 1981 to 1993, researchers completed biennial cardiovascular risk factor (CVRF) surveys in two cities of randomly selected residents who were 18 to 64 years old. The purpose was to test the hypothesis that CVRF intensity or prevalence would decrease significantly in the city that provided multilevel education, screening, and counseling (regarding risk factor, behavior change, and community activation).[27] Small, but nonsignificant, positive differences were noted in the intervention community for blood cholesterol and blood pressure. A significant increase was seen for body-mass index in the comparison community. The predicted cardiovascular disease rates were 16% (significant) and 8% less in the intervention community than in the comparison community during and after the education. These findings suggest the need for sustained, consistent effort within the community, along with national directives and policies from the outside, to reinforce the importance of the intervention.[27]

Etiological Factor Exploration

Data from epidemiologic studies cannot prove a causal association between a factor and a disease. Data can identify risk factors of a disease that require further testing to prove a cause-and-effect relationship. The data can effect change in behavior, norms, and public policy. The Framingham Heart Study and the Bogalusa Heart Study are examples of adult and pediatric community assessments using cohorts and cross-sectional samples, respectively, to identify risk factors for cardiovascular disease.[7,8]

The Bogalusa Heart Study (BHS) is a community-based program that examines the distribution and secular trends of CVRF variables in youth, the interrelationships of the variables, and genetic and environmental determinants (such as dietary and biobehavioral factors). The investigation is a prospective survey with a mixed epidemiologic design to study the early natural history of atherosclerosis in a biracial pediatric population. Cross-sectional studies linked with longitudinal observations of specific age cohorts (groups whose members were all born in the same year) permit collection of data over an extended range of ages from birth to over 30 years of age, but within a short observational time period. The biracial population is 65% Caucasian and 35% African American (see Appendix 1–B).[8]

The Framingham Heart Study began in 1948 as a survey of 2,366 men and 2,873 women 30 to 62 years old. Survivors of this original cohort have been monitored every two years for their risk factor status. Data from offspring and spouses of participants in the Framingham Heart Study showed that certain characteristics can aggregate in families and that these characteristics can be called *risk factors* for coronary heart disease (CHD). The study identified the major risk factors and established a database that provided rates for CHD separately for men, their children, and their grandchildren.

Community Nutrition Assessment

Assessing the initial awareness among community members about nutrition and then supporting community nutrition needs and services are essential if changes in behavior, norms, and public policy are to be evaluated. Table 1–2 presents a subjective data assessment grid that can be used to evaluate the knowledge of nutrition, perceived need for nutrition, and attitude of health care professionals and other important community members. These data, along with data that characterize the community's health status, are needed to develop programs for a healthier living environment.

Types of Analysis

Assessment and monitoring provide measures of disease frequency and yield data to evaluate the effectiveness and efficiency of programs or interventions. *Effectiveness* means producing positive results, and *efficiency* means producing positive results at the lowest cost.

Rates can numerically express effectiveness and efficiency. They can be used to define the risk of disease in populations in specific geographic areas (such as cities, states, and countries) and in population subgroups by age, sex, ethnicity, and occupation. Rates can be defined for a specific time, such as a month or a year. As rates are monitored, change over time can be defined. Location defines a geographic unit, such as urban versus rural or institutionalized versus free-living. Community characteristics can be informative, such as socioeconomic, marital, or educational status.

Rates are essential to compare or contrast groups or to establish whether a characteristic of the host is associated with a health event. Clarifying whether factors relate or do not relate, and examining the extent of the relationship establishes an analytical approach to the epidemiologic process.

A rate is a single, statistical expression that defines the proportion of individuals who have experienced a specific health event. The proportion of disease occurrence is called *morbidity rate*

Table 1–2 A Community Nutrition Assessment Worksheet to Acquire Subjective Data about Nutrition Needs, Attitudes, and Knowledge—Possible Responses

Community Members	Perceived Nutrition Needs in the Community	Attitude toward Nutrition Services			Knowledge of Nutrition		
		+	0	-	+	0	-
Clients/patients	Weight management		0			0	
Public	Weight management		0			0	
Media	Overeating, nutrition education for seniors		0			0	
Government officials	None			-			-
Agency administrators	None			-			-
Physicians/dentists	Lower fat and sugar	+			+		
Hospital administrators	Weight management		0			0	
Nurses	Work with teens, train diabetics, education about fat	+			+		
Health educators	Lifestyle	+			+		
Nutritionists/dietitians	Food selection	+			+		
Agency board members	Limited			-			-
Principals/teachers	Improve school meals		0			0	
Social workers	Provide better choices		0			0	
Clergy	Focus on homeless	+				0	

Key: + = positive, supportive attitude toward nutrition and health services.
0 = neutral or apathetic attitude toward nutrition.
- = negative attitude toward nutrition.

Source: Adapted from *Nutrition in Public Health: A Handbook for Developing Programs and Services* by M. Kaufman, p. 52, Aspen Publishers, Inc., © 1990.

and the proportion of deaths is called *mortality rate.* The number of individuals in the group who have a disease or have experienced a health event at a given point in time constitutes the *numerator.* The *denominator* is the population at risk of experiencing a health event. For example:

$$\text{Incidence rate} = \frac{\text{\# of new cases of a disease}}{\text{population at risk}} \text{ per time period}$$

$$\text{Prevalence rate} = \frac{\text{\# of existing cases of a disease}}{\text{total population}} \text{ at a time point}$$

Point prevalence refers to the number of cases present at a specified moment of time; period prevalence refers to the number of cases that occur during a specified period of time—for example, a year. Period prevalence consists of the point prevalence at the beginning of a specified period of time plus all new cases that occur during that period.[1]

Rates not only identify groups in the community at high risk of disease but also designate groups needing further assessment or monitoring. The high-risk group may be selected for intervention to alter risk factors that relate to the health event. Risk factor profiles of high-risk groups aid decision makers who set program priorities.[4]

To compare rates in different groups, a standardized denominator for a specified time period is needed (e.g., 100,000 in 1994). *Crude rates* are calculated by dividing the total number of events by the total population and multiplying by 1,000, 10,000, or 100,000. The crude birth rate in the United States in 1990 was 16.7 live births per 1,000 population,[28] and in 1991 it was 16.2 live births per 1,000 population.[29] The crude birth rate for 1992 (based on provisional data) is estimated to be 15.9 live births per 1,000 population.[30]

A common rate used by epidemiologists is the death rate. The crude death rate reflects deaths among the entire US population of about 260 million individuals. For the United States, crude death rate was 861.9 deaths per 100,000 population in 1990[28] and 854.0 deaths per 100,000 population in 1991.[29] A standardized birth or death rate is a rate that is adjusted for different age and sex distributions. This adjustment is necessary because the US composition and population profile change with time. Basic epidemiology or demography texts describe how to adjust data. This is beyond the scope of this text, but an important aspect of community health.

If any two or more populations are compared for a health outcome, and they differ on a characteristic that may relate to the health outcome or to a risk factor, then an adjustment must be made. This adjustment is necessary because the characteristic may confound the comparison. For example, US mortality rates increase rapidly beginning at 55 years of age. When rates are distinctly different for different ages (e.g., cancer deaths are low among children but high among older adults), one should adjust the rates for differences in the study population by calculating age-specific rates.

Age-adjusted death rates for the United States reduce the effect of age. In 1990, the overall age-adjusted mortality rate per 100,000 population was 515,[28] compared with 508 per 100,000 population in 1991.[29] Looking at death rates from any cause—referred to as *all-cause* mortality—age-adjusted rates demonstrate a *J*-shaped curve that shows a slight elevation in infancy, low rates from 5 to 14 years, and a slow persistent increase thereafter. Mortality from accidents, homicides, and suicides reflect age patterns influenced by societal factors.[31]

Infant mortality rate (IMR) measures death during the first year of life. IMR is calculated by dividing the number of infant deaths in a year by the number of live births for the same time. IMR is presented as a rate per 1,000 or per 100,000 live births. This rate is commonly used to compare health care among countries. Table 1-3 shows high IMRs for the United States in 1983, 1984, and the average of the years 1985 to 1987. Rates for different ethnic groups are also listed. The health of a country is reflected in the level of care and quality of life afforded its youngest members. In the United States, lowering the IMR among minorities is a major challenge. The 1992 IMR in the United States was 8.5 per 1,000 live births.[5]

IMR equals the sum of the neonatal plus postneonatal mortality rates. *Neonatal mortality rate* is the number of deaths among infants less than 28 days old, divided by the number of live births during the same year. The 1992 neonatal mortality rate in the United States was 5.4 deaths per 1,000 live births. *Postneonatal mortality rate* is the number of deaths in children between 28 days and 11 months of age, divided by the number of live births. The 1992 rate was 3.1 deaths per 1,000 live births. *Maternal mortality rate* is the number of women dying from complications of pregnancy or childbirth, divided by the number of live births in the same year. *Case-fatality rate* is the number of cause-specific deaths divided by the number of cases.[5]

TYPES OF EPIDEMIOLOGIC STUDIES

Health data are collected for various reasons and use various methods. Studies using epidemiologic techniques are either controlled (experimental) or uncontrolled (observational). *Controlled* studies mean that an artificial or planned situation exists. One or more independent variables are selected and controlled or remain static. *Uncontrolled* studies are natural observations. The type of epidemiologic approach depends on the research question being asked and the time perspective (current, past, or future). Uncontrolled and controlled studies are described below, and the pros and cons of each type of study are detailed (see Figure 1-3).

Table 1-3 Infant, Neonatal, and Postneonatal Mortality Rates by Ethnic Group in 23 US States and the District of Columbia Using the Linked Birth and Infant Death Data, 1983–1987

Ethnic Group	IMR 1983	IMR 1984	IMR (NMR+PMR) 1985–1987 NMR	IMR (NMR+PMR) 1985–1987 PMR
African American	18.9	17.9	5.5	12.0
American Indian	14.4	12.5	6.1	7.2
Asian	8.4	8.8	4.7	2.9
Latino	9.5	9.3	5.5	3.0
Mexican	9.1	8.9	5.2	2.9
Puerto Rican	12.9	12.9	7.3	3.7
Cuban	7.5	8.1	5.5	2.2
Central/South American	8.5	8.3	5.2	2.6
Other Latino	8.5	8.3	5.7	3.4
White	10.9	10.4	5.5	3.1

Note: IMR = infant mortality rate, NMR = neonatal mortality rate, PMR = postneonatal mortality rate.

Source: Data from National Center for Health Statistics: Annual summary of births, marriages, divorces, and deaths: 1990. *Monthly Vital Statistics Report*, 1991;39(13):8-28-1991; US, MCH Bureau, Health Resources & Services Adm., Rockville, Md, August, 1995.

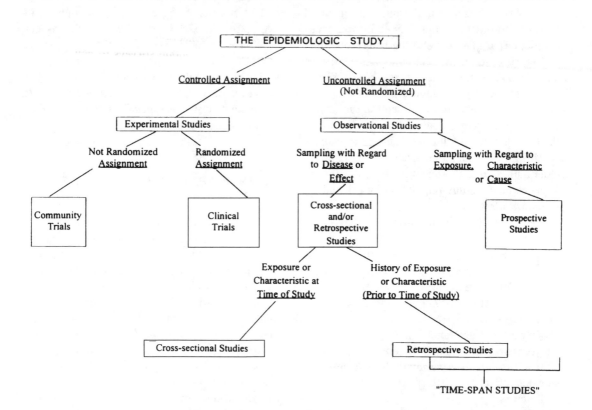

Figure 1-3 The anatomy of the epidemiologic study. *Source:* Reprinted from *Foundations of Epidemiology*, 3rd ed., by D.E. Lilienfeld and P. Stolley, p. 152, with permission of Oxford University Press, © 1994.

Uncontrolled Assignment Studies

Cross-Sectional Studies

Cross-sectional studies define the distributions of health-related characteristics in populations by taking a snapshot look at the population at one point in time. Cross-sectional studies generally represent a sample from a population. Statistical inferences drawn from a sample relate to the method of sample selection. High- and low-risk groups can be identified, and hypotheses can be tested regarding the association of one variable to another.[32]

Each individual in a cross-sectional study is measured once. The same types of data are collected for all individuals in a standardized manner following protocols. Data generated create large databases for statistical analysis.

Cross-sectional studies cannot explore or test cause and effect. They can assist with formulating public health education and intervention programs. For example, one of the largest nutrition-based, cross-sectional studies in the United States is the National Health and Nutrition Examination Survey (NHANES). The first NHANES began in 1960, and NHANES III was completed in 1994. Direct interviews and medical examinations were included. Lipoprotein levels and prevalence rates were determined.[33,34]

Cross-sectional studies provide data to calculate prevalence rates. *Prevalence* is the number of existing health events and becomes a rate when expressed as the proportion of individuals in a population who have a certain trait.

In a cross-sectional study, associations between variables are often explored for one independent variable and one dependent variable. A *dependent variable* is the health outcome, such as blood pressure. An *independent variable* is one of several characteristics being measured, such as sodium or potassium intake. The association of independent and dependent variables can be tested with correlational data analysis.

The pros of the cross-sectional study are as follows:

- Provides quick "snapshot" look.
- Has low cost.
- Defines prevalence.
- Determines associations between variables.
- Generates hypotheses.

The cons of the cross-sectional study are as follows:

- Cannot establish cause and effect.
- Uses "live" individuals.
- Is insensitive to rare characteristics.
- Requires a sample or subsample of a population.
- Describes current, not past or future events.

The Behavioral Risk Factor Survey is an example of a cross-sectional study. It has been conducted since 1981 by the Centers for Disease Control and Prevention. Researchers have conducted a telephone survey of adults in 47 states and the District of Columbia about their health behaviors.[35]

Telephone surveys have been used for cross-sectional data collection.[36,37] Van Horn and colleagues used telephone surveys to collect food intake data of preadolescents.

Pros of telephone surveys are as follows:

- speed of data collection
- less expensive than face-to-face interview
- less supervision
- ease of administration
- centralized procedure
- direct observation of data collection

The cons of telephone surveys are as follows:

- limited to individuals with phones
- may not reach lower socioeconomic status individuals
- decreased accuracy with self-report
- impersonal

Case-Control Studies

A retrospective approach called the case-control study compares cases and controls for the presence of antecedent variables. The flashback approach requires that cases and controls come from similar populations. Similarity of characteristics before the study begins ensures that cases and controls have the same exposure and that their health outcome is not related to one or more confounder. However, cases should differ from controls in one respect: cases must have the health outcome (the disease). Defining cases and controls requires objective criteria and their rigid application. Once cases and controls are identified, differences in antecedent exposure are investigated.

Accurate assignment or labeling as a case or control involves sensitivity and specificity (see Table 1–4).

Sensitivity is the percent of individuals who have the disease and are confirmed by the test:

$$\text{Sensitivity (\%)} = \frac{A}{A + C} \times 100$$

Specificity is the percent of individuals who do not have the disease and are confirmed by the test:

$$\text{Sensitivity (\%)} = \frac{D}{B + D} \times 100$$

Individuals testing positive who have the disease are called *true positives*, those testing positive who do not have the disease are *false negatives*, and those testing negative who do not have the disease are *true negatives*.[1]

$$\text{Sensitivity} = \frac{\text{True positives}}{\text{True positives plus false negatives}} = \frac{\text{True positives}}{\text{All those without the disease}}$$

$$\text{Sensitivity} = \frac{\text{True negatives}}{\text{True negatives plus false positives}} = \frac{\text{True negatives}}{\text{All those without the disease}}$$

The confounding effect of a variable can be avoided by selecting cases and controls of the same age, ethnicity, and gender. This is termed *matching* and sounds easy. However, the more variables to be matched, the larger the number of cases and controls needed. For example, to match on age, sex, and socioeconomic class, a control must be similar to the case on all three variables (e.g., males, 24 to 30 years old, middle socioeconomic status).

Several factors must be considered when selecting cases. If case-control studies include patients receiving treatment, these patients may differ from controls on residence, income, etc. Cases may be limited to survivors, which demonstrates the selective-survival concept. Because only survivors are included, and not newly diagnosed cases or cases with known outcome of death, result and interpretation can be influenced.

A statistic commonly used in case-control studies is *relative risk*. It can be determined easily and is also called the odds ratio or relative odds. It is calculated as follows:

Table 1–4 Indicators of the Accuracy of a Test or Diagnostic Exam—Sensitivity and Specificity

Test or Exam	With Disease	Without Disease
Positive (indicating disease is probably present)	A (true positives)	B (false positives)
Negative (indicating disease is probably absent)	C (false negatives)	D (true negatives)
Totals	A + C	B + D

Source: Reprinted from *Foundations of Epidemiology*, 3rd ed., by D. Lilienfeld and P. Stolley, p. 151, with permission of Oxford University Press, © 1994.

$$\frac{a \times d}{b \times c}$$

where *a* equals the number of cases who have a characteristic, *d* is the number of controls who do not have the characteristic, *b* is the number of controls with the characteristic, and *c* is the number of cases who do not have the characteristic.

A *confidence interval* is the probability (e.g., 95%) that the true value would be within a range. Confidence intervals are statistically significant if they do not include 1.0. For example, if a confidence interval for a relative risk of 2.5 is 2.1 to 3.7, it would be significant. This means that the risk is significantly greater for individuals not exposed to the variable.

Pros of the case-control study are as follows:

- Cases are easily available in clinical settings.
- It is relatively quick and inexpensive.
- Results support, but do not prove, causal hypotheses.
- Secondary analyses are possible, as clinical records are available and no further information from the cases or controls is needed.
- Sample size is small.
- Study of rare diseases is possible.

Cons of the case-control study are as follows:

- Data are from memory, which increases bias (an error that occurs in unknown ways but can produce an over- or underestimate).
- Records may be inadequate.
- Criteria for diagnoses may vary among clinicians.
- Cases are selective survivors.
- Cases may not be representative because they have come for treatment.
- Antecedent data reflect only living cases.

Cohort Studies

This type of observational study can confirm causal associations and establish secular trends between antecedent characteristics and outcomes. Cohort studies are prospective studies and can project risk estimates for future events. Results of cohort studies can be provided to decision makers who are responsible for planning and evaluating intervention, education, and treatment programs. Specifically, cohort studies confirm causation and present decision makers with specific health-related factors to modify for community wellness.[5]

A cohort study begins with a group of people who have known characteristics. The cohort is selected by virtue of an exposure or innate characteristic. Each member of the cohort is identified as free of the health event at the beginning of the study. The cohort is followed over time, maybe several years, to record health events. The number of individuals who develop the outcome are counted, creating prevalence rates that can be reported any time during the study. Any new cases reported within a select time period, such as a year, provide incidence rates.

An example of an observational cohort study is one conducted by Folsom and colleagues. Folsom et al observed the body-fat distribution and the five-year risk of death in older women. They tested the hypothesis that both body mass index (the ratio of weight in kilograms to height in meters squared) and the ratio of waist circumference to hip circumference are positively associated with risk of death in older women.[38] A cohort of 41,837 Iowa women from 55 to 69 years old was followed for five years. During this time 1,504 deaths occurred. Body mass index was associated with mortality following a *J*-shaped curve. This means that death was highest among two groups—the leanest and the most obese women. Waist/hip circumference ratio had a significant, positive association with mortality, which increased in increments. A 0.15-unit increase in waist/hip circumference ratio was associated with a 60% greater relative risk of death. This occurred after adjustment for age, marital status, body mass index, smoking, alcohol and estrogen use, and education. Waist/hip circumference ratio emerged as a better marker of risk of death among older women than body mass index.

Relative risk, which can be calculated in this type of study, determines the extent of risk for a health event when individuals have certain characteristics. As explained earlier, it is determined by dividing the incidence rate among individuals exposed by the incidence rate among individuals not exposed. For example, in the Framingham Heart Study, white men with high cholesterol were 2.04 times more likely to develop coronary heart disease (CHD) than white men with low cholesterol; the study results show that high serum total cholesterol is an antecedent characteristic that increases the probability of developing CHD.[5]

The potential for an association between an antecedent variable and a health outcome is increased if a larger dose produces higher rates. This concept is called "dose-response" and is applicable to the association of serum total cholesterol level and CHD incidence. Again using Framingham Heart Study data, at higher cholesterol levels, higher CHD incidence rates occur. In fact, given four groups, extremely high, high, moderate, and lowest, the relative risks for individuals at extremely high serum total cholesterol levels are about three times that for individuals at the lowest level. Accordingly, relative risk is two times greater for the extremely high to moderate group, and 1.7 times that of the high group.

An interesting question is whether cholesterol levels of a community could be reduced to the point of preventing or lowering the incidence of CHD. The answer is yes, if a community intervention could lower all high cholesterol levels to low cholesterol levels. Further, the result could be expressed in terms of incidence rate.

For example, say IR_e is the incidence rate for the exposed group (high cholesterol), and IR_o is the incidence rate for the nonexposed group (low cholesterol). If IR_e = 154 per 1,000 and IR_o = 73 per 1,000, a reduction in the CHD rate could be realized. The risk attributed to high cholesterol equals the difference (81 per 1,000). This is called the *attributable risk*.

If an eating behavior and exercise intervention could successfully reduce every high cholesterol level to a low cholesterol level, a population's attributable risk fraction could be calculated. This is the proportion or fraction of the rate in a community that the exposed group represents. The total community rate minus the rate in the risk-free group would equal the risk contributed by individuals at risk. This is the proportion of the total rate yielding the community attributable risk proportion. For example, say the incidence rate for the total community is 73 per 1,000. For the low cholesterol group, it is 28 per 1,000. The proportion of the total population rate is calculated as 28/73 or 0.384. The interpretation is that 38% of the new cases of disease among the population would be prevented if all had low cholesterol levels.[5]

Because population attributable risk percent specifies the reduction in health events expected if a risk factor is removed, the percent in risk reduction can be determined for each potential factor. The cost and practicality of risk reduction can then be determined. This allows decision making based on extent of short-term risk reduction and long-term disease outcome.

Cohort studies do not prove beyond a doubt that a risk factor causes a health event. Inferences are possible and can be obtained by comparing secular trends.

Pros of the cohort study are as follows:

- Increases potential for confirmation of cause and effect.
- Quantifies extent of effect due to risk factor.
- Provide baseline rates for new cases in a community.
- Estimates prevalence.
- Allows for hypothesis testing.
- Participant cooperation is high.
- Reduces information bias.
- Minimizes selection factors, since all members of the cohort are disease-free.
- Follows original cohort even if individuals relocate.

Cons of the cohort study are as follows:

- It requires a long observation period.
- Loss to follow-up occurs, which creates selection bias.
- It is expensive.

- Ecological changes can affect and/or create associations and outcomes.
- Rare diseases cannot be studied.

Controlled Assignment Studies

The unique characteristic of an experimental study is the investigator's control over assignment of individuals to groups (random assignment). Randomization ensures comparability of individuals and groups to all known and unknown factors except the one studied. It also avoids bias and increases comparability.[1] The phrase *ceteris paribus*, meaning "all things equal," is germane. Clinical trials require randomized assignment.

An experiment evaluates what occurs after exposure to a risk factor. An intervention group receives an intervention, and a control group does not. The two groups are then compared. For example, a clinical trial is an experiment. A trial could test if antihypertensive drugs lower blood pressure and reduce strokes, or it could evaluate the impact of exercise or eating behavior on CHD mortality rates in a community.[5]

Experimental studies determine factors that confound a cause-and-effect association. These findings increase confidence in future studies that focus on or control known risk factors. Such an approach increases the internal validity of the study.

The basic types of experimental studies[1] are as follows:

- *Therapeutic*: An agent or procedure is given to relieve symptoms or improve survival (i.e., secondary or tertiary intervention).
- *Intervention*: Intervention occurs either before a disease has developed, after, or during a disease expression.
- *Prevention*: Intervention occurs to determine the efficacy of an agent (i.e., primary prevention).

One nonrandomized community trial involved physical fitness as an intervention. The relationship between physical fitness and risk of mortality was studied over an eight-year period among 10,224 men and 3,120 women. There were 110,482 person-years of observation. A maximal treadmill exercise test indicated physical fitness. The observed decline in mortality from any cause occurred for men and women due to their fitness level and lower rates of cardiovascular disease and cancer.[5]

Fitness quintiles were determined and ranged from the highest degree of fitness, quintile 5, to the lowest degree of fitness, quintile 1. An age-adjusted mortality from all causes of death declined across fitness quintiles from lowest to highest. Low physical fitness emerged as the most important risk factor attributing to death. This was true for both men and women. The least fit men had 64.0 deaths per 10,000 person-years, compared to 18.6 deaths per 10,000 person-years among the most fit men. The least fit women had 39.5 deaths per person-years, compared to only 8.5 deaths per person-years among the most fit women. These declines in death rates occurred even after controlling for age, smoking, serum cholesterol, blood pressure, blood glucose, and parental history of CHD.[39]

From 1974 to 1982, a randomized, primary prevention trial in CHD called the Multiple Risk Factor Intervention Trial involved 20 clinical centers and 12,000 men, 37 to 50 years old. The primary objective was to determine whether men at high risk of CHD death would have a significant reduction in mortality if they participated in a special intervention. A "usual care" group received basic information from private physicians, and the intervention group received intense counseling from a multidisciplinary team of physicians, nutritionists, smoking cessation specialists, and behavioral scientists. This trial provided useful but somewhat alarming data about CHD mortality. Not only did high mortality occur among participants who had high levels of cholesterol (>200 mg%), but relatively high mortality occurred among participants with very low total cholesterol levels (<140 mg%).[40]

THE LINK BETWEEN EATING BEHAVIOR AND CHRONIC DISEASE

The growing body of epidemiologic, clinical, and laboratory data demonstrate that what a population or sample of people eats is one of the many important factors involved in the etiology of chronic diseases. During the past 40 years, scientists have been challenged with identifying dietary factors that influence specific disease and defining their pathophysiological mechanisms. Simultaneously, public health policy makers, the food industry, consumer groups, and others have been debating how much and what kind of evidence justifies giving dietary advice to the public and how best to mitigate risk factors on which there is general agreement among scientists.[41]

Prior reports have not been sufficiently comprehensive. They have not crossed the boundary separating the simple assessment of dietary risk factors for single chronic diseases from the complex task of determining how these risk factors influence the entire spectrum of chronic diseases—atherosclerotic cardiovascular diseases, cancer, diabetes, obesity, osteoporosis, dental caries, and chronic liver and kidney diseases.

Diet and Health[42] complements the *Surgeon General's Report on Nutrition and Health*[43] and other efforts of government agencies and voluntary health and scientific organizations by providing an in-depth analysis of the relationship between diet and the full spectrum of major chronic diseases.

Diet and Health focuses on risk reduction rather than on management of clinically manifest disease. The distinction between prevention (or risk reduction) and treatment may be blurred in conditions for which dietary modification might delay the onset of clinical diseases (e.g., the cardiovascular complications in diabetes mellitus) or slow the progression of impaired function. Risk reduction focuses on decreased morbidity as well as mortality from chronic diseases, and proponents of risk reduction believe that dietary modification should be considered to reduce the risk for both.

Ecological correlations of dietary factors and chronic diseases among human populations provide valuable data but cannot be used alone to estimate the strength of the association between diet and diseases. The effect of diet on chronic diseases has been most consistently demonstrated in comparisons of populations with substantially different dietary practices, possibly because it is more difficult to identify such associations within a population whose eating pattern is fairly homogeneous. Generally, case-control and prospective cohort studies underestimate the association within populations. In intervention studies, long exposure is usually required to manifest the effect of eating behavior on chronic disease risk. The strict criteria for selecting participants in epidemiological studies may result in more homogeneous study samples, which limit the application of results to the general population. Despite the limitations of various types of studies in humans, the committee writing *Diet and Health* concluded that repeated and consistent findings of an association between certain dietary factors and diseases are likely to be real and indicative of a cause-and-effect relationship, even though the epidemiologic data do not provide "proof beyond a reasonable doubt."[42]

Experiments on dietary exposure of different animal strains can account for genetic variability and permit more intensive observation. However, extrapolation of data from animal studies to humans is limited by the ability of animal models to simulate human diseases and the comparability of absorption and metabolic phenomena among species.[44]

Six criteria can be used to evaluate the association between eating pattern and chronic diseases. There are strength of association, dose-response relationship, temporally correct association, consistency of association, specificity of association, and biologic plausibility. The strength, consistency, and amount of data and the agreement among epidemiologic, clinical, and laboratory evidence influenced the conclusions and recommendations in *Diet and Health*.[42] This report reviews the epidemiologic, clinical, and experimental data pertaining to each nutrient or dietary factor and specific chronic diseases—including cardiovascular diseases, specific cancers, diabetes, hypertension, obesity, osteoporosis, hepatobiliary disease, and dental caries—along with nutrient interactions and mechanisms of action.[42]

The evidence relating nutrients to specific chronic diseases and diet-related conditions clearly defines the role of dietary patterns in the etiology of the diseases and assessment of the potential for reducing their frequency and severity. Conclusions can be drawn directly either from the research data, where the evidence pertains to dietary patterns of foods and food groups, or from extrapolations taken from data on individual nutrients. Individuals must mature in their thinking—that is, people must change from only considering individual nutrients to considering in a stepwise manner, foods, then food groups, and then dietary patterns as they relate to the spectrum of chronic diseases:

Pathway linking food and health:
Dietary component → Food → Food group
→ Pattern → Disease

Proof beyond a reasonable doubt is generally accepted as a standard for making decisions and taking action. A food and health paradigm can be constructed using the strength of the evidence as one criterion for determining the course of action. Other factors include the likelihood and severity of an adverse effect, the potential benefits of avoiding the hazard, and the feasibility of reducing exposure. Current evidence supports (1) a comprehensive effort to inform the public about the likelihood of certain risks and the possible benefits of dietary modifications and (2) the use of technology and other means (e.g., production of leaner animal products) to facilitate dietary change.[42]

Synergistic and antagonistic effects of dietary interactions must be considered. Assessing potential competing risks and benefits and nutrient interactions is simplified by an inherent consistency in dietary recommendations to maintain good health.

Quantitative guidelines should be proposed when warranted by the strength of the evidence and the potential importance of recommendations to public health. Such guidelines can take into account nutrient interactions. These guidelines are less susceptible to misinterpretation when translated into food choices, and they provide specific targets that can serve as a basis for nutrition programs and policy.

Two complementary approaches[42] to reducing risk factors in the target population are as follows:

- the public health or population-based approach, targeting the general population
- the high-risk or individual-based approach, targeting individuals with defined risk profiles

Most chronic diseases etiologically associated with nutritional factors (e.g., atherosclerotic cardiovascular diseases, hypertension, obesity, many cancers, osteoporosis, and diabetes mellitus) also have genetic determinants, and genetic-environmental interactions play an important role in determining disease outcome. For many diseases, it is not yet possible to identify susceptible genotypes and risks to specific individuals. Major chronic disease burden, however, falls on the general population. Approximately 70% of all deaths in the US population are due to cardiovascular diseases and cancer. The greatest benefit is likely to be achieved by a public health prevention strategy to reduce dietary risk factors by means of dietary recommendations to reduce chronic disease risk in the general population.[42] By so doing, the United States may realize an increased rectangularization of the survival curve (see Figure 1–4).[44]

The public health approach to prevention recognizes that even though reduction of risk for individuals with average risk profiles might be small or negligible, people with average risk represent the great majority of the population. High-risk persons need special attention (i.e., secondary and tertiary prevention), but an effective primary prevention strategy should be aimed at the general public and, where knowledge permits, it should be complemented with recommendations for those at high risk.

Over the past decade, clinical practice guidelines have been published to assist practitioners who detect, evaluate, and manage various diet-related diseases. The importance of medical nutrition therapy is emphasized in the report of the Joint National Committee on High Blood Pressure,[45] and the expert panel reports of the National Cholesterol Education Program regarding adults[46] and children and adolescents.[47] Prevention goals are stated in the U.S. Department of Health and Human Services' *Healthy People 2000*,[41] which calls for expansion of nutritional

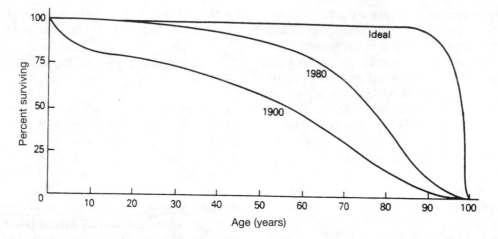

Figure 1-4 Increasing rectangularization of the survival curve. *Source:* Reprinted from Haylick L., The Cell Biology of Human Aging. *Scientific American*, Vol. 242, p.60, with permission of Scientific American, Inc., © 1980.

counseling by primary care providers. Practical recommendations for dietary instruction, monitoring, and follow up are available to physicians who wish to incorporate nutritional counseling into their daily practices. The client's or patient's failure to adhere to a recommended regimen is a major obstacle for achieving the preventive and therapeutic nutritional goals set for the nation.[41]

RESEARCH DIRECTIONS

How can nutritional epidemiology and medical nutrition therapy become natural companions to health promotion and disease prevention? A conceptual framework for planning interdisciplinary collaborative research has been proposed in Exhibit 1-1. Seven categories are identified. The framework encompasses different kinds of investigations: short- and long-term experiments in vitro and in vivo, food consumption surveys, food composition analyses, uncontrolled and controlled epidemiologic studies, metabolic studies, clinical trials in humans, and social and behavioral research.[42]

Current approaches to medical nutrition therapy, important research data linking eat-

Exhibit 1-1   Research Categories Proposed by the Committee on Diet and Health, National Research Council

- Identify foods and dietary components that alter the chronic disease risk, and identify their mechanisms of action.
- Improve dietary assessment methods.
- Identify markers of exposure and early indicators of the disease risk.
- Quantify both adverse and beneficial effects of diet; determine optimal dietary ranges of macro- and microcomponents.
- Conduct intervention studies to assess risk reduction potential.
- Conduct community-based programs that apply current knowledge of eating behavior and disease.
- Expand molecular and cellular nutrition research.

Source: Adapted with permission from *Diet and Health: Implications for Reducing Chronic Disease Risk.* Copyright © 1989 by the National Academy of Sciences. Courtesy of the National Academy Press, Washington, D.C.

ing behavior with disease prevention as well as onset, and ways community nutrition professionals can integrate and remain a vital part of health care, are all explored in the following chapters.

REFERENCES

1. Lilienfeld AM, Lilienfeld DE. *Foundations of Epidemiology*. 2nd ed. New York, NY: Oxford University Press Inc; 1980.

2. Last JM. *Dictionary of Epidemiology*. 2nd ed. New York, NY: Oxford University Press Inc; 1988.

3. Green LW. *Community Health*. 6th ed. St. Louis, Mo: Times Mirror/CV Mosby Co; 1990.

4. *Principles of Epidemiology: An Introduction to Applied Epidemiology and Biostatistics*. 2nd ed. Atlanta, Ga: Centers for Disease Control and Prevention; 1992.

5. Page R, Cole G, Timmrock T. *Basic Epidemiologic Methods and Biostatistics*. Boston, Mass: Jones and Bartlett Publishers; 1993.

6. Doll R, Hill AB. Smoking and carcinoma of the lung. *Br Med J*. 1950;1:739-748.

7. Dawber TR, Kannel WB, Lyell LP. An approach to longitudinal studies in a community: The Framingham study. *Ann NY Acad Sci*. 1963;107:539-556.

8. Berenson GS, McMahan CA, Voors AW, et al. A summing up, In: Hester AC, ed. *Cardiovascular Risk Factors in Children—The Early Natural History of Atherosclerosis and Essential Hypertension*. New York, NY: Oxford University Press Inc; 1980:381-396.

9. Blackburn H, Luepker RV, Kline FG, et al. The Minnesota Heart Health Program: A research and demonstration project in cardiovascular disease prevention. In: Matarazzo JD, Weiss SM, Herd JA, et al, eds. *Behavioral Health: A Handbook of Health Enhancements and Disease Prevention*. New York, NY: John Wiley & Sons Inc; 1984:1171-1178.

10. Farquhar JW, Fortmann SP, Maccoby N, et al. The Stanford Five City Project: An overview. In: Matarazzo JD, Weiss SM, Herd JA, et al, eds. *Behavioral Health: A Handbook of Health Enhancements and Disease Prevention*. New York, NY: John Wiley & Sons Inc; 1984:1154-1165.

11. Puska P, Tuomilehto J, Salonen J, et al. *The North Karelia Project: Evaluation of a Comprehensive Communication Programme for Control of Cardiovascular Disease in North Karelia, Finland, 1972-1977*. Copenhagen, Denmark: World Health Organization-EURO; 1981.

12. Caggiula AN, Christakis G, Farrand M, et al. The Multiple Risk Factor Intervention Trial (MRFIT): IV. Intervention on blood lipids. *Preventive Med*. 1981;10:443-475.

13. MacMahon B, Pugh TF. *Epidemiology: Principles and Methods*. Boston, Mass: Little, Brown, & Company; 1970.

14. *Public Health Reports*. Atlanta, Ga: Centers for Disease Control; 1923;38:2361-2368.

15. Myers GW. History of the Massachusetts General Hospital, June 1872 to December, 1900. 1929. Unpublished manuscript. Available in: Mary C Egan Reference Collection, National Center for Education in Maternal and Child Health, Arlington, Va.

16. Hunt CL. *The Life of Ellen H. Richards*. Washington, DC: American Home Economics Association; 1958.

17. Egan MC. Public health nutrition: a historic perspective. *J Am Diet Assoc*. 1994;94:298-304.

18. Getting V. A modern nutrition program in a state health department. *Milbank Q*. 1947;25:3.

19. Eliot MM, Heseltine MM. Nutrition in maternal and child health programs. *Nutr Rev*. 1947;5:33-35.

20. Massachusetts Department of Public Health. Conference on standardization of qualifications and salaries of nutritional workers. 1920. Unpublished report. Available in: Mary C Egan Reference Collection, National Center for Education in Maternal and Child Health, Arlington, Va.

21. Association of State and Territorial Public Health Nutrition Directors. Application for a research grant. 1960. Unpublished report. Available in: Mary C Egan Reference Collection, National Center for Education in Maternal and Child Health, Arlington, Va.

22. Kaufman M. *Nutrition in Public Health—A Handbook for Developing Programs and Services*. Gaithersburg, Md: Aspen Publishers Inc; 1990:570.

23. Frank GC. Primary prevention in the school arena: A dietary approach. *Health Values*. 1983;7:14-21.

24. Thacker SB, Berkelman RL. Public health surveillance in the United States. *Epidemiol Rev*. 1988;10:164-190.

25. Orenstein WA, Bernier RH. Surveillance information for action. *Pediatr Clin North Am*. 1990;37:709-734.

26. Belloc NB, Breslow L. Relationship of physical health status and health practices. *Preventive Med*. 1972;1:409-421.

27. Carleton RA, Lasater TM, Assaf AR, et al. The Pawtucket Heart Health Program: Community changes in cardiovascular risk factors and projected disease risk. *Am J Public Health*. 1995;85:777-785.

28. *Annual Summary of Births, Marriages, Divorces, and Deaths: United States, 1990. Monthly Vital Statistics Report*. Washington, DC: National Center for Health Statistics; August 28, 1991;39:13.

29. *Annual Summary of Births, Marriages, Divorces, and Deaths: United States, 1991. Monthly Vital Statistics Report*. Washington, DC: National Center for Health Statistics; September 30, 1992;40:13.

30. *Births, Marriages, Divorces, and Deaths for 1992. Monthly Vital Statistics Report*. Washington, DC: National Center for Health Statistics; May 19, 1993;41:12.

31. Rosenberg HM, Curtin LR, Maurer J, et al. Choosing a standard population: Some statistical considerations. In:

Feinleib M, Zarate AO, eds. *Reconsidering Adjustment Procedures. Vital and Health Statistics.* Washington, DC: US Department of Health and Human Services, Public Health Service; 1984:29–67. DHHS publication 93-1466, Series 4.

32. Paffenbarger RS. Conditions of epidemiology to exercise science and cardiovascular health. *Med and Sci in Sports and Exercise.* 1988;20:426–438.

33. Sempos CT, Cleeman JI, Carroll MD, et al. Prevalence of high blood cholesterol among US adults: An update based on guidelines from the Second Report of the National Cholesterol Education Program Adult Treatment Panel. *JAMA.* 1993;269:3009–3014.

34. Johnson CL, Rifkind BM, Sempos CT, et al. Declining serum total cholesterol levels among US adults: The National Health and Nutrition Examination Surveys. *JAMA.* 1993;269:3002–3008.

35. Frazier EL, Franks AL, Sanderson LM. Behavioral risk factor data. In: *Using Chronic Disease Data: A Handbook for Public Health Practitioners.* Atlanta, Ga: Centers for Disease Control and Prevention; 1992.

36. Van Horn L, Gerrhofer N, Moag-Stahlberg A, et al. Dietary assessment in children using electronic methods: Telephones and tape recorders. *J Am Diet Assoc.* 1990;90:412–416.

37. Groves RM, Kahn RL. *Surveys by Telephone.* New York, NY: Academic Press; 1979.

38. Folsom AR, Kaye SA, Sellers TA, et al. Body fat distribution and 5-year risk of death in older women. *JAMA.* 1993;269:483–487.

39. Blair SN, Kohl HW, Paffenbarger RS, et al. Physical fitness and all-cause mortality: A prospective study of healthy men and women. *JAMA.* 1989;262:2395–2401.

40. Jacobs D, Blackburn H, Higgins M, et al. Report of the conference on low blood cholesterol: mortality associations. *Circulation.* 1992;86:1046–1060.

41. *Healthy People 2000: National Health Promotion and Disease Prevention Objectives.* Washington, DC: US Department of Health and Human Services; 1991. Public Health Service publication 91-50212.

42. National Research Council. *Diet and Health: Implications for Reducing Chronic Disease Risk.* Washington, DC: National Academy Press; 1989.

43. *Surgeon General's Report on Nutrition and Health.* Washington, DC: US Department of Health and Human Services; 1988. Public Health Service publication 88-50210.

44. Haylick L. The cell biology of human aging. *Scientific American.* 1980;242:60.

45. Joint National Committee. The 1988 report of the Joint National Committee on Detection, Evaluation, and Treatment of High Blood Pressure. *Arch Intern Med.* 1988;148:1023–1038.

46. National Cholesterol Education Program. *Report of the Expert Panel on Detection, Evaluation, and Treatment of High Blood Cholesterol in Adults.* Bethesda, Md: US Department of Health and Human Services, Public Health Service, National Institutes of Health, National Heart, Lung, and Blood Institute; January 1988. Publication 88-2925.

47. National Cholesterol Education Program. *Report of the Expert Panel on Blood Cholesterol Levels in Children and Adolescents.* Bethesda, Md: US Department of Health and Human Services, Public Health Service, National Institutes of Health, National Heart, Lung, and Blood Institute; April 1991. NIH Publication 91-2732.

Design of the Minnesota Community Prevention Program for Cardiovascular Diseases

Community Pair Type	Year								
	1	2	3	4	5	6	7	8	9
Small towns (N = 60,000)									
Educated	A–C ———————————————→								F
	D	E	E						
Comparison	A–C ———————————————→								F
Large Towns (N = 200,000)									
Educated	A–C ———————————————→								F
		D	E	E					
Comparison	A–C ———————————————→								F
Suburbs (N = 100,000)									
Educated	A–C ———————————————→								F
			D	E	E				
Comparison	A–C ———————————————→								F

Note: A = mortality surveillance, B = morbidity surveillance, C = population survey, D = community analysis, E = mass screening, F = data analysis.

Courtesy of the National Heart, Lung and Blood Institute, 1980.

Appendix 1–B

Bogalusa Heart Study

The design (Table 1–B1) of the first phase of the Bogalusa Heart Study involved cross-sectional and longitudinal studies of all infants and children from birth to 17 years of age. Cardiovascular risk factor variables were the focus.

The variables that were collected sequentially in cross-sectional and longitudinal surveys included the following:

- Demographic
  1. Age, years

- Anthropometric
  1. Body height, cm
  2. Body weight, kg
  3. Skinfold thickness at various body sites, mm
  4. Upper arm length and circumference, cm
- Blood pressure
  1. Mean of 6 systolic and diastolic (4th phase) by mercury sphygmomanometer, mm Hg

---

Table 1–B1 Study Design

| | Age (years) | | | | | | | | | | | | | | | | | | |
| | Preschool Children | | | School Children | | | | | | | | | | | | | | |
Year	0	0.5	1	2	3	4	5	6	7	8	9	10	11	12	13	14	15	16	17
1973–1974	0			2	3	4	5	6	7	8	9	10	11	12	13	14			
1974–1975		0.5	1					6			9			12			15		
1975–1976				2					7			10			13			16	
1976–1977					3		5	6	7	8	9	10	11	12	13	14	15	16	17

Note: Diagonal entries are longitudinal cohorts; horizontal entries comprise cross-sectional surveys.

Source: Data from Frank, G.C. Dietary Studies of Infants and Children, *Cardiovascular Risk Factors in Children: The Early Natural History of Atherosclerosis and Essential Hypertension*, A.C. Hester, ed., pp. 289–307, New York: Oxford University Press © 1980.

2. Mean of 3 systolic and diastolic (4th phase) by physiometrics automatic, mm Hg
- Laboratory
  1. Fasting serum lipids and lipoproteins, mg/dL
  2. Fasting plasma glucose and insulin, mg/dL

The basic examination flow (Figure 1–B1) included orientation for students whose parents had given written consent to their participation; collection of a blood sample for fasting serum total cholesterol, triglycerides, lipoprotein concentrations, and hemoglobin determination. Four randomly chosen children, 10% per day, provided an additional aliquot for blind duplicate analyses to assess the laboratory measurement error. Students were served a light brunch before physical examination by a physician, who also graded for maturation. All variables were obtained using standard protocols and trained observers.

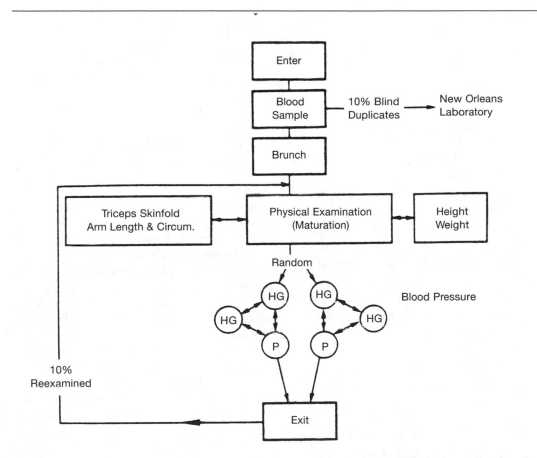

Figure 1–B1 Flow of examination in the cross-sectional components of the Bogalusa Heart Study. *Source:* Data from Frank, G.C., Dietary Studies of Infants and Children, *Cardiovascular Risk Factors in Children: The Early Natural History of Atherosclerosis and Essential Hypertension,* A.C. Hester, ed., pp. 289–307, Oxford University Press, © 1980.

2

Nutrition in the United States

- Enumerate the major nutrition guidelines for Americans.
- Explain the diet and health associations existing in the United States that set the stage for the *Healthy People 2000* initiative.
- Identify the role, components, and benefits of the National Nutrition Monitoring System.
- Describe the three levels employed by US Department of Agriculture (USDA) to monitor food and nutrient consumption in the United States.
- Describe how the Centers for Disease Control and Prevention provide nutrition surveillance data.
- Explain how the Recommended Dietary Allowances (RDAs) integrate with nutrition surveillance, programming, and policy development.
- Detail aspects of the Nutrition Labeling and Education Act (NLEA) regarding food labels and health claims.
- Define biotechnology and discuss its benefits and resulting new food products.
- Discuss the alternative medicine approach that uses nutraceuticals.

- Delineate the components of nutrition misinformation and disinformation.

High Definition Nutrition

Bionutrition—a vision for research that integrates the study of how genetics, molecular biology, and cell biology interact with nutrients of other environmental influences to shape more complex levels of biological organization and, ultimately, health.

Biotechnology—food engineering based on biology that benefits the quantity, value, safety, nutritional quality, desirable characteristics, and variety of foods. Examples of products are chymosin for cheese making and bovine somatotropin (BST) for milk productivity.

Erogenics—performance-enhancing nutritional supplements. These may include but are not limited to amino acids, anabolic steroids, trace minerals, herbs, glandulars, vitamin-mineral supplements, and stack-packs or variety packs of five to ten or more tablets in one plastic pack for daily intake.

Growth retardation—defined as height-for-age below the fifth percentile of children in the National Center for Health Statistics' reference population.

Nutraceutical—any substance that may be considered a food or part of a food and provides medical or health benefits, such as the prevention and treatment of disease.

Nutrition assessment–selecting indicators of nutritional status and collecting those indicators among a sample or population.

Nutrition monitoring–intermittent assessment to identify change in nutritional risk of a group or community.

Nutrition screening–focused assessment generally available to a total community or group to identify at-risk individuals.

Nutrition surveillance–a sequential, community-based assessment to identify a change in the distribution or occurrence of indicators. This assessment is often used to determine a trend.

Registered dietitian (RD)–a nutrition expert in the health care profession. RDs provide reliable therapeutic and wellness counseling and help individuals achieve a total food intake that tastes good and ensures good health. RDs have met the requirements for credentialing by the American Dietetic Association. This involves at least a bachelor's degree, a supervised training program in an accredited/approved institution, a national registration examination, and continuing postgraduate study. A registered dietitian can be located by calling 1-800-234-RD4U.

Recommended Dietary Allowances (RDA)–the levels of intake of essential nutrients that are adequate to meet the known nutrient needs of practically all healthy persons. *The Recommended Dietary Allowances*, 10th revised edition, 1989, is available from the National Academy Press for $19.95 (prepaid); telephone 1-800-624-4242 or 202-334-3323.

POPULATION CHANGE

In the United States the changing proportions of young and old persons in the population can be represented in a population pyramid. Figure 2-1 contrasts the population pyramid for 1987 with the projected pyramids for the years 2000, 2010, and 2030. Each horizontal bar in these pyramids represents a ten-year birth cohort (i.e., people born within the same ten-year period). By comparing these bars, one can determine the relative size of each birth cohort. In the first graph, the distribution of the population in 1987 had already moved from a true pyramid to one with a bulge. The bulge represents the baby boomers. This pyramid will become column-like over time.

Changes in the pyramid reflect the changes and demands on health care (e.g., the aging of babies who later need care when they are adults with chronic or long-term conditions). In the 1990s, death from acute diseases is rare. Maternal, infant, and early childhood death rates have declined considerably since the early 1900s. As a result, an increasing number of individuals survive to old age, often with clustered illness requiring long-term care.[1]

Each cohort in a population pyramid represents individuals with different health care needs, lifestyles, and nutrient intakes. Part II of this book addresses the lifestyles and health care needs of each age cohort in greater detail.

Healthy People 2000 (HP2K), published by the US Department of Health and Human Services, established three overarching goals amid the complex health challenges of the 1990s.[2] They are: (1) increase the span of healthy life for Americans, (2) reduce health disparities among Americans, and (3) achieve access to preventive services for all Americans.

Basic to these goals is the premise that dietary factors are associated with five of the ten leading causes of death: coronary heart disease, some types of cancer, stroke, non-insulin-dependent diabetes mellitus, and atherosclerosis. Three other major causes of death have been associated with excessive alcohol intake: cirrhosis of the liver, unintentional injuries, and suicides (see Table 2-1).[2] Health status objectives linked with nutrition are listed in Exhibit 2-1.

Inadequate and/or excessive intake of several dietary components fuel the diet and health relationships. *The Surgeon General's Report on Nutrition and Health* acknowledged that in the United States there is a disproportionate consumption of foods high in fats. This high fat intake is generally at the expense of foods high in complex carbohydrates and dietary fiber that may be more conducive to health.[3] The *Dietary Guide-*

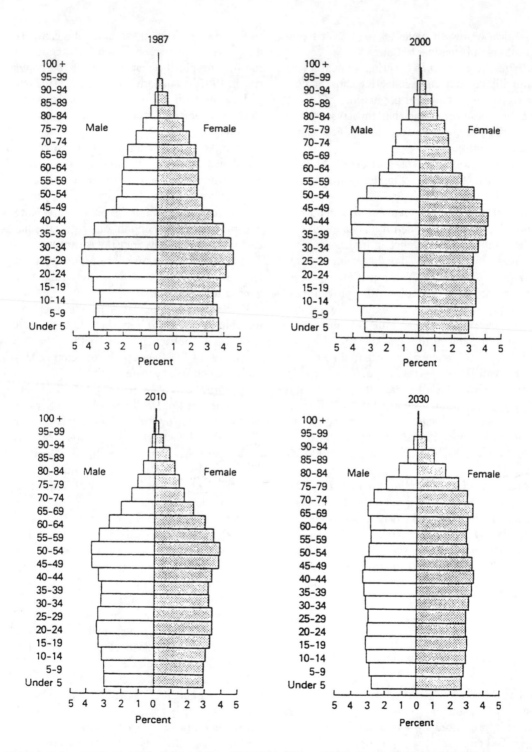

Figure 2–1 Age distribution of the US population: 1987, 2000, 2010, and 2030. *Source:* Reprinted from U.S. Bureau of the Census, Projections of the Population of the U.S. by Age, Sex, and Race: 1988–2080. *Current Population Reports*, Series P-25, No. 1018, U.S. Department of Commerce, 1984.

Table 2–1 The Ten Major Causes of Death in the United States: 1977, 1987, and 1992

1977	*1987*	*1992*
Coronary heart disease	Coronary heart disease	Coronary heart disease
Cancer	Cancer	Cancer
Stroke	Accidents	Stroke
Accidents	Stroke	Chronic lung disease
Chronic lung disease	Chronic lung disease	Accidents
Pneumonia/influenza	Pneumonia/influenza	Pneumonia/influenza
Suicide	Suicide	Diabetes
Liver disease	Diabetes	Human immunodeficiency virus (HIV)
Diabetes	Liver disease	Suicide
Atherosclerosis	Atherosclerosis	Homicide

Source: Data from *Healthy People 2000: National Health Promotion and Disease Prevention Objectives*. U.S. Department of Health and Human Services; 1991. DHHS (PHS) Publication No. 91-50212, p.3; and from *Monthly Vital Statistics Report*, 43, 6S, p. 5. DHHS (PHS) Publication 95-1120, 4-2415, December, 1994.

lines for Americans[4] are based on the premise that staying healthy means eating a variety of foods; maintaining healthy weight; choosing a diet low in fat, saturated fat, and cholesterol; choosing a diet with plenty of vegetables, fruits, and grain products; using sugars only in moderation; using salt and sodium only in moderation; and, if alcoholic beverages are consumed, drinking in moderation.[4]

US adults consume about 36% of their total calories from fat and about 13% of calories from saturated fat. Estimates are that 26 to 32% of the adult population is overweight. This is considerably above the 1990 objective of no more than 10% of men and 17% of women being overweight. At the same time that obesity is widespread, stunted growth is seen in more than 10% of young, low-income children. In 1985, US adult men consumed about 18 grams of dietary fiber, and women 19 to 50 years old consumed about 12 grams. This is only one-half the amount recommended by the National Cancer Institute to reduce the risk for some types of cancer.

Approximately 9% of the total population consumes more than two alcoholic beverages each day. Low calcium intake is common for women and presents a special concern because the median daily intake is well below the 1989 Recommended Dietary Allowances (RDAs).[5]

For low-income women and children, a reduction in iron deficiency anemia remains a priority.

There are other broad-based nutrition concerns, but data are currently unavailable for some special groups at an increased nutritional risk. These concerns include the nutritional status of individuals in hospitals, nursing homes, and convalescent centers. The concerns extend to the physically, mentally, and developmentally disabled individuals in community settings; children with stunted growth; children in child care facilities; Native Americans on reservations; populations in correctional facilities; and the homeless. Additional data are also needed on the old (i.e., 75–84 years) and oldest-old (i.e., 85 years and older), and Americans living alone.

No national database exists for individuals with eating disorders such as anorexia nervosa and bulimia. Hunger is a major societal issue, but definitions of and measurements for hunger status are still evolving (see Chapter 4). Nutrition fraud has increased greatly due to increasing interest in diet and health. The costs, uses, and harms caused by fraud warrant a more careful assessment and monitoring.

With this canvas existing in the United States, national health objectives to reduce medical problems by targeting nutrition have been developed (see Exhibit 2–2). Successful achievement of the

Exhibit 2-1 Health Status Objectives That Link with Nutrition

2.1   Reduce coronary heart disease deaths to no more than 100 per 100,000 people.
2.2   Reverse the rise in cancer deaths to achieve a rate of no more than 130 per 100,000 people.
2.3   Reduce overweight to a prevalence of no more than 20% among people aged 20 and older and no more than 15% among adolescents aged 12 through 19.

Special Population Targets

Overweight Prevalence		*2000 Target*
a	Low-income women aged 20 and older	25%
b	Black women aged 20 and older	30%
c	Hispanic women aged 20 and older	25%
d	American Indians/Alaska Natives	30%
e	People with disabilities	25%
f	Women with high blood pressure	41%
g	Men with high blood pressure	35%

2.4   Reduce growth retardation among low-income children aged 5 and younger to less than 10 percent.

Special Population Targets

Prevalence of Short Stature		*2000 Target*
a	Low-income black children <age 1	10%
b	Low-income Hispanic children <age 1	10%
c	Low-income Hispanic children aged 1	10%
d	Low-income Asian/Pacific Islander children aged 1	10%
e	Low-income Asian/Pacific Islander children aged 2-4	10%

Source: Reprinted from *Healthy People 2000: National Health Promotion and Disease Prevention Objectives.* U.S. Department of Health and Human Services, DHHS (PHS) Publication 91-50212, 1991.

Healthy People 2000 nutrition objectives depends on four factors:

1. marked improvement in accessibility of nutrition information and education for the general public
2. the maintenance and improvement of a strong national program of basic and applied nutrition research
3. further development of the scope and magnitude of the National Nutrition Monitoring System
4. development of a sustained program to implement and evaluate the objectives

Objectives for specific services and protection of the public are outlined in Exhibit 2-3. Knowing the health status and health needs of the population is a basic function of community nutrition and basic to improving the nutritional well-being of American communities.[2] *Healthy People 2000* (HP2K) objectives relevant to the chapters in this book are written at the end of each chapter, beginning in Chapter 3.

Since the 1940s, food guidance for healthy eating has concentrated on grouping foods and recommending serving sizes and the number of servings needed for nutrient adequacy. Government guidance systems have included the Seven

Exhibit 2-2 Risk Reduction Objectives

2.5 Reduce dietary fat intake to an average of 30% of calories or less and average saturated fat intake to less than 10% of calories among people aged 2 and older.

2.6 Increase complex carbohydrate and fiber-containing foods in the diets of adults to 5 or more daily servings for vegetables (including legumes) and fruits, and to 6 or more daily servings for grain products.

2.7 Increase to at least 50% the proportion of overweight people aged 12 and older who have adopted sound dietary practices combined with regular physical activity to attain an appropriate body weight.

2.8 Increase calcium intake so at least 50% of youth aged 12 through 24 and 50% of pregnant and lactating women consume 3 or more servings daily of foods rich in calcium, and at least 50% of people aged 25 and older consume 2 or more servings daily.

2.9 Decrease salt and sodium intake so at least 65% of home meal preparers prepare foods without adding salt, at least 80% of people avoid using salt at the table, and at least 40% of adults regularly purchase foods modified or lower in sodium.

2.10 Reduce iron deficiency to less than 3% among children aged 1 through 4 and among women of childbearing age.

Special Population Targets

	Iron Deficiency Prevalence	*2000 Target*
a	Low-income children aged 1–2	10%
b	Low-income children aged 3–4	5%
	Mothers Feeding Infants Age 5–6 Months	
c	Low-income women of childbearing age	4%
	Anemia Prevalence	
d	Alaska Native children aged 1–5	10%
e	Black, low-income pregnant women (third trimester)	20%

2.11 Increase to at least 75% the proportion of mothers who breastfeed their babies in the early postpartum period and to at least 50% the proportion who continue breastfeeding until their babies are 5 to 6 months old.

Special Population Targets

	Mothers Breastfeeding in Early Postpartum	*2000 Target*
a	Low-income mothers	75%
b	Black mothers	75%
c	Hispanic mothers	75%
d	American Indian/Alaska Native mothers	75%
	Mothers Feeding Infants Age 5–6 Months	
a	Low-income mothers	50%
b	Black mothers	50%
c	Hispanic mothers	50%
d	American Indian/Alaska Native mothers	50%

2.12 Increase to at least 75% the proportion of parents and caregivers who use feeding practices that prevent baby bottle tooth decay.

continues

Exhibit 2-2 continued

	Special Population Targets	
	Appropriate Feeding Practices	*2000 Target*
a	Parents and caregivers with less than high school education	65%
b	American Indian/Alaska Native parents and caregivers	65%

2.13   Increase to at least 85% the proportion of people aged 18 and older who use food labels to make nutritious food selections.

Source: Reprinted from *Healthy People 2000: National Health Promotion and Disease Prevention Objectives.* U.S. Department of Health and Human Services, DHHS (PHS) Publication 91-50212, 1991.

Exhibit 2-3 Services and Protection Objectives

2.14   Achieve useful and informative nutrition labeling for virtually all processed foods and at least 40% of fresh meats, poultry, fish, fruits, vegetables, baked goods, and ready-to-eat carry-away foods.

2.15   Increase to at least 5,000 brand items the availability of processed food products that are reduced in fat and saturated fat.

2.16   Increase to at least 90% the proportion of restaurants and institutional food service operations that offer identifiable low-fat, low-calorie food choices, consistent with the *Dietary Guidelines for Americans.*

2.17   Increase to at least 90% the proportion of school lunch and breakfast services and child care food services with menus that are consistent with the nutrition principles in the *Dietary Guidelines for Americans.*

2.18   Increase to at least 80% the receipt of home food services by people aged 65 and older who have difficulty in preparing their own meals or are otherwise in need of home-delivered meals.

2.19   Increase to at least 75% the proportion of the nation's schools that provide nutrition education from pre-school through 12th grade, preferably as part of quality school health education.

2.20   Increase to at least 50% the proportion of work sites with 50 or more employees that offer nutrition education and/or weight management programs for employees.

2.21   Increase to at least 75% the proportion of primary care providers who provide nutrition assessment and counseling and/or referral to qualified nutritionists or dietitians.

Source: Adapted from *Healthy People 2000: National Health Promotion and Disease Prevention Objectives.* U.S. Department of Health and Human Services, DHHS (PHS) Publication 91-50212, 1991.

Food Group plan and now the Food Guide Pyramid. Each of these blueprints has met with debate during development. Advocates, nutritionists, and researchers have interacted with government agencies to improve the eating guides prior to their use.

THE FOOD GUIDE PYRAMID

The Food Guide Pyramid (FGP) was born, died, and born again. Political and nonpolitical groups battled to identify the most appropriate food groups—and names of the groups—to fill the pyramid.

The resulting FGP outlines graphically what to eat each day (see Figure 2-2). The foundation is comprised of breads, cereals, rice, and pasta. Moving up the pyramid one finds vegetables and fruits as two distinct groups. The third level reflects the milk, yogurt, and cheese group adjacent to the meat, poultry, fish, dry beans, eggs, and nuts group. The tip of the pyramid contains fats, oils, and sweets.[6]

Food Guide Pyramid

A Guide to Daily Food Choices

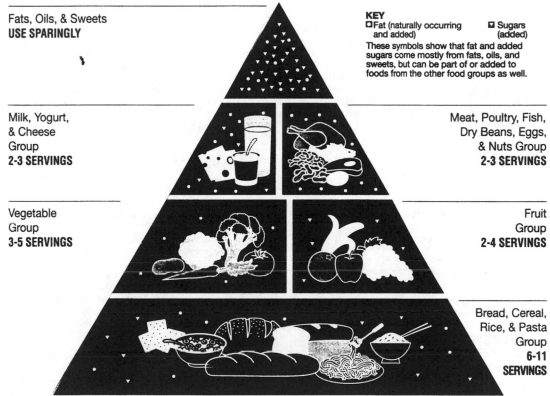

Fats, Oils, & Sweets
USE SPARINGLY

KEY
□Fat (naturally occurring and added)   ☑ Sugars (added)
These symbols show that fat and added sugars come mostly from fats, oils, and sweets, but can be part of or added to foods from the other food groups as well.

Milk, Yogurt, & Cheese Group
2-3 SERVINGS

Meat, Poultry, Fish, Dry Beans, Eggs, & Nuts Group
2-3 SERVINGS

Vegetable Group
3-5 SERVINGS

Fruit Group
2-4 SERVINGS

Bread, Cereal, Rice, & Pasta Group
6-11 SERVINGS

SOURCE: U.S. Department of Agriculture/U.S. Department of Health and Human Services

Use the Food Guide Pyramid to help you eat better every day. . .the Dietary Guidelines way. Start with plenty of Breads, Cereals, Rice, and Pasta; Vegetables; and Fruits. Add two to three servings from the Milk group and two to three servings from the Meat group.

Each of these food groups provides some, but not all, of the nutrients you need. No one food group is more important than another — for good health you need them all. Go easy on fats, oils, and sweets, the foods in the small tip of the Pyramid.

To order a copy of "The Food Guide Pyramid" booklet, send a $1.00 check or money order made out to the Superintendent of Documents to: Consumer Information Center, Department 159-Y, Pueblo, Colorado 81009.

U.S. Department of Agriculture, Human Nutrition Information Service, August 1992, Leaflet No. 572

continues

Figure 2-2 The USDA Food Guide Pyramid outlines the type and number of foods to eat daily for a healthy eating pattern. *Source:* Reprinted from U.S. Department of Agriculture/U.S. Department of Health and Human Services, Human Nutrition Information Service, Leaflet No. 572, August 1992.

How to Use The Daily Food Guide

What counts as one serving?

Breads, Cereals, Rice, and Pasta
1 slice of bread
1/2 cup of cooked rice or pasta
1/2 cup of cooked cereal
1 ounce of ready-to-eat cereal

Vegetables
1/2 cup of chopped raw or
  cooked vegetables
1 cup of leafy raw vegetables

Fruits
1 piece of fruit or melon wedge
3/4 cup of juice
1/2 cup of canned fruit
1/4 cup of dried fruit

Milk, Yogurt, and Cheese
1 cup of milk or yogurt
1-1/2 to 2 ounces of cheese

Meat, Poultry, Fish, Dry Beans, Eggs, and Nuts
2-1/2 to 3 ounces of cooked lean
  meat, poultry, or fish
Count 1/2 cup of cooked beans,
  or 1 egg, or 2 tablespoons of
  peanut butter as 1 ounce of lean
  meat (about 1/3 serving)

Fats, Oils, and Sweets
LIMIT CALORIES FROM THESE
especially if you need to lose weight

> The amount you eat may be more than one serving. For example, a dinner portion of spaghetti would count as two or three servings of pasta.

How many servings do you need each day?

	Women & some older adults	Children, teen girls, active women, most men	Teen boys & active men
Calorie level*	about 1,600	about 2,200	about 2,800
Bread group	6	9	11
Vegetable group	3	4	5
Fruit group	2	3	4
Milk group	**2-3	**2-3	**2-3
Meat group	2, for a total of 5 ounces	2, for a total of 6 ounces	3 for a total of 7 ounces

*These are the calorie levels if you choose lowfat, lean foods from the 5 major food groups and use foods from the fats, oils, and sweets group sparingly.

**Women who are pregnant or breastfeeding, teenagers, and young adults to age 24 need 3 servings.

A Closer Look at Fat and Added Sugars

The small tip of the Pyramid shows fats, oils, and sweets. These are foods such as salad dressings, cream, butter, margarine, sugars, soft drinks, candies, 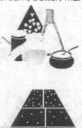 and sweet desserts. Alcoholic beverages are also part of this group. These foods provide calories but few vitamins and minerals. Most people should go easy on foods from this group.

Some fat or sugar symbols are shown in the other food groups. That's to remind you that some foods in these groups can also be high in fat and added sugars, such as cheese or ice cream from the milk group, or french fries from the vegetable group. When choosing foods for a healthful diet, consider the fat and added sugars in your choices from all the food groups, not just fats, oils, and sweets from the Pyramid tip.

Figure 2–2 continued

The number of servings recommended from each group is based on the number of calories an individual needs. In formulating the number of servings, three calorie levels were defined.

- *1,600 calories*–bread group (6 servings), vegetable group (3 servings), fruit group (2 servings), milk group (2 to 3 servings), meat group (2 servings, for a total of 5 ounces), fats/sweets (6 teaspoons).
- *2,200 calories*–bread group (9 servings), vegetable group (4 servings), fruit group (3 servings), milk group (2 to 3 servings), meat group (2 servings, for a total of 6 ounces), fats/sweets (12 teaspoons).
- *2,800 calories*–bread group (11 servings), vegetable group (5 servings), fruit group (4 servings), milk group (2 to 3 servings), meat group (3 servings, for a total of 7 ounces), fats/sweets (18 teaspoons).

A range for the number of servings for each food group was determined. Each individual should eat the minimum number of servings. Active adults and adolescents should consume the higher number. Children need variety among fewer servings and may need smaller portions–except for milk, where a minimum of two servings is essential.[6]

Several alternatives to the FGP have been developing. One of the most visible is discussed below to give a sense of the difference of opinions between professionals in the fields of public health, medicine, and nutrition.

In June 1994, the Oldways Preservation and Exchange Trust, in Boston, Massachusetts, introduced an alternative to the FGP–the Traditional Healthy Mediterranean Diet Pyramid. The Exchange Trust joins the World Health Organization (WHO) European Regional Office, the WHO, and the Food and Agriculture Organization Collaborating Center in Nutrition at Harvard School of Public Health in presenting the pyramid for comment. The pyramid is accompanied by a list of ten characteristics of the diet and acknowledges the need for further research and consideration.[7]

The Traditional Healthy Mediterranean Diet Pyramid is based on the dietary traditions of Greece, southern Italy, and much of the rest of the Mediterranean region in approximately 1960. The diet is structured in light of current nutrition research. The Mediterranean Pyramid and its accompanying notes describe a diet that was collectively much higher in food from plant sources–fruits and vegetables, breads and grains, legumes, nuts, and seeds–than the dietary pattern suggested by the US Food Guide Pyramid. Other apparently health-promoting aspects of the traditional Mediterranean diet include the following:

- Red meat was consumed only a few times per month, or somewhat more often in very small amounts. Other foods from animal sources were used on a sparing to moderate basis.
- Most of the fat in the diet was monounsaturated-rich olive oil. Total fat ranged from less than 25% to over 35% of total energy (calories).
- Wine was consumed on a moderate basis, usually with meals and in a family context.
- Foods were, for the most part, minimally processed.

Reflecting the importance of regular physical activity in the traditional, healthy Mediterranean lifestyle, the Mediterranean Pyramid also includes an illustration of a male and female figure exercising.

EATING HABITS OF AMERICAN FAMILIES

What do Americans eat? How do they make their food selections? How can we monitor the food habits and nutrient intakes of US residents using epidemiologic techniques?

A 1994 national survey of 1,000 representative adults responded to a telephone interview about their families' food practices and eating habits. The study was conducted by the Food Marketing Institute and *Prevention* magazine. Respondents had primary or equally shared responsibility for food shopping for their households. A stratified, random digit dialing was used to avoid listing bias. The number of telephone numbers randomly sampled from within a county was proportional to the county's share of telephone households in the state. Four attempts were made to complete each interview.[8]

The final sample was 27% male and 73% female; 37% were 25 to 39 years old, 20% were 40 to 49 years old, 20% were 50 to 64 years old, 9% were less than 25, and 12% were over 64 years old. Of the respondents, 38% were high school graduates and another 29% were college graduates. Regarding income, 33% earned $25,000 or less, and 21% earned more than $50,000.

A brief summary of results[8] reveal the following:

- Of shoppers, 45% say they have changed a food-buying decision in the last month because they read the food label.
- Nearly 50% agree that they are concerned about fat but uncertain how to cut back on fat.
- Of the respondents, 26% have high-fat foods (e.g., hamburger, bacon, chicken with skin, or eggs) at least 1 time a day; an additional 7% have them 15 or more times each week.
- African Americans are much more likely than whites to consume high-fat meats; 60% have unhealthy eating patterns compared with 29% of whites.
- Of the respondents, 60% report that a major change occurred in their eating habits during the past 10 years due to health.
- Changes in eating patterns are more common among women over 40 years old and among more affluent consumers.
- The most common changes are lowering fat (63%) and increasing fruit and vegetable intake (30%).
- Overweight shoppers have particular concerns about obesity, high cholesterol, and hypertension.
- African Americans are more motivated than whites to change food patterns due to high blood pressure rather than to heart disease.
- Only 20% of respondents believe their eating pattern is healthy, and only 7% consider it as healthy as possible.

- Of the respondents, 69% are overweight (i.e., over their recommended weight using Metropolitan Life Insurance Company tables). Of 18-to-39 year olds, 57% are overweight, and of respondents 40 years and older, 79% are overweight.
- Over one-third of those who are heavy believe they are within the proper weight range.
- Of the respondents, 43% report regular, strenuous exercise; fewer than one in ten spent time in the hospital the prior year.

Because all sample surveys are subject to sampling error, the researchers provided recommended allowances or a range in percentage points or +/- points at a 95% confidence interval. A partial listing is provided in Appendix 2–A.

Info Line

The 1995 Food Marketing Institute and *Prevention* magazine survey included a special oversampling of 500 African-American shoppers to contrast their views with eating habits of the total sample. The major findings were: (1) these shoppers were not different in trying to make healthful changes; (2) they experienced a higher level of confusion and frustration when making choices; (3) they were more likely to make poor food choices; and (4) they had unhealthy eating patterns more often.

For further information contact The Research Department, Food Marking Institute, 800 Connecticut Avenue NW, Washington, DC, 20006.

SURVEILLANCE AND MONITORING

The National Nutrition Monitoring and Related Research (NNMRR) Act (Public Law 101-445) became law on October 22, 1990 to provide timely data about food and nutrient intake and the resulting nutritional status of the public.[9]

Lack of timely nutrition data has been a persistent problem when program planners and decision makers are at the discussion and planning table. One outcome is that decisions are often made on assumptions and insufficient information. The real problems may not be addressed. Even though goals may be achieved, they may likely fall short of addressing the major problems. Nutrition data that are accurate and current are essential.

Five measurement elements spearhead the monitoring and research activities. They are as follows:

1. nutrition and health-related assessment
2. food and nutrient intake
3. knowledge, attitude, and behavior measures
4. databases about nutrients and composition of foods
5. adequacy and quality of food supply

Over 45 surveys and surveillance systems will comprise the monitoring effort in the United States between 1992 and 2002 to address the existing inadequate system.[10] Table 2-2 details 22 nutrition and health-related assessments. Food and nutrient intakes will be monitored in 13 surveys outlined in Table 2-3. For the decade 1992

Table 2-2 Nutrition and Related Health Assessments, 1992–2002

Date	Survey	Target	Department	Agency
1988–1994	Third National Health and Nutrition Examination Survey (NHANES)	US noninstitutionalized, civilian population, aged 2 months or older; oversampling of blacks and Mexican Americans, children up to age 5 years, and individuals aged 60 years and older	DHHS	CDC/NCHS
1988–1994	NHANES III Supplemental Nutrition Survey of Older Persons	Individuals aged 50 years and older examined in NHANES III, in households with telephones	DHHS	CDC/NCHS, NIH/NIA
1991–1992	Navajo Health and Nutrition Survey	Persons aged 12 years and older residing on or near the Navajo reservation in Arizona, New Mexico, and Utah	DHHS	IHS
1992	National Home and Hospice Care Survey	A sample of home health agencies and hospices along with a subsample of patients	DHHS	CDC/NCHS
1992	NHANES I Epidemiologic Followup Survey	Individuals examined in NHANES I who were 25–74 years old at baseline	DHHS	CDC/NCHS
1992	NHIS on Cancer Epidemiology and Cancer Control	Individuals aged 18 years and older	DHHS	CDC/NCHS, NIH/NCI
Annual	National Health Interview Survey (NHIS)	Civilian, noninstitutionalized individuals	DHHS	CDC/NCHS
Annual	National Hospital Discharge Survey	Discharges from nonfederal, general, and short-stay specialty hospitals	DHHS	CDC/NCHS
Continuous	Vital Statistics Program	Total US population	DHHS	CDC/NCHS
Continuous	Pregnancy Nutrition Surveillance System	Low-income, high-risk, pregnant women	DHHS	CDC/ NCCDPHP

continues

Table 2–2 continued

Date	Survey	Target	Department	Agency
Continuous	Pediatric Nutrition	Low-income, high-risk children	DHHS	CDC/NCCDPHP
Annual	National Ambulatory Medical Care Survey Surveillance System	Office visits to nonfederal, office-based physicians from birth to 17 years	DHHS	CDC/NCHS
1992 (continuous)	NHANES II Mortality Followup Survey	Individuals examined in NHANES II who were 35–75 years old at baseline	DHHS	CDC/NCHS
1992 (continuous)	Hispanic Hanes (HHANES) Mortality Followup Survey	Individuals interviewed in HHANES who were 20–74 years old at baseline	DHHS	CDC/NCHS
1992 (annual)	National Hospital Ambulatory Medical Care Survey	Visits to hospital emergency and outpatient departments of nonfederal, short-stay, general, and specialty hospitals	DHHS	CDC/NCHS
1992 (continuous)	NHANES III Longitudinal Followup Survey	Individuals interviewed and examined in NHANES III who were aged 20 years or older at baseline	DHHS	CDC/NCHS
1993	National Mortality Followback Survey	Individuals aged 25 years and older	DHHS	CDC/NCHS
1994	National Survey of Family Growth	Women aged 15 to 44 years	DHHS	NCHS
1994 (continuous)	Adult Nutrition Surveillance System	Adults aged 18 years and older who were participating in local public health programs	DHHS	CDC/NCCDPHP
1995	NHIS on Health Promotion/ Disease Prevention	Individuals aged 18 years and older	DHHS	CDC/NCHS
1995	NHANES I Epidemiologic Followup Study	Individuals examined in NHANES I who were 55 to 74 years old at baseline	DHHS	CDC/NCHS
1997+	National Health and Nutrition Examination Survey (NHANES 1997+)	US noninstitutionalized population	DHHS	CDC/NCHS

Notes: DHHS = US Department of Health and Human Services
CDC = Centers for Disease Control and Prevention
NCHS = National Center for Health Statistics
NIH = National Institutes of Health
NIA = National Institute on Aging
IHS = Indian Health Service
NCI = National Cancer Institute
NCCDPHP = National Center for Chronic Disease Prevention and Health Promotion

Source: Adapted from Kuczmarski M.F., Moshfegh A., and Briefel, R., Update on Nutrition Monitoring Activities in the U.S., *Journal of the American Dietetic Association,* Vol. 94, pp. 753–760, with permission of the American Dietetic Association, © 1994.

Table 2–3 Food and Nutrient Intake, 1992–2002

Date	Survey	Target	Department	Agency
1988–1994	NHANES III and NHANES III Supplemental Nutrition Survey of Older Persons	Representative US population; elderly	DHHS	CDC/NCHS, NIH/NIA
1991–1992	Development of a National Seafood Consumption Survey Model	Individuals residing in eligible households and recreational/ subsistence fishermen	DOC	NMFS/NOAA
1992	School Nutrition Dietary Assessment Study	School-aged children in grades 1 through 12	USDA	FNS
1992	School Food Authority Menu Modification Demonstration Projects	Students in elementary schools	USDA	FNS
1992	Adult Day Care Program Study	Adult day care centers and adults participating and not participating in the Child and Adult Care Food Program	USDA	FNS
Annual	Total Diet Study	Representative diets of specific age-sex groups	DHHS	FDA
Continuous	Nutritional Evaluation of Military Feeding Systems and Military Populations	Enlisted personnel of the Army, Navy, Marine Corps, and Air Force	DOD	USARIEM
Continuous	Consumer Expenditure Survey	Civilian, noninstitutionalized population and a portion of the US institutionalized population	DOL	BLS
Continuous	Survey of Income and Program Participation	Civilian, noninstitutionalized US population	DOC	Census
1994–1996 (annual)	Continuing Survey of Food Intakes by Individuals (CSFII)	Individuals of all ages residing in eligible households nationwide; oversampling of individuals in low-income households	USDA	HNIS
(1997+)	NHANES 1997+	US noninstitutionalized civilians	DHHS	CDC/NCHS
1997–1998	Household Food Consumption Survey	Civilian households and individuals residing in eligible households	USDA	HNIS
1997–1998	Low-Income Nationwide Food Consumption Survey	Low-income civilian households and individuals residing in eligible households	USDA	HNIS

Notes: DHHS = US Department of Health and Human Services
CDC = Centers for Disease Control and Prevention
NCHS = National Center for Health Statistics
NIH = National Institutes of Health
NIA = National Institute on Aging
DOC = US Department of Commerce
DOD = US Department of Defense
NMFS = National Marine Fisheries Service

NOAA = National Oceanic and Atmospheric Administration
USDA = US Department of Agriculture
FNS = Food and Nutrition Service
FDA = Food and Drug Administration
USARIEM = US Army Research Institute of Environmental Medicine
DOL = US Department of Labor
BLS = Bureau of Labor Statistics
HNIS = Human Nutrition Information Service

Source: Adapted from Kuczmarski M.F., Moshfegh A., and Briefel, R., Update on Nutrition Monitoring Activities in the U.S., *Journal of the American Dietetic Association,* Vol. 94, pp. 753–760, with permission of the American Dietetic Association, © 1994.

to 2002, seven surveys will document knowledge, attitudes, and behaviors (see Table 2–4). Surveys related to nutrient databases are listed in Table 2–5. Two surveys will determine adequacy and quality of the food supply (Table 2–6).

Title I of the NNMRR Act established a 22-member agency board (see Exhibit 2–4). The secretaries and undersecretaries of the US Department of Agriculture (USDA) and the US Department of Health and Human Services (DHHS)

serve as chairpersons to implement and to report to the US President and to Congress. Title II established a National Nutrition Monitoring Advisory Council with nine nonfederal members who have expertise in public health, nutrition monitoring research, or food production and distribution. This group gives scientific and technical advice and evaluates the effectiveness of the program.[10]

A ten-year comprehensive plan is mandated by PL 101-445. National, state, and local objectives

---

Table 2–4 Knowledge, Attitude, and Behavior Measures, 1992–2002

Date	Survey	Target	Department	Agency
Biennial	Youth Risk Behavior Survey	Civilian, noninstitutionalized adolescents, aged 12 to 18 years	DHHS	CDC/ NCCDPHP
1992	Infant Feeding Practices Survey	New mothers and healthy, full-term infants from birth to 1 year old	DHHS	FDA
1992	Consumer Food Handling Practices and Awareness of Microbiological Hazards Screener	Individuals aged 18 years and older in households with telephones	DHHS	FDA
1992	NHIS on Youth Risk Behavior	Civilian, noninstitutionalized adolescents, aged 12 to 21 yrs	DHHS	CDC/NCHS CDC/ NCCDPHP
Continuous	Behavioral Risk Factor Surveillance System	Individuals aged 18 years and older residing in participating states in households with telephones	DHHS	CDC/ NCCDPHP
Biennial	Health and Diet Survey	Civilian, noninstitutionalized individuals aged 18 years and older in households with telephones	DHHS	FDA
1994–1996	Diet and Health Knowledge Survey	Selected adults aged 20 years and older in households and noninstitutionalized group quarters participating in the CSFII	USDA	HNIS

Notes: DHHS = US Department of Health and Human Services
CDC = Centers for Disease Control and Prevention
NCCDPHP = National Center for Chronic Disease Prevention and Health Promotion
FDA = Food and Drug Administration
NCHS = National Center for Health Statistics
HNIS = Human Nutrition Information Service

Source: Adapted from Kuczmarski M.F., Moshfegh A., and Briefel, R., Update on Nutrition Monitoring Activities in the U.S., *Journal of the American Dietetic Association,* Vol. 94, pp. 753–760, with permission of the American Dietetic Association, © 1994.

Table 2–5 Nutrient Databases and Composition of Foods, 1992–2002

Date	Survey	Target	Department	Agency
Annual	Total Diet Study	Representative diets of specific age-sex groups	DHHS	FDA
Biennial	Food Label and Package Survey	NA	DHHS	FDA
Continuous	Langual	NA	DHHS	FDA
Continuous	National Nutrient Data Bank	NA	USDA	HNIS
Continuous	Survey Nutrient Data Base	NA	USDA	HNIS

Notes: NA = Not applicable
DHHS = US Department of Health and Human Services
FDA = Food and Drug Administration
HNIS = Human Nutrition Information Service
USDA = US Department of Agriculture

Source: Adapted from Kuczmarski M.F., Moshfegh A., and Briefel, R., Update on Nutrition Monitoring Activities in the U.S., *Journal of the American Dietetic Association,* Vol. 94, pp. 753–760, with permission of the American Dietetic Association, © 1994.

Table 2–6 Adequacy and Quality of Food Supply, 1992–2002

Date	Survey	Target	Department	Agency
Annual	Fisheries of the US	NA	DOC	NOAA/NMFS
Annual	US Food and Nutrition Supply Series Estimate of Food Available and Estimate of Nutrients	NA	USDA	ERS/HNIS

Notes: NA = not applicable
DOC = US Department of Commerce
HNIS = Human Nutrition Information Service
NMFS = National Marine Fisheries Service
NOAA = National Oceanic and Atmospheric Administration
USDA = US Department of Agriculture
ERS = Economic Research Service

Source: Adapted from Kuczmarski M.F., Moshfegh A., and Briefel, R., Update on Nutrition Monitoring Activities in the U.S., *Journal of the American Dietetic Association,* Vol. 94, pp. 753–760, with permission of the American Dietetic Association, © 1994.

are required.[10] To assist with achievement of the national objectives, the comprehensive plan outlines activities for each of the five measurement elements. National objectives are as follows:

- ensure a comprehensive, continuous, and coordinated program

- improve comparability and quality of data
- strengthen the research base

The state and local objectives are as follows:

- improve capacity for complementary data collection

Exhibit 2-4 Members of the Interagency Board for Nutrition Monitoring and Related Research, United States, 1990

- Agency of International Development (AID)
- Agricultural Research Service, USDA
- Bureau of the Census, DOC
- Bureau of Labor Statistics, DOL
- Cooperative State Research Service, USDA
- Department of Defense
- Department of Education
- Department of Veterans Affairs
- Economic Research Service, USDA
- Environmental Protection Agency
- Extension Service, USDA
- Food and Drug Administration, DHHS
- Food and Nutrition Service, USDA
- Food Safety and Inspection Service, USDA
- Health Resources and Services Administration, DHHS
- Human Nutrition Information Service, USDA
- Indian Health Service, DHHS
- National Center of Chronic Disease Prevention and Health Promotion, CDC, DHHS
- National Center for Health Statistics, CDC, DHHS
- National Institutes of Health, DHHS
- National Marine Fisheries Service, National Oceanic and Atmospheric Administration, DOC
- Substance Abuse and Mental Health Services Administration, DHHS

Source: Adapted from Kuczmarski M.F., Moshfegh A., and Briefel, R., Update on Nutrition Monitoring Activities in the U.S., *Journal of the American Dietetic Association,* Vol. 94, pp. 753-760, with permission of the American Dietetic Association, © 1994.

- create more sophisticated methods of promoting comparability of data across levels
- enhance the quality of monitoring data

Surveillance and data systems can support improvement of nutrition in the United States, but will they? The National Nutrition Monitoring System intends to provide timely detection and measurement of nutritional problems, dietary practices, and nutrition-related knowledge and behaviors. Data can be collected not only for the US population in general, but also for specific high-risk groups.[11,12] One challenge is to ensure that national and state operational objectives are met. Enthusiastic and effective management must occur at both levels, as well as sufficient funding for staff, training, and the necessary technology.

The nutrient intakes and nutritional status of the US population are periodically documented by several surveys (Exhibit 2-5). The Ten State Nutrition Survey—the first comprehensive US survey—focused primarily on low-income populations in California, Kentucky, Louisiana, Massachusetts, Michigan, New York, South Carolina, Texas, Wash-

ington, and West Virginia. Documentation that children and adults were experiencing hunger and malnutrition provided an essential shot in the arm for nutrition surveillance. Serial surveys now include the National Health and Nutrition Examination Surveys (NHANES) conducted by the National Center for Health Statistics (NCHS) of the Centers for Disease Control and Prevention (CDC) and the Nationwide Food Consumption Surveys (NFCS). The NFCS include the Continuing Surveys of Food Intakes by Individuals (CSFII) conducted by the Human Nutrition Information Service (HNIS) of USDA.

Information about nutrition and health status of specific population groups, consumer knowledge and behavior, and food and diet composition is provided by other data sources. These include the Pregnancy and the Pediatric Nutrition Surveillance Systems by CDC, the National Health Interview Surveys (NHIS) by NCHS, the Diet and Health Knowledge Survey by HNIS/USDA, and the Total Diet Study and Health and Diet Surveys by the Food and Drug Administration (FDA). The Pediatric Nutrition Surveillance System in-

Exhibit 2-5 Highlights of US Nutrition Surveys and Nutrition Surveillance

Ten State Nutrition Survey, 1968
    Sample: 24,000 low-income families
    Results: Malnutrition was highest among low-income families.
               Iron-deficiency anemia was a problem.
               As many as 50% of women were obese at some ages.
               Poor dental health was a problem.
Preschool Nutrition Survey, 1968-1970
    Sample: 3,400 children 1-6 years of age
    Result: Malnutrition and low birth weight was associated with low income.
National Health and Nutrition Examination Survey: NHANES I (1971-1975), II (1976-1980), and III (1988-1994)
    Sample: 21,000 people, ages 6 months to 74 years
    Results: This survey represented the first assessment of nutritional status over time.
               Iron levels were most often found below standard.
Hispanic Health and Nutrition Examination Survey: HHANES (1984)
    Sample: Probability sample of Puerto Ricans in New York City, Mexican Americans in the Southwest, and Cuban Americans in Florida
    Result: This was the first national survey of health and nutrition parameters targeting these ethnic groups.
Nationwide Food Consumption Surveys (NFCS), every year
    Sample: Varies
    Results: (1978 and 1988 comparison) Calcium was low, especially in females over 12 years; calories decreased, vitamin C increased; iron intake in females 12-50 years was at 35-40% of RDA.

cludes every state. The Pediatric Nutrition Surveillance System and the Behavioral Risk Factor and Youth Risk Behavior Surveillance Systems are also conducted by CDC. The National Institutes of Health (NIH) and the Agricultural Research Service of USDA provide the primary research base for these nutrition-monitoring activities.

The National Nutrition Monitoring System provides data at intervals to assess progress toward the HP2K objectives.[2] However, new data collection is needed to identify the nutritional status of several groups not routinely surveyed. New survey methods are needed that not only increase and refine the current epidemiologic database but also identify the relationships between dietary patterns and chronic diseases. As the number and type of surveys increase to establish the surveillance system, consistent methods *must* be used. Governmental agencies must remain vigilant. Standardized, valid, and reliable assessment instruments and protocols are essential across all surveys, or analysts will be forced to "adjust" or "correct" data for comparison. One persistent question is whether surveillance provides the accurate, useful data needed to profile the nutritional status of American people.

The timeliness of the data are also an issue. Researchers are attempting to make all data more readily available at both the state and local levels for program planning, evaluation, and research policy formation (see Figure 2-3).[12] Important questions are: Will the data be available when they are needed for decision making? Will the data answer our future questions, or will we always be playing "catch-up" because no techniques currently provide on-line assessment? Are new methods or adaptations of established methods needed to meet the technology and state of the nutrition science for the 21st century?

NATIONWIDE FOOD CONSUMPTION

USDA surveys are used to describe food consumption behavior and to assess the nutrient composition of eating patterns.[13] Findings influence policies relating to food production and marketing, food safety, food assistance, and nutrition education. As part of the National Nutrition Monitoring System, USDA monitors food and nutrient consumption at three levels[13]:

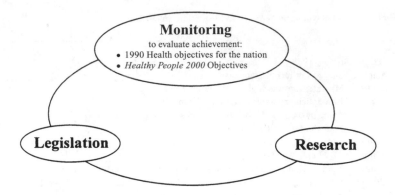

Figure 2-3 The interaction of nutrition monitoring, research, and legislation. Products resulting from the interaction include knowledge of the achievement of national objectives and formulation of recommendations. *Source:* Adapted from Kuczmarski M.F., Moshfegh A., and Briefel, R., Update on Nutrition Monitoring Activities in the U.S., *Journal of the American Dietetic Association*, Vol. 94, pp. 753–760, with permission of the American Dietetic Association, © 1994.

- *Food available to the US civilian population (food supply or food disappearance):* Data on production, imports and exports, military use, and beginning and year-end inventories are aggregated to describe the US food supply. Per capita data are used with tables of food composition to estimate the nutrient intake of each individual. These data have been available since 1909.

- *Food purchased and consumed by households:* Every ten years the cost and amount of food consumed by households over a seven-day period are surveyed. The quantities of foods reported are converted to pounds and merged with nutrient composition to estimate household nutrient content.

- *Individual food profile:* Every ten years a national survey is complemented with smaller, ongoing surveys to assess foods eaten at home and away from home. The individual food profile reflects actual food ingested and provides nutrient intakes most suitable for dietary assessment purposes (see Table 2-7). The 1987 database was expanded to provide fatty acid, antioxidant, B-vitamin, and mineral data of increasing scientific interest.[14,15]

Data from the household and individual food profiles comprise the USDA Nationwide Food Consumption Surveys. With each new but recurrent survey, various steps are taken to create a timely description of US food patterns.[13,16,17] These steps include the following:

- A review is conducted to establish why the USDA needs the data and how the data are used by other federal agencies, food industry analysts, nutrition specialists, home economists, agricultural economists, state and local governments, and academicians. Exhibit 2-6 identifies potential uses of the data.

- A review and evaluation are completed of food consumption and related surveys conducted by the USDA, federal departments, states, and the private sector.

- Definitions, questions, and assumptions used previously (e.g., in Nationwide Food Consumption Surveys or the National Health and Nutrition Examination Surveys) are reviewed to improve comparability and linkages across surveys.

- Methodological studies are reviewed to identify procedures appropriate for large national surveys and to demonstrate techniques for improved validity and reliability, such as whether to increase the number of 24-hour dietary recalls per respondent. Because the 24-hour recall is commonly used, the trend is to collect multiple days of dietary data to

Table 2–7 USDA Nutrient Database for Nationwide Food Consumption Surveys

	Database	
Dietary Component	*1977–1978*	*1987*
Food energy	*	*
Protein	*	*
Total fat	*	*
Saturated fatty acids		*
Monounsaturated fatty acids		*
Polyunsaturated fatty acids		*
Cholesterol		*
Carbohydrate	*	*
Vitamin A (IU)	*	*
Vitamin C	*	*
Thiamin	*	*
Riboflavin	*	*
Niacin	*	*
Vitamin B_6	*	*
Vitamin B_{12}	*	*
Carotenes		*
Vitamin E		*
Calcium	*	*
Phosphorus	*	*
Magnesium	*	*
Iron	^	*
Folate		*
Zinc		*
Copper		*
Sodium		*
Potassium		*

*Dietary component is present in the nutrient database.

Source: Adapted from Peterkin, B.B., Rizek, R.L., and Tippett, K.S. Nationwide Food Consumption Survey, 1987. *Nutrition Today,* Vol. 18, p. 24, with permission of Williams & Wilkins, © 1988.

accurately assess usual food intake (see Exhibit 2–7).

- Research using new technology for data collection and processing is explored (e.g., evaluating the advantages of using microcomputers during household interviews or automating food coding of individual interviews).
- The USDA nutrient database that is used to profile nutrient composition of foods reported in the surveys is reviewed.
- Recommendations of committees within the National Research Council, the President's Task Force on Food Assistance, and the Joint Nutrition Monitoring Evaluation Committee of Congress are considered.

- Emerging diet and health associations are identified.
- Lifestyles altering eating patterns (e.g., increased physical activity or increased television watching) are evaluated.

The Continuing Survey of Food Intakes by Individuals (CSFII) has occurred on an annual basis since 1989.[13] CSFII monitors the dietary status of small national samples of women and young children in the general population (N = 1,500 households) and low-income population (N = 750 households) during interim years. Although the CSFII uses the 24-hour recall method similar to that used by the Nationwide Food Consumption Surveys (NFCS) in

Exhibit 2-6 Potential Applications for Data from Nationwide Food Consumption Surveys

DIETARY INTAKE PROFILES

- Provide baseline data on food and nutrient intake of the population.
- Monitor the nutritional content of eating patterns.
- Project the size and nature of high-risk populations.
- Identify intervention (food assistance, fortification, or education) most appropriate for populations at risk.
- Identify socioeconomic factors associated with diets.

ECONOMICS OF FOOD INTAKE

- Determine agricultural product, marketing facility, and service needs.
- Define the interplay of socioeconomic factors on the food demand and cost.
- Establish the importance of home gardens.
- Identify frequency and outcome of eating out.

FOOD PROGRAMS AND GUIDANCE

- Specify factors and the effect of participation in entitlement food programs on food cost and quality.
- Determine the effect of entitlement programs on food needs and requests.
- Select nutritional high-risk populations.

- Monitor the effect of eating pattern changes on health risk.
- Develop realistic food plans that address food preferences, dislikes, and restricted incomes.
- Enumerate adequate and practical amounts of foods for food entitlement programs.

FOOD SAFETY CONSIDERATIONS

- Quantify intake of contaminants, additives, and natural toxic substances in foods.
- Identify extraordinary eating patterns that include additives and other specific components.
- Recommend foods that might serve as suitable substrates for additives.
- Monitor food regulations and suggest changes.
- Determine the exposure or contact with certain foods and food products that increase one's nutritional risk.

HISTORICAL TRENDS

- Analyze the association between food intake, nutrient profile, and disease prevalence and incidence.
- Track food intake patterns from birth to elder ages.
- Forecast food intake and nutrient profiles resulting from various economic, technical, and societal changes.

Source: Adapted from Peterkin, B.B., Rizek, R.L., and Tippett, K.S. Nationwide Food Consumption Survey, 1987. *Nutrition Today,* Vol. 18, p. 24, with permission of Williams & Wilkins, © 1988.

Exhibit 2-7 Rationale for Collecting Multiple Days of Dietary Data

- To estimate interindividual and intraindividual variability
- To estimate an individual's usual eating patterns, including amount and type of foods consumed
- To evaluate prevalence of eating patterns against dietary recommendations

- To describe the distribution of nutrient intakes in different subgroups (e.g., children, ethnic groups)
- To identify intake of uncommon foods
- To encompass the variety and the consistency of different foods in an individual's eating pattern
- To control for weekday and weekend biases

1977–1978, modifications regarding fat and salt patterns, smoking, and physical activity were made. The nutrient database was expanded to include 28 food components. Results are reported annually using a "moving average" approach. A snapshot look at the 1987 NFCS demonstrates features of the survey design, data collection, and data management elements[13] (see Exhibit 2-8).

The NFCS is designed to obtain data from two probability samples: (1) the general population or basic survey, which acquires data from 6,000 households and 15,000 members, and (2) the low-income survey, comprised of 3,600 households with 10,100 members.

Both household data and individual data are collected via household interview with trained and experienced interviewers. Each household

Exhibit 2-8 Data Elements in the Nationwide Food Consumption Survey (NFCS), 1987

HOUSEHOLD COMPONENT

Questions appear on the screen of a laptop computer. An interviewer first asks the question and then enters the participant's response directly into the computer.

- Household composition and meal data for each family member
  1. sex, age
  2. pregnancy/lactation status
  3. number of meals or snacks during the previous week
     (a) at home
     (b) away from home
     (c) as guest or purchased
  4. cost of food
- Household food during the past week
  1. quantity of each food
  2. source (e.g., purchased, home-produced, or gift)
  3. purchase unit and price
  4. drinking water source
- Food entitlement program participation
  1. WIC (Special Supplemental Food Program for Women, Infants and Children)
  2. school lunch and breakfast
  3. food stamps
  4. direct distribution of cheese and butter
- Household characteristics
  1. race
  2. ethnicity
  3. income previous month
  4. income previous year
  5. cash assets
  6. size
  7. food shopping practices
  8. education of male and female heads
  9. age of male and female heads
  10. employment of male and female heads
  11. description of dwelling
  12. kitchen equipment

INDIVIDUAL COMPONENT

An interviewer asks each participant to recall the types and amounts of each food eaten during the 24-hour period before the interview. Information is entered onto a form. Each participant is asked to record all foods and beverages eaten on the interview day and the next day. The resulting food records are reviewed and collected the day after the records are completed.

- Three-day food records:
  1. time
  2. eating contact (breakfast, snack, etc.)
  3. situation (alone, with family, etc.)
  4. description of food (descriptors in an easy-to-use instruction book are used)
  5. quantity consumed (measuring utensils are provided)
  6. food source (foods at home versus from restaurant, etc.)
  7. preparation additions (salt, fat, etc.)
  8. water intake
- Other pertinent information:
  1. regarding food
     (a) how typical
     (b) healthfulness (self-evaluation)
     (c) added salt at table
     (d) special restrictions
     (e) vegetarian
     (f) supplement use
     (g) calcium-rich foods
     (h) alcohol intake
  2. regarding respondent
     (a) height and weight (self-reported)
     (b) health status (self-evaluation)
     (c) smoking
     (d) disability, handicap
     (e) diagnosed disease
     (f) problem chewing food and why
     (g) leisure physical activity

Note: To obtain more information on the NFCS instrumentation, contact Nutrition Monitoring Division, Human Nutrition Information Service, USDA, Federal Building, Hyattsville, Maryland 20782.

Source: Adapted from Peterkin, B.B., Rizek, R.L., and Tippett, K.S. Nationwide Food Consumption Survey, 1987. *Nutrition Today,* Vol. 18, p. 24, with permission of Williams & Wilkins, © 1988.

---

is contacted a week before a two-to-three-hour interview with the person most knowledgeable about meal planning and preparation. This household food manager is asked to retain store receipts, recipes, menus, or calendars that will increase the accuracy of the interview. Data collection has three components:

- *Household food use component:* Using a laptop computer, the food manager is asked to recall the types and amounts of food that have disappeared from home food supplies over the previous seven days. This includes food that was prepared, eaten, discarded, leftover, or fed to pets. The cost of each food is recorded.

- *Individual intake component:* At the close of the household interview, the respondent is asked to recall the foods eaten during the previous 24 hours.
- *Follow up:* The interviewer leaves three-day food diaries for the respondent and any children in the household. Teenagers and other adults recall and record their own food intakes. Two days later the interviewer returns to review and to collect all food records.

The data management component addresses the system by which the collected data are converted into nutrient profiles:

- *Household food use component:* Each food is given one of more than 4,000 food codes linked to a food group and price. Mean prices are recorded for foods consumed, and foods are converted to pounds. A nutrient profile with 28 food components is calculated with the nutritive value of the household eating pattern compared with the RDA values. This profile indicates whether the household food was sufficient to meet RDAs for all members.
- *Individual food intake component.* Each food is assigned a food code, and the amount consumed is converted to grams of edible portion. Individuals nutrient intake for a three-day period is determined and compared to sex- and age-specific RDAs.

In 1989, DHHS's Food and Drug Administration and USDA's Food Safety and Inspection Service assisted the Human Nutrition Information Service with a telephone survey of consumer knowledge and attitudes about certain diet/ health and safety issues. The data will serve as a foundation for future exploration of food intake behavior, knowledge, and attitudes using a national sample.[13]

BENEFITS AND DISADVANTAGES OF SURVEYS

Combining large, decennial surveys of household food use with the smaller, continuous surveys is beneficial. Decennial surveys yield cross-sectional household and food intake data, identify differences among population segments, and elucidate factors associated with food consumption and nutritional quality of diets. Concerns include changes over time (e.g., changes in nutrient databases and food composition), potential lack of standardization due to different interviewers and training techniques, and the analytical problems of merging the data. Cost remains a concern.

Smaller surveys enable continuous monitoring of food intakes by all sex/age groups, provide data for two subgroups (the general public and low-income groups), are economical and flexible, and yield a format to explore issues and methodological investigations. Although small surveys are less expensive than larger surveys, concerns about them include the tendency to rely on the data for decision making because it is available sooner and the potential change or deviation in methods because the measurements are closer and observers may become lax.

The continuing survey will occur throughout most of the six years of NHANES III, allowing for comparisons of dietary data across surveys for validity checks and other purposes. To date, various target surveys have been conducted and others are still needed (e.g., surveys on recent immigrants, seniors, homeless persons, drug users) in the United States to establish the general health of the nation. In general, the resulting data from surveys have provided baseline profiles and temporal changes to direct policy, programs, and further surveys.[13]

THE RECOMMENDED DIETARY ALLOWANCES

Nutrition surveillance and monitoring can detect nutritional problems by comparing intakes against standards. In the United States, the most common standards are the Recommended Dietary Allowances (RDAs).[13]

The RDA publication serves as a principal guide for developing nutrition programs and policies in the United States. The 10th edition of the National Research Council's *Recommended Dietary Allowances* in 1989 was the first update of the nutrient intake recommendations in nearly a decade.[5] This edition was issued by a five-member subcommittee of the Food and Nutrition Board. RDAs for two nutrients (vitamin K and selenium) were added, and RDAs were changed for several vitamins and minerals.

Role of the RDAs

The first RDAs were published in 1941 and served as a guide for advising the federal government about nutrition problems related to national defense, especially the dietary needs of US troops during World War II. Various uses of the RDAs are listed in Table 2–8. The RDAs are based on the nutritional needs of groups rather than individuals, but they are often used to evaluate adequacy of an individual's food pattern. Until an improved standard is identified, community nutrition professionals should use RDAs for assessment of groups, employ multiple days of assessment to evaluate an individual's intake, and expand beyond dietary data (e.g., biochemical and anthropometric data) to characterize a group. RDA reference points (see Figure 2–4) provide a systematic way to organize scientific research data[18]:

- *Deficient*–level of intake of a nutrient below which almost all healthy people can be expected, over time, to experience deficiency symptoms of a clinical, physical, or functional nature.
- *Average requirement*–mean level of intake of a nutrient or food component that appears, on the basis of experimental evidence, sufficient to maintain the desired biochemical/physiological function in a population. It is also important to know the variation in the mean requirement.

- *Recommended Dietary Allowance* (RDA)–level of intake of an essential nutrient or food component considered on the basis of available scientific knowledge to be adequate to meet the known nutritional needs of practically all healthy persons. There will be a continuing need to redefine numerical recommendations. For some nutrients, other functional endpoints might be defined and included as criteria for the definition of recommended intakes.
- *Upper safe*–level of intake of a nutrient or food component that appears to be safe for most healthy people and beyond which there is concern that some people will experience symptoms of toxicity over time.

The USDA uses the RDAs to evaluate adequacy of the US food supply, to establish standards for food assistance programs, and to determine the nutritional status of the US population. The FDA uses the RDAs to prepare product labels and to evaluate new food products.

The 1989 RDAs include protein, 11 vitamins, and 7 minerals (see Tables 2–9 through 2–12). Recommended allowances are not given for each known nutrient because compositional data are insufficient. By eating a variety of foods that meet the RDAs, adequacy of other nutrients is likely. Otherwise, if a deficiency is observed, such as iron deficiency in women, fortification and possibly individual supplementation appears appropriate.

The RDAs are time-averaged goals, not daily objectives. When planning meals or food supplies, individuals should design eating patterns to meet all the RDAs over a five-to-ten-day interval.

Major RDA Changes: 1980 to 1989

The National Health and Nutrition Examination Survey (HANES) data and research conducted since 1980 provided evidence for making important revisions in the RDAs. RDAs for adults

Table 2–8 Uses of the RDAs

Use	Model	Suggestion
Food planning and procurement	Use to develop plans for feeding groups of healthy people.	Use as an appropriate nutrient standard for a period of at least a week, but also use as one of many food-planning criteria; this should be adjusted as group varies from RDA reference individual.
	Use for food purchasing, cost control, and budgeting.	Use as an appropriate nutrient standard with knowledge of such factors as food composition, availability, acceptability, and storage changes and losses.
Food programs	Serve as a basis for the nutritional goal for feeding programs.	Use as a standard for nutritional quality of meals, along with other food-selection criteria.
	Provide the nutritional standard for the Thrifty Food Plan, the basis for allotments in the Food Stamp Program.	Use as a guideline, along with other food-selection criteria.
	Provide nutritional guidelines for food distribution programs.	Use as a standard for nutritional quality of food packages.
Evaluating dietary survey	Evaluate dietary intake of individuals.	Use as a standard for data evaluating dietary status, but not for evaluating individual nutritional status.
	Evaluate household food use.	Use as a benchmark to compare households and to identify nutrient shortfalls.
	Evaluate national food supply (food disappearance data).	Use only as a benchmark for comparison over time and to identify nutrient shortfalls.
Guides for food selection	Develop and evaluate food guides and family food plans.	Use along with other food-selection criteria.
Food and nutrition information and education	Provide guidelines for obtaining nutritious diets.	Use as a point of reference; this information becomes more useful to consumers when translated into food-selection goals.
	Use as a basis for educators to discuss individuals' nutrient needs.	Use in combination with information in the text accompanying the RDA table and with recognition that the RDAs are for reference individuals.
	Evaluate an individual's diet as a basis for recommending specific changes in food patterns and/or dietary supplements.	Use to identify nutrient shortfalls and as a tool to assess nutrient contribution of diet; do not use in prescriptive manner.
Food labeling	Provide basis for nutritional labeling of foods.	Use as a basis for labeling standards; such standards should not be used to determine nutritional intake of individuals or groups.

continues

Table 2–8 continued

Use	Model	Suggestion
Food fortification	Serve as a guide for fortification for general population.	Use as a guide, but such other factors as food-consumption patterns and contribution to the total diet also must be considered.
Developing new or modified food products	Provide guidance in establishing nutritional levels for new food products.	Use in combination with information or probable products; use within the context of the total diet.
Clinical dietetics	Develop therapeutic diet manuals.	Use to assess the nutritional quality of modified diets.
	Plan modified diets.	Use as a starting point along with information on the patient's nutritional status and individual needs.
	Counsel patients who require modified diets.	Use as one basis for advice on food selection.
	Plan menus and foods served in institutions for the developmentally disabled.	Use as a starting point, but modify for individual's developmental status and body size.
Nutrient supplements and special dietary foods	Use as a basis to formulate supplements and special dietary foods.	Use as a basis in developing infant formulas and other oral supplements or foods, but also consider nutrient bioavailability and nutrient balance; RDAs cannot be used as the only guide for parenteral feeding products.

Source: Adapted with permission from *How Should the Recommended Dietary Allowances Be Revised?* Copyright © 1994 by the National Academy of Sciences. Courtesy of the National Academy Press, Washington, D.C.

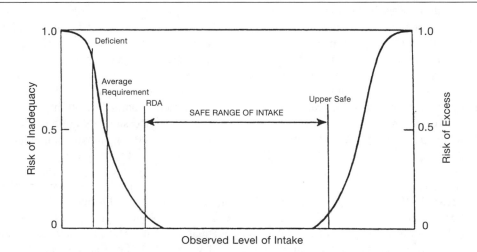

Figure 2–4 The concept of a safe intake range. The safe intake range is associated with a very low probability of either inadequacy or excess for an individual selected at random from the population. *Source:* Adapted from Health and Welfare, Canada, 1983.

Table 2–9 Recommended Dietary Allowances[a]

Category or Condition	Age (years)	Weight[b] (kg)	(lb)	Height[b] (cm)	(in)	Protein (g)
Infants	0.0–0.5	6	13	60	24	13
	0.5–1.0	9	20	71	28	14
Children	1–3	13	29	90	35	16
	4–6	20	44	112	44	24
	7–10	28	62	132	52	28
Males	11–14	45	99	157	62	45
	15–18	66	145	176	69	59
	19–24	72	160	177	70	58
	25–50	79	174	176	70	63
	51+	77	170	173	68	63
Females	11–14	46	101	157	62	46
	15–18	55	120	163	64	44
	19–24	58	128	164	65	46
	25–50	63	138	163	64	50
	51+	65	143	160	63	50
Pregnant						60
Lactating 1st 6 months						65
2nd 6 months						62

[a]The allowances, expressed as average daily intakes over time, are intended to provide for individual variations among most normal persons as they live in the US under usual environmental stresses. Diets should be based on a variety of common foods in order to provide other nutrients for which human requirements have been less well defined.

[b]Weights and heights of Reference Adults are actual medians for the US population of the designated age, as reported by NHANES II. The median weights and heights of those under 19 years of age may not be ideal.

Source: Reprinted with permission from *Recommended Dietary Allowances,* 10th ed., Copyright © 1989 by the National Academy of Sciences. Courtesy of the National Academy Press, Washington, D.C.

in the 1989 edition were based on actual heights and weights in the population; thus, some RDAs differed from the 1980 recommendations.

Observations of adult populations in the United States and Canada show adults can maintain good health by consuming less folate (e.g., about 200 µg a day). Therefore, the RDA was not maintained at 240 µg for men and 190 µg for women. Folate is found in liver, leafy vegetables, and some fruits; severe deficiency causes anemia. The RDA for Vitamin B_{12} was reduced from 3 µg a day. Vitamin B_{12} assists with normal metabolism and function of the blood-forming organs and is found in animal products.

Vitamin K aids normal blood clotting; 80 and 65 µg a day are recommended for men and women, respectively. Green leafy vegetables are the best source. The RDAs for selenium are 70 µg for men and 55 µg for women.

An additional 10 g of protein a day was recommended for women during pregnancy. The RDA for iron was lowered from 18 to 15 mg for adolescent girls and premenopausal women, and increased for pregnant women by 15 mg to 30 mg. There was no change in the RDA for vitamin C, which remained at 60 mg for men and women. Cigarette smokers are advised to consume at least 100 mg daily of vitamin C, due to their rapid loss of the vitamin.

An average daily intake of 1,200 mg of calcium is recommended for adolescents through age 24, rather than through 18 years as previously recommended. The scientific belief is that adequate calcium intake throughout the adolescent years offers the best nutritional approach to reduce osteoporotic risk in later life. The calcium allowance for women 25 years of age and older remained at 800 mg.

Table 2–10 Recommended Dietary Allowances—Fat-Soluble Vitamins

Category or Condition	Age (years)	Fat-Soluble Vitamins			
		Vitamin A (μg RE)[a]	Vitamin D (μg)[b]	Vitamin E (mg alpha-TE)[c]	Vitamin K (μg)
Infants	0.0–0.5	375	7.5	3	5
	0.5–1.0	375	10	4	10
Children	1–3	400	10	6	15
	4–6	500	10	7	20
	7–10	700	10	7	30
Males	11–14	1,000	10	10	45
	15–18	1,000	10	10	65
	19–24	1,000	10	10	70
	25–50	1,000	5	10	80
	51+	1,000	5	10	80
Females	11–14	800	10	8	45
	15–18	800	10	8	55
	19–24	800	10	8	60
	25–50	800	5	8	65
	51+	800	5	8	65
Pregnant		800	10	10	65
Lactating 1st 6 months		1,300	10	12	65
2nd 6 months		1,200	10	11	65

[a]Retinol equivalents. 1 retinol equivalent = 1 microgram retinol or 6 micrograms beta-carotene.
[b]As cholecalciferol. 10 micrograms of cholecalciferol = 400 IU of vitamin D.
[c]Alpha-tocopherol equivalents. 1 mg d-alpha-tocopherol = 1 alpha-TE.

Source: Reprinted with permission from *Recommended Dietary Allowances,* 10th ed., Copyright © 1989 by the National Academy of Sciences. Courtesy of the National Academy Press, Washington, D.C.

RDAs for magnesium are decreased not only for children but also for women during pregnancy and lactation. The RDA for zinc was lowered to 12 mg a day for adult women, but remained at 15 mg for adult men. RDAs for Vitamin B_6 were reduced for adult men and women.

Changing the RDAs

The Food and Nutrition Board organized a symposium called "Should the Recommended Dietary Allowances Be Revised?" which was held June 28–29, 1993. Various groups of individuals demanded further discussion about food labels, vitamins, and dairy and meat products. Nutrition became a basketball in the political arena.

The scientific and advocacy communities voiced opinions in response to five general questions. The questions and a summary of the responses follow[18]:

1. *What has been the experience applying the RDAs in different situations, and what factors limit their usefulness?*
   - incompleteness of the scientific base used for the RDAs
   - uncertainties about the biological variability in requirements that exist among individuals
   - limitations that result from the focus on the traditional concern of preventing deficiency disorders
   - lack of additional age-specific recommendations for individuals over the age of 51
   - lack of sufficient emphasis on the range of appropriate macronutrient intakes
   - lack of relevance to chronic disease and the concomitant need to address dietary fat, fiber, and some vitamins

Table 2–11 Recommended Dietary Allowances—Water-Soluble Vitamins

Category or Condition	Age (years)	Water-Soluble Vitamins						
		Vitamin C (mg)	Thiamin (mg)	Riboflavin (mg)	Niacin (mg NE)[a]	Vitamin B$_6$ (mg)	Folate (µg)	Vitamin B$_{12}$ (µg)
Infants	0.0–0.5	30	0.3	0.4	5	0.3	25	0.3
	0.5–1.0	35	0.4	0.5	6	0.6	35	0.5
Children	1–3	40	0.7	0.8	9	1.0	50	0.7
	4–6	45	0.9	1.1	12	1.1	75	1.0
	7–10	45	1.0	1.2	13	1.4	100	1.4
Males	11–14	50	1.3	1.5	17	1.7	150	2.0
	15–18	60	1.5	1.8	20	2.0	200	2.0
	19–24	60	1.5	1.7	19	2.0	200	2.0
	25–50	60	1.5	1.7	19	2.0	200	2.0
	51+	60	1.2	1.4	15	2.0	200	2.0
Females	11–14	50	1.1	1.3	15	1.4	150	2.0
	15–18	60	1.1	1.3	15	1.5	180	2.0
	19–24	60	1.1	1.3	15	1.6	180	2.0
	25–50	60	1.1	1.3	15	1.6	180	2.0
	51+	60	1.0	1.2	13	1.6	180	2.0
Pregnant		70	1.5	1.6	17	2.2	400	2.2
Lactating	1st 6 months	95	1.6	1.8	20	2.1	280	2.6
	2nd 6 months	90	1.6	1.7	20	2.1	260	2.6

[a]1 NE (niacin equivalent) is equal to 1 mg of niacin or 60 mg of dietary tryptophan.

- lack of information that addresses nutrient needs over the life cycle
- little consideration of nutrient interactions and varying activity levels
- potential overestimation of actual requirements, making it difficult to determine at what levels of intake a population is truly at risk
- existence of several levels of dietary allowances to address different needs and purposes
- development of a separate set of RDAs for use in food labeling
- the need for additional documentation to explain the derivation of the numbers and to facilitate their appropriate application
- the need to merge dietary guidelines with the RDAs to promote one consistent message to the public and to provide this information for the public's use in a less scientific and more accessible publication.

2. *What new evidence would argue for a change from the present values or a reexamination of the evidence?*
   - recommendations for an increase in an existing RDA (e.g., folic acid, calcium, vitamin D, and the antioxidant vitamins [ascorbic acid and vitamin E]) for a least some age and sex categories
   - recommendations for a decrease in an existing RDA (e.g., caloric intake, protein, and iron)
   - recommendations for establishing a new RDA for a particular nutrient or food component not currently covered (e.g., beta-carotene, omega-3 fatty acids, sodium, potassium, choline, dietary fiber, or macronutrients)

3. *Should concepts of reduction of risk of chronic disease be included in the devel-*

Table 2–12 Recommended Dietary Allowances—Minerals

Category or Condition	Age (years)	Calcium (mg)	Phospho- rus (mg)	Magnesium (mg)	Iron (mg)	Zinc (mg)	Iodine (µg)	Selenium (µg)
Infants	0.0–0.5	400	300	40	6	5	40	10
	0.5–1.0	600	500	60	10	5	50	15
Children	1–3	800	800	80	10	10	70	20
	4–6	800	800	120	10	10	90	20
	7–10	800	800	170	10	10	120	30
Males	11–14	1,200	1,200	270	12	15	150	40
	15–18	1,200	1,200	400	12	15	150	50
	19–24	1,200	1,200	350	10	15	150	70
	25–50	800	800	350	10	15	150	70
	51+	800	800	350	10	15	150	70
Females	11–14	1,200	1,200	280	15	12	150	45
	15–18	1,200	1,200	300	15	12	150	50
	19–24	1,200	1,200	280	15	12	150	55
	25–50	800	800	280	15	12	150	55
	51+	800	800	280	10	12	150	55
Pregnant		1,200	1,200	320	30	15	175	65
Lactating	1st 6 months	1,200	1,200	355	15	19	200	75
	2nd 6 months	1,200	1,200	340	15	16	200	75

Source: Reprinted with permission from *Recommended Dietary Allowances,* 10th ed., Copyright © 1989 by the National Academy of Sciences. Courtesy of the National Academy Press, Washington, D.C.

opment of allowances? The majority said that concepts of risk reduction for chronic disease should be included in developing the RDAs. Others argued that the RDAs should remain distinct from dietary guidelines for reducing the risk of chronic disease, because the purposes of the RDAs and the dietary guidelines are very different. A nutrient standard for narrower nutritional applications, like food labeling, was mentioned.

4. *How should recommended levels of intake be expressed?* Ranges rather than single values were favored because ranges allow differences among individuals and groups, give more recognition to the biological heterogeneity among individuals, and dispel the notion that the numbers recommended represent exact requirements.

5. *Is knowledge of relationships among nutrients sufficient to consider when estab-*

lishing the RDAs? Very few comments were received on this question. Use of bioavailability algorithms in establishing the RDAs may be considered.

NUTRIENT INFORMATION ON FOOD LABELS

The best guide for individuals to evaluate how well their eating pattern meets the RDAs is found on the food label. In addition, the most visible and accessible format for nutrition education for the public is the food label. The regulatory authority for food labeling rests with the FDA, USDA, and the Federal Trade Commission (FTC). USDA regulates poultry according to the Poultry Products Inspection Act and regulates meat under the Federal Meat Inspection Act. Under the Food, Drug and Cosmetic (FD&C) Act, FDA regulates the labeling of all other foods. Manufacturers must obtain prior approval by USDA for any label.[19] The FTC challenges product claims when products cross state boundaries.

FDA can challenge mislabeled products, and it maintains persistent monitoring. A committee sponsored by both FDA and USDA met in 1989 and published recommendations in 1992 about how food labels could be improved to help consumers with healthy eating. One recommendation was that FDA and USDA adopt mandatory and uniform nutrition labeling requirements. A second recommendation was that Congress endorse the authority of FDA and USDA to mandate nutritional labeling.

President George Bush signed the Nutrition Labeling and Education Act (NLEA) on November 8, 1990.[20,21] On January 6, 1993, the FDA issued the Final Rule implementing the NLEA.[20,21] Provisions became effective May 8, 1993.[22]

NLEA is considered the most powerful piece of legislation about food and labeling since the 1938 FD&C Act.[23-25] It is a landmark effort because it requires standard food labels and nutrition information on practically all foods produced and sold in the United States. NLEA mandated the following:

- nutrition labeling for conventional foods
- FDA regulation of claims about health (e.g., low fat to prevent cancer and heart disease, low sodium to prevent hypertension, and calcium to prevent osteoporosis)

The nutrition label is required to include information on total calories, calories from fat, total fat, saturated fat, cholesterol, sodium, total carbohydrates, dietary fiber, sugars, protein, vitamin A, vitamin C, calcium, and iron (see Figure 2–5).[22] Manufacturers may volunteer information on calories from saturated fat and on amounts of polyunsaturated and monounsaturated fat, soluble and insoluble fiber, sugar alcohol, other carbohydrate, potassium, additional vitamins and minerals with established Reference Daily Intakes (RDIs), and the content of vitamin A as beta-carotene. The nutrition label information must characterize the packaged product accurately prior to consumer preparation.

The final FDA rule establishes a standard format for nutrition information on food labels.[22,26] This information includes the quantitative amount per serving for each nutrient except vitamins and minerals, the amount of each nutrient as a percentage of the Daily Value for a 2,000-calorie diet, a footnote with reference values for selected nutrients based on 2,000-calorie and 2,500-calorie diets, and caloric conversion information.

Some foods are exempt from mandatory nutrition labeling requirements. These include foods offered for sale by small businesses; foods sold in restaurants or other establishments in which food is served for immediate human consumption; foods similar to restaurant foods (e.g., ready-to-eat but not for immediate consumption), but primarily prepared on site and not offered for sale outside the premise; foods that contain insignificant amounts of all nutrients subject to this rule (e.g., coffee and tea); dietary supplements, except those in conventional food form; infant formula; medical foods; custom-processed fish or game meats; foods shipped in bulk form; and donated foods.[22] Manufacturers that make a nutrient content claim or health claim on an exempted food forfeit the exemption.

Some food products are not required to include food label information due to special labeling provisions. These include foods in small packages with less than 12 square inches available for labeling (an address or telephone number is required for consumers to obtain nutrition information); packages with 40 square inches or less (these may list the required information in tabular or linear fashion if the package shape cannot accommodate the other information in the specified format); food for children less than two years of age (these products must not declare information concerning calories from fat, fatty acids, and cholesterol); foods for children less than four years of age (these must not include Daily Value information); raw fruits, vegetables, and fish (these should follow voluntary nutrition labeling guidelines); packaged single-ingredient fish or game meat (these may provide information on an "as prepared" basis); foods sold from bulk containers and game meat products (these may provide information on labeling); shell eggs (these

LEAN·POCKETS®

Fast & Healthy™

COOKING DIRECTIONS:
MICROWAVE HEATING: Lean Pockets are specially formulated to come out crisp in the microwave.

QUANTITY	HEATING TIME (frozen)
1 Lean Pockets	Heat 2½-3½ minutes
2 Lean Pockets	Heat 4-5 minutes

*Individual ovens heat differently, cooking time is approximate

1. Unwrap frozen Lean Pockets and insert into crisping sleeve. Microwave on HIGH according to chart*. Using pot holder, rotate ½ turn once during heating

2. CAUTION: Product will be hot. Using pot holder, remove from crisping sleeve and serve. Do not re-use crisping sleeve. NOTE: For softer crust, do not use crisping sleeve. Instead, place on a paper towel and microwave on high 2-3 minutes.

3 MINUTES TO GREAT TASTE!
Treat yourself and your family to the taste that has made Lean Pockets America's favorite.

Lean Pockets are the quick-and-easy "Hot Meal in a Pocket" — perfect for busy lifestyles. Lean Pockets fits into a healthy balanced diet.

TRY ALL LEAN POCKETS —
FAST & HEALTHY —
GREAT TASTE —
♦ Turkey, Broccoli & Cheese
♦ Sausage & Pepperoni Pizza Deluxe
♦ Chicken Fajita
♦ Chicken Parmesan
♦ Beef and Broccoli
♦ Glazed Chicken Supreme

TOASTER OVEN OR REGULAR OVEN:
1. Remove Lean Pockets from wrapper. Throw away sleeve. (Sleeves are for microwave use only.)
2. Place on aluminum foil or baking sheet. Bake at 350° F in heated oven for 20-25 minutes*.

Nutrition Facts

Serving Size 1 Sandwich (128g)
Servings Per Container 2

Amount Per Serving

Calories 260   Calories from Fat 70

	% Daily Value*
Total Fat 8g	**12%**
Saturated Fat 3g	**16%**
Cholesterol 40mg	**13%**
Sodium 770mg	**32%**
Total Carbohydrate 36g	**12%**
Dietary Fiber 3g	**13%**
Sugars 4g	
Protein 12g	

Vitamin A 8%	•	Vitamin C 4%
Calcium 20%	•	Iron 4%

*Percent Daily Values are based on a 2,000 calorie diet. Your daily values may vary higher or lower depending on your calorie needs:

		Calories	2,000	2,500
Total Fat	Less than		65g	80g
Sat. Fat	Less than		20g	25g
Cholesterol	Less than		300mg	300mg
Sodium	Less than		2,400mg	2,400mg
Total Carbohydrate			300g	375g
Dietary Fiber			25g	30g

Diet Exchanges † Per Serving: 1 Medium Fat Meat, 2 Bread/Starch, 1 Fat.
†Exchange calculations based on the Exchange Lists for Meal Planning. ©1989 the American Diabetes Association, The American Dietetic Association.

Figure 2–5 Label of a convenience food giving preparation instructions, nutrition facts, and diet exchange profile. Courtesy of Chef America, Inc., Chatsworth, California.

---

may provide the required nutrition information inside the egg carton); multi-unit packages (only the outer package of unit containers must provide nutrition information); and gift packs of food (manufacturers may provide information on labeling according to the special requirements).[22]

Reference Daily Intakes and Daily Reference Values

The final FDA rule establishes the reference values for the food label. The Dietary Supplement Act of 1992[22] requires FDA to retain current US Recommended Daily Allowance values for vita-

mins and minerals (i.e., values that had been developed chiefly by selecting the highest RDA value from among the various sex/age groups listed in RDA tables published in 1968). The Dietary Supplement Act of 1992 establishes label reference values for 19 vitamins and minerals. The description for those values changes from US Recommended Daily Allowance to Reference Daily Intake (RDI). The Dietary Supplement Act of 1992 did not establish reference values for infants, children less than four years of age, pregnant women, or lactating women.

The FDA regulation expands the label reference values to include eight other nutrients, including fat, cholesterol, and fiber. These values are called Daily Reference Values (DRVs) and are established for nutrients of public health importance. They serve as a point of reference for adults and children four years of age and older.[22] An energy intake of 2,000 calories per day is used as the basis for reference values. The resulting nutrients with DRVs are: fat (65 g), saturated fat (20 g), cholesterol (300 mg), total carbohydrate (300 g), fiber (25 g), sodium (2,400 mg), potassium (3,500 mg), and protein (50 g). To reduce confusion, all reference values on food labels are called Daily Values or DVs.

Serving Sizes

A serving size regulation was established that does the following:

- It defines serving size based on the amount of food usually consumed per eating occasion.
- It establishes reference amounts usually consumed for 139 specific food product categories and establishes a petition process of modifying the list.
- It provides rules for using the reference amounts to determine serving sizes for specific food products.
- It requires both common household and metric measures on the label (e.g., 1 cup [240 mL] for milk, 1 slice [28 g] for sliced bread).
- It permits optional declaration of serving size in US measures (ounces or fluid ounces) in addition to the household and metric measures (e.g., 1 cup [240 mL/8 fl oz]).
- It allows a second column on the nutrition label to express the nutrition content per 100 g or 100 mL or per 1 oz for all products; per unit for products in discrete units (e.g., sliced products such as bread, muffins, cookies, ice cream bars, etc.); and per cup popped for popcorn.
- It defines a "single-serving container" as any package that contains less than 200% of the reference amount for the food product category. The reference amount for soft drinks is 8 fl oz. A 12 fl oz can of soft drink is a single-serving container. Its nutrient content

must be based on the entire contents of the can. If products contain more than 150% but less than 200% of the reference amount when the reference amount is 100 g or 100 mL or larger, the manufacturer may determine whether to declare one or two servings. If 245 g is the reference amount for soups, a 15-oz can of soup may be labeled as two servings.

- It defines a unit of product in discrete segments (e.g., sliced bread or a single muffin). If multiserving containers are sold, a single serving is allowed on the label if the unit weighs more than 50% but less than 200% of the reference amount. For bread, the reference amount is 50 g and the serving size of sliced bread is 1 slice if a slice weighs more than 25 g.
- It allows claims such as "low sodium" if the product qualifies based on the reference amount for the product category. When serving size differs from the reference amount but the product qualifies for the claim, the claim must be followed by the criteria (for example, "very low sodium, 35 mg or less per 240 mL or 8 fl oz")[22]

Definition of Descriptor Terms

FDA defines the terms *free, low, light* or *lite, reduced, less,* and *high,* along with selected synonyms. The terms *good source, very low* (for sodium only), *lean, extra lean, fewer, more,* and *added* (or *fortified* or *enriched*) are also identified. The terms *healthy* and *fresh* are defined, but *natural* is not. A partial list of terms and definitions is given in Table 2–13.

Free equates to an amount that is nutritionally insignificant. The following can be labeled as zero: sodium, less than 5 mg; calories, less than 5 calories; sugars, less than 0.5 g; saturated fat, less than 0.5 g; and trans fatty acids not exceeding 1% of total fat; and cholesterol, less than 2 mg. Foods that do not undergo a special process to reduce the nutrient are basically free and must be labeled as such (e.g., "leaf lettuce, a sodium-free food").

Table 2–13 Partial Listing of Key Words and Health Claims on Food Labels Regulated by FDA

Key Word	Meaning
Fat Free	Less than 0.5 g fat per serving
Low Fat	3 g fat (or less) per serving
Lean	Less than 10 g fat, 4 g saturated fat, and 95 mg cholesterol per serving
Light (Lite)	1/3 less calories or no more than 1/2 the fat of the higher-calorie, higher-fat version; or no more than 1/2 the sodium of the higher-sodium version
Cholesterol Free	Less than 2 mg cholesterol and 2 g (or less) saturated fat per serving

Source: Data from Food and Drug Administration. The FDA's final regulations on health claims for foods. *Nutr Rev.* March 1993;51:90–93. (Editor's article.)

A *cholesterol-free* claim is only allowed on foods containing 2 g or less of saturated fat per reference serving. Foods having more than 13 g total fat per reference serving must list the total fat content per serving immediately adjacent to the cholesterol claim.

Criteria for the term *low* are based on reference serving sizes. The values for different components include: sodium, less than 140 mg; calories, less than 40 calories; fat, less than 3 g; saturated fat, less than 1 g and not more than 15% of calories from saturated fat; and cholesterol, less than 20 mg. If the food is naturally low in a nutrient, the label must explain that all similar foods are low (e.g., "frozen bagel, a low-fat food," or "very low sodium describes a food with a sodium value less than or equal to 35 mg of sodium").

High and *good source* are based on a percentage of the Daily Value of the specific nutrients in a reference serving. *High* means 20% or more of the daily amount, whereas *good source* is between 10% and 19% of the daily amount.

For *light, reduced,* and *added,* the reference food must be similar to the product bearing the claim (e.g., a *lite* potato chip must be similar to regular potato chips). The terms *added, fortified,* and *enriched* are used interchangeably. All related claims must be accompanied by information on the identity of the reference food and the percentage or fraction by which the nutrient has been modified. The amount of the nutrient in the labeled product compared to the amount in the reference food must appear on the information panel.

The terms *reduced, less,* or *fewer* refer to a food with at least 25% less of the nutrient than the reference food; *more* or *added* defines a food with 10% or more of the Daily Value per reference serving. *Light* or *lite* means a food has at least 50% less calories from fat if the reference food has 50% or more of its calories from fat. Reference foods with 50% of calories from fat require the *light* foods be reduced in fat by at least 50% or in calories by at least one-third.

A food labeled *light in sodium* must have at least a 50% reduction in sodium content compared to an appropriate reference food. The words, *light in sodium* must be printed in the same size, style, color, and prominence as the remaining label. *Light* may also be used to describe an organoleptic quality if specific (e.g., "light in color").

Descriptions of percentage and amount for nutrients may be given on a food label, if such statements are truthful and not misleading (e.g., "6 g fat per serving, but not a low-fat food").

Lean describes fish or game meat if the food contains less than 10 g fat, less than 4 g saturated fat, and less than 96 mg cholesterol per reference serving and per 100 g. *Extra lean* defines a product with less than 5 g fat, less than 2 g saturated fat, and less than 95 mg cholesterol per reference serving and per 100 g.

Meal and main-dish product definitions are similar to single-nutrient definitions of *free. Free* is based on the specific nutrient value per 100 g.

High and *good source* are not applicable to meal-type products. These terms refer to a single food in the meal that meets the definition. The term *low calorie* means 120 calories per 100 g. To use the word *light*, the product must show which component the meal meets (e.g., "light, a low-fat meal," or "light in sodium").

The term *fresh* implies that a food is unprocessed, in its raw state, and never frozen or thermally processed. "Fresh bread" and "fresh milk" are not affected by this regulation.

The terms *lightly salted, no added sugar*, and ___% *fat free* are allowed on food labels if specific definitions are used. Implied claims are restricted. The term *healthy* can be printed on foods with less than 480 mg sodium or less than 60 mg cholesterol per serving.

Definition of *Healthy* Finalized

FDA and USDA published final rules defining the term *healthy* and its derivatives, *healthful* or *healthier*, as a nutrient content claim in food labeling effective May 8, 1994. Existing products are expected to comply by January 1, 1996. The rule that applies to meat and poultry product labels became official November 10, 1995. The term *healthy* may be used as an implied nutrient content claim on individual, FDA-regulated foods if the food complies with the following:

- contains 3 g fat or less per reference amount
- contains 1 g or less of saturated fatty acids per reference amount, which accounts for no more than 15% of calories
- contains at least 10% of the RDI or DRV of one of the following micronutrients per reference amount and per serving: vitamin A, vitamin C, protein, calcium, iron, and fiber (except for raw fruits and vegetables)
- contains 480 mg or less of sodium per reference amount and per serving prior to January 1, 1998, and 360 mg or less after that date

Restaurant menus are not within the scope of the regulations. If claims are made, restaurant foods must meet these definitions, but the claims can be based on nutrient database calculations. Restaurants have additional time to comply with the regulations.

Standardized Foods

A product with a nutrient content claim must have performance characteristics similar to those of the standardized food. The product must contain the ingredients used in the standardized food and any other safe and suitable ingredients. Water and approved fat substitutes can replace fat and calories.[22]

Declaration of Ingredients

The ingredient list on a food label lists all ingredients in order by weight, with the most predominant ingredient listed first. All certified color additives and protein hydrozylates must be identified by their common name (e.g., FD&C Blue No. 1, or hydrolyzed soy protein). Commonly used flavor enhancers may be added as a parenthetical term (e.g., "contains glutamate"). All ingredients in foods that are identified by a standard of identity must be listed. A sulfating agent having a functional effect or present at at least 10 parts per million must be identified.[22]

Preservative coatings on fresh fruits and vegetables can be listed by a generic name. Caseinate must be identified as a milk derivative if it is an ingredient and the food label states that the product is nondairy.

The standard of identity of canned tuna requires the words "includes soybeans" in the name, if soybeans are a vegetable extract in the broth.[22] The delimiter "and/or" can be used for sweeteners in soft drinks (e.g., "sugar and/or high-fructose corn syrup").

Juice Beverages

The ingredient statement on beverages containing fruit or vegetable juice must include the percentage of total juice. Criteria for naming juice beverages include the following:

- A beverage with less than 100% juice is a *juice beverage* or *juice drink*, not a *juice*.
- A multijuice beverage can list the names of the juices present, but if minimal in amount, the label must describe and give a 5% range (e.g., "strawberry-flavored juice blend" or "juice blend, 2–7% strawberry juice").

A 100% juice beverage must state *from concentrate* if it is made from concentrated juice. Modified juice beverages must describe their modification and accurately calculate the percentage of total juice present.[22]

GENERAL REQUIREMENTS FOR HEALTH CLAIMS ON FOOD LABELS

The Nutrition Labeling and Education Act mandates nutrition labels for conventional foods and requires FDA to regulate any claims printed on labels.[20,21,27,28] Several key words on labels have specific, defined meanings. If a health claim is made, then the food must have a certain composition (see Table 2–14).

The term *health claim* is defined for food labels to encompass both explicit and implied claims. Food labeling can include health claims, but the claims must be supported by valid and substantial scientific evidence. The claims must also be those FDA has specifically identified by regulation. The final rules exist for the following health claims: calcium and osteoporosis, dietary saturated fat and cholesterol and risk of coronary heart disease, dietary fat and cancer, sodium and hypertension, fiber-containing foods and cancer, fiber-containing foods and coronary heart disease, and folic acid and neural tube defects. Health claims that are not authorized include zinc and immune function in the elderly, and omega-3 fatty acids and coronary heart disease.[27,28]

A general health claim rule exists. It defines *disqualifying nutrient levels* and refers to specified levels of total fat, saturated fat, cholesterol, and sodium. A food will be disqualified from making any health claim if it contains one or more of these nutrients in amounts above widely accepted guidelines for reducing the risk. A higher value is allowed for main dish and meal products.[27,28]

A food bearing a health claim must be a good source of either vitamin A, vitamin C, iron, calcium, protein, or fiber before addition of other nutrients. Claims on infant and toddler foods are prohibited unless under a special permit. The final rule identifies the FDA process to review food label petitions and the information required for the review.[27,28] Rationale for and examples of model health claims are presented below.

Table 2–14 Health Claims and Required Composition on Labels

Health Claims Regarding:	Required Composition
Heart disease and fats	Low in fat, saturated fat, and cholesterol
Blood pressure and sodium	Low in sodium
Heart disease and fruits, vegetables, and grain products	A fruit, vegetable, or grain product low in fat, saturated fat, and cholesterol, that contains at least 0.6 g soluble fiber, without fortification, per serving

Source: Adapted from *How to Read the New Food Label* by the U.S. Food and Drug Administration and the American Heart Association, 1993.

Fiber-Containing Grain Products, Fruits, and Vegetables, and Cancer

Food labeling health claims relating low-fat, high-fiber foods and cancer are allowed. Research data show an association between fiber-containing grain products, fruits, and vegetables and below-normal rates of some cancers. The exact role of total dietary fiber and fiber components is not fully understood.

To have a health claim for fiber-containing grains, fruits, and vegetables and a reduced risk of cancer, a food must qualify as a low-fat food and contain, without fortification, a "good source" of dietary fiber. The claim cannot give any credit for cancer risk reduction to low-fat and fiber-rich foods, and it cannot specify types of dietary fiber that may relate to cancer risk.[22]

> *Model Health Claim:* "Low-fat diets rich in fiber-containing grain products, fruits, and vegetables may reduce the risk of some types of cancer, a disease associated with many factors."[22]

Fruits, Vegetables, and Grain Products That Contain Fiber, Particularly Soluble Fiber, and Risk of Coronary Heart Disease

Sufficient scientific evidence and scientific agreement exist that show that an eating pattern low in saturated fat and cholesterol and rich in fruits, vegetables, and grain products with certain dietary fibers may enhance coronary heart disease (CHD) risk reduction. Numerous scientific and professional organizations recommend that Americans consume foods low in saturated fat and cholesterol and rich in fruits, vegetables, and grain products. These foods are rich sources of soluble fiber, which is associated with lowering blood cholesterol. This claim clearly exemplifies applied nutritional epidemiology. That is, epidemiologic data provided the foundation linking food with nutrition and health; the science of nutrition identified the specific "protective" foods to promote health; and nutrition education of the public about food selection at the point of purchase has become the channel to communicate the message. Nutrition and epidemiology thereby became essential partners in the identification of the problem and the promotion and prevention of disease.

To bear a health claim relating fiber-rich fruits, vegetables, and grain products to CHD, a food must contain, without fortification, at least 0.6 g of soluble fiber in the common serving. The claim cannot give a numeric value to the potential risk reduction.[22]

> *Model Health Claim:* "Diets low in saturated fat and cholesterol and rich in fruits, vegetables, and grain products that contain some types of dietary fiber may reduce the risk of heart disease, a disease associated with many factors."[22]

Calcium and Osteoporosis

Sufficient scientific evidence exists to demonstrate an association between inadequate calcium intake and osteoporosis. Risk factors include the following:

- increased age
- being a female of the Caucasian or Asian race
- menopausal women experiencing loss of the hormone estrogen
- an inadequate amount of calcium throughout life
- lack of regular exercise
- an unhealthy eating pattern

For individuals at greatest risk of osteoporosis, an adequate calcium intake can increase bone mass during the teens and early adult life. Bone loss begins at about age 35; however, women and men with higher bone mass before age 35 delay their bone loss and pending bone fractures.[22]

To list a calcium-osteoporosis health claim, a food or supplement must contain at least 20% (at least 200 mg) of the calcium RDI. The food or supplement should not contain excess amounts of other nutrients (e.g., fat or sodium) that are contrary to overall good health. The form of the calcium in the food must be bioavailable and dissolve well. In addition, the amount of phosphorus cannot exceed the amount of calcium. Labels of products having more than 40% of the RDI or 400 mg must indicate that a total dietary calcium intake greater that 200% of the RDI for calcium (2,000 mg) does not give additional benefit to bone health. This claim is another excellent example of applied nutritional epidemiology.

> *Model Health Claim Appropriate for Most Conventional Foods:* "Regular exercise and a healthy diet with enough calcium helps teens and young adult white and Asian women maintain good bone health and may reduce their high risk of osteoporosis later in life."[22]

Dietary Fat and Cancer

Scientific data show a significant association between dietary fat and some cancers. Eating behaviors, heredity, and exposure to environmental factors are the major risk factors for cancer. Scientific data support a link between high fat intake and some cancers, but not specific fatty acids and cancer. Individuals at risk for cancer cannot be clearly identified; however, the public in general is at risk due to the high average fat intake. A lower fat intake is preventative and advised.[22]

To have a health claim, a food must be a "low fat" food. This health claim is the third excellent example of applied nutritional epidemiology.

> *Model Health Claim:* "Development of cancer depends on many factors. A diet low in total fat may reduce the risk of some cancer."[22]

Dietary Saturated Fat and Cholesterol and Risk of CHD

The data linking (1) an eating pattern high in saturated fat and cholesterol with an increased risk of heart disease, and (2) an eating pattern low in saturated fat and cholesterol linked with decreasing CHD risk are strong, convincing, and consistent. Excessive intakes of saturated fat and cholesterol are the major determinants of total cholesterol, low-density-lipoprotein cholesterol (LDL cholesterol), and an increased risk of CHD.

Foods that are low saturated fat, low cholesterol, and low fat can have a health claim. Fish and game meats must be extra lean. The health claim must state that eating patterns low in saturated fat and cholesterol "may" or "might" reduce the risk of heart disease and that CHD has many causal factors.[22]

The effects of dietary changes in saturated fat and cholesterol on the total and LDL cholesterol levels of blood vary among individuals. However, most individuals will benefit from diets low in saturated fat and cholesterol. Acceptable recommendations for all Americans are to follow eating patterns with less than 30% of calories from total fat, less than 10% from saturated fat, and less than 300 mg of cholesterol per day. Each individual recommendation and the aggregate of all the recommendations exemplify applied nutritional epidemiology.

> *Model Health Claim:* "While many factors affect heart disease, diets low in saturated fat and cholesterol may reduce the risk of this disease."[22]

Fruits and Vegetables and Cancer

Foods that are low in fat and are a good source of dietary fiber, vitamin A as beta-carotene, or vitamin C, can lower an individual's cancer risk. Health claims linking antioxidant vitamins themselves to reduced cancer risk are not authorized. FDA has concluded that, based on the totality of scientific evidence, there is significant scientific agreement that eating patterns low in fat and high in fruits and vegetables reduce the risk of cancer.[22]

The health claim must say that low fat and high fruit and vegetable intakes "may" or "might" reduce the risk of "some cancers" or "some types of cancer." No specific level of cancer risk reduction can be stated. Each food with a claim must be or contain a fruit or vegetable, be a low-fat food and a natural "good source" of vitamin A, vitamin C, or dietary fiber. This link between fruits, vegetables, and cancer prevention again demonstrates applied nutritional epidemiology.

> *Model Health Claim:* "Low fat eating patterns rich in fruits and vegetables and low in fat but high in dietary fiber, vitamin A, or vitamin C may reduce the risk of some types of cancer, a disease associated with many factors. Broccoli is high in vitamins A and C, and is a good source of dietary fiber."[22]

Sodium and Hypertension

High blood pressure is correlated to a family history of hypertension, aging, obesity, excess alcohol intake, and an eating pattern high in sodium. Sodium chloride, commonly known as table salt, is 40% sodium. Sodium occurs naturally in many foods, but an excess intake is unnecessary and potentially harmful. Individuals need only 500 mg of sodium each day. A total intake of 2,400 mg of sodium per day exceeds basic needs, even though a typical intake is between 3,000 and 6,000 mg.

Foods with a claim must state that a low-sodium eating pattern "may" or "might" reduce high blood pressure risk and that high blood pressure is multifactorial. A specific statement about the magnitude of risk reduction expected with a low-sodium eating pattern is not allowed. Foods eligible for the sodium claim must be low sodium and have acceptable levels of fat, saturated fat, and cholesterol.[22] Applying the nutritional science to the selection of foods to reduce high blood pressure is yet another example of how nutrition can be applied in the community to improve the health of the nation.

> *Model Health Claim:* "Diets low in sodium may reduce the risk of high blood pressure, a disease associated with many factors."[22]

Folic Acid and Neural Tube Defects

For most women who have problems due to inadequate folate intake, these problems develop before they are aware they are pregnant. Adequate folate protects unborn babies from spina bifida, in which the backbone does not fully form around the nerves of the spinal cord. The spinal cord is exposed and may be damaged when the child is born. This can result in paralysis. Foods that are fortified with 140 µg of folic acid per 100 g of bread and grain product can make a health claim.

> *Model Health Claim:* Daily consumption of folate by women of child-bearing age may reduce the risk of neural tube defects in their offspring.[22]

RESEARCH NEEDS

Food and nutrition are integrative disciplines that invite other specialties to join their research and program agenda. Together these disciplines develop new avenues of thought when presented with human nutrition problems facing both individuals and groups. The problems may surface from surveillance or monitoring or from development or adaptation of products for human use. A recurrent challenge is to keep the research agenda for food and nutrition invigorated by innovations in the biological sciences.[29] Exhibit 2–9 highlights major research themes of the Institute of Medicine (see Chapter 3). The committee recognizes that food and nutrition policies involve social, economic, and biological issues.[29-32]

Exhibit 2-9 Key Research Themes Identified by the Committee on Opportunities in Nutrition and Food Sciences, Food and Nutrition Board, Institute of Medicine

- nutrients in human development
- genes, food, and chronic disease
- determinants of food intake
- enhancing the food supply
- food and nutrition policies

Source: Adapted from Dwyer J. Nutrition research for the year 2000 and beyond. *Contemporary Nutr.* 1993;18(6):1-2.

Efforts are being taken to evaluate the efficacy of nutrition research. Uniform and up-to-date reporting methods of research costs include the Human Nutrition Research and Information Management System. This is an on-line retrieval system to identify and categorize federally funded human nutrition research projects in all government agencies.[33]

Analysis of the cost-effectiveness of the research shows whether investments in nutrition are worthwhile. Research investments and their benefits, especially for basic research, are difficult to measure.[34] Nutrition research can provide the best available knowledge to address national problems and goals and to help the United States maintain a leadership position in technologies that affect industrial and economic performance.[35]

The Relationship between Nutrition and Disease

In today's food-selection environment, the roles of several dietary factors in the etiology and prevention of chronic diseases—including cancer, osteoporosis, and stroke—have been elucidated. We have a fairly clear understanding of the childhood dietary patterns that will best provide adequate intake of calories and nutrients essential for growth and development, yet prevent the early onset of chronic diseases. The effects of maternal nutrition on the health of the developing fetus remains pivotal for young mothers in their teen years as well as for women over 20 years of age. Nutrient and energy requirements of older adults need to be extended to include the effects of nutrition on age-related impairment of organ system functions (e.g., cardiovascular, gastrointestinal/oral cavity, immune, musculoskeletal, and nervous systems). In addition, comprehensive dietary recommendations for older adults should reflect common comorbidity patterns.[29]

The relationship of total body fat and body fat distribution to health outcomes (i.e., a health-related definition of obesity) needs further study. Research efforts could be directed toward the epidemiology of weight gain and successful weight loss, the health effects of weight loss and regain (weight cycling), and the healthy nutritional practices that best promote weight loss.

Conversely, the etiology, epidemiology, prevention, and treatment of eating disorders such as anorexia nervosa and bulimia need exploration. Nutrition-to-drug interaction research and delineation of the definition and measurement of hunger are needed.

Determining valid and reliable biochemical markers of dietary intake remains a challenge, yet credible markers will improve the ability of community nutrition professionals to monitor the effectiveness of dietary intervention.

Research efforts are needed to translate nutrient requirements and dietary recommendations into healthful dietary patterns. How to achieve appropriate food choices and sustained behavioral changes for various subpopulations needs further exploration. Creating, evaluating, and communicating information about food by using labels that are more informative can be a part of social research efforts to evaluate behavior change. The goal of creating healthy foods rather than changing eating habits has fostered the development of biotechnology.[29,30,36]

Biotechnology

Traditional biotechnology involves plant and animal breeding and mutation, collection, selection, and natural products. New biotechnology produces genetic modification at the molecular level. The American Medical Association and the American Dietetic Association both support biotechnology for food uses,[37,38] while others oppose it.[39] Surveys of consumer awareness and acceptance of biotechnology demonstrate the greatest consumer trust in independent health organizations, such as the American Medical Association, and least trust in grocery stores, activist groups, and chefs.[40,41]

In molecular biotechnology or genetic engineering, genes are isolated and chemically characterized and the protein produced by the gene and its function are known.[42] Appendix 2-B is a modern case study involving a tomato gene and a new Flavr Savr™ tomato.[43-48]

Molecular biotechnology allows genes to be moved from one unrelated organism to another to produce a *transgenic* organism. The gene for chymosin, the milk coagulant used in cheese production, has been isolated in pure form from calves and introduced into *Escherichia coli* K 12. This enhances fermentation and isolation of pure chymosin. An impure renin from the stomachs of slaughtered calves does not have to be used. The chymosin is identical in form and function to the chymosin from calves.[36] Another transgenic product, bovine somatotropin (BST), has increased efficiency of milk production of cows by 10% to 20%. Several organizations provide position papers, pamphlets, and information sheets on biotechnology (see Table 2-15).

Other food products are being developed as a result of advances in biotechnology. Microbial *Bacillus thuringiensis* toxin (BT) is a biological insect control agent[49] that produces a protein that is toxic to insects but not to mammals.[50] Transgenic potato contains the BT gene and eliminates the use of synthetic chemical pesticides.[45,51]

Some transgenic plants have improved nutritional and healthful qualities. Potatoes with a higher starch content produce french fries and potato chips that absorb less fat.[52] Vegetable oils in transgenic plants have less saturated fats and can eliminate hydrogenation.[53] Transgenic corn or soybeans contain a balance of essential amino acids producing a higher quality animal feed. In time, researchers may be able to remove allergens from foods.[54] Vaccines using transgenic bananas for oral immunization to children in developing countries may become available, costing less than two cents per "vaccine" fruit.[55] BST has been approved for use with dairy cows, but the process has met opposition (see Exhibit 2-10).

Nutraceuticals

An alternative medicine movement has begun in the United States. This has in part occurred as more foods and specific nutrients are linked to disease prevention and promotion (e.g., linking high-fat foods with heart disease and cancer) via epidemiologic studies. As individuals take an increasing responsibility for their health, health-preventing behaviors include the use of alternative approaches. The term *nutraceuticals* is being used in today's health care arena. The term was coined by the Foundation for Innovation in Medicine (FFIM) in 1989.[56] *Nutra* comes from the Latin word for "nourish," and *pharmaceutical* is derived from the Greek term meaning "a medicinal drug." (*Note*–Unpublished position papers are available from FFIM, 411 North Avenue East, Cranford, NJ 07016.)

Nutraceuticals range from isolated nutrients, to dietary supplements, to real food and even diet plans (see Table 2-16). Genetically engineered "designer" foods, herbal products, and processed foods such as cereals, soups, and beverages are also included.[57]

In Japan, nutraceuticals are known as functional foods or foods derived from naturally occurring substances that are consumed as part of a daily diet or that regulate or affect certain body processes. The Japanese have instituted new rules for food for specified health use. The first approvals were to occur in 1993, although tension between the food and pharmaceutical industries influenced these approvals. The new rules deal with products that fall between traditional drugs and foods. It is predicted that this market will rocket from $58 billion in the next few years to more than $500 billion by the year 2010.[56]

The definition of nutraceuticals in the United States has created a real dilemma for regulatory agencies. Many of the nutraceutical products make a health claim. The FDA regulates products based on claims, not on their manufacture. Biopharmaceuticals are judged by their safety and effectiveness for the intended use claimed by their

Table 2–15 Abbreviated List of Resources about Food Biotechnology

Organization Name	Address	Resources
American Council on Science and Health, Inc.	1995 Broadway, 2nd Floor New York, NY 10023-5860 (212) 362-7044	• "Public Perception of Food Safety," *Priorities for Long Life & Good Health*, Summer 1991 • "Leaner Meat: A Product of Biotechnology," *Priorities for Long Life & Good Health*, Summer 1992 • "Biotechnology—The New Designer Genes," *Priorities for Long Life & Good Health*, Spring 1993
American Culinary Federation, Inc.	10 San Bartola Road St. Augustine, FL 32085-3466 (904) 824-4468	• "Biotechnology: Beyond the Hysteria," *The National Culinary Review*, November 1992
The American Dietetic Association	216 W. Jackson Blvd. Suite 800 Chicago, IL 60606-6995 (312) 899-0040	• "Position of the American Dietetic Association: Biotechnology and the Future of Food," *Journal of the American Dietetic Association*, February 1993
Council on Scientific Affairs, The American Medical Association	515 N. State St. Chicago, IL 60610 (312) 422-2922	• "Biotechnology and the American Agricultural Industry," *Journal of the American Medical Association*, March 20, 1991
Food and Drug Administration	5600 Fishers Lane Rockville, MD 20857 (301) 443-3170	• "Genetically Engineered Foods: Fears & Facts—An Interview with FDA's Jim Maryanski," *FDA Consumer*, January-February 1993 • Question and answer sheet, "FDA's Statement of Policy: Foods Derived from New Plant Varieties"
International Food Information Council	1100 Connecticut Ave. NW Suite 430 Washington, DC 20036 (202) 296-6540	• "Consumers Support Use of Food Biotech," *Food Insight*, September-October 1992
Institute of Food Technologists	221 N. LaSalle St. Chicago, IL 60601 (312) 782-8424	• *Journal of the Institute of Food Technologists*
Produce Marketing Association	1500 Casho Mill Road P.O. Box 6036 Newark, DE 19714-6036 (302) 738-7100	• "Position Paper on Biotechnology," October 1992
Science Magazine	1333 H St. NW Washington, DC 20005 (202) 326-6500	• "The Safety of Foods Developed by Biotechnology," *Science*, June 26, 1992, 48:36.

Source: List compiled from *School Food Service Journal*, Vol. 48, No. 8, p. 36, American School Food Service Association, © 1994.

Exhibit 2-10 Executive Summary of the use of Bovine Somatotropin (BST) in the United States: Its Potential Effects

The US Food and Drug Administration (FDA) approved the metabolic protein hormone, bovine somatotropin (BST), for commercial use in the United States on November 5, 1993. BST increases milk production in dairy cows. Key findings of experts who reviewed scientific evidence are presented below.

SAFETY

- There is no evidence that BST poses a health threat to humans or animals. There is no legal basis requiring the labeling of BST milk, which is indistinguishable from non-BST milk. Voluntary labeling is permitted.

THE DAIRY INDUSTRY

- Income for individual farmers who adopt BST is likely to increase. Productivity and profit per cow should rise.
- BST use will increase US milk production by about 1% through FY 1999, leading to a 2% decline in prices over the next six years. A 1% decline in aggregate dairy farm income is expected.
- Lower milk prices may contribute to higher federal government dairy price-support costs, but decreased federal costs for Food Stamps and the Special Supplemental Food Program for Women, Infants and Children (WIC).
- Federal dairy price-support program costs may increase by approximately $150 million in FY 1996 and decline in later years. This represents a 1.8% increase in total projected federal farm commodity subsidies in 1996.

- Cost savings for federal feeding programs would begin in FY 1997 and may completely offset the increased cumulative costs over 10 years.

CONSUMERS

- Consumers benefit from the lower price for milk. Net national economic impact of BST usage is expected to be positive.
- No significant reduction of demand for milk and dairy products is expected to occur. Some surveys reveal strong consumer resistance to BST; others indicate confidence in the US milk supply. There appears to be a need for nutrition education on BST's effects.

THE ENVIRONMENT

- BST is expected to have a minor, but beneficial net impact on the environment leading to a slightly smaller US dairy herd, less pollution from decreased use of fertilizers for feed production, and less cow manure and methane production.

EXPORTS

- BST should have minimal effect on US dairy exports. Nearly half of US dairy export volume goes to countries that have approved the use of BST, and more countries are expected to do so.

BIOTECHNOLOGY INDUSTRIES

- US leadership in biotechnology is enhanced by approval of the use of BST.

Source: Reprinted from *Executive Summary—Use of BST in the United States,* U.S. Department of Health and Human Services/ Food and Drug Administration, 1994.

manufacturer. The same is true for foods created by biotechnology. Health claims for foods have therefore become one of the main regulatory issues of the day.[58] The federal Food, Drug and Cosmetic Act defines drugs as substances used in the diagnosis, cure, treatment, or prevention of disease in man and animals. Drugs are also considered any article other than food that is intended to affect the structure or function of the body. Foods are subject to the drug laws if therapeutic claims are made.

A nutraceutical may be considered a food additive. If so, it must be shown to be safe by the

"generally recognized as safe" regulation. Nutraceuticals may also be considered a medical product with intended use only under medical supervision.

Medical Foods

FDA requires that *medical foods* be used for oral or tube feeding and make a therapeutic claim. They must be labeled if intended for dietary management of a specific condition (Section 5[b] of the Orphan Drug Act [21 USC 360 ee(b)]).[59] Medi-

Table 2–16 Nutraceutical Foods to Prevent Illness

Food	Action
Carrots, sweet potatoes, orange squash	Contain beta-carotene to prevent cancer.
Chili peppers	Contain capsaicin to treat arthritis pain.
Cranberry juice	Prevents urinary tract infections by killing bacteria and increasing acidity of urine.
Cruciferous vegetables (broccoli, brussel sprouts, cabbage) and fish oil	Contain vitamin A to fight cancer, omega-3 fatty acids to prevent heart disease by lowering blood triglyceride levels.
Garlic	Lowers cholesterol and reduces blood clotting.
Green tea	Contains tannins and suppresses tumors in mice.
Licorice root	Contains prostaglandin inhibitors to inhibit cancer, ulcers, and tooth decay.
Soybeans	Contain genistein to stop tumor growth.

Source: Adapted from Dunkin, A., Eat Nine Cloves of Garlic, and Call Me in the Morning from the February 25, 1993 issue of *Business Week* by special permission, © 1993 by McGraw-Hill, Inc.

cal foods do not require premarket approval. They are distinguished from conventional foods that make health claims. Medical foods are not foods simply recommended by a health care provider to reduce disease risk or medical condition.

Medical foods are not all foods fed to patients, rather they are specially formulated and processed foods. This contrasts with naturally occurring foodstuffs used in their natural state. Medical foods were considered drugs prior to 1972, when FDA reclassified them as foods. They are used today for the dietary management of lung, kidney, heart, and liver diseases. Information about medical foods is important for community nutrition professionals, as more individuals are being cared for at home during rehabilitation. These individuals must draw from community services to meet their needs. Home care is a growing, progressive field, and community nutrition services in health departments and health maintenance organizations are beginning to expand home health services.

Many questions remain. Bran can lower serum cholesterol in blood. Is bran a drug? Is psyllium, a biopolymer that reduces blood cholesterol and glucose levels, a drug?

Amino acids used for total parenteral nutrition are used therapeutically in hospitals and fall into the health claims controversy. The same prob-lem exists for L-dopa in Parkinson's disease, and beta-carotene for cancer prevention.

A 1992 legislative action, the Hatch-Richardson Bill, defined a *dietary supplement* as different from a food additive or a drug. It permits health claims without government approval if there are adequate data to support the claim.[60]

MISINFORMATION/DISINFORMATION

A constant consumer challenge is to decipher the volumes of nutrition information beaming from magazines, television, billboards, and product advertisements. Often the media take bits and pieces of nutrition data from epidemiologic studies and extrapolate it to mass application, creating mass confusion. Or manufacturers adapt a nutrition finding such as the benefit of a vitamin by creating a new product or "magic bullet." The truth about the benefit of the vitamin may be stretched or taken out of context. Ironically, the public may not view the fields of nutrition, epidemiology, and nutritional epidemiology as credible due to the confusion, and the public may view business and industry as the knowledgeable group responding to help the consumer.

Disinformation is a term that describes statements, testimonials and messages given to the public but unsubstantiated by scientific research or credible sources.[61] Seven situations or statements that should be questioned are as follows[61]:

1. Beware of a dramatic or unusual statement that is not supported by a recognized organization, such as advice cited by a single individual speaking on his/her own behalf or a single individual speaking alone about his/her specific research that does not fit into mainstream research. The advocate may claim to be "ahead of the times." Be concerned about a small, unknown or little-known advocacy group that could be representing facts or statements with no consensus agreement from a reputable organization. For example, "Milk is bad for all children" is not a valid claim.

2. Beware of a story that covers very diverse subjects and then leads to an overall conclusion that represents a very narrow interpretation of the information.

3. Beware when the spokesperson is a "star" figure whose expertise is not in the subject area that he or she is discussing. Testimonial and anecdotal nutrition statements by Hollywood stars, such as protest statements regarding Alar on apples, should make you suspicious.

4. Beware of promises or implications that there will be dramatic benefits from the use of a product or regimen. Be wary of statements implying that individuals can eat anything they want when using a particular substance or regimen, promising dramatic weight loss or renewed vigor, or claiming that use of a familiar food can alter a behavior. Review situations that carefully encourage the purchase of special products, involve an expensive regimen, or claim that products contain a unique nutritional ingredient unavailable in the normal food supply (for example: "Wheatgrass cleanses the body of toxins," "Sugar causes hyperactivity in children," or "These particular fish oils and oat bran lower risk of heart disease and cancer").

5. Beware of nutrition advice that does not meet the Dietary Guidelines for Americans. Question recommendations that advocate eating very small or very large amounts of specific foods or that recommend exclusion of all foods from one or more food groups (for example: the Stillman Diet, Beverly Hills Diet, Scarsdale Diet, and the Physicians' Committee for Responsible Medicine's new four food groups).

6. Beware of nutrition recommendations that come from politically based environmental groups rather than from a health or medicine perspective. For example, the Physicians' Committee for Responsible Medicine decries all children's consumption of cow's milk without offering reasonable nutrient alternatives. This is an animal rights group, representing less than 1% of all physicians in this country.

7. Beware of nutrition recommendations that leave no room for differences in life stages, such as for pregnant or lactating women, seniors, adolescents, and children. For example, question an unsupervised vegan diet for young children or pregnant women without referral to a medical or trained health care specialist for guidance.

The public can believe the following nutrition messages[61]:

- Messages that comment on reputable confirmed research or represent the consensus opinion of a recognized professional organization or government agency, including DHHS, FDA, and USDA. Volunteer health organizations, such as the American Cancer Society, the American Diabetes Association, and the American Heart Association, are credible sources of nutrition information. Reputable consumer organizations include the Better Business Bureau, the Consumers Union, and the National Council Against Health Fraud. Credible scientific and professional organizations include the American Dietetic Association and any state dietetic association, the Society for Nutrition Education, the American Medical Association, and the American Academy of Pediatrics.

- Messages that suggest a range of food choices based on the food grouping system represented by the USDA food guide pyramid.
- Messages can describe a special diet that severely restricts food groups in the USDA food group pyramid, but they should be backed by a recognized professional organization that provides specific, practical food recommendations for adequate nutrients normally provided by the missing food groups.
- Messages that identify children's nutrient needs and eating habits as different from adults.
- Messages about new, preliminary research using 50 to 100 or more participants and a rigorous research design.

FRAUD AND QUACKERY

Obstacles to optimal health habits and positive eating behaviors include nutrition misinformation, fraud, and quackery.[62] An epidemic of quick cures, magic foods, perfect diets, and easy remedies overshadow simple truths about healthy eating. Certain situations appear to fuel nutrition quackery[63]:

- *"Magic bullets":* These include just about anything that can be sold and generally labeled as a dietary supplement.
- *Nutrition publications:* These are numerous and protected by the First Amendment of the US Constitution.
- *The title "nutritionist":* This can be used to describe one who assumes he or she is an expert because he or she likes to eat, one who likes to cook, or one who completes a college degree.
- *Premature presentation of research:* The practice of presenting research findings is

very common when only preliminary work is completed and not replicated or validated. Although findings may contradict a science base, they may seem just as important to novice consumers as a volume of sound research.

One of the greatest areas of nutrition quackery relates to sports nutrition. A competitive edge is sought by athletes and health-conscious individuals, who may believe that the potential for success is greater with ergogenics.[63] As many as 50% of team members may use ergogenics.[64]

The array of ergogenic items includes more than 700 brands, products, or ingredients.[64] The buyer is receptive and unaware of the potential danger of the products. Deceptive tactics include the following[63]:

- selecting only pieces of published research to prove a point
- displaying unauthorized endorsement or support of professional organizations
- falsely stating that research has been conducted or is continuing
- providing inaccurate documentation of research
- substituting testimonials as research
- patenting products without evaluating them
- using mass media to publicize and to promote products

Another area where fraud and quackery are common is the weight-loss industry. Fraudulent products and programs are unscrupulous and persuasive[65] (see Exhibit 2–11). Many registered dietitians (RDs) work in weight-loss programs and decipher the fraudulent practices and products for their clients.

Community nutrition professionals must be astute in recognizing the demands of competitive athletes for a winning edge and health-conscious adults for vitality, and the role played by pseudonutrition products.[63,66,67] Continuing education provides professionals who are not athletes with some of the necessary back-

Exhibit 2-11 Weight Loss Fraud and Quackery—Guidelines for Identification

MESSAGE

- Claims or implies a large, fast weight loss—often promised as easy, effortless, guaranteed, or permanent.
- Implies weight can be lost without restricting calories or exercising, and discounts the benefits of exercise.
- Uses typical quackery terms such as: miraculous, breakthrough, exclusive, secret, unique, ancient, accidental discovery, doctor-developed.
- Claims to get rid of cellulite.
- Relies heavily on undocumented case histories, before-and-after photos, and testimonials by "satisfied customers."
- Misuses medical or technical terms, refers to studies without giving complete references, claims government approval.
- Professes to be a treatment for a wide range of ailments and nutritional deficiencies as well as for weight loss.

PROGRAM

- Promotes a medically unsupervised diet of less than 1,000 calories per day.
- Diagnoses nutrient deficiencies with computer-scored questionnaire and prescribes vitamins and supplements. Recommends them in excess of 100% of Recommended Dietary Allowance.
- Requires special foods purchased from the company rather than conventional foods.
- Promotes aids and devices such as: body wraps, sauna belts, electronic muscle stimulators, passive motion tables, ear stapling, aromatherapy, appetite patches, and acupuncture.
- Promotes a nutritional plan without relying on at least one author or counselor with nutrition credentials.
- Fails to state risks or recommend a medical exam.

INGREDIENTS

- Uses unproven, bogus, or potentially dangerous ingredients such as dinitrophenol, spirulina, amino acid supplements, glucomannan, human chorionic gonadotrophin (HCG) hormone, diuretics, slimming teas, echinacia root, bee pollen, fennel, chickweed, and starch blockers.
- Claims ingredients will block digestion or surround calories, starches, carbohydrates, or fat, and remove them from the body.

MYSTIQUE

- Encourages reliance on a guru figure who has the "ultimate answers."
- Grants mystical properties to certain foods or ingredients.
- Bases plan on faddish ideas, such as food allergies, forbidden foods, or "magic combinations" of foods.
- Declares that the established medical community is against this discovery and refuses to accept its miraculous benefits.

METHOD OF AVAILABILITY

- Is sold by self-proclaimed health advisors or "nutritionists"—often door-to-door, in health food stores, or a chiropractor's office.
- Distributes through hard-sell mail order advertisements or through ads that list only an 800 number without an address, indicating possible Postal Service action against the company.
- Demands large advance payments or long-term contracts.
- Uses high-pressure sales tactics, one-time-only deals, or recruitment for a pyramid sales organization. Displays prominent money-back guarantee.
- Available at popular locations such as fitness centers, beauty salons, spas, health food stores, drug stores, and grocery stores.

Source: Adapted from Berg FM. *Healthy Weight Journal*, p. 2, © 1995.

ground to organize workshops or group presentations for parents, coaches, and athletes. It is necessary to counter quick results and "magic bullet" products, which are attractive but may present risks. Informed presentations and media messages with alternatives that are science-based may correct faulty nutrition knowledge and improve approaches to athletic training and performance. This arena is growing, and methods are needed to label products with accurate claims about their composition and benefit much in the same way NLEA functions.

<table>
<tr><td>

Info Line

The National Council Against Health Fraud, Inc.
Post Office Box 1276
Loma Linda, California 92354-1276

</td></tr>
</table>

HEALTHY PEOPLE 2000 ACTIONS

Community nutrition professionals must be actively involved in developing and implementing programs to help consumers and their clients become nutrition smart. The knowledge base of the public influences its ability to make healthy food choices (see Exhibit 2-12). Kaufman has

Exhibit 2-12 *Healthy People 2000* Objectives for Informed Consumers

2.13 Increase to at least 85% the proportion of people aged 18 and older who use food labels to make nutritious food selections. (Baseline: 74% used labels to make food selections in 1988.)

2.15 Increase to at least 5,000 brand items[a] the availability of processed food products that are reduced in fat and saturated fat. (Baseline: 2,500 items reduced in fat in 1986.)

2.16 Increase to at least 90% the proportion of restaurants and institutional food service operations that offer identifiable low-fat, low-calorie food choices, consistent with the Dietary Guidelines for Americans. (Baseline: About 70% of fast food and family restaurant chains with 350 or more units had at least one low-fat, low-calorie item on their menu in 1989.)

2.20 Increase to at least 50% the proportion of work sites with 50 or more employees that offer nutrition education and/or weight management programs for employees. (Baseline: 17% offered nutrition education activities, and 15% offered weight-control activities in 1985.)

22.1 Develop a set of health status indicators appropriate for federal, state, and local health agencies and establish use of the set in at least 40 states. (Baseline: None existed in 1990.)

22.2 Identify, and create where necessary, national data sources to measure progress toward each of the year 2000 national health objectives. (Baseline: 77% of the objectives have baseline data in 1990.)

<table>
<tr><td colspan="3" align="center">**Type-Specific Target**</td></tr>
<tr><td></td><td>*1989 Baseline*</td><td>*2000 Target*</td></tr>
<tr><td>22.2a Obtain state-level data for at least two-thirds of the objectives</td><td>23 states*</td><td>35 states</td></tr>
</table>

*Measured using the 1989 Draft Year 2000 national health objectives.

22.3 Develop and disseminate among federal, state, and local agencies procedures for collecting comparable data for each of the year 2000 national health objectives and incorporate these into Public Health Service data collection systems. (Baseline: Although such surveys as the National Health Interview Survey may serve as a model, widely accepted procedures did not exist in 1990.)

22.4 Develop and implement a national process to identify significant gaps in the nation's disease prevention and health promotion data, including data for racial and ethnic minorities, people with low incomes, and people with disabilities, and establish mechanisms to meet these needs. (Baseline: No such process existed in 1990.)

22.5 Implement in all states periodic analysis and publication of data needed to measure progress toward objectives for at least ten of the priority areas of the national health objectives. (Baseline: 20 states reported that they disseminate the analyses they use to assess state progress toward the health objectives to the public and to health professionals in 1989.)

continues

Exhibit 2-12 continued

	Type-Specific Target	
	1989 Baseline	*2000 Target*
22.5a Periodic analysis and publication of state progress toward the national objectives for each racial or ethnic group that makes up at least 10% of the state population	0 states	25 states

22.6 Expand in all states systems for the transfer of health information related to the national health objectives among federal, state, and local agencies.[b] (Baseline: 30 states reported that they have some capability for transfer of health data, tables, graphs, and maps to federal, state, and local agencies that collected and analyzed data in 1989.)

22.7 Achieve timely release of national surveillance and survey data needed by health professionals and agencies to measure progress toward the national health objectives. (Baseline data available in 1993.)

[a]A brand item is defined as a particular flavor and/or size of a specific brand and is typically the consumer unit of purchase.
[b]Information related to the national health objectives includes state- and national-level baseline data, disease prevention/health promotion evaluation results, and data generated to measure progress.

Source: Reprinted from *Healthy People 2000: National Health Promotion and Disease Prevention Objectives.* U.S. Department of Health and Human Services, DHHS (PHS) Publication 91-50212, 1991.

Exhibit 2-13 Model Nutrition Objectives for Reduced Risk Factors

By 19__, the following contaminants will not be present in the state food supply above toxic/hazardous levels as defined by state or federal agencies:

- Agricultural: pesticides, fertilizers, growth regulators
- Drugs: antibiotics, steroids/hormones, growth regulators
- Environmental: organics, inorganics/heavy metals

- Food additives: preservatives, colors, flavors, sweeteners, stabilizers
- Industrial: organics, inorganics/heavy metals, radioactives
- Microbial: bacteria, molds, fungi, virus, protozoa, and related toxins
- Naturally occurring toxins: carcinogens, mutagens, neurotoxins

Source: Adapted from *Model State Nutrition Objectives,* The Association of State and Territorial Public Health Nutrition Directors, 1988.

Exhibit 2-14 Model Nutrition Objectives for Increased Public and Professional Awareness

By 19__, there will be an ongoing interdisciplinary information program for public health and food industry professionals on food safety, labeling, health claims, nutrition fraud, and the reporting of food-borne illness.

Source: Adapted from *Model State Nutrition Objectives,* The Association of State and Territorial Public Health Nutrition Directors, 1988.

formulated model nutrition objectives for reducing risk factors for disease and for increasing public and professional awareness[68] (Exhibits 2-13 and 2-14). Acronyms commonly used in community nutrition are listed in Appendix 2-C.

REFERENCES

1. Hooyman NR, Kiyak, HS. *Social Gerontology*. 3rd ed. Needham Heights, Mass: Simon & Schuster, Inc; 1993.

2. *Healthy People 2000: National Health Promotion and Disease Prevention Objectives*. Washington, DC: US Department of Health and Human Services; 1991. Public Health Service publication 91-50212.

3. *The Surgeon General's Report on Nutrition and Health*. Washington, DC: US Department of Health and Human Services; 1988. Public Health Service publication 88-50210.

4. *Dietary Guidelines for Americans*. Washington, DC: US Department of Agriculture and US Department of Health and Human Services, Human Nutrition Information Service; 1994. Home and Garden Bulletin 253-1 to 253-8.

5. National Research Council. *Recommended Dietary Allowances*. 10th ed. Washington, DC: National Academy Press; 1989.

6. *The Food Guide Pyramid*. Washington, DC: US Department of Agriculture, Human Nutrition Information Service; August 1992. Leaflet no. 572.

7. Oldways Preservation and Exchange Trust. *The Traditional Healthy Mediterranean Diet Pyramid*. Boston, Mass: Oldways Preservation and Exchange Trust; 1993.

8. Food Marketing Institute and *Prevention* Magazine. *Shopping for Health, 1994; Eating in America: Perception and Reality*. Washington, DC: Food Marketing Institute and *Prevention* Magazine; 1994.

9. Public Law No. 101-455.

10. Kuczmarski MF, Moshfegh A, Briefel R. Update on nutrition monitoring activities in the US. *J Am Diet Assoc*. 1994;94:753-760.

11. *Nutrition Monitoring in the United States: A Progress Report from the Joint Nutrition Monitoring Evaluation Committee*. Washington, DC: US Department of Health and Human Services and US Department of Agriculture; 1986:356.

12. US Department of Health and Human Services and US Department of Agriculture. *Joint Implementation Plan for a Comprehensive National Nutrition Monitoring System*. Report to Congress; August 1981:59.

13. Peterkin BB, Rizek RL, Tippett KS. Nationwide Food Consumption Survey, 1987. *Nutr Today*. 1988;18:24.

14. *Nationwide Food Consumption Survey, Continuing Survey of Food Intakes by Individuals: Women 19-50 Years and Children 1-5 Years, 1 Day, 1985*. Washington, DC: US Department of Agriculture, Human Nutrition Information Service; 1985:102.

15. *Nationwide Food Consumption Survey, Continuing Survey of food Intakes by Individuals: Women 19-50 Years and Children 1-5 Years, 4 Days, 1985*. Washington, DC: US Department of Agriculture, Human Nutrition Information Service; 1987:182.

16. *Research on Survey Methodology: Proceedings of a Symposium Held at the 71st Annual Meeting of the Federation of American Societies for Experimental Biology, April 1987*. Washington, DC: US Department of Agriculture, Human Nutrition Information Service; 1987:77. Administrative report 382.

17. US Department of Health and Human Services and US Department of Agriculture. *Operational Plan for the National Nutrition Monitoring System*. Report to Congress; August 1987:47.

18. Food and Nutrition Board, Institute of Medicine. *How Should the Recommended Dietary Allowances Be Revised?* Washington, DC: National Academy Press; 1994.

19. McNamara SH. New food labeling legislation enacted. *Regulatory Affairs*. 1990;2:483-487.

20. 21 *CFR* Part I, *Federal Register*. January 6, 1993;58 Book II:2302-2964.

21. Tillotson JE. United States nutrition labeling and education act of 1990. *Nutr Rev*. 1991;49:273-276.

22. The FDA's final regulations on health claims for foods. *Nutr Rev*. 1993;51:90-93. Editorial.

23. Shank FR. "The Nutrition Labeling and Education Act of 1990." *Food and Drug Law J*. 1992;47:247-252.

24. Final rule mandatory status of nutrition labeling and nutrient content revision, formal for nutrition label. *Federal Register*. January 6, 1993;58:2079.

25. Kessler DA. Restoring the FDA's preeminence in the regulation of food. *Food Drug Cosmetic J*. 1991;46:391-394.

26. *How To Read the New Food Label*. Dallas, Texas: Food and Drug Administration and American Heart Association; 1993.

27. Final rule: General requirements for health claims for foods. *Federal Register*. January 6, 1993;58:247.

28. Mandatory nutrition labeling–FDA's final rule. *Nutr Rev*. 1993;51(special report):101-105.

29. Dwyer J. Nutrition research for the year 2000 and beyond. *Contemporary Nutr*. 1993;18:1-2.

30. National Institutes of Health. *Ad Hoc Bionutrition Group, NIH Bionutrition Initiative Nutrition Notes: Draft Guidance Document April 29, 1993*. Bethesda, Md: American Institute of Nutrition; 1993;29:7-9.

31. Taylor H, Voivodas G. *The Bristol-Myers Report: Medicine in the Next Century.* New York, NY: Louis Harris and Assoc.; 1986.

32. Shafter MO, Story M, Houghton B. *Report: Survey of the Association of Graduate Faculty Programs in Public Health Nutrition.* Minneapolis, Minn; 1993. Unpublished manuscript.

33. National Institutes of Health. *Fourteenth Annual Report of the NIH Program in Biomedical and Behavioral Nutrition Research and Training, Fiscal Year 1990.* Bethesda, Md: National Institutes of Health; 1990. NIH publication 91-2092.

34. Office of Technology Assessment, US Congress. *Research Funding as an Investment: Can We Measure the Returns?* Washington, DC: US Government Printing Office; 1986.

35. Committee on Science, Engineering and Public Policy of the Academies and the Institute of Medicine. *Science, Technology and the Federal Government: National Goals for a New Era.* Washington, DC: National Academy of Sciences; 1993.

36. Hardy RWF. Biotechnology and food. *Contemporary Nutr.* 1994;19:2.

37. Council on Scientific Affairs, American Medical Association. Biotechnology and the American agricultural industry. *JAMA.* 1991;265:1429-1436.

38. Kunkel ME. Position of the American Dietetic Association—Biotechnology and the future of food. *J Am Diet Assoc.* 1993;93:189-192.

39. Vines G. Guess what's coming to dinner. *New Sci.* 1992;136:13-14.

40. Hoban TJ, Woodrum E, Czaia R. Public opposition to genetic engineering. *Rural Sociol.* 1992;57:476-493.

41. Hoban TJ. *Consumer Awareness and Acceptance of Bovine Somatotropin (BST).* Raleigh, NC: NC State University; 1994:15.

42. National Research Council. *Field Testing Genetically Modified Organisms.* Washington, DC: National Academy Press; 1989:170.

43. Kramer MG, Sheehy, RE, Hiatt Wr. Progress toward the genetic engineering of tomato fruit softening. *Trends Biotechnol.* 1989;7:191-194.

44. Kramer MG. *NABC 2.* Ithaca, NY: Boyce Thompson Institute; 1990:127-130.

45. Hiatt WR, et al. *Genetic Engineering.* New York, NY: Plenum Publications; 1989;11:49-63.

46. National Cancer Institute. *Frequently Consumed Vegetables.* Washington, DC; 1993.

47. Redenbaugh K, Berner T, Emlay D, et al. Regulatory issues for commercialization of tomatoes with an antisense polygalacturonase gene. *In Vitro Cell & Dev Biol.* 1993;29:17-26.

48. Redenbaugh K, Hiatt W. Field trials and risk evaluation of tomatoes genetically engineered for enhanced firmness and shelflife. *Acta Hort.* 1993;336:133-146.

49. Marrone PG, Sandmeier R. *NABC 3.* Ithaca, NY: Boyce Thompson Institute; 1991:228-237.

50. Goldburg RJ, Tjaden G. Are BTK plants really safe to eat? *Bio/Technology.* 1990;8:1011-1015.

51. Perlak FJ, Fischhoff DA. *Advanced Engineered Pesticides.* New York, NY: M. Dekker; 1993:199-211.

52. Stark DM, Timmerman KP, Barry GF, et al. Regulation of the amount of starch in plant tissues by ADP glucose pyrophosphorylase. *Science.* 1992;258:287-292.

53. Ohlrogge JB. Design of new plant products—engineering of fatty acid metabolism. *Plant Physiol.* 1994; 104:821-826.

54. Flora F, ed. *Naturally Occurring Substances in Traditional and Biotechnologically Derived Foods.* Washington, DC: US Department of Agriculture, CRS; 1992:29.

55. Arntzen CJ, et al. *Vaccines '94.* Cold Springs Harbor, NY: Cold Springs Harbor Publications; 1994.

56. *Marketletter Monitor.* February 8, 1993.

57. Dunkin A. Eat nine cloves of garlic, and call me in the morning. *Data Business Week.* February 15, 1993.

58. Chew NJ. Nutraceuticals: Using food to treat disease. *BioPharm.* July-Aug. 1993:18-19.

59. Pub. Law. No. 101-535, 104 Stat 2353 (1990), preprinted in *Regulatory Affairs Volume 2.* 1990:488-504.

60. LaBell F. Experts ask policy change on health claims. *Food Processing.* April 1993:52-57.

61. California Dietetic Association. *Help or Harm.* San Diego, Calif: California Dietetic Association; 1992:2.

62. Position of the American Dietetic Association: Identifying food and nutrition misinformation. *J Am Diet Assoc.* 1988;88:1589-1591.

63. Short SH. Health-quackery: Our role as professionals. *J Am Diet Assoc.* 1994;94:607-611.

64. Philen RM, Ortiz DI, Auerbach SB, et al. Survey of advertising for nutritional supplements in health and bodybuilding magazines. *JAMA.* 1991;268:1008-1011.

65. Berg FM. *Obesity and Health.* Hettinger, ND: Healthy Living Institute; 1990.

66. Stare FJ. Combating misinformation—A continuing challenge for nutrition professionals. *Nutr Today.* 1992;27:43-46.

67. Marquart LF, Sobal J. Vitamin/mineral supplement use among athletes. *J Am Diet Assoc.* 1992;92(suppl):A56. Abstract.

68. Kaufman M. *Nutrition in Public Health—A Handbook for Developing Programs and Services.* Gaithersburg, Md: Aspen Publishers, Inc; 1990:570.

Appendix 2-A

Sampling Error

The recommended allowance for sampling error was determined in a telephone survey of American eating habits. The allowance was given in percentage points at the 95% confidence level.

Percentages near	Sample Size			
	700	600	500	400
10	3	3	5	3
20	3	4	4	4
30	4	4	5	5
40	4	5	5	5
50	4	5	5	5
60	4	5	5	5
70	4	4	5	5
80	3	4	4	4
90	3	3	5	3

Source: Food Marketing Institute/*Prevention. Shopping for Health, 1994; Eating in America: Perception and Reality.* Food Marketing Institute and *Prevention* magazine. Washington, DC and Emmaus, Pa; 1994, 40 pgs.

Appendix 2–B

Biotechnology: Modern Case Study

The Flavr Savr™ tomato is a food product of molecular biotechnology. Although fruit and vegetable intake may not be the recommended "five a day" for each US resident, there are favorites (see Table 2–B1) for a list of the most frequently consumed vegetables in the United States).

Many fruits and vegetables are not available for domestic consumption all year around. Tomatoes have been common in the United States since the colonies were formed. In a typical month, about 55 million consumers purchase at least three pounds of fresh tomatoes. To meet the market demand, tomatoes are picked when they are green to allow for transportation to local vendors. The taste of the store tomato does not reflect the full, mature vegetable due to the early harvest.

Scientists at Calgene Fresh, Inc., discovered a type of tomato gene that softens tomatoes in reverse. This slows the softening process. Tomato polygalacturonase (PG) is a key enzyme in tomatoes that causes them to soften and eventually

Table 2–B1 Frequently Consumed Vegetables in the United States

Rank	Vegetable	Number of Individuals Consuming Vegetable (per 10,000)
1	Potatoes	4,171
2	Green Salad	4,030
3	**Tomatoes (raw and cooked)**	**2,552**
4	Dried peas and beans	1,070
5	Green beans	992
6	Cole slaw, cabbage	944
7	Corn	852
8	Carrots	811
9	Green peas	553
10	Onions	385
11	Broccoli	249
12	Greens, collards	244
13	Spinach	237
14	Sweet potatoes	158
15	Cooked green peppers	129

Source: Adapted from *Frequently Consumed Vegetables* by the National Cancer Institute. National Institutes of Health, 1993.

NRC/NAS	National Research Council/National Academy of Science
NSF	National Science Foundation
ODPHP	Office of Disease Prevention and Health Promotion
OMB	Office of Management and Budget
OTA	Office of Technology Assessment
PAHO	Pan American Health Organization
PHS	Project Head Start
PPO	preferred provider organization
PSRO	Professional Standards Review Organization
RDA	Recommended Dietary Allowance
RUMBA	quality assurance criteria (acronym for relevant, understandable, measurable, behavioral, achievable)
SOAP	subjective data, objective data, assessment, and plan
SNE	Society for Nutrition Education
SSA	Social Security Administration
UNESCO	United Nations Economic and Social Council
UNICEF	United Nations Children's Emergency Fund
USDA	US Department of Agriculture
USDHHS	US Department of Health and Human Services
USPHS	US Public Health Service
WHO	World Health Organization
WIC	Special Supplemental Food Program for Women, Infants and Children

3

The Community Nutrition Professional

Learning Objectives

- Define community nutrition and community nutrition research and how it fits within the scope of research, from basic research to community application.
- List the vocabulary common to professionals in community nutrition research.
- Describe various communication skills needed to relate effectively with the media and the viewing audience.
- Enumerate the educational needs and skills of individuals functioning as community nutrition educators or researchers.
- Identify the factors that motivate community nutrition research.
- Identify the characteristics of defendable nutrition research methods.
- Outline a nutrition research agenda for the year 2000 for community nutrition and for manpower-related research.

High Definition Nutrition

Distance learning—any formal instruction process in which the educator and the student are in different locations.

Entrepreneurialship—a tenor that reflects a creative spirit, a dedication to persist, and a problem-solving nature.

Nutrition counseling—an extension of nutrition teaching to assist individuals to change old and to maintain new eating behaviors.

Nutrition education—the process of imparting knowledge for improved nutritional status of the public.

Nutrition information—information about food and nutrition and their relationship to good health and disease.

Nutrition teaching—providing information through nutrition instruction to individuals or groups.

Nutrition education research—a five-stage process often using a number of methodologies to increase a knowledge content base.

Technology—the types of equipment and methods used to perform tasks.

AVENUES OF OPPORTUNITY IN COMMUNITY NUTRITION

Community nutrition activities form an umbrella needed to implement many objectives stated in *Healthy People 2000*.[1] Although the nutrition field in general and community nutrition specifically are considered primarily service professions, community nutrition professionals perform multiple services, including high-quality research.

Community nutrition professionals are challenged to use scientific methods to study, interpret, promote, and apply findings to remediate public health problems. To do so, community nutrition professionals need requisite skills (e.g., research skills, the ability to critique and to determine the usefulness of research, a broad knowledge base, and an entrepreneurial tenor). Requisite skills involve a focused education about public health problems, training and technical skill development, and first-hand experience with people and organizations that function at the community level.

Knowledge is essential and must include not only a general base, but a level of expertise in a chosen area (e.g., the needs of pregnant women, older individuals, or migrant individuals). A creative spirit and a dedication to persist and to solve problems are both essential.

There are many relevant issues for community nutrition as a practice and as a research effort. In the 1990s and beyond the year 2000, meeting multiethnic needs is a major issue in community nutrition. Using computer technology efficiently, choosing defendable research methods, and using valid and reliable instrumentation are also major issues. Further, community nutrition professionals must understand nutritional needs across the life cycle when planning, implementing, evaluating, and reporting programs and research efforts. To venture down the community nutrition research path, individuals should pause to appreciate the scenery and the human road signs along the way. Each contact enriches the community nutritionist's art of creating ways to improve the world through nutrition.[2]

The flow of research as defined by the National Heart, Lung, and Blood Institute (NHLBI) in 1988 identifies how the research community moves from basic research to application (see Figure 3-1).[3] In basic, applied, or clinical research, the individual—a plant or an animal—is generally the unit of intervention and analysis. If a sufficient number of units have been observed and tests have been conducted, researchers can document the failures and successes. If success is linked to either a therapy or an approach to remediate disease morbidity or mortality, then research efforts may move from individual units of experimentation to a broader human application. This may include demonstration and education research to integrate a successful treatment into a public health domain.

Community nutrition research is usually identified at the level of demonstration and education research in the NHLBI model, because community implies groups of individuals linked by a commonality. On the other hand, community nutrition research often evolves as either a product of knowledge transfer, application, and inquiry, or of evaluation research (see Figure 3-2). Baseline data are often collected on a group participating in a nutrition program or intervention. The end-point data may be a repetition of the same data elements to see if a change has occurred because of the intervention. Using this repeat or test-retest approach as a model, evaluation defines a format for nutrition research: develop a nutrition intervention, select a target population or high-risk group, collect baseline data, apply the intervention, and then repeat the baseline assessment.

Another way to look at community nutrition is as a sophisticated, community-oriented program akin to a research effort. There is a strong belief that eating behavior still remains insignificant and is not a powerful intervention to bring about health change. Pharmacological approaches continue to have a leading edge and certainly re-

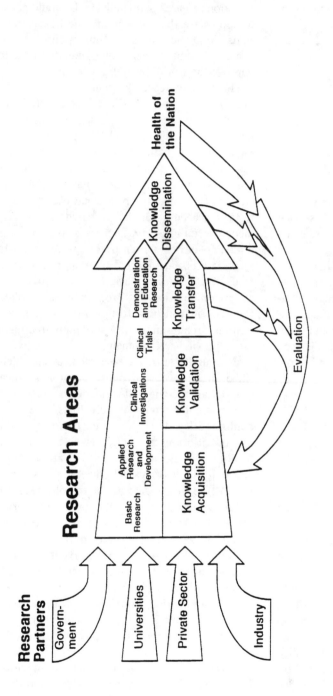

Figure 3-1 The flow of research from basic research to application. *Source:* Adapted from Stone, E., Obtaining an NIH Grant: Basic Building Blocks, *Cardiovascular Nursing, Vol.* 25, No. 2, pp. 7-11, with permission of the American Heart Association, © 1989.

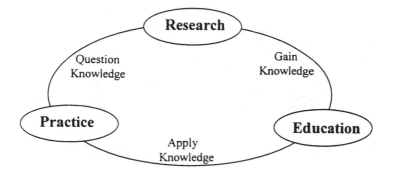

Figure 3-2 A conceptual framework linking community nutrition research, education, and practice via different levels of knowledge transfer

quire more of the health care dollar than dietary intervention. Current technological advances and surgical procedures appear more effective than dietary intervention as a modality for health change, but it doesn't need to stay that way.

It is important to establish the point at which a nutrition program begins. Nutrition intervention that precedes the onset or the diagnosis of a disease is called *primary prevention*. Programs that are implemented after a diagnosis as a result of services given to a target group are called *secondary prevention* or *secondary intervention*. Nutrition programs provided to an individual or group after disease symptoms appear and the disease expresses itself with increasing morbidity and pending mortality are known as *tertiary care*. Tertiary care or intervention is an attempt to offset early mortality.

WHAT MOTIVATES COMMUNITY NUTRITION RESEARCH?

Three major motivational forces for community nutrition research are:

1. the public health problems that exist in our society (These are often termed the *morbidity* and *mortality* within a population and quantified with *rates*, such as the number of new cases of hypertension in a given year. See Chapter 1.)

2. the scientific and professional consensus regarding relevant needs, severity of a disease, and resulting health goals (*Objectives for the Nation* and *Healthy People 2000* are two major documents identifying a research agenda for community nutrition in the United States.[1,4])

3. advocacy as demonstrated by research involving women's health issues, which has lagged behind research on men until recently

In addition, resource dollars motivate community nutrition research. Generally, funding agencies, called *sponsors*, must be addressed when planning nutrition research projects or evaluating the state of health of a community. Sponsors may select certain topics or health problems as priorities and earmark only these for research dollars. Federal or state funding is often received in the form of block grants. Community nutrition research is often based on soft moneys that may be available only for a period of one, two, or three years and may focus on only certain health concerns. Because the major governmental or sponsorship concerns will shift, the community nutrition research focus must be flexible.

Healthy People 2000 is the current national directive to increase a healthy life span, reduce disparities among groups within the population, and increase access to service. The directive lists 289 specific objectives within 22 priority areas, including nutrition. The objectives are quantifiable and specific, and give the rationale for a community nutrition research agenda.[1] These objectives create the ideal research opportunity for community nutrition professionals.

In addition, *Healthy Youth 2000*, a directive of the American Medical Association, focuses on priorities for youth, 10 to 24 years of age. These priorities include many that are related to nutrition, such as the need to address obesity, inadequate calcium intake, iron deficiency anemia, and inability to choose foods using food labels.[5]

An astute community nutrition professional serving a target group can create a research agenda by focusing on and advocating for one or two priorities related to nutrition of this target group. For example, the professional may choose to reduce obesity to less than 20% of the youth; to have at least 50% of children receiving adequate calcium intakes; to decrease iron deficiency anemia to less than 3%; or to increase the use of food labels in making nutritious choices among 85% of the youth.

REQUIREMENTS FOR CONDUCTING COMMUNITY NUTRITION RESEARCH

Community nutrition professionals need skills, knowledge of research techniques, advanced knowledge, and an entrepreneurial tenor to conduct quality research.

Knowledge of Research Techniques

To conduct community nutrition research, individuals need technical training to acquire "field" or "hands-on" experience. A common vocabulary aids communication.[2] Important terms are divided into three general domains: design, implementation, and analysis.[6] All three domains overlap, but what is important is that students understand and apply them correctly.

Design
- *Population*—the target group that receives the program, is involved in the research, or

is in greatest need for nutritional intervention (*N*).
- *Sample*—denotes a subset within a population (*n*).
- *Sampling frame*—the collection area and description of the population from which the sample is chosen.
- *Randomization*—the process by which individuals in a group have an equal chance of being selected.
- *Matching*—a statistical procedure to control for potential confounders and to ensure that individuals are alike on important characteristics before they are assigned to treatment or control conditions.

Implementation

- *Methods*—procedures, techniques, and instruments.
- *Protocols*—procedures for assessing, implementing, or evaluating the program or research.
- *Quality control*—a reflection of how carefully data collection, interventions, or methods are conducted. Examples include protocols for each technique, training of interviewers or observers in a standardized fashion, duplicate measures, and data editing prior to computer entry.
- *Timelines (Gantt charts)*—a formal delineation of activities across time. One can track progress and clearly show the order of specific events. For example, a timeline states *when* researchers do something, *what* they are doing, and in *what order* they are doing it.
- *Coalitions*—combinations of organizations and individuals with a common goal. Coalitions might involve groups such as the American Cancer Society, a district dietetic association, the Cooperative Extension Service, or a nursing agency addressing a colon cancer screening and education program.
- *Sponsors*—those who fund a program or research study.

Analysis

- *Statistics*—analysis of data. Descriptive statistics, such as measures of central tendency (mean, mode, and median) are quite different than inferential statistics, such as reporting how well two or more variables relate (correlation) or if one variable predicts another.
- *Confounder*—a characteristic that appears to have an influential role in the nature of an outcome. Potential confounders must be controlled in the sampling or analysis.
- *Evaluation/accountability*—a process for comparing a measure against a standard or objective. If a *Healthy Youth 2000* objective was chosen, the evaluation research could analyze how close the baseline and end-point measures were to the objective (e.g., less than 20% of youths overweight); or analysts could evaluate effectiveness (e.g., whether a change from 30% overweight to 25% overweight was achieved with the program); or analysts could evaluate *efficiency* (if a change from 30% to 25% was achieved spending $1,200 per child).
- *Paradigm*—defines a design, how different components link (O = observation, X = intervention), and if a random (R) or quasi-experimental design is being used (e.g., R. . .O. . .X. . .O).
- *Framework*—the organization of work. Models such as PRECEDE and PROCEED are examples.[7]

Qualifications

Experience helps professionals to develop their skills. Community nutrition professionals find that each year of experience strengthens their basic skills, alerts them to improved techniques, and allows them to streamline their efforts in the community to enlarge their population or study sample.

Since 1920, various professional groups have met to review the functions and qualifications of community nutrition professionals.[8] The University of Tennessee was the first graduate training program in nutrition to receive Title V Maternal and Child Health Services funding for public health nutrition training grants. This funding was followed by awards to the University of California Berkeley, Case Western Reserve University, the University of Michigan, the University of North Carolina, and Harvard University. The training awards were expanded with Title VII of the Public Health Act in the mid-1970s.[9]

During the past 75 years, qualifications of community nutrition professionals have been carefully documented and demonstrate a commitment to high educational standards in an evolving field that responds to the nutritional needs of individuals and the community. Chronologically, educational qualifications are briefly outlined as follows[9]:

- 1937—minimum qualifications for home economists and nutritionists were identified for health and welfare agencies.
- 1950—objectives for preparation of public health nutritionists were enumerated.
- 1962—educational qualifications of nutritionists in health care agencies were listed.
- 1989—a description of personnel in public health nutrition for the 1980s was outlined.
- 1990—strategies for successful graduate programs in public health nutrition were identified.

Competencies

Today, standard entry-level skills for minimal knowledge and understanding of community nutrition can be acquired through a didactic program in dietetics, a dietetic internship, or an Approved Preprofessional Practice Program.[10] All Approved Preprofessional Practice Programs will convert to accredited internships by the year 2000. At the completion of these programs, entry-level competencies should include the following:

- knowledge of and ability to apply the scientific research method across all age and ethnic groups for primary, secondary, and tertiary prevention

- a basic understanding of how to work with and communicate with groups to recruit and retain research and program participants
- an understanding of how to target and pinpoint high-risk individuals for assessment and intervention
- the ability to develop, program, and delegate responsibilities to a variety of trained individuals during research, implementation, and analysis stages

These competencies are needed to implement the community nutrition program that may be the center of the research endeavor. Specific educational needs of an individual who plans to conduct research in the community require a minimum of an M.P.H. or M.S. degree with courses in research methods, statistics, sampling, interpretation, and communication. A doctoral program with an emphasis in research would refine these skills. A Dr.P.H. or a Ph.D. program that includes coursework in research methods, statistics, sampling, communication, accounting, and ethics is important in today's world (see Appendix 3-A), because community nutrition professionals are managers. Their positions require skills in managing staff as well as managing delivery programs, implementing research objectives, and conducting research studies.

Knowledge of multinutrient databases and the ability to establish complex data management systems to articulate and integrate collected data are important. Familiarity with the personal computer versions of statistical packages for data management and with simple, user-friendly, educational software packages is essential.

Several terms are commonly used by educators of practitioners in public health/community nutrition and nutrition research. Students would benefit from learning and applying these terms in written and verbal communications[11] (see Appendix 3-B).

Future Training

A current concern of nutrition professionals is the continual training of students to meet the changing community nutrition environment. One avenue for training public health/community nutritionists is the Approved Preprofessional Practice Program. Representatives of the Food and Nutrition Service, the National Association of WIC Directors, and the Association of State and Territorial Public Health Nutrition Directors convened in June 1992 to study the issue of recruitment and retention of qualified nutritionists in public health/community nutrition programs. The working group solicited the assistance and support of the American Dietetic Association (ADA) in developing effective recruitment strategies.

A meeting was held with ADA and other interested national agencies on May 11, 1993, to identify specific actions to be taken. Eleven actions were proposed, of which two were specific to Approved Preprofessional Practice Programs sponsored by public health/community nutrition programs:

1. *Increase the number of Approved Preprofessional Practice Programs in public health/community nutrition programs.* The Food and Nutrition Service is committed to the development of more Approved Preprofessional Practice Programs in WIC (Special Supplemental Food Program for Women, Infants and Children). The sponsoring of a practice program by a public health/community nutrition program can serve as a training program for WIC nutritionists to improve their skills and, at the same time, to acquire professional credentials. Further, the sponsoring of an Approved Preprofessional Practice Program by a WIC agency can serve as an effective recruitment/retention tool for state and local programs. There are currently 144 Approved Preprofessional Practice Programs listed in the ADA *1994–1995 Directory of Dietetic Programs.* About a dozen of these programs are sponsored by either a state or local health department. Interest continues as these programs are developed within state WIC agencies.

2. *Develop a prototype of the Approved Preprofessional Practice Program self-*

study for use by health departments. The Food and Nutrition Service is developing a national self-study prototype for development of Approved Preprofessional Practice Programs, which will be adaptable for use by state and local WIC directors. The prototype could be expanded and applicable for other child nutrition programs.

PROFESSIONALISM

A *professional* has certain distinct characteristics. The professional is generally employed full-time in an occupation, possesses strong motivation for making a particular career choice, and possesses a specialized body of knowledge and skills acquired in a set academic course. A professional has a service orientation, interprets client needs without moral judgment, and allows peers to judge his or her knowledge and performance. Participating in a professional association, following a code of ethics, and demonstrat-

ing both leadership and status in an area of expertise further distinguish a professional from a nonprofessional.[12-15]

To measure differences between professional attitudes of dietetics students and practitioners, Spears et al[16] developed a five-item questionnaire with a Likert response scale. The professional statements that loaded at a 0.36 or greater level using factor analysis were considered significant. The researchers identified 12 scales, and noted differences in the way students versus experienced members responded. For example, the score for social service orientation, which assessed responsibility and commitment to help others, was higher for younger respondents than for experienced practitioners.[16] Table 3–1 provides an index for individuals to evaluate the extent of their professionalism.

Community nutrition professionals can continue their education in a specific direction or they can enlarge their knowledge base by joining professional organizations such as the Society of Nutrition Education, the American Public Health Association, or a council in the American

Table 3–1 Professional Self-Assessment Form

Belief	Level of Agreement[a] Strongly Disagree ◄———► Strongly Agree				
I believe the profession of dietetics is important.	1	2	3	4	5
I believe continuing education for dietitians is important.	1	2	3	4	5
I believe dietitians have a responsibility to help others.	1	2	3	4	5
I believe that it is important for dietitians to be active in the political process.	1	2	3	4	5
I believe that it is important for dietitians to be active in professional organizations.	1	2	3	4	5
I believe that a career in dietetics provides intellectual growth and job challenges.	1	2	3	4	5
I believe dietetics is important to society.	1	2	0	4	5
I believe dietitians should have professional autonomy.	1	2	3	4	5
I believe dietitians have an obligation to uphold the profession's code of ethics.	1	2	3	4	5
I believe dietitians make a substantial contribution to the provision of quality health care.	1	2	3	4	5

[a]Agreement codes are 1 = strongly disagree, 2 = disagree, 3 = not sure, 4 = agree, 5 = strongly agree.

Source: Adapted from Spears, M.C., Simonis, P.L., and Vaden, A.G., Professional Attitudes of Dietetics Students and Practitioners, *Journal of the American Dietetic Association*, Vol. 92, pp. 1522–1526, with permission of the American Dietetic Association, © 1992.

Heart Association. Professionals may also join one or more dietetic practice groups (DPGs) of the American Dietetic Association (see Appendix 3–C). The focus of the DPGs ranges from Public Health Nutritionists, a large US network composed primarily of practicing community nutritionists; to the Hunger and Malnutrition DPG, which enrolls nutrition professionals from across the United States; to the Nutrition Research DPG, whose members range from university professors conducting research to clinical registered dietitians (RDs) involved in randomized trials. These professionals may or may not work directly with social problems. They may contribute ideas, volunteer time in their own communities, or incorporate messages into their writings or newsletters for other groups to aid campaigns.

A description of personnel in public health nutrition reflects a corp of dedicated, trained professionals.[17] In the year 2000, community nutrition professionals will continue to serve the public; however, the nature of their service may be more research-based. Community nutrition professionals must strengthen their research skills and remain vigilant about improving their basic tasks to plan, assess, define, target, develop, train, implement, monitor, evaluate, and report community nutrition activities.

IMPORTANT ISSUES RELEVANT TO COMMUNITY NUTRITION RESEARCH

Six important issues related to community nutrition research must be addressed:

1. Participants must be informed prior to consent. They need to understand the risks and benefits of participating in research or demonstration studies. Written, signed, and witnessed documents are essential.
2. Studies should focus on multiethnic groups, children, women, and older adults during the next decade. For example, in San Francisco, a study of the hypertension morbidity among the Vietnamese community has challenged the efforts of nutrition professionals and produced important information regarding the influence of beliefs and structure on medical and health decisions of this population, including youth and adult (i.e., "Suc Khoe la Vang!" or "Health is Gold!").[18]
3. It is important to conduct surveys of various groups across the age spectrum to understand the needs of individuals in different stages of the life cycle. Instruments that identify and characterize eating behaviors of children and seniors should be developed.[19]
4. Methods and instruments should be developed and evaluated so they can be used to assess multicultural population patterns, eating behaviors, physical activities, and decision-making patterns. Methods and instruments must be clearly defined and defendable. Four characteristics of defendable methods are as follows[6]:
   - *Reliable*—relates to how well a method can be repeated in a similar setting and give the same answer.
   - *Valid*—relates to whether an instrument measures what one is trying to measure.
   - *Comparable*—means being able to contrast results for two or more different studies.
   - *Transportable*—means that an approach tested or applied in one setting can be transferred and applied to another setting. Transportability reduces the need to "reinvent" the wheel.

An example of a defendable method is the fat-cholesterol avoidance scale, a quick, handy tool with a relative validity to assess the extent of fat avoidance in a study sample. Researchers validated the instrument in both adult and pediatric populations. They reported differences between Mexican-American and Anglo samples in two different states.[20,21]

Frequency tools are evolving and allow researchers to assess multiple days of intake including a representative group of 50 to 80 foods to characterize an overall pattern.[22,23] Frequencies are valuable when categorizing individuals into broad groups (e.g., low-fat versus high-fat consumers). One-to-one interview techniques or individual self-reports involve shorter time periods. Three-day or seven-day food records are essential for identifying specific nutrient intake instead of food group intakes.[19]

5. Because community nutrition research is fluid, researchers must learn to ask questions and integrate new questioning techniques for mass data collection (e.g., telephone surveys).[24] Interactive video, use of computer networks, and E-mail and the "Net" are new but viable options for data collection, transfer, and communication.

6. Community nutrition professionals must quantify their value in any nutrition research study. One way is to establish a value or cost for each task and the value of professional time to complete each task. Individual costs can be aggregated to establish total project cost. Community nutrition managers must document staff responsibilities for program implementation, data collection, and analysis. Knowledge of the cost or value of a task can assist with salary negotiations. Establishing competitive salaries also helps to maintain high-quality staff. Salary differential should be real for experienced compared with new researchers. Women in research positions and with varying degrees of experience should evaluate and seek salary equity compared to male peers in similar positions and with similar education and experience.

RESEARCH AGENDA FOR THE YEAR 2000

Nutrition research in the United States can address national problems and identify national goals. Nutrition research strengthens technology, which affects the US industrial and economic agenda.[25]

Food science and nutrition are integrative disciplines that incorporate other specialties into their research and program agendas. New avenues of thought develop when researchers confront human nutrition problems that face both individuals and groups. A recurrent challenge is to keep the research agenda for food science and nutrition invigorated. One recommendation is to infuse the field with innovations from the biological sciences by developing a field of bionutrition.[26] Bionutrition is integrative and concerns the interaction of genetics, molecular biology, and cell biology with dietary components, and environmental influences and the outcome in terms of more complex levels of biological organization and human health.[27]

The Committee on Opportunities in the Nutrition and Food Sciences, the Food and Nutrition Board, and the National Academy of Sciences have published a landmark report that identifies nutrition research opportunities for health promotion and disease prevention.[28] Major research themes are listed in Exhibit 3–1. Others have identified social, economic, and biological issues.[29,30] In addition, the Human Nutrition Research and Information Management System is an on-line retrieval system that identifies and categorizes federally funded human nutrition research projects in all government agencies.[31]

Research must be considered worthwhile and show cost-effectiveness. This is often difficult for nutrition research, where examples of both cost-benefit and cost-effectiveness are lacking and needed.[32-34]

There are numerous opportunities for research on issues related to dietetic manpower.[35,36] Specific opportunities can be identified for community nutrition. Several terms are useful to understand the research opportunities and approaches[36]:

- *Distance learning* describes formal instruction in which a majority of teaching and learning occurs while the educator and the student are at a distance from one another.
- *Nutrition counseling* is an extension of nutrition teaching that is intended to help an individual adjust to change required to achieve and to maintain new eating behaviors. It can be an individualized process by which a client is helped to acquire the abil-

Exhibit 3-1 Key Research Themes for the Year 2000

- Nutrients in stages of human development spanning from conception to death (specific areas are cell differentiation, growth, aging, physiological functions, and wellness)
- Genetic mapping, food, and degenerative disease
- Determinants of eating patterns in multicultures
- Development of new health-promoting, high-quality economic and wholesome foods that are environmentally safe
- Effective food and nutrition policies for improved access to and acceptance of food programs and surveillance of nutritional status across the life cycle

Source: Adapted from Dwyer J. Nutrition Research for the Year 2000 and Beyond, *Contemporary Nutrition*. Vol. 18, No. 6, pp. 1-2 with permission of General Mills, Inc., © 1994.

---

ity to manage nutritional care, and it requires a relationship between a professionally trained, competent nutritionist/dietitian and an individual. It may also involve a group of individuals who seek help in following a special diet, gaining knowledge or self-understanding, improving decision-making skills, or changing behavior.

- *Nutrition education* is the process of imparting knowledge to the public aimed at the general improvement of nutritional status through elimination of unsatisfactory dietary practices, promotion of adequate food habits and better food hygiene, and more efficient use of food resources.
- *Nutrition information* is a generic term that refers to routine information that meets an individual's or group's need for knowledge about food and nutrition, and their relationship to good health and disease. Its purpose is generally to improve the ability of an individual or group to self-manage any dietary change.
- *Nutrition teaching* involves providing instruction and information that seeks to promote specific changes in eating behaviors and improved self-management of dietary treatment.

- *Nutrition education research* is a process that can be described in five stages: (1) hypothesis development; (2) methods development and message focus; (3) intervention-effectiveness test; (4) efficacy in the real world; and (5) dissemination of the intervention. A number of methodologies can be used for achieving a better understanding of a knowledge content base.
- The *level of technology* is defined by the types and patterns of activity, equipment, material, and knowledge or experience used to perform tasks.

Seven major arenas of change in the United States and the relevance for community nutrition professionals involved in nutrition education and research are briefly discussed below. Potential researchable questions are listed for each arena of change.

Societal Change

The Institute of Medicine identifies two factors that will affect the future demand for nutrition services: (1) consumer desire for nutrition information and direction, and (2) the potential willingness of the consumer to pay for the service.[37] In both 1988 and 1992, the strategic plan for the American Dietetic Association identified the following influential societal trends[38,39]:

- cost containment
- lifestyle and demographic changes
- awareness of the relationship of diet to health
- governmental influence on health care
- changing technology
- environmental issues
- nutrition information channels

One of the most important demographic trends is the aging of the US population and the extended longevity of the aging cohort. One result is an increased use of medical services by individuals over 65 years of age. In 1982–1983, health care expenses equaled 4.4% of the total expenditures of all consumer units. This contrasts with 9.9% of the total expenditures for consumer units with heads of household over 65 years of age.[40] Further, an increase in the number of 85-year-old individuals living independently will challenge home health services.

Potential manpower-related research questions for community nutrition research are as follows:

- What community nutrition services will be essential due to the increasing number of consumer units over 65 years of age?
- What educational opportunities or hands-on experiences are currently available to train community nutrition professionals to work with individuals over 65 years of age?
- Are community nutrition professionals currently providing nutrition services to individuals in their homes? If so, what are the services? If not, what services are needed?

Changes in Lifestyle

Two changes that are important for community nutrition professionals are: (1) the restructuring of careers (i.e., no more 25-year careers in one position or setting[40]); and (2) the mobility of the work force on a daily basis, resulting in an increasing demand for quick, convenient foods that bear nutrition information (e.g., point-of-choice nutrition information).[41]

Researchable questions include the following:

- What new career paths are of interest to and within the reach of established community nutrition professionals?
- How well do community nutrition professionals practice healthy eating behaviors on a daily basis?
- What types of information do community nutrition professionals use to make their own food choices?

Technological Change

Increased skill in the use of nutritional databases, communication and retrieval systems, and robotics is needed. Timely strategies for training professionals in communication skills are needed.[42] This includes expanded use of computer-assisted instruction, videotapes, distanced education, telephone menus for messages and hot lines, television programming (both live and cable-access), and immediate information regarding nutritional content of foods at the point of choice.[43-49]

Researchable questions include the following:

- Are community nutrition professionals aware of and using contemporary computerized nutritional analysis systems?
- What costs are involved in using up-to-date technology in nutrition information transmission?
- What skills are needed for community nutrition professionals to use robotics, computer-assisted instruction, videos, and live television?
- What is the effectiveness of these methods in changing eating behaviors of groups and communities?

Changes in Business and Industry

Technological changes generally challenge community nutrition professionals to become actively involved in business and industry, which are likewise experiencing their own changes. The demands for community education are due in large part to the Nutrition Labeling Education Act, the appeal of radio and television for entertaining education, and innovative marketing and advertising approaches of the food and nutrition supplement industries. Community nutrition professionals with a broad knowledge base can become skilled management consultants and open new fields of employment and new outreach techniques, such as self-employment, working at home, and telephone conferencing.[50]

Researchable questions include the following:

- What employment opportunities exist for community nutrition professionals who wish to develop a business-oriented career track?
- What marketing and communication skills are part of the training of community nutrition professionals?

Changes in Health Care

Several new target groups have been identified for community nutrition programs, including individuals who have tested positive for HIV (human immunodeficiency virus), pregnant teens, adolescents with alcohol problems, and children and adults with eating disorders and vascillating weight-management skills.[51] Segmented health care delivery and shifts from hospital to clinic-, outpatient-, and worksite-based health care all influence the community nutrition approach.[50] Specialization of health care professionals and the need for certification (e.g., Certified Health Education Specialists and state licensure for community nutrition professionals) create new continuing education demands.[52]

Researchable questions include the following:

- What are the differences in effectiveness and cost of delivering community nutrition services in various health and employment settings?
- Are community nutrition professionals ready and willing to practice their profession in a variety of settings from physicians' offices to community-based clinics, and from school-based clinics to worksites?

Changes in Dietetic Education

The fairly small pool of doctoral-trained academicians in community nutrition may face retirement within the next decade.[53] Early retirement due to university downsizing negatively influences the educational arena. Refining undergraduate programs and merging similar programs (e.g., health education, community nursing, epidemiology, public health nutrition, etc.) may redefine the education of community nutrition professionals.

Researchable questions include the following:

- What is the magnitude of the timeline for retirement of current university professors in community nutrition?
- Are specific strategies in place to strengthen a new pool of community nutrition professionals?
- Why are men not entering the community nutrition profession as rapidly as women?
- What are the similarities between programs in nutrition, nursing, sociology, health education, and epidemiology? Are there untapped areas of overlap that could be strengthened to allow interdisciplinary and multicultural training?

Changes in Student Profile

The community nutrition professional is often female and white.[54,55] Men have not entered the field as quickly as women. Many universities are opening their doors to adult reentry students who are changing their careers or finishing ones they began before they started families.[56] Communities are becoming more culturally diverse, and skilled professionals from all cultural groups are needed to improve communication and acceptance of nutrition programs by the diverse US population.[57]

Researchable questions include the following:

- Are university training programs preparing a multiethnic cadre of professionals to mirror the US population?
- Do training programs acknowledge and address the differing needs of male, adult reentry, and minority students?

PROFESSIONAL SKILL DEVELOPMENT

A community nutrition practitioner needs certain skills to function effectively, including creativity, communication skills, and developing a professional presence. Covey has defined seven habits of highly effective people.[58] Professionals in a community nutrition practice or research setting can practice these habits to strengthen their skills and performance. The habits are as follows[58]:

1. *Be proactive.* The habit of being proactive, or the habit of personal vision, means taking responsibility for one's attitudes and actions.
2. *Begin with the end in mind.* The habit of personal leadership means to begin each day with a clear understanding of the desired direction and destination.
3. *Put first things first.* The habit of personal management involves organizing and managing time and events according to the personal priorities identified in habit 2.
4. *Think win-win.* Win-win is the habit of interpersonal leadership. In families and businesses, effectiveness is largely achieved through the cooperative efforts of two or more people. Win-win is the attitude of seeking mutual benefit. Win-win thinking begins with a commitment to explore all options until a mutually satisfactory solution is reached, or to make no deal at all. It begins with an "abundance mentality," a belief that by synergistically increasing the "pie," there are pieces enough for everybody.
5. *Seek first to understand, then to be understood.* The habit of communication is one of the master skills in life, the key to building win-win relationships, and the essence of professionalism.
6. *Synergize.* "Synergize" is the habit of creative cooperation or teamwork. For those who have a win-win abundance mentality and exercise empathy, differences in any relationship can produce synergy, where the whole is greater than the sum of its parts.
7. *Sharpen the saw.* The habit of self-renewal is the foundation for the first six habits of successful people. The habit of sharpening the saw regularly means having a balanced, systematic program for self-renewal in the physical, mental, emotional-social, and spiritual components of life.

Creativity

A creative edge is needed to enhance both individual and organizational innovation and bring them to their fullest potential.[59] New ways of solving problems, handling situations and relationships, and managing change must be considered. To overcome barriers to creativity, restricted mindsets must be guided to use linear and intuitive techniques. These techniques promote new approaches and new questions.

Every idea should be communicated and encouraged. Linear methods redirect how information is organized (e.g., information is examined from a new angle). A linear model begins at one point and moves in small steps toward a goal. A linear approach called matrix analysis uses a two- or three-dimensional matrix to explore new ideas. It is constructed like a crossword puzzle or spreadsheet. One axis is labeled "market needs" and the other is labeled "available technology." Intersections between market needs and available technology establish or mark a new goal or position.

Intuitive techniques draw upon stored data to synthesize solutions. Often imagery is used as a window to intuitive, creative thought. Brainstorming is an intuitive technique in which one states the problem and then participants give random ideas to solve the problem. Meditation is not only an intuitive technique but also a focused state of related attention. A mind in a quiet state can give quick, new responses to questions that otherwise seem puzzling.

Creativity within an organization should ideally evolve in the context set by the organization's vision. Strategies can then be identified that will propel an individual or an organization toward its goals. Effective change addresses all groups and processes and occurs under the guidance of a committed leadership.[59]

Individuals can propose creative processes and a creative climate by opening their minds and making contributions. If an organization is to have a creative edge, four activities must occur[59]:

1. promotion of the organization's status in a market or with a service
2. confrontation of the frontiers of marketing technology and health care
3. participation in change
4. exploration and development of each employee's creativity

When individuals are creative, they tend to possess one or more of the following distinct characteristics[59]:

- *Spontaneous*: is fresh, curious, willing to take risks; has sense of humor.
- *Persistent*: is energetic, courageous, assertive, independent, determined.
- *Inventive*: looks at problems in new ways, likes challenge, is sometimes skeptical, is comfortable with ambiguity.
- *Rewarding*: is willing to share credit, values personal satisfaction and peer recognition over money.
- *Inner openness*: is intuitive, easily switches from logic to fantasy, is open to emotions, can think/act/create/innovate in different modes.
- *Transcendent*: sees situations realistically, fantasizes how he/she wants things to be, is confident he/she can effect change, chooses growth over fear.
- *Evaluative*: is discerning, discriminating, judgmental at appropriate times.
- *Democratic*: values and respects people, seeks stimulation from variety of people, is responsible, promotes highest benefits of all concerned.

Creativity can be blocked due to a variety of reasons. The more common ones are emotional patterns including guilt and anger over previous experiences, personal or cultural perceptions that evoke narrow-mindedness, and social blocks such as fear of rejection or the unwillingness to collaborate. Creativity can also be blocked by an individual's or group's preference for how to solve problems, skills or training, stress, or lack of imagination.[59]

Within an organization, creativity is spurred by external forces. These include the economy, which is both global and information-based; competition; technical evolution; changes in social mores and demographics; and a growing awareness of the relationships between lifestyle and health.[59] However, a basic tenet of a successful individual or organization is the need to possess a sense of purpose and vision. Purpose is related to values; vision shows the path for achieving the purpose. Statements of purpose and vision set the standard for evaluating day-to-day and year-to-year success and give direction to actions. The American Dietetic Association periodically articulates and updates its mission and vision[60] (see Exhibit 3–2).

Highly effective community nutrition professionals realize that their creativity can be demonstrated and enhanced by communicating with the public and that skills are needed to communicate in several media.

Speaking Effectively

Community nutritionists are frequently called upon to give formal presentations to public and professional groups as a recruitment technique. Developing verbal and nonverbal skills increases their effectiveness and improves their chance of becoming popular speakers. Community awareness, nutrition education, and coalition-building rely on the communication skills of professionals[60] (see Table 3–2).

Preliminary steps are essential for preparing an effective presentation. Learn about the organization and audience. Analyze the situation by asking about the purpose of the talk and who and what else is on the program. Find out where the talk will be given and check out the physical environment of the room. Is it classroom or theater style? Ask if there will be a head table, a podium, a microphone, and visual projection equipment.

Analyze the audience, includings its size, age, education, and gender. Decide what the audience has in common. Does the audience know the

Exhibit 3-2 The American Dietetic Association Mission and Vision

Mission	The American Dietetic Association is the advocate of the dietetics profession serving the public through the promotion of optimal nutrition, health, and well-being.
Vision	Members of The American Dietetic Association will shape the food choices and impact the nutritional status of the public.
Philosophy	Members of The American Dietetic Association serve the profession best by serving the public first.
Values	• Excellence in the identification, development, and delivery of quality programs, services, and products • Leadership in significant food, nutrition, and related health issues • Integrity in all professional and personal actions • Respect for diverse viewpoints and individual differences • Communication that is timely and effective • Collaboration for action on critical issues • Fiscal responsibility in effectively providing and managing human and financial resources • Action that is timely and strategic

Source: Adapted with permission from the American Dietetic Association Membership brochure, p. 2.

Table 3-2 Verbal and Nonverbal Skills

Skill	*Point*
Rate and volume of voice	Vary the volume of your voice and rate of speech, using a slightly louder voice when opening, closing, and when emphasizing important points. Making slash marks in the text will remind you to pause or change volume.
Articulation	Pronounce words precisely, but not artificially. Use formal or informal language depending upon the situation. Do not sacrifice simplicity and clarity for formality.
Vary sentence length	Use short statements to emphasize key points. Avoid reading to the audience. This will eliminate monotony.
Be concise	The more concise you are, with memorable statements, the more impact you will have. Don't try to fill a one-hour time slot if what you have to say takes only 45 minutes.
Eye contact	Establish eye contact; move your eyes around the room, but don't let them roam. It is helpful to focus your attention on a few interested and responsive people in various areas of the room.
Body language	Maintain an open and natural style, using gestures and enthusiasm to give meaning to your words. Avoid handling paper clips, rubberbands, or other items when you are speaking. Avoid placing your hands in your pockets, clenching them in front or back of you, or keeping them glued to your sides. Try to keep your hands at waist level in a natural position. If there is a podium, do not clutch it or hide behind it. Remember that your message is important—the audience came to hear you!
Maintain interest	Use funny stories or jokes when appropriate, if it feels natural. Ask the audience questions to garner interest. Inject personal anecdotes to make your point come alive.

Source: Data from Ambassador Roundtable, American Dietetic Association annual meeting, Anaheim, California, 1993.

topic? Use a speaker's checklist (Table 3–3) to assist in planning and evaluating the talk.

When sitting down to write a speech, think about how to write a persuasive talk but keep it entertaining and informative. Plan the speech with three components.

1. *Introduction*. Get your audience's attention. Give them a clue that what you have to say will be "good." The primary objective in the introduction is to capture your audience's attention and establish rapport. Keep it simple. The statement of purpose should be short. Let your audience know what they can expect to get from the meeting. Include a few objectives and goals, a statement of the problem or situation, and your solution.
2. *Body*. In the body of the talk, support themes or points with evidence that is clear and easy to follow.
3. *Conclusion*. The conclusion becomes the message an audience leaves with and re-members. Summarize the key objectives or messages. For example, "If there's one thing I'd like to leave with you today, it is the feeling of confidence and skill in being an effective speaker."

Keep visual aids simple by limiting each slide or overhead to seven lines per page. Make visuals easy to read and understand. Use large lettering and styles that have eye appeal.

Allow the audience to ask questions at the close of the talk. Repeat the question in your own words, and then give evidence to support your point. End on a positive note and never demean a question or the person asking the question.

Developing and Nurturing Media Relations

Community nutritionists must learn techniques to build and maintain positive and productive media relationships. The media is a channel for

---

Table 3–3 Speaker's Checklist

Do You . . .	Action
_____	Check room, equipment, podium, and lighting, prior to speech?
_____	Focus on communications objectives?
_____	Keep control of: _____self?
	_____environment?
	_____materials?
_____	Project a strong, positive image?
_____	Maintain direct eye contact with audience?
_____	Use gestures effectively for emphasis and to convey feeling?
_____	Eliminate distracting body language (swaying, clutching podium, etc.)?
_____	Remain calm and relaxed?
_____	Exhibit enthusiasm?
_____	Project voice adequately?
_____	Smile and use humor?
_____	Vary tone, pitch, volume, and pace?
_____	Avoid undue dependence on notes (script, outline)?
_____	Enunciate clearly?
_____	Maintain sincerity, credibility?
_____	Avoid nervous habits (clearing throat, shuffling papers)?
_____	Maintain clarity in providing technical information?
_____	Use personal examples, anecdotes?
_____	Use visual aids appropriately and effectively?
_____	Anticipate questions?

communicating, educating, and recruiting for nutrition programs and research. Key elements of a positive media relationship include building a media resource inventory, becoming a reliable media source, understanding time pressures, and keeping track of the media (see Exhibit 3-3).

Build a media resource inventory. Check with your local Chamber of Commerce, United Way, or government public information office to see if a compiled list of local media exists. If not, abstract information from the yellow pages or media directories in libraries. For newspapers, the managing editor's office can supply names of specialized reporters. Check newspapers for lifestyle, health and fitness, food, medical, science, and consumer writers. Editors' names may appear on articles as bylines. Food sections often appear midweek (e.g., Tuesday, Wednesday, or Thursday), and community calendars usually run weekly.

For radio programming opportunities, include public service announcements, community calendar announcements, public affairs shows, daily news reports, call-in shows (question-answer format), and specialty shows (health/fitness). For television, the challenge is to identify the gamut of air opportunities and not only learn how to access them but to achieve a positive media presence and high marks for meeting the public's needs (see Figure 3-3).

Exhibit 3-3 Keys to Becoming a Reliable Media Source

1. Keep current. Be dynamic, consumer-oriented, informed, and reliable.
2. Stay "tuned in" to media happenings. Know what allies and adversaries say.
3. Provide your business card. Ensure that you are in reporters' resource files.
4. Send an occasional pitch letter. Provide articles or leads that will be of interest to a reporter.
5. Offer background information, recipes, graphics, audiovisual materials, or other contacts (health professionals, consumers) to make a story more exciting.
6. Do the interview if at all possible. Too many obstacles and too many "NOs" are sure to exclude you from a reporter's resource file.
7. Be honest. Take the interview only if you can handle it, refer the request to another media resource if you cannot handle it.

Source: Data from Ambassador Roundtable, American Dietetic Association annual meeting, Anaheim, California, 1993.

Info Line

The early methods used to describe the audience that listened to radio were crude. Usually the announcer's closing remarks would be something like, "to keep this fine program coming your way, send a postcard to our sponsor and let him know how much you enjoyed the program." Once the postcards were received and sorted, they were weighed. The weight reflected the popularity and audience size.

A.C. Nielsen, Sr, sought a more reliable method and purchased a patent for a radio meter developed for the Lever Brothers Company. Between 1938 and 1945 the meter was modified and tested, and it finally entered the market as the *Nielsen Rating*. Today a small electronic computer called a "People Meter" is installed in a cross-sectional sample of 4,000 households.

Each Nielsen audiometer links by telephone to a central computer, which polls the sample responses nightly. Ratings are calculated and transmitted to the subscribers early the following morning. Reports using slightly different methods are also produced for tracking the television-viewing audience for 210 major metropolitan areas.

Subscribers include broadcasters, advertisers and their agencies, program producers, and talents. The goal of the service is to determine fair and equitable prices for the broadcasts and commercials, based upon the size and demographics of the sample tracked by the audiometer. The Nielsen method is used not only in the United States but in many other countries where television is an important advertising medium.

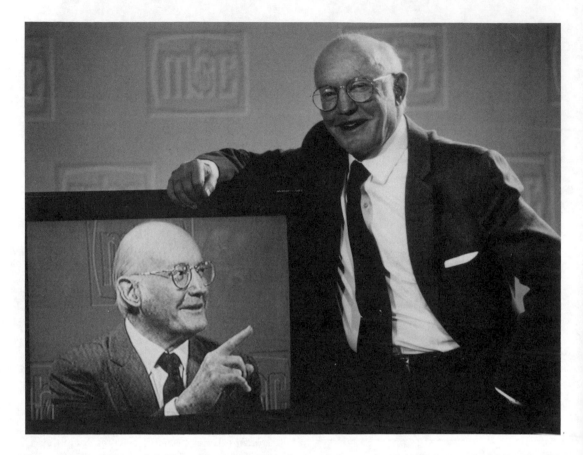

Figure 3-3 The Nielsens. A.C. Nielsen, Jr, and his father developed the popular Nielsen's Ratings for television, which reflect the importance of meeting the public's interest. RDs on television are not evaluated by the Nielsen Ratings, but they are sensitive to the power of this media. Courtesy of A.C. Nielsen, Jr, Northbrook, Illinois.

Phone or write the television station's public service director. Request a local programming schedule and personnel guide. Watch the station to identify the style and topics discussed. Focus on opportunities such as community calendar announcements, public service announcements, daily news reports (consumer, medical, or health), weekly public affairs shows, and entertainment talk programs.

Understand time pressures because the media, both print and electronic, work on a minute-to-minute basis. Being sensitive to their time crunch strengthens your chance to serve as a resource.

Being a resource means responding to a reporter's questions on the spot (your education and experience should enable you to respond to many nutrition issues without major research) or referring the reporter to the appropriate expert.

To track the media, use data sheets and document who you work with and the final outcome of your contact. As you widen your circle of media contacts, you become more adept at responding to inquiries and you become more visible to the community as a valuable resource.

Working Effectively with Print

To work effectively with the media, story angles that sell are a must! Five tips for success are outlined in Exhibit 3–4. Creative topics for print media are topics that hold a reader's interest or explore a hot issue. Food trends, food myths, and

Exhibit 3-4 Five Tips for Success with Print Interviews

1. Understand that interviews will be edited, so interviewee may say a lot but only be quoted a little. It's important to be relaxed and friendly but stay with the agenda. If answers are concise, there is less chance of being misquoted.
2. Provide solid, well-researched information. Reporters are usually unfamiliar with the subject and rely on the nutritionist's expertise. Explain technical terms in lay language. Answer irrelevant questions, but learn to "bridge" to a more relevant topic.
3. If pressed due to a reporter's deadline, ask reporter to call back so interviewee can collect thoughts, write a brief outline, and then honor the interview.
4. A negative impression is difficult to change. Think of the reporter as a live microphone. Only say what you wouldn't mind having quoted.
5. Make yourself available for follow up and fact checking. Ask for a copy of the published article, and send a thank you note after publication.

Source: Data from Ambassador Roundtable, American Dietetic Association annual meeting, Anaheim, California, 1993.

food and health never grow old. Every January, print media address weight loss and how to rebound from the holiday overload. Sports nutrition and fitness occupy most summer issues, and the fall turns to packing healthy school lunches, after-school snacks, and dormitory food. Winter thrives on holiday and food pleasures. Community nutritionists can provide local angles to any story and help the reader to identify with real-life events.

When working with print media, especially newspaper, create a health calendar and pitch story ideas accordingly. For example, November is Diabetes Month and April is Cancer Month. Link preventive care or medical nutrition therapy with eating behavior. Your choice of topics depends on which area you feel most well versed.

Working Effectively with Television

The purpose of television interviews is to inform, provide a service, promote, or entertain.[60]

To work successfully with television, nutritionists should differentiate between the types of interviews they may experience and decide which ones will most effectively present their message to the community. The most common types of interviews for television are news shows, talk shows, consumer-interest segments, and public service announcements.

News shows can include hard news, such as two-to-four-minute segments on timely issues, or 15-second interviews to represent specific viewpoints. Talk shows are generally entertainment-oriented. Visuals are frequently used and can help "sell" a viewpoint. Consumer-interest segments are one-to-seven-minute spots that are presented as regular news features for a brief discussion of a current topic.

Public service announcements are 10 to 60 seconds in length and pretaped as educational segments. These announcements are informative and are not commercials.

Prior to the television interview, it is important to profile the audience by watching similar shows. Specifically identify who is listening and what their interests are. Consider visuals to support the message. The media professional thinks about the audience while the amateur thinks about the topic!

Clarify on paper your key messages before beginning. Define your "Single Overriding Communication Objectives" (SOCOs). Focus on these objectives and don't wait for the right question to be asked. Bridge the questions to fit your objective. When the interview begins, address the interviewer by his or her first name. Reiterate each message two to three times during the interview. Help to build the story. Don't leave it up to the interviewer to make the points understood, because that allows the interviewer to direct the story (see Exhibit 3–5).

Working Effectively with Radio

Five formats are used for programming in the radio broadcast media. The community nutritionist needs to match his or her message and style to the radio medium.[60]

Exhibit 3-5 General Guidelines for Television Interviews

- *Behavior*: Be punctual. At the end of the show, keep still until you hear the "all clear" signal from the director. Maintain correct posture and gestures for television interviews.
- *Chairs*: As the guest, lean forward in your chair to show involvement and interest. Sit at a 45-degree angle to the interviewer. This will cause you to lean slightly to one side, resting your elbow on the armrest and freeing your hands for gesturing. Don't swivel.
- *Hands*: Use gestures constructively. They look natural and illustrate your speech.
- *Legs*: Cross your legs at the ankles. If you do cross your legs at the knees, be sure to avoid bouncing your foot up and down.
- *Eyes*: The audience will unconsciously be studying your eyes in search of confidence, credibility, and enthusiasm. Have regular eye contact with the interviewer. This makes you appear interested and attentive. When two people are being interviewed, look at the guest who is speaking, but bring your eyes directly back to the interviewer afterward.
- *Speech*: Before the show, the audio person may ask for a "sound check." At this time, say the alphabet or count to ten at normal speaking volume. Speak clearly and distinctly. Mumbling sounds worse on television than it does in real life. Speak with a normal volume, but don't be afraid to be excited or animated. Remember that you're answering the questions; therefore, you hold the advantage over the interviewer and audience since the answers given will dictate what type of message is being communicated.

Source: Data from Ambassador Roundtable, American Dietetic Association annual meeting, Anaheim, California, 1993.

When giving nutrition information on the radio, the community nutritionist is allowed more time for verbal illustration of points. Audience retention is better than with television. Radio stations have an ongoing need for guests with timely, interesting, and controversial topics, and nutrition remains one of those "hot" topics. The radio host is usually prepared for the interview with some knowledge of the topic; however, the host's knowledge base may not always be accurate, or the host may have a strong opinion. Being prepared and specific is the best preparation. Learn to provide facts and examples without being defensive.

Five radio formats are as follows:

1. *News shows*. Scripts that are 30 to 60 seconds long are common. Hard news outlines research, an occurrence, or a discovery. The purpose is to inform the listener about current information in a timely manner. It is best to address the issues from the public's point of view and to keep it simple. The first 85 words are the ones most likely to be included in a taped interview. People tend to remember the first thing that is said in an interview, not the last.
2. *Talk shows*. Time slots of 10, 30, or 60 minutes are frequently used to discuss topics of broad interest to inform and entertain listeners. The show may be live or taped. The host is usually well informed and/or opinionated and includes himself or herself in the discussion. Use the host's first name, and don't be afraid to ask the host a question.

   Use hooking, bridging, and flagging techniques to help direct the conversation and to allow important points to be covered. If there are other guests, know the credentials, place of employment, areas of interest and expertise, and published works of these individuals. Avoid being scheduled head to head on a controversial topic.
3. *Call-in shows*. This format provides the longest time slot of 30 to 120 minutes since there are many interruptions and breaks. The time of day the show airs determines the audience. Programming is almost always live, and guests are generally scheduled a few weeks in advance.

   Keep the discussion on target, but be flexible enough to handle varied questions from the callers. Consumer information is typically dealt with in an entertaining manner. Plan to speak in personal terms and use the caller's first name. Prepare an out-

Exhibit 3-6 *Healthy People 2000* Health Status Objectives Targeting Professionals

2.21   Increase to at least 75 percent the proportion of primary care providers who provide nutrition assessment and counseling and/or referral to qualified nutritionists or dietitians. (Baseline: Physicians provided diet counseling for an estimated 40 to 50 percent of patients in 1988.)

8.13   Increase to at least 75 percent the proportion of local television network affiliates in the top 20 television markets that have become partners with one or more community organizations around one of the health problems addressed by the *Healthy People 2000* objectives. (Baseline data available in 1991.)

21.8   Increase the proportion of all degrees in the health professions and allied and associated health profession fields awarded to members of underrepresented racial ethnic minority groups as follows:

Degrees Awarded To	1985–86 Baseline	2000 Target
Blacks	5%	8%
Hispanics	3%	6.4%
American Indians/Alaska Natives	0.3%	0.6%

Note: Underrepresented minorities are those groups consistently below parity in most health profession schools—blacks, Hispanics, and American Indians and Alaska Natives.

Source: Reprinted from *Healthy People 2000: National Health Promotion and Disease Prevention Objectives*, U.S. Department of Health and Human Services, Public Health Service, Publication No. 91-50212, 1991.

line and rehearse by practicing in front of a mirror. Smile frequently to make you more relaxed and to project a more personable voice.

4. *Public affairs programs.* This programming format may be 10, 30, or 60 minutes in length and usually airs on Sundays or off-hours. The purpose of this format is to inform, educate, or provide a service. Generally the shows are taped.

5. *Editorial or rebuttal segments.* A single issue is covered in this 30-to-60-second spot. Facts are presented in a concise, direct manner, and the segment is often pretaped.

HEALTHY PEOPLE 2000 ACTIONS

Community nutrition professionals are the focus of several *Healthy People 2000* objectives and the driving force to achieve them (see Exhibit 3-6). Objectives are defined for working with the media, maintaining continuing educa-tion at the professional level, and increasing multiethnic representation among health care professionals.

REFERENCES

1. *Healthy People 2000: National Health Promotion and Disease Prevention Objectives.* Washington, DC: US Department of Health and Human Services; 1991. Public Health Service publication 91-50212.

2. Frank GC. On the road to research: Avenues of opportunity in community nutrition. Presented at American Dietetic Association Annual Meeting; October 1991; Dallas, Texas.

3. National Heart, Lung, and Blood Institute. *National Institutes of Health Conceptual Model for Research.* Bethesda, Md. NHLBI; 1991.

4. US Department of Health and Human Services. *Promoting Health/Preventing Disease: Objectives for the Nation.* Washington, DC: US Government Printing Office; 1980.

5. American Medical Association. *Healthy Youth 2000.* Chicago, Ill: American Medical Association; December 1990.

6. Miller DC. *Handbook of Research Design and Social Measurement.* 5th ed. Los Angeles, Calif: Sage Publications; 1991.

7. Green LW, Kreuter MW, Deed SG, et al. *Health Education Planning: A Diagnosis Approach*. Palo Alto, Calif: Mayfield; 1980.

8. Massachusetts Department of Public Health. Conference on standardization of qualifications and salaries of nutritional workers. Unpublished report. 1920. Available in Mary C Egan Reference Collection, National Center for Education in Maternal and Child Health, Arlington, Va.

9. Egan MC. Public health nutrition: A historic perspective. *J Am Diet Assoc*. 1994;94:298-304.

10. Directory of Dietetic Programs. Chicago, Ill: American Dietetic Association; 1994.

11. University of Tennessee. *Guide for Field Experiences in Community and Public Health Nutrition*. Knoxville, Tenn: University of Tennessee Press; 1978.

12. Vollmer HM, Mills DL. *Professionalization*. Englewood Cliffs, NJ: Prentice-Hall; 1966.

13. Wilensky HL. The professionalization of everyone? *Am J Sociol*. 1964;70:137-158.

14. Laramae SH. Entry-level practice: Challenges, obligations, and opportunities. *J Am Diet Assoc*. 1989;89:1247-1249.

15. Hill L. Women's changing work roles: implications for the progress of the dietetic profession. *J Am Diet Assoc*. 1991;91:25-27.

16. Spears M, Simonis PL, Vaden AG. Professional attitudes of dietetics students and practitioners. *J Am Diet Assoc*. 1992;92:1522-1526.

17. Dodds JM, Kaufman M, eds. *Personnel in Public Health Nutrition for the 1990's*. Washington, DC: The Public Health Foundation; 1991.

18. McPhee SJ, Hung S, Suc Khoe La Vang. *Health is Gold!* Health Program for the Vietnamese. San Francisco, Calif: Department of Health Services and the University of California, San Francisco, 1990-1993.

19. Frank GC. Taking a bite out of eating behavior: Food records and food recalls of children. *J School Health*. 1991;61:198-200.

20. Knapp JA, Hazuda HP, Haffner SM, et al. A saturated fat/cholesterol avoidance scale: Sex and ethnic differences in a biethnic population. *J Am Diet Assoc*. 1988;88:172-177.

21. Frank GC, Zive M, Nelson J, et al. Fat and cholesterol avoidance among Mexican American and Anglo preschool children and parents. *J Am Diet Assoc*. 1991;91:954-961.

22. Frank GC, Nicklas TA, Webber LS, et al. A food frequency questionnaire for adolescents: Defining eating patterns. *J Am Diet Assoc*. 1992;92:313-318.

23. Willett W, Sampson LS, Stampfer MJ, et al. Reproducibility and validity of a semi-quantitative food frequency questionnaire. *Am J Epidemiol*. 1985;122:51-65.

24. Van Horn L, Gernhofer N, Moag-Stahlberg A, et al. Dietary assessment in children using electronic methods: telephones and tape recorders. *J Am Diet Assoc*. 1990;90:412-416.

25. Committee on Science, Engineering and Public Policy of the Academies and the Institute of Medicine. *Science, Technology and the Federal Government: National Goals for a New Era*. Washington DC: National Academy of Sciences; 1993.

26. Dwyer J. Nutrition research for the year 2000 and beyond. *Contemporary Nutr*. 1994;18(6):1-2.

27. Ad Hoc Bionutrition Group. *NIH Bionutrition Initiative Nutrition Notes*. Bethesda, Md: American Institute of Nutrition; 1993. National Institutes of Health, Draft Guidance Document. April 29, 1993;29:7-9.

28. Committee on Opportunities in the Nutrition and Food Sciences. *Opportunities in the Nutrition and Food Sciences: Research Challenges and the Next Generation of Investigators*. Washington, DC: National Academy Press; 1993.

29. Taylor H, Voivodas G. *The Bristol-Myers Report: Medicine in the Next Century*. New York, NY: Louis Harris and Associates, Inc; 1986.

30. Shafer MO, Story M, Houghton B. Survey of the association of graduate faculty programs in public health nutrition. Unpublished report. Minneapolis, Minn; 1993.

31. National Institutes of Health. *Fourteenth Annual Report of the NIH Program in Biomedical and Behavioral Nutrition Research and Training, Fiscal Year 1990*. Bethesda, Md: National Institutes of Health; 1990. NIH publication 91-2092.

32. Office of Technology Assessment, US Congress. *Research Funding as an Investment: Can We Measure the Returns?* Washington, DC: US Government Printing Office; 1986.

33. Raiten DJ, Berman SM. *Can the Impact of Basic Biomedical Research Be Measured? A Case Study Approach*. Bethesda, Md: Life Sciences Research Office, Federation of Associated Societies for Experimental Biology; 1993.

34. National Institutes of Health. *Cost Savings Resulting from NIH Research Support*. Bethesda, Md: National Institutes of Health; 1990. Publication 90-3109.

35. Cassell J. Professional supply and demand of dietetic practitioners. In: *The Research Agenda for Dietetics: Conference Proceedings ADA, May 14-15, 1992*; 104-117. Chicago, Ill: American Dietetic Association; 1993.

36. American Dietetics Association. *The Research Agenda for Dietetics: Conference Proceedings*. Chicago, Ill: American Dietetics Association; 1993.

37. Institute of Medicine. *Allied Health Services: Avoiding Crises*. Washington, DC: National Academy Press; 1989.

38. *Dietetics in the 21st Century: A Strategic Plan for the American Dietetic Association*. Chicago, Ill: American Dietetic Association; 1988.

39. *Achieving Competitive Advantage: The American Dietetic Association 1992 Strategic Thinking Initiative.* Chicago, Ill: American Dietetic Association; 1992.

40. Kutscher RE. Overview and implications of the projections to 2000. In: *Projections 2000.* Washington, DC: US Dept of Labor; 1988:1-7. Bureau of Labor Statistics bulletin 2302.

41. Mayer JA, Dubbert PM, Elder JP. Promoting nutrition at the point of choice: A review. *Health Ed Q.* 1989; 16:31-43.

42. Gillespie A, Shafer L. Position of the American Dietetic Association: Nutrition education for the public. *J Am Diet Assoc.* 1990;90:107-110.

43. Disbrow D. The cost-benefit of nutrition services. In: *The Research Agenda for Dietetics: Conference Proceedings ADA, May 14–15, 1992;* 118-126. Chicago, Ill: American Dietetic Association; 1993.

44. Dennison KF, Dennison D, Ward JY. Computerized nutrition program: Effect on nutrient intake of senior citizens. *J Am Diet Assoc.* 1991;91:1431-1433.

45. Luker KA, Caress AL. The development and evaluation of computer assisted learning for patients on continuous ambulatory peritoneal dialysis. *Computer in Nursing* 1991,9.15-21.

46. Bethea CD, Stallings SF, Wolman PG, et al. Comparison of conventional and videotaped diabetic exchange lists instruction. *J Am Diet Assoc.* 1989;89:405-406.

47. NCND launches consumer hotline. *ADA Courier.* 1992;31:1.

48. Levine J, Gussow JD. Better than we think? A reassessment of "Feeling Good." *J Nutr Ed.* 1991;23:296-302.

49. Shannon B, Mullis RM, Pirie PL, et al. Promoting better nutrition in the grocery store using a game format: The Shop Smart Game Project. *J Nutr Ed.* 1990;22: 183-188.

50. Personick VA. Industry output and employment through the end of the century. In: *Projections 2000.* Washington, DC: US Dept of Labor; 1988:28-43. Bureau of Labor Statistics bulletin 2302.

51. Sargent J, Pfleeger J. The job outlook for college graduates to the year 2000. *Occupational Outlook Quarterly.* 1990;34(2):2-8.

52. National Commission for Health Education Credentialing. Certification Examination for Certified Health Education Specialists. New York, NY.

53. Bryk JA, Kornblum TH. Report on the 1990 membership data base of the American Dietetic Association. *J Am Diet Assoc.* 1991;91:1136-1141.

54. Kaufman M, Heimendinger J, Foerster S, et al. Survey of nutritionists in state and local public health agencies. *J Am Diet Assoc.* 1986;86:1566-1570.

55. *Minorities and Women in the Health Fields.* Washington, DC: US Dept of Health and Human Services, Public Health Service; 1990.

56. Sawyer TR. Re-entry and second career. In: *Abstracts of the American Dietetic Association 71st Annual Meeting.* Chicago, Ill: American Dietetic Association; 1988:21.

57. Gitchell R, Fitz PA. Recruiting minority students into dietetics: An outreach and education project. *J Am Diet Assoc.* 1985;85:1293-1295.

58. Covey S. *The Seven Habits of Highly Effective People.* New York, NY: Simon & Schuster, Inc; 1989.

59. Miller WC. The creative edge. In: *Executive Book Summaries.* Bristol, Vt: Sandview Executive Book Summaries; 1988;10, no. 1, part 3:1-8.

60. American Dietetic Association. ADA ambassador roundtables. Presented at ADA annual meeting; 1993; Anaheim, CA.

Appendix 3–A

Partial Listing of US Universities with Schools of Public Health Offering Advanced Nutrition Degrees Blending Public Health, Epidemiology, and Nutrition

University	Department or School	Degrees	Emphasis
The University of North Carolina at Chapel Hill	Department of Nutrition, School of Public Health 2201 McGarran-Greenberg Hall University of North Carolina, Chapel Hill Chapel Hill, NC 27599 919-966-7210	M.P.H. in nutrition Ph.D. in nutrition Dr.P.H. in nutrition (minor in epidemiology)	Science and practice of public health Teaching and research Policy analysis and leadership
University of Minnesota	School of Public Health Box 197 420 Delaware St, SE Minneapolis, MN 55455 612-624-6669	M.S. in epidemiology (nutritional epidemiology concentration) Ph.D. in epidemiology (nutritional epidemiology concentration)	Teaching, research, and administration Teaching, research, and administration
University of Pittsburgh	Graduate School of Public Health 114 Parran Hall Pittsburgh, PA 15261 412-624-3002	M.P.H. in nutritional epidemiology (for RDs) Ph.D./Dr.P.H.	Nutritional factors related to disease, nutritional assessment, and intervention skills Disease and health behavior
Emory University	School of Public Health 1599 Clifton Road, NE Atlanta, GA 30329 404-727-3956 404-727-0190	M.P.H. (behavioral science or health education)	Evaluation skills and application of theory into practice
Tulane University	School of Public Health and Tropical Medicine Tulane University Medical Center 1501 Canal Street, Suite 700 New Orleans, LA 70112-2699 504-588-5387	M.P.H.	Community nutrition, health promotion, disease prevention, clinical nutrition

University	Department or School	Degrees	Emphasis
Johns Hopkins University	Division of Human Nutrition 615 North Wolfe Street Baltimore, MD 21205 410-955-3543	Sc.D. Dr.P.H. Ph.D.	Nutritional assessment, biochemical and metabolic processes, and effective prevention strategies
Harvard School of Public Health	Department of Nutrition 677 Huntington Ave. Boston, MA 02115 617-432-1031	M.P.H.	Public health management, community health
		S.D./D.P.H.	Nutritional epidemiology, international nutrition
		Ph.D.	Nutritional biochemistry
Saint Louis University	Department of Nutrition and Dietetics School of Allied Health Professions 1504 S. Grand Blvd. St. Louis, MO 63104 314-577-8523	M.P.H. M.H.A. Ph.D.	Community health Health administration Health sciences research

Note: Universities cited are those with a school of public health who responded to a request for information; originally sent to 20 universities.

Appendix 3-B

Key Terms of Educators in Public Health and Community Nutrition

- *Agency advisor/preceptor*–the member of the nutrition unit/program assigned the responsibility for the overall planning and guidance of an undergraduate or graduate student while he or she is training or receiving field experience at an agency.
- *Block field experience*–segment of an educational program within a field agency for an uninterrupted, extended time period of about 12 full-time work weeks.
- *Chief of nutrition unit*–the nutritionist administratively responsible for the generalized nutrition program and services of the field agency.
- *Community dietitian/community nutritionist*–a professional with baccalaureate education and training in community nutrition and/or dietetics including nutrition in health and disease, community health, behavioral sciences, and communication sciences. He or she begins at an entry-level staff position, working under the guidance of a public health nutritionist.
- *Concurrent field experience*–component of an educational program that takes place in a field agency simultaneously with support of classroom instruction.
- *Contractual/written agreement*–a legal transaction jointly prepared and signed by the educational institution and the field agency that defines the provision of field experiences for students in community/public health nutrition.
- *Dietetic intern*–an individual who has completed the didactic academic program of professional education in dietetics as approved by the American Dietetic Association and is enrolled in an accredited dietetic internship or an Approved Preprofessional Practice Program to: (1) fulfill planned experiences in clinical, management, and community dietetics; and (2) achieve competency in the ADA standards of practice for an entry-level dietitian.
- *Dietetic/nutrition graduate student*–an individual enrolled in a university graduate program to fulfill the academic and supervised field experience required for completion of the M.S. or M.P.H. degree in dietetics or nutrition.
- *Dietetic/nutrition undergraduate student*–a person enrolled in an undergraduate college to fulfill the didactic program of academic and supervised field experiences required for the B.S. degree in dietetics or nutrition.
- *Educational institution*–an institution of higher education offering a program of study in food and nutrition, dietetics, food service management, food science, public health, and/or community nutrition.
- *Faculty advisor/faculty field coordinator*–the member of the faculty of an educational institution responsible for facilitating and coordinating the field experience component of the

community and/or public health nutrition curriculum.

- *Field agency*—an agency or organization (official, volunteer, state, regional, or local) providing field experiences for an undergraduate or graduate student in community and/or public health nutrition.
- *Field course*—block field experience with additional university requirements for credit.
- *Field experience*—participation in an education program that takes place in a field agency.
- *Field observation*—observing or viewing a service or program within the field agency or a related agency for the purpose of helping the student to identify and interpret the components of the service or program and, therefore, extending the student's understanding of how the service or program supports the overall goals of the agency.
- *Field orientation*—introducing the student to the mores and customs of the field agency. This occurs by attending formal orientation conferences regularly scheduled for new employees of the agency and/or conferences with administrative personnel responsible for the agency's nutrition program.
- *Field practice*—developing and carrying out a specific nutrition activity or service under guidance.
- *Field supervisor*—the staff member of the nutrition unit/program to whom the agency advisor/preceptor may delegate responsibility for supervision of activities.
- *Nutrition unit*—the administrative unit (or individual) responsible for the generalized nutrition program and services of the field agency.

- *Nutritional epidemiologist*—a professional trained in both nutrition and epidemiology who investigates the role of eating behavior on health outcomes in populations of people, develops programs to evaluate or remediate with nutritional therapies, trains staff with standardized protocols and instruments, analyzes data with technical skill, and reports findings to the scientific community.
- *Public health nutritionist*—a professional with a master's and/or doctoral degree; training in advanced nutrition, public health, health education, behavioral sciences, or education; and experience in nutrition or a related field. The public health nutritionist is a member of a health team who assesses community nutrition needs and plans, and administers, coordinates, and evaluates the nutrition component of the agency program.
- *Public health nutrition graduate student*—a person enrolled in a graduate public health nutrition program to fulfill the didactic and supervised field experience requirements. The goal of the student is to become a practicing public health nutritionist meeting criteria established by public health graduate faculties.
- *Registered dietitian*—an individual who has completed the didactic program in dietetics with a B.S. degree followed by completion of a preprofessional experience. After passing the Registration Examination for Dietitians, this professional accrues 75 hours of continuing education every five years.

Appendix 3-C

Dietetic Practice Groups of the American Dietetic Association

Dietetic Practice Group	Group Number*	Group Dues
Public Health Nutrition	DP 10	$15.00
Gerontological Nutritionists	DP 11	$15.00
Dietetics in Developmental and Psychiatric Disorders	DP 12	$18.00
Vegetarian Nutrition	DP 14	$10.00
Hunger and Malnutrition	DP 15	$20.00
Environmental Nutrition	DP 16	$10.00
Oncology Nutrition	DP 20	$15.00
Renal Dietitians	DP 21	$20.00
Pediatric Nutrition	DP 22	$20.00
Diabetes Care and Education	DP 23	$20.00
Dietitians in Nutrition Support	DP 24	$20.00
Dietetics in Physical Medicine and Rehabilitation	DP 25	$20.00
Dietitians in General Clinical Practice	DP 27	$18.00
Perinatal Nutrition	DP 28	$20.00
Nutrition Entrepreneurs	DP 30	$25.00
Consultant Dietitians in Health Care Facilities	DP 31	$20.00
Dietitians in Business and Communications	DP 32	$25.00
Sports and Cardiovascular and Wellness Nutritionists	DP 33	$22.00
Management in Health Care Systems	DP 41	$25.00
School Nutrition Services	DP 42	$20.00
Clinical Nutrition Management	DP 44	$20.00
Technical Practice in Dietetics	DP 45	$25.00
Dietetic Educators of Practitioners	DP 50	$20.00
Nutrition Educators of Health Professionals	DP 51	$15.00
Nutrition Education for the Public	DP 52	$20.00
Nutrition Research	DP 54	$20.00

*DP = Dietetic Practice.

Source: Reprinted with permission from the American Dietetic Association Professional Membership pamphlet, p. 3, © 1993.

4

Working with Special Groups in a Complex Environment

Learning Objectives

- Define the ways community nutrition professionals can acquire cultural competence.
- Identify how to develop and to evaluate nutrition education materials for multiethnic groups.
- Describe the wasting syndrome common among individuals with HIV and how secondary infections affect morbidity and mortality of HIV-positive individuals.
- Enumerate unproven nutritional therapies and unconventional diets used by individuals with HIV infection
- Discuss the historic development of the US policy to identify and alleviate hunger.
- Describe the composition of a vegetarian eating pattern, and explain the health benefits of such a pattern.

High Definition Nutrition

Acculturation—repeated exposure to influences from a different culture. The process is related to age, education, frequency of interaction, and income and occurs on a continuum.

Cachectin factor—the ability to promote catabolism in fat cells; cytokines exhibiting this property include interleukin-1 and interferons alfa, beta, and gamma. The factor has also been called the cytokine tumor necrosis factor.

Cultural broker—an individual who arbitrates and mediates on behalf of individuals from different cultures.

Cultural competence—the ability to increase one's understanding and appreciation of cultural differences and commonalities by developing knowledge and interpersonal skills.

Cultural sensitivity—recognition that cultural differences and similarities exist.

Cultural universal—structures and functions common to every culture (i.e., a family unit, marriage, parental roles, education, health care, and occupations).

Cultural values—standards that characterize groups.

Culturally appropriate—an entity that is sensitive to cultural differences and commonalities and often uses cultural symbols to communicate a message.

Culture—Unique values, customs, language, and history. It can transcend time or change with time.

Enculturation—the process of learning the beliefs, attitudes, and behaviors of a group.

Ethnic—the commonality of a group expressed by its nationality, language, or race.

Ethnocentric—perception or belief that one's own values, beliefs, and practices are superior to those in another culture.

Food deprivation—an inability of individuals to obtain sufficient food to meet their nutrient needs.

Food poverty—an incapacity of households to obtain access to food (as opposed to a national scarcity of food).

Food security—level of assurance in which any individual could obtain a culturally acceptable and nutritionally adequate eating pattern from nonemergency food sources at any time.

Homeless person—an undomiciled individual unable to secure permanent and stable housing without special assistance.

Household—the basic socioeconomic unit that decides how and when investments, including the acquisition of food, are made for its members.

Lacto-vegetarian—an individual who eats a diet of fruits, vegetables, grains, dairy foods, and eggs.

Malnutrition—the consequence of changes in any of the processes involved in nutrition or in those factors affecting it (i.e., over- or under-nutrition). Undernutrition, associated with deficiencies of one or more nutrients, is caused by one or more primary causes, such as inadequate ingestion, absorption, or utilization, or increased excretion and requirement.

Multicultural—composed of two or more unique cultures.

Nationality—the homeland of an individual or group.

Nutrition—the sum total of the processes involved in the ingestion and use of nutrients that are involved in the growth, repair, and maintenance of the body's components and their functions. These processes include ingestion, digestion, absorption, metabolism, and functional use of nutrients. Accessibility of a balanced diet is influenced by an array of physical, sociocultural, economic, behavioral, genetic, and medical factors.

Race—a genetically linked population.

Religion—a structure involving worship and beliefs about a higher power.

Society—people unified by a common culture and geography.

Subculture—the knowledge, beliefs, and values common to a segment of a society (e.g., socio-economic or age groups).

Vegan—an individual who does not eat meat, fish, fowl, eggs, or dairy products.

COMMUNITY NUTRITION PROFESSIONALS AND DIVERSITY

The United States is a land of beautiful diversity—diversity of peoples, religions, educations, and work experiences, to name a few[1] (see Table 4-1). The richness of this mosaic creates challenges for community nutrition professionals who attempt to meet the various nutritional needs of diverse individuals and groups.

The needs of a multiethnic society differ from the needs of subgroups with risk factors for and complications of devastating disease such as acquired immune deficiency syndrome (AIDS). The potential nutritional cures or remedies for the complications and the wasting syndrome experienced by individuals who test positive for the human immunodeficiency virus (HIV) challenge community nutrition professionals to present accurate information and interpretation of these remedies.

In another arena, community nutrition professionals who work with multiethnic groups need cultural competence to assess eating behavior and nutritional status as part of nutritional epidemiology, and also to provide effective nutrition education as a primary, secondary, or tertiary intervention. A nutrition professional may formulate a program to alleviate hunger one day, and the next day instruct pregnant vegetarian mothers how to plan nutritionally adequate meals for themselves and their families. These women and their families may come from any one of several ethnic groups.

These real-life situations demand new skills, increased knowledge, and sincere efforts by community nutrition professionals to practice their profession. Working in a culturally diverse environment is not new, but it remains a daily challenge.

Table 4–1 Dimensions of Diversity

Primary	Secondary
Age	Educational background
Ethnicity	Geographic location
Gender	Income
Physical ability	Marital status
Race	Military experience
Sexual/affectional	Parental status
orientation	Religious beliefs
	Work experience

Source: List compiled from *Workforce America!: Managing Employee Diversity as a Vital Resource* by M. Loden and J.B. Rosener, Irwin Professional Publishing, © 1990.

WORKING IN A MULTICULTURAL ENVIRONMENT

The US population today is one of multiethnic groups living in geographic areas that do not resemble their homelands. Working successfully in a multicultural environment demands an understanding of the culture of each group.

California, for example, is projected to be the first US mainland state with a majority of "minorities," possibly by the year 2005.[2] To address the challenge, strategies for California and companion states facing multiethnic majorities must include intra-assessment. This assessment must identify factors influencing health and illness specific to population groups other than middle-income whites, the usual standard. Gaps in health status may then be reduced, and US health statistics may then be improved. Central to the endeavor is understanding the various cultures.

Culture has been defined as the accumulation of a group's beliefs, assumptions, customs, and values that direct the lifestyle of the group's members.[3,9] Beliefs stem from the knowledge, opinions, and faith individuals or groups have and often precipitate customs or common practices. Values are beliefs deemed important by an individual or group, whereas assumptions are statements that are taken for granted. Values expressed by one culture may not be honored in another culture.[3]

Cultural sensitivity is awareness of one's own cultural beliefs and the ability to understand and to acknowledge the values and customs of another culture. Cultural sensitivity during nutrition education sessions or programs may simply mean that nutrition professionals do not express their personal bias about individuals from ethnic groups different than their own.[10]

One early cultural group immigrating to the United States consisted of white, Anglo-Saxon Protestants (WASPs), who remain distinct by their eye, skin, and hair colors.[11] Current immigrants to the United States range from Southeast Asians to South and Central Americans. Each group embodies their own customs, languages, beliefs, and appearances.[6-7]

Cultural competence is the acquisition of knowledge and requisite skills to identify and appreciate differences and commonalities of various groups.[12] Knowledge alone does not produce cultural competence. Understanding the codes and mores of a group and its numerous subgroups equips nutritionists with powerful communication and evaluation skills. As professionals recruit participants into studies and programs, develop assessment tools, interpret data, and employ staff to complete projects, cultural competence is essential. A self-evaluation instrument is given in Exhibit 4–1.[13]

Info Line

E. Randall-David's *Strategies for Working with Culturally Diverse Communities and Clients* (1st ed, 1989, U.S. DHHS; Washington, D.C.: Office of Maternal and Child Health) is designed to assist health care providers by increasing their understanding of the cultural aspects of health and illness so they can work effectively with clients and families from culturally diverse communities. The book is available from the Association for the Care of Children's Health, 7910 Woodmont Avenue, Suite 300, Bethesda, Maryland 20814, 301-654-6549.

Exhibit 4–1 Community Nutritionist Self-Evaluation about Diversity Awareness

Do I . . .

- Know about the rules and customs of different cultures?
- Know and admit that I hold stereotypes about other groups?
- Feel equally comfortable with people of all backgrounds?
- Actively associate with those who are different from me?
- Find it satisfying to work on a multicultural team?
- Find change stimulating and exciting?
- Like to learn about other cultures?
- Show patience and understanding with individuals who speak limited English?
- Find that more gets done when I spend time building relationships?
- Feel that both newcomers and society need to make an effort to change?

Source: Adapted from Gardenswartz L, Rowe A. "What's your diversity quotient?" *Working World*. August 31, 1992, with permission of Rhodes Publications, Inc., © 1992.

To respect and accept a cultural group's beliefs and behaviors, the community nutritionist may have to study individuals and their broader community-based structure. Incorporating community leaders into decision-making positions, forming coalitions, and employing residents from within the community are actions a community nutritionist can take to acquire cultural sensitivity and respect.[11]

Four stages identify the process of acquiring cultural competence. These are (1) *cultural awareness* of one's own values by self-assessment; (2) *cultural knowledge* of the target group using books, lectures, film, and personal contact; (3) *cultural skill* in communication, interpretation, and definition of the target group's beliefs and customs; and (4) an increased frequency of *cultural encounters* that expand understanding and ease communication while enhancing respect.[3] A checklist for gathering information about culturally diverse communities to aid organizations that wish to work with diverse groups is presented in Exhibit 4–2. A quick guide to assist community nutrition and other health professionals who counsel multicultural groups was developed by the US Department of Agriculture (Exhibit 4–3).

The guide addresses activities to prepare for counseling, enhance communication, and promote positive change.[14] See Appendix 4–A for a list of questions for clients to evaluate their eating environment.

A framework for counseling different ethnic groups is called LEARN (listen, explain, acknowledge, recommend, and negotiate). Using this framework, nutrition educators can improve their communication skills.[15] The components include listening to the client's statement of his or her problems, explaining what was heard, acknowledging similarities and differences, projecting a common understanding, recommending changes, and negotiating an action plan.

PREPARING INFORMATION FOR AND COUNSELING MULTIETHNIC GROUPS

All information intended to reach people of a particular culture must pass through cultural filters before it is received and acted upon. As information goes through these filters, it is colored by social norms, values, traditions, and history. This filtering process is essential for information directed toward any ethnic group living in the United States. When working on prevention and treatment programs among various ethnic groups, community nutritionists must understand cultural filters that influence the comprehension and, ultimately, the behavior of the group. Professionals who are sensitive to the values and traditions of the multiethnic groups are more likely to overcome barriers that may exist to prevention, intervention, or treatment.[16]

Two good resources are Randall-David's *Stategies for Working with Culturally Diverse Communities and Clients*, Office of Maternal and Child Health, US Department of Health and Human Services; and Sue and Sue's *Counseling the Culturally Different: Theory and Practice*.[9,17]

Hispanics/Latinos

The Hispanic/Latino population in the United States includes Mexican Americans, Puerto Ricans, and Cuban Americans; recent immigrants from El Salvador, Nicaragua, and the Dominican Republic; and immigrants from other Central and South American countries. The people in each

Exhibit 4-2 Checklist for Information Gathering

Check the items as you complete the important steps to your own satisfaction.

- Have you gathered information on and increased your understanding of the following?
  - _____ The demographics of the target community
  - _____ The major historical issues of the community
  - _____ The community's economic and political concerns
  - _____ The major cultural beliefs, values, and practices of the target community
  - _____ The health problem as it can be addressed within the cultural context(s) of this community
  - _____ Other questions you have chosen to explore
- Have you also consulted the following sources?
  Library resources, such as the following:
  - _____ Census data, government documents, reports, and statistics
  - _____ Public health literature
  - _____ Behavioral and social science literature
  - _____ Local newspapers
  Experts, such as the following:
  - _____ Academicians with knowledge or experience working with specific ethnic or cultural groups

  - _____ Health professionals who work in similar communities or with similar problems
  - _____ Other professionals working in diverse communities or in the target community
  - _____ Individuals from the target community
- Have you prepared your staff to work in the community through the following activities?
  - _____ Summary of research findings in a report for your staff
  - _____ Discussion of this information with staff's input
  - _____ Exploration of staff's cultural attitudes and beliefs and how these might influence staff members' behavior in the community
  - _____ Assessment of your and your staff's past experiences in working with diverse communities to determine who has the necessary skills
  - _____ Training and/or ongoing support for staff to help them resolve personal and professional issues as they arise in the community

Source: Adapted from Health Promotion Section, Multi-Ethnic Health Promotion Task Force Reports, California Department of Health and Human Services, 1991.

Hispanic/Latino subgroup have different needs and experiences that have shaped their attitudes toward health, family, and nutrition. Lack of awareness and sensitivity to this fact can build formidable barriers in reaching Hispanic/Latino audiences.[16]

According to US Census Bureau statistics, Hispanics/Latinos in the continental United States number nearly 20 million, not counting Puerto Rico's 3 million inhabitants. Approximately 62% are Mexican Americans; 13% are mainland Puerto Ricans; 5% are Cuban Americans; 12% are of predominantly Central and South American origins; and 8% are of other Hispanic origins. Undocumented laborers and illegal immigrants are not included.[16]

Hispanics/Latinos constitute the second largest minority in the United States, after African Americans. They represent 8% of the total US population and are expected to become the largest minority group early in the next century. The Hispanic/Latino population is increasing three times faster than the non-Hispanic US population and may account for one-quarter of the nation's growth during the next 20 years. They are the fastest-growing and the youngest minority, with a median age of 25. About 40% are under 21.[16]

Hispanics/Latinos are difficult to reach primarily because of language and cultural barriers. Program planners or community nutritionists can learn Spanish and become sensitive to the myriad of ethnic nuances that can make or break interpersonal relationships. Subgroups may differ by education, income level, health status, and degree of assimilation to mainstream American culture. Professionals can also employ, train, and guide local community paraprofessionals whose fluency and acceptance by the subgroup may be greater than that of the professional.

A potential reason the Hispanic/Latino population may neglect health care is that money is often scarce. About 26% of all Hispanic families in the United States live below the poverty line. Many do not have the basic insurance to cover treatment. In addition, as a rule, Hispanics/Latinos are very proud and very private when it comes to family problems. It is difficult for a fami-

Exhibit 4-3 Quick Guide for Cross-Cultural Counseling

Preparing for Counseling

- Understand your own cultural values and biases.
- Acquire basic knowledge of cultural values, health beliefs, and nutrition practices for client groups you routinely serve.
- Be respectful of, interested in, and understanding of other cultures without being judgmental.

Enhancing Communication

- Determine the level of fluency in English and arrange for an interpreter, if needed.
- Ask how the client prefers to be addressed.
- Allow the client to choose seating for comfortable personal space and eye contact.
- Avoid body language that may be offensive or misunderstood.
- Speak directly to the client, whether an interpreter is present or not.

- Choose a speech rate and style that promotes understanding and demonstrates respect for the client.
- Avoid slang, technical jargon, and complex sentences.
- Use open-ended questions or questions phrased in several ways to obtain information.
- Determine the client's reading ability before using written materials in the process.

Promoting Positive Change

- Build on cultural practices, reinforcing those that are positive, and promoting change only in those that are harmful.
- Check for client understanding and acceptance of recommendations.
- Remember that not all seeds of knowledge fall into a fertile environment to produce change. Of those that do, some will take years to germinate. Be patient and provide counseling in a culturally appropriate environment to promote positive health behavior.

Source: Adapted from *Cross-Cultural Counseling: A Guide for Nutrition and Health Counselors*, U.S. Department of Agriculture, 1986.

---

ly to stop a member who has problems, such as with alcohol, and still more difficult to recommend external help. For Hispanic/Latino families, revealing secrets and looking for answers outside the strong family unit is adverse to their culture.[16]

Hispanic/Latino families work as a team with their focus on the good of the whole or the good of others. Interdependence, rather that independence, is encouraged. This value influences receptivity to community nutrition programs and printed materials. Community nutrition programs may be more attractive if advertisements appeal to individual members' commitment for the common good of the family. A publication might start out with the appeal that "It will benefit your husband . . . children . . . sister, if you learn more about healthy eating."

The Hispanic/Latino family bond, or *carino*, evokes a deep sense of unqualified caring and protection. All family members are equal, unconditionally accepted, and valued simply because they are, not because of what they have done or not done. Machismo among Hispanics/Latinos is accepted, and men are expected to be dominant, protective, and authoritarian. Hispanic/Latino women are expected to conform to the female ideal of purity, discipline, and self-sacrifice in body, mind, and spirit.

General recommendations for working with Hispanic/Latino populations are[16]:

- Target prevention and intervention efforts to the entire family and their religious leaders.
- Help Hispanic/Latino fathers recognize how important their role is to their children. Encourage mothers to learn strategies for including their spouses in family interactions.
- Educate mothers and daughters to reduce the shame associated with asking for help.
- Emphasize the family as a unit in printed materials. Tailor separate versions for males and females.
- Emphasize participation in healthy eating and exercise programs to adjust to the American culture without abandoning their own.
- Reach Hispanic/Latino audiences through Spanish-speaking, community-level organizations and leaders.

- Educate community nutritionists and assistants about traditional gender roles to aid their efforts.

Nontraditional religions are very powerful, especially in Puerto Rican and Cuban-American communities. Two popular nontraditional religions draw heavily from the traditions of the Catholic church and mix the belief in saints with psychic powers and the spirit world. *Espiritismo* is popular among Puerto Ricans, and *santeria* is likely to be found in Cuban-American communities. The believers regularly follow spiritual leaders called *espiritistas* and *santeros/santeras*, respectively, who are supposedly born with or develop psychic powers and knowledge of spells, charms, and incantations.[16]

Nutrition education and prevention program planners must explore the demographic characteristics and religions of their target group. This translates into several tasks:

- Obtain approval of the local *espiritistas* or *santeros/santeras*, because they may tell their followers that the prevention program is not good and thereby destroy a community effort.
- Do not attempt to hold joint meetings, seminars, or fund-raisers with different religious groups.
- Ensure that learning about the different religions is a part of the planning process, because insulting religious beliefs due to ignorance may be fatal for a community-based program.

Several national centers are available to assist health professionals who work with Hispanic/Latino families.

Info Line

- **The Office of Minority Health Resource Center**, Director of Information and Programs, PO Box 37337, Washington, DC 20013-7337, 1-800-444-6472 (toll free). Established by the US Department of Health and Human Services' Office of Minority Health, the center provides health professionals with information aimed at minorities, including Hispanic/Latino youth and families. It maintains listings of prevention programs operating at the national, state, and community levels.

- **Spanish Catholic Center (Centro Católico)**, Washington Archdiocese, Father Julio Alvarez-Garcia, Executive Director, Mary Lynn Mercado, Social Services Coordinator, 2700 27th St, NW, Washington, DC 20008, (202) 483-1520 (8:30 A.M.–5:00 P.M., Monday–Friday). This is a national center that refers (Spanish-English) Hispanic/Latino parents to counselors and social services and assists Hispanic/Latino families seeking help for alcohol and other drug problems. The center also offers parental guidance on other issues. A brochure is available on the services, which include Hispanic youth recreational and educational centers, English as a second language, and other subjects.

- **The National Clearinghouse for Alcohol and Drug Information** (NCADI) can provide a national listing of Diocesan Directors and a Directory of Community Minority Organizations for Hispanic Affairs when requested.

- **Directory of Community Minority Organizations**, National Heart, Lung, and Blood Institute Minority Program Information Center, 4733 Bethesda Avenue, Suite 530, Bethesda, MD 20814, (301) 951-3260. This directory of minority organizations was created to support the dissemination of health information to minorities. The directory includes groups such as the following:

Hispanic Health Council
96–98 Cedar Street
Hartford, CT 06106
(203) 527-0856

Latino Caucus of the APHA
Midwest Hispanic AIDS Coalition
1725 W North Avenue, Room 4C
Chicago, IL 60622
(312) 772-8195

African Americans

Nutrition counseling for individuals eating African-American/soul foods requires knowledge of and sensitivity to a "spiritual" actuating principle of nutriment in solid form.[18] This belief stemmed from a slave culture that identified an escape and means of nourishing the tired and weary.[19-22] The types of foods that embody "soul food" reflect West African fare, limited resources in the United States, seasoning to improve taste, and extended boiling to tenderizing tough and course foods[23] (see Table 4-2).

Table 4–2 Traditional versus Contemporary Food Choices of Multiethnic Groups

Ethnic Group	Traditional	Contemporary
Hispanic	Breakfast • Corn tortillas, eggs with chorizo (sausage), salsa • Mexican sweet bread and fruit • Hot chocolate or coffee with milk	Breakfast • Traditional foods or Americanized choices such as bacon, eggs, and toast, or cold cereal with milk • Milk, fruit juice, or coffee with milk
	Lunch • Corn tortillas; rice and beans; beef, chicken, or pork stewed with chilis and tomatoes • Soft drinks or coffee with milk	Lunch • Traditional foods at home or fast food including pizza, hamburgers, burritos, and sandwiches • School lunch for most children • Milk, fruit juice, or soft drinks
	Dinner • Enchiladas, rice, and beans • Cactus with pork and onion, beans, and corn tortillas • Soft drinks or coffee with milk	Dinner • Traditional food choices such as rice, beans, a meat dish, and tortillas • Typical Americanized food choices such as spaghetti or barbecued chicken, corn, salad, and bread • Fruit juice, soft drinks, or coffee with milk
African American	Breakfast • Eggs, country ham with red-eye gravy, biscuits, and fried potatoes or grits • Coffee or milk	Breakfast • Much lighter than traditional • May include toast; eggs and bacon; cream of wheat, oatmeal, or grits
	Dinner (the traditional luncheon meal) • Fried chicken or catfish, boiled cabbage and potatoes • Beef-vegetable stew with cornbread • Fruit cobbler • Buttermilk and fruit-flavored drinks	Lunch • Typical fast-food choices: hamburgers, hot dogs, sandwiches, pizza • School lunches for most children • Milk, fruit juice, or coffee
	Supper (the traditional dinnertime meal) • Boiled legumes or greens with ham hocks, coleslaw, and cornbread • Buttermilk or fruit-flavored drinks	Dinner • Baked chicken with bread stuffing, green beans, green salad, bread and butter • Macaroni and cheese • Cobblers • Coffee, tea, fruit-flavored drinks, or milk
Filipino	Breakfast • Broiled fish, leafy vegetables with fish sauce, rice • Dried salty fish, rice, and fruit • Coffee with milk and sugar	Breakfast • Rice with egg or meat dish • Toast or cold cereal with milk • Coffee with milk

continues

Table 4–2 continued

Ethnic Group	Traditional	Contemporary
	Lunch • Bamboo shoots with shrimp and coconut milk, eggplant sauce, rice, and fruit • Stir-fried rice with leftover meat and vegetables • Coffee with milk and sugar	**Lunch** • Meat dish with vegetables and rice • School lunch for most children • Milk and fruit juice
	Dinner • Dried, salted fish, sauteed okra, rice, and fruit • Beef or chicken and vegetable stew with rice • Soy milk, coffee with milk and sugar, or tea	**Dinner** • Sauteed meat, long green beans, and rice • Typical westernized meals: roast beef with vegetables and bread, barbecued meats, corn, salad, and bread • Soft drinks, fruit drinks, or coffee with milk
Chinese	**Breakfast** • Rice porridge seasoned with small amounts of meat or fish • Bowl of noodles with vegetables and meat	**Breakfast** • Similar to traditional choices but may include westernized selections of cold cereal with milk, or eggs with toast
	Lunch • Rice or fried noodles, Chinese greens, and a seasoned meat dish with clear soup • Tea	**Lunch** • Traditional choices including rice with leftovers • Sandwiches and other take-out foods • School lunch for most children • Tea, fruit juice, or milk
	Dinner (a larger version of lunch) • Rice, tofu with sausage, several vegetable dishes, and clear soup • Tea (In northern China, soup is usually the beverage at meals; in southern China the beverage is usually tea.)	**Dinner** • Most similar to traditional pattern including rice, meat or fish dishes, sauteed vegetables with soy sauce or oyster sauce, and clear soup • Tea, fruit juice, or milk
Vietnamese	**Breakfast** • Soup with rice noodles, sliced meat, bean sprouts, and mustard greens • Boiled egg with meat and pickled vegetables on French bread	**Breakfast** • French bread with fried eggs • Toast with butter and sugar sprinkled on top • Instant noodles
	Lunch • Rice, fish with lemon grass, string beans, clear soup with vegetables, and fruit	**Lunch** • Rice with seasoned beef, sauteed vegetables, and clear soup • School lunch for most children
	Dinner • Rice, sauteed pork, leeks, clear soup, and fruit • Coffee with sweetened condensed milk, tea, or fruit drinks (drunk after meal)	**Dinner** • Similar to the traditional dinner with rice, a meat or fish dish, stir-fried vegetables, clear soup, fruit for dessert • Coffee with sweetened condensed milk, tea, or soft drinks

Source: Data from *A Celebration of Culture: A Food Guide for Educators,* Dairy Council of California, 1994.

The basics of soul food are inconsistent with three of the guidelines found in the *Dietary Guidelines for Americans*[24]:

- Guideline 3: Choose a diet low in fat (30% or less), saturated fat (10% or less), and cholesterol (300 mg or less).
- Guideline 4: Choose a diet with plenty of vegetables, fruits, and grain products.
- Guideline 6: Use salt and sodium only in moderation.

Young African Americans have high-fat eating patterns, and African Americans in general consume about 36% of total calories from fat and exceed 300 mg of cholesterol each day.[25] On the other hand, African Americans enjoy many nutrient-rich, cruciferous vegetables and fruits high in vitamins A and C. Intakes of high-fiber cereal and grain products are not common.[26] Use of cured and salted meats and the addition of salt during cooking and eating are common, resulting in a high sodium intake.[27] Counseling for African Americans should address the following points to improve healthy eating and reduce health risk (see Exhibit 4-4)[18]:

- Lower total fat, animal or saturated fat, and cholesterol intake.
- Try new cooking procedures and new tastes; attend cooking demonstrations.
- Taste food before seasoning with salt, order unsalted fast foods.

Exhibit 4-4   Food Preparation Techniques to Lower Fat, Cholesterol, and Sodium in African-American or Soul Foods

Breakfast

- Substitute fat-free mayonnaise in biscuits for regular mayonnaise.
- Serve turkey ham or homemade turkey sausage with sage and seasonings instead of bacon.
- Use "light" or sugar-free syrup or fruit; use egg substitute in pancake, waffle, and biscuit recipes.
- Measure all fats added to foods: mayonnaise, margarine, oil.

Frying

- Use nonstick skillet lightly coated with vegetable oil spray for egg, fish, and vegetables.
- Substitute "low saturated fat" oils instead of white shortening or bacon drippings.

Flavoring

- Cook vegetables with smoked but not cured lean meat, such as turkey necks.
- Add flavor without fat or sodium by using liquid smoke sparingly.
- Use low-potassium salt substitute.
- Season with onion, garlic, peppers, or hot sauce to lower the amount of salt.

Source: Adapted from Bronner, Y., Burke, C., and Joubert, B., African-American Soul Foodways and Nutrition Counseling, *Topics in Clinical Nutrition*, Vol. 9, No. 2, pp. 20–27, Aspen Publishers, Inc., © 1994.

Native Americans

It is estimated that 20,000 to 50,000 years ago the Bering Strait provided the entrance for about 400 Indian and Alaskan nations to enter North America. Many moved to the territory we now call the United States. Their languages were only verbal, not written, so the record of early food habits is scarce. What is known is that several centers of Indian culture flourished (for example, the Cherokees, Chickasaws, Choctaws, Creeks, and Seminoles in the southeast; the Iroquois in the northeast or New York state; and the Pueblo community near the Rio Grande and the Little Colorado Rivers in the southwest).[28]

The socioeconomic status of Native Americans declined dramatically with forced migration in the 19th century. This was most notable when tribal nations moved to areas with limited agricultural resources. Indian food habits reflect the land and its climate and vegetation. Much of the daily endeavor of traditional American Indians focused on hunting, gathering, and preparing food.

Staples common to most American Indians were beans, corn, and squash. Traditional foods included blueberries, cranberries, grapes, beans, corn, pumpkins, lobster, moose, pigeon, rabbit, squirrel, and turkey on the east coast; peanuts, potatoes, sweet potatoes, and tomatoes in the south; salmon and fruit on the Pacific; chili peppers, melons, and squash in the southwest; and buffalo and wild rice on the plains.

Only a few US cities serve most residents of the Native-American population today. These include in descending order of importance: Los Angeles, San Francisco, Tulsa, Minneapolis-St. Paul, Oklahoma City, Chicago, and Phoenix. The remaining American Indians live in rural areas and on reservations[28] (see Figure 4-1).

American Indians hold food in high spiritual regard and link physical health, balance, and harmony with food. Corn has a special healing significance; agave leaves assist with wound healing, chilis remediate arthritis and warts, and mint tea eases gastrointestinal ailments. Certain tribes practice dietary restrictions to correct health problems. For example, cabbage, eggs, fish, onions, organ meat and other meats, and milk may be restricted in general; cod, halibut, and certain types of salmon are restricted for a short period after childbirth.

Traditional foods are not as visible in the eating patterns of American Indians today. If the food gatekeeper (i.e., the individual who plans, purchases, and cooks the meals) inherited traditions, then these are reflected in foods; however, native greens, wild game meats, cornmeal mush, hominy, and wild sumac berry pudding are rare today.[29-32] Meal patterns may be repetitive, with fried foods for breakfast and lunch, and boiled meat for dinner. Today, fast foods are purchased and consumed with more frequency by each new generation.[29]

Over the past few decades, the total energy, protein, and fiber intakes, as well as calcium, iron, phosphorus, vitamins A and C, and riboflavin intakes of American Indians have declined among certain tribes.[31] With lifestyle changes, health changes have also been identified. Infant mortality and maternal mortality rates for American Indians are 2.5 and 4 times the US average, respectively. Obesity, diabetes, heart disease, and alcoholism are the major health problems. There

have been dramatic increases for diabetes, heart disease, and hypertension among American Indians[28] (see Figure 4-2).

Health care providers who counsel American Indians must recognize traditional beliefs and practices. For example, all individuals speak for themselves, as no other can speak for them; "yes" and "no" are considered complete responses, and explanations are not thought to be warranted (see Appendix 4-B). In-depth interviews are not consistent with the belief in personal autonomy in the American Indian culture, and direct eye contact is not common.[28]

Info Line

For further information, contact the Indian Health Service (IHS), US Department of Health and Human Services, Washington, DC.

Asians

Asian immigrants to the United States include people from China, Japan, Korea, and Southeast Asian countries, such as Thailand, Taiwan, Laos, Burma, Cambodia, Vietnam, Philippines, and Malaysia. The major Chinese immigration began in the 1850s with the gold rush to California. Koreans immigrated beginning in the mid-1950s, and refugees from Vietnam and Cambodia arrived in the United States beginning in the 1970s.[28]

Chinese

Chinese enjoy a broad range of foods; however, dairy products are not common, and polished white rice is the staple. Wheat is used for crepes and wrappers of many foods, noodles, and wontons. Meat, fish, and poultry are common but generally served in small portions reflecting food habits originating in generations of famine in China. Soybeans are considered the "poor man's cow," because they are transformed into many milk-type products, soy milk, bean curd/tofu, black beans, soy sauce, and hoisin and oyster

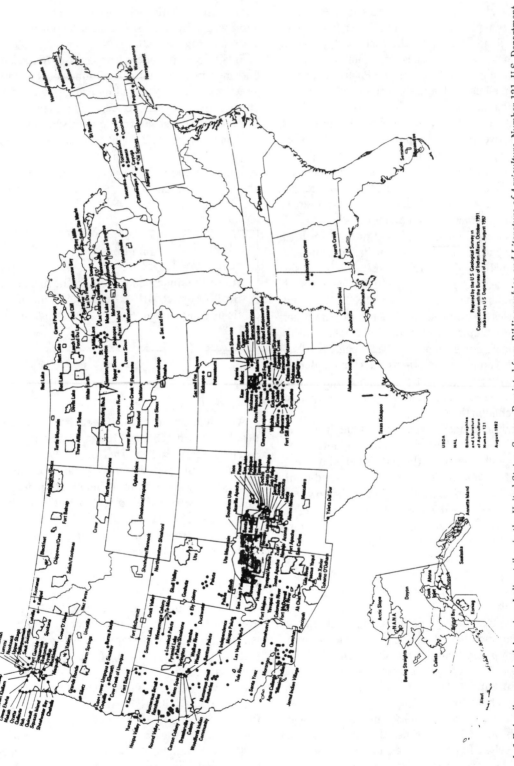
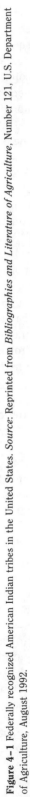

Figure 4–1 Federally recognized American Indian tribes in the United States. *Source:* Reprinted from *Bibliographies and Literature of Agriculture,* Number 121, U.S. Department of Agriculture, August 1992.

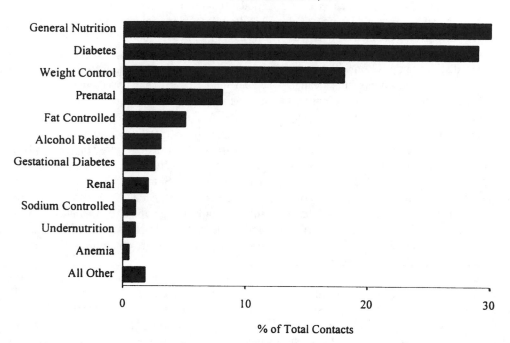

Total Number: 140,414

% of Total Contacts

Figure 4-2 Major clinical nutrition patient/client contacts among Native Americans, FY 1992. Of the clinical nutrition counseling contacts made by the nutrition and dietetics program in FY 1992, the majority were for general nutrition (30%) and diabetes (29%) nutrition counseling. *Source*: Reprinted from *1993 Trends in Indian Health*, U.S. Department of Health and Human Services, Public Health Service, Indian Health Service, p. 105, 1993.

sauces. Hot soup and tea are common accompaniments. Wines, beers, and distilled alcohols are made from starches, such as bamboo-leaf green, hua diao, and red rice wine. Raw fruits, often unripe, are served for dessert. Stir-frying and deep-fat frying of bite-size portions is common.[28]

Meal patterns for Chinese generally reflect three meals and several snacks. A *yin* (cold) and *yang* (hot) balance is complemented with a *fan* and *ts'ai* balance. *Fan* refers to foods made of grains and served in individual dishes; *ts'ai* is the meat/vegetable combination served on a platter for all to pass and take a serving. It is proper to raise the rice bowl to the mouth when using chopsticks, and the *ts'ai* is served in small portions on the rice with the sauce flowing to the bottom.[33]

Food among the Chinese symbolizes harmony of the body with the *yin/yang* and the *fan/ts'ai*

foods. Tiredness and early winter postpartum months signal use of hot foods; dry lips, irritability, and summer months evoke consumption of cold foods. Disease is considered either a hot disease (e.g., measles and sore throats) and treated with cold foods, or a cold disease (e.g., anemia) and treated with hot foods.[33]

Japanese

Japanese immigration to the United States began after 1890. Basic beliefs and practices include a strong sense of family and community commitment, suppression of emotions, visibility of politeness and respect, and care of elders.[28,34] Japanese food preparation is unique, but it includes the traditional *yin* and *yang* concepts. Identification of all ingredients in meals and visual pleasure are most important. Basic foods are soybeans, rice, and tea. Sushi is rice mixed with a vinegar. Teriyaki sauce is comprised of soy sauce and a sweet rice wine called mirin. Seaweed and algae are common and used as either seasoning or made into a wrapping.[28]

Meals have a distinct composition with a traditional pattern of three meals plus a snack called an *oyatsu*; breakfast has a salty sour plum and rice soup, and pickled vegetables; lunch often includes rice and leftovers from the night before; dinner consists of rice, soup, a main dish of fish or shellfish, and pickled vegetables (*tsukemono*). Sweets, rice crackers, and fruit comprise the snacks; sweet bean jelly and dumplings are common.[28] Japanese believe that certain foods have harmful or beneficial effects. For example, they believe that cherries and milk cause illness; they use hot tea and pickled plums therapeutically to alleviate constipation.

Even though traditional Japanese foods are low in fat and cholesterol, increased incidence of several chronic diseases have signified the impact of Western food fare on coronary heart disease (CHD) and cancer mortality rates. Japanese experienced a progressive increase in CHD mortality and colon cancer as they migrated to Hawaii and then to the United States, primarily the San Francisco area. High sodium intakes, low red meat and iron intakes, and insufficient calcium intakes are common among older persons. Lactose intolerance is frequent.[35]

Southeast Asians

Large numbers of individuals from the Philippines, Vietnam, Cambodia, and Laos have immigrated to the United States. Many "boat people" arrived in the United States, fleeing from political conflicts and wars in their countries. They arrived with no material or financial resources. Vietnamese live primarily in urban areas in extended families; Cambodian and Laotian refugees are often dependent on US government services until they obtain employment. All groups have a high regard for family, respect elders, and rely on families for support.[36]

Traditional food habits include rice, soybeans, and tea as staples, and rich desserts (e.g., cream-filled French pastries or custard flan). Filipino food preparation is based on three principles: (1) do not cook any food alone, (2) use garlic in olive oil or lard to fry foods, and (3) prepare foods with a sour-cool taste. The French introduced many ingredients and foods into the Southeast Asian food pattern that have remained: strong coffee, asparagus, French bread, meat pâtés, and pastries. A Chinese influence is noted in the use of chopsticks, stir-frying, individually served foods, long-grain rice, and *yin-yang* concepts. A fermented fish paste or sauce is substituted for salt throughout Southeast Asia. Coconut is a common food in the Pacific Islands. Soy milk, tofu, uncooked vegetables, fish, shellfish, pork, and fresh herbs and spices including basil, ginger, mint, and lemon are common in Vietnamese foods.

Filipinos enjoy three meals and two snack breaks with fritters, sweets, or an egg roll. Vietnamese likewise eat three meals but an optional snack. A traditional Vietnamese breakfast has a soup with noodles, and perhaps an egg or pickled vegetables on French bread. Lunch and dinner are comprised of a soup, rice, fish/meat, and vegetable. Coffee with sugar and condensed milk is common. Holidays in the Philippines involve midnight suppers, fiestas, parties, and celebrations, with food central to the event.[28]

Folklore regarding foods is common in the Philippines; Vietnamese believe that eating organ meats benefits that organ. Lifestyle changes have occurred as the immigrants have become westernized. Health screening identifies diabetes mellitus, gout, and hypochromic microcytic anemia among Filipinos. Low-birth-weight infants and poor maternal weight gain are noted among Vietnamese.[37]

When counseling individuals from these ethnic groups, it is important to understand that they do not use direct eye contact unless to express anger or sexuality. Relatives are important to the success of rehabilitation, treatment, or dietary behavior change. Social harmony is important, yet grouping all Southeast Asians into one room or one interview area may be unproductive and offend the individuals.

Translating Nutrition Materials

Literal translation of nutrition materials does not work. For example, the Spanish-speaking population in the United States includes at least seven Hispanic/Latino subgroups. It is ideal to adapt/test to a neutral, simple, and grammatically correct language that can be understood by the subgroups of the region.

Once a publication has been adapted to the comprehensive language, it should be tested with focus groups to ensure that the text does not contain inappropriate language or insulting expressions. To provide effective nutrition education to different ethnic groups, consider assessing their current food purchasing and preparation procedures. Use of a rapid assessment tool (see Appendix 4–A) can form the basis for understanding how the group is currently making food choices and how westernized they have become.

NUTRITION AND HIV INFECTION

A new challenge facing nutrition professionals is the need to understand and work effectively with the growing population of people with HIV infection. These high-need men and women reside in many US towns and cities. Many need nutritional counseling to maintain their health and well-being.[38]

> "The enormous burden of grief and loss that AIDS will impose on our society has yet to be felt fully, and the work in care, prevention, and research must be not merely sustained but accelerated just to keep pace. . . . The human immunodeficiency virus (HIV) has profoundly changed life on our planet. America has not done well in acknowledging this fact or in mobilizing its vast resources to address it appropriately. Many are suffering profoundly because of that failure, and America is poorer because of this neglect." [38]

The clinical course of HIV infection in adults varies greatly from one individual to the next. Usually, there is a sudden onset of a mononucleosis-like syndrome. The onset is about one to two weeks in length and relates to the seroconversion process. Referred to as a *primary* HIV infection, the condition occurs between two and four weeks after exposure and may include various neurological, dermatological, and other pathophysiological problems.[39] The next period is asymptomatic and may include a persistent, generalized lymphadenopathy. This stage is often followed by the early manifestations of HIV infection, which include fatigue, seborrhea, eczema, fevers, diarrhea, muscle pain, night sweats, weight loss, oral candidiasis, herpes zoster, and other opportunistic infections. None of these conditions are life threatening. The cluster of these signs and symptoms is referred to as AIDS-related complex (ARC) and is the antecedent of AIDS.

The Centers for Disease Control and Prevention (CDC) has developed a classification system for HIV infection and AIDS surveillance among adolescents and adults[40] (see Table 4–3). The 1993 revision of adult and adolescent case definitions for AIDS for surveillance purposes is found in Appendix 4–C.

Considerations for HIV-Infected Pediatric Patients

HIV infection in infants and children may result in children who are asymptomatic or critically ill. Most children experience lymphadenopathy, hepatosplenomegaly, oral candidiasis, low birth weight, failure to thrive, weight loss, diarrhea, chronic eczematoid dermatitis, or fever.[41] Serious bacterial infections with *Streptococcus* pneumonia, *Hemophilus* influenza, salmonella, and other organisms are common manifestations of AIDS.

Many HIV-infected children are more susceptible to various opportunistic and pathogenic microorganisms because they never developed appropriate immunity prior to infection. A majority are partially affected by a common encephalopathy that causes developmental delay or reduced motor and intellectual function.[41] Lymphocytic interstitial pneumonitis is rare in adults, but common in children; the reverse is

Table 4–3 1993 Revised Classification System for HIV Infection and Expanded AIDS Surveillance Case Definition for Adolescents and Adults*

	Clinical Categories		
CD4+ Cell Categories	A Asymptomatic or PGL**	B Symptomatic, Not A or C Conditions	C AIDS-Indicator Conditions
(1) ≥ 500/mm³	A1	B1	C1
(2) 200–499/mm³	A2	B2	C2
(3) < 200/mm³	A3	B3	C3

AIDS-indicator cell count
    *Persons in Category C are reportable to every health department. Individuals in Categories C1/C2/C3/A3/B3 are reportable as AIDS cases in the United States and Territories.
    **PGL = persistent generalized lymphadenopathy. Category A includes acute (primary) HIV infection.

Source: Reprinted from HIV Classifications, Centers for Disease Control and Prevention, Atlanta, Georgia, 1992.

---

true of Kaposi's sarcoma and HIV-associated lymphomas.[40]

Some infants are born with passively acquired antibodies from their HIV-infected mothers.[42] Conventional tests cannot detect the difference between passively acquired antibodies and those that have been endogenously produced. A diagnosis for HIV infection in very young children should include direct identification of live virus, HIV-specific nucleic acids, or HIV-specific antigens.[42]

Nutrition Concepts and HIV

Data derived from experimental studies regarding the role of nutrition in HIV infection and AIDS is limited but increasing. The involuntary weight loss or wasting indicative of severe protein-energy malnutrition observed in many patients with HIV infection demands nutritional care.[43] Nutrition and specific nutrients play an intimate and inextricable role in immunocompetence.[44] For many diseases, the nutritional status of the individual will have an impact on morbidity and mortality, irrespective of the disease process.[45,46] Several questions remain unanswered regarding the relationship between nutrition and HIV disease:

- What is the impact of nutritional status or specific nutrients on the progression of the HIV infection?
- What is the impact of the HIV virus and subsequent infections and/or neoplasms on general or specific nutritional needs?
- What are the potential iatrogenic effects of current treatments on nutritional status?

Community nutrition health workers must recognize the importance of a conceptual framework based on an understanding of fundamental concepts of nutrition and nutritional assessment in order to address these issues and to develop effective secondary and tertiary prevention programs.

To interpret studies relating nutrition to any disease, including HIV infection, it is necessary to use appropriate nutritional assessment methodologies to identify the stage of a nutritional deficiency.[47] A deficiency may progress from manifestations such as weight loss or lethargy, to specific biochemical and anatomic lesions and eventual death. In HIV, clinical assessments should progress from general, nonspecific, sensitive indicators of overall nutrient intake and nutritional status to specific, sensitive biochemical measures. Further, the method should document if the result reflects immediate food intake or long-term eating status. Interpretation of the biochemical assessment must address dietary intake, dietary supplements, and drug use (both recreational and therapeutic).

> "The term AIDS is obsolete. HIV infection more correctly defines the problem. The medical, public health, political, and community leadership must focus on the full course of HIV infection rather than concentrating on the later stages of the disease (ARC and AIDS). Continual focus on AIDS rather than the entire spectrum of HIV infection has left our nation unable to deal adequately with the epidemic." (Report of the Presidential Commission on Human Immunodeficient Virus Epidemic; 1988)

AIDS is a generic term. Some research studies focus only on very ill AIDS patients, while other studies include patients who are HIV positive and asymptomatic or patients who have AIDS. The physiology, immunocompetence, and nutritional status of patients who are HIV positive and asymptomatic vary greatly from those with terminal stages of AIDS. Generalizations should not be made about changes observed in AIDS patients or the application of treatment to all HIV-positive patients.

In addition, most published studies have examined adult males with AIDS; about one-third are from peer-reviewed, refereed scientific journals. Studies are rarely prospective and tend to have inadequate sample sizes and inappropriate control groups. Many reported studies are preliminary abstracts or letters to the editor, reflect small samples, and are observational rather than investigative.

Wasting is a major cause of morbidity and mortality in people with AIDS.[48-50] To understand the wasting process, it is important to understand the mismatch between energy intake and total energy expenditure, as well as the processes that accelerate negative nitrogen balance or protein wasting.

In both the absence of disease and in AIDS, starvation leads to death when body weight is 66% of ideal.[49,51-54] Studies suggest that it is the degree of wasting rather than its specific cause

that leads to death. Thus, theoretically, therapies that maintain body cell mass could prolong life. Many studies document that even after AIDS-related illnesses begin, wasting is not inevitable. This finding suggests that wasting is not a component of immunodeficiency.[48,55-58] AIDS differs from simple starvation in that the metabolic disturbances prevent nitrogen sparing and allow adipose tissue conservation.[48,53,54,59] Body cell mass may be lost, but there may be minimal body fat loss.[48,49]

The host response to infection appears to cause the changes in metabolism. It is now generally accepted that cytokines mediate the host immune response and metabolic changes.[60-65]

Each metabolic disturbance must be considered in the context of total energy balance.[66-70] Animals that eat more to compensate for metabolic disturbances maintain weight, whereas animals that do not, lose weight.[71] Numerous studies suggest that synergistic interactions between cytokines may be necessary for the wasting syndrome to develop.[72] Plasma triglyceride concentrations are very high in patients with AIDS and slightly elevated in HIV-positive individuals compared with controls,[55,73] and they may persist for a long time without substantial wasting.[55]

In one study, increased levels of tumor necrosis factor were reported for patients with AIDS.[74] It has been proposed that tumor necrosis factor (cachectin) is responsible for the cachexia of AIDS.[74-76] Numerous follow-up studies have observed no significant differences in tumor necrosis factor levels between patients with AIDS and appropriate controls.[57,73,77-79]

Patients with AIDS have persistently high serum levels of interferon alfa.[78] In AIDS, triglyceride levels correlate positively with circulating levels of interferon alfa.[73,78,80] There is an even stronger correlation between levels of interferon alfa and both the decrease in triglyceride clearance and the increase in hepatic synthesis of fatty acids while fasting.[73]

AIDS and Energy Balance

To maintain weight, total energy expenditure must equal food energy (caloric) intake. Total energy expenditure equals resting energy expenditure plus dietary thermogenesis plus energy expenditure in activity. If energy intake exceeds total energy expenditure, the excess calories are stored as either body cell mass or fat. On the other hand, if total energy expenditure exceeds the energy absorbed, an energy deficit results. This promotes the breakdown of protein or fat for use as energy. Energy deficiency can be due to a decrease in consumed or absorbed energy, an increase in total energy expenditure, or both. In AIDS, a malfunction may occur for each component of the energy-balance equation. To understand the wasting process in AIDS, both the metabolic disturbances due to HIV infection itself and those due to secondary infections must be analyzed.

In one study, the average weight of randomly selected patients with HIV infection or full-blown AIDS was stable in the absence of active secondary infections.[55] Patients with AIDS and active secondary infections had an average weight loss of 5% within 28 days.[58] Data suggest that accelerated protein breakdown and negative nitrogen balance occur in patients with AIDS who also have active secondary infections. Levels of interferon alfa are chronically elevated in AIDS. Tumor necrosis factor, interleukin-1, and related cytokines are thought to be activated during secondary infection. The synergy between these cytokines may mediate the accelerated weight loss.[57,58]

In industrialized countries, most patients with AIDS do not experience continuous wasting.[55-58] They experience stable weight interspersed with rapid wasting, which generally occurs during active secondary infections. In developing countries, such as those in Africa, treatment is usually not available for disease caused by indigenous pathogens or opportunistic infections. Wasting then becomes relentless, and AIDS is known as the "slim disease."[81]

Decreased physical activity may conserve body cell mass by countering the metabolic disturbance. Physical activity helps to maintain muscle mass. Inactivity and the stressful symptoms of an infection cause both a decrease in muscle mass and an inability to rebuild the muscle after a period of wasting.[82]

HIV infection creates a series of metabolic disturbances (i.e., increased resting energy expenditure and decreased rate of protein synthesis). Secondary infection in the presence of cancer leads to anorexia. A limited food intake and an elevated resting energy expenditure create rapid weight loss and negative nitrogen balance. Debilitation and weight loss set the individual back after each weight loss episode. The result is progressive debilitation, along with increased morbidity and mortality.[73] Figure 4–3 outlines the flow of these processes.

In search of a cure, many common, unproven nutritional therapies and unconventional diets are used by patients with HIV-infection. These include the following[38]:

- *AL 721*. This compound of active lipids (AL) is 70% neutral lipid, 20% phosphatidylcholine (lecithin), and 10% phosphatidylethanolamine, creating the "721." AL 721 can slow or stop HIV infection of lymphocytes in vitro[74] and was approved by the Food and Drug Administration (FDA) for clinical trials.[75] A clinical trial in 40 patients with ARC reported minor toxicity; no consistent trends in T-cell or HIV cultures; and increases in body weight, serum total, high-density lipoprotein (HDL), and low-density lipoprotein (LDL) cholesterol levels.[76]

- *Beta-carotene*. Clinical trials sponsored by the National Cancer Institute are testing megadoses for chemoprevention.

- *Butylated hydroxytoluene (BHT)*. BHT has stopped the growth of HIV in vitro.[77] Efficacy of inhibiting the HIV virus growth is not known,[78] and supplementation with BHT is questioned.[79]

- *Coenzyme Q*. Called ubiquinone, it concentrates in cardiac muscle. It is effective for treating cardiovascular disease[80] and can stimulate the immune system.[81] Improvement in AIDS and ARC patients has been reported.[78]

- *Dr. Berger's Immune Power Diet*. This diet is based on the premise that "immune hypersensitivity" to cow's milk, wheat, corn, yeast, soy, sugar, and eggs produces poor

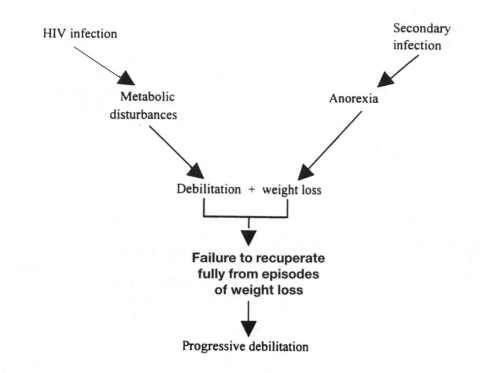

Figure 4-3 Debilitation and wasting in AIDS. Pathways of progressive debilitation and wasting are shown. In addition, primary HIV infection may lead to relative anorexia, and secondary infection may cause other metabolic disturbances. Malabsorption may also decrease the intake of nutrients. *Source*: Reprinted from Grunfeld, C., and Feingold, R.R., Metabolic Disturbances and Wasting in the Acquired Immunodeficiency Syndrome, *Seminars in Medicine*, Vol. 327, No. 5, p. 334, Massachusetts Medical Society, with permission of the New England Journal of Medicine, © 1992.

health. A three-week elimination of foods that cause allergies, followed by a reintroduction and a maintenance diet is promoted. The goal is to revitalize the immune system; efficacy is not known.[82]

- *Gerson method.* This is a procedure that limits all foods except oatmeal and uncanned fresh fruits and vegetables. Regular enemas (e.g., coffee enemas) are common, and efficacy is uncertain.[83]

- *Herbal remedies.* Herbs are proposed as a way to strengthen the immune system.[84,85] Garlic is thought to have an antiviral, antiparasitic potential.[86] Seven HIV patients consumed 5 g/day of an aged garlic extract for six weeks, followed by 10 g daily for an additional six weeks.[87] Results indicated natural killer-cell activity and some improvement in the helper-suppressor cell ratio.

- *Glycyrrhizin.* A component of licorice, glycyrrhizin has been used to inhibit HIV-induced plaque formation in a preliminary study of three patients with AIDS and hemophilia.[88] Doses of 400 to 1600 mg of glycyrrhizin were given six times during a one-month period. Viral replication in vivo was stopped without serious side effects.[89] Glycyrrhizin (150 to 225 mg) was given daily in oral doses to 10 asymptomatic HIV-positive patients for 12 to 24 months, and the disease did not progress.[90]

- *Kelley regime.* Meat, milk products (except yogurt), and peanuts are eliminated to compensate for a pancreatic enzyme deficiency. Vitamins and mineral supplements are recommended, but protein and calcium deficiencies, fluid and electrolyte losses, and vitamin A toxicity are possible.[83]

- *Laetrile.* The efficacy of laetrile for individuals who follow a strict vegan diet and vitamin supplements is not known. Inadequate calcium, iron, niacin, and vitamin B_{12} amid excess thiamin, vitamin C, vitamin A, and zinc is possible.[83]

- *Lecithin.* This phospholipid is the active ingredient of AL 721. It is thought to destroy HIV by "membrane fluidization."[78]

- *Macrobiotic diet.* The diet is based on creating balance and harmony between *yin* and *yang* forces to eliminate the HIV infection.[91] The diet is comprised of 50% whole-grain cereals, 20% to 30% vegetables, 10% to 15% cooked beans or seaweed, and 5% miso (fermented soy paste) or tamari broth soup. Protein-energy malnutrition and calcium deficiency among children and adults is possible.

- *Maximum immunity diet.* Megadoses of vitamin C may strengthen the immune system, but efficacy is not known.[92]

- *Megadoses of vitamins A, E, C, and B_{12}; selenium; and zinc.* The purpose is to restore immunity by increasing T-cell number and activity. Efficacy and outcome has not been established in controlled testing. Toxicity may develop from chronic intakes of vitamin A greater than 50,000 IU per day and large single doses.[93] HIV virus gene growth was stopped in cultured cells using retinoids, ascorbic acid, and tocopherol.[94] High doses of vitamin A enhanced survival of mice.[95,96] Vitamin C in combination with usual treatments for secondary infections has also been promoted.[97] Zinc salts are recommended due to their known antiviral capabilities.[98]

- *Yeast-free diet.* The diet is planned to prevent opportunistic yeast infections such as candidiasis by excluding high-carbohydrate and yeast-containing foods.[99,100] Undernutrition is possible.

An abbreviated case study conducted with an AIDS patient is presented in Appendix 4-D. It characterizes the role of nutrition amid the belief in "magic" foods.

In light of the unconventional diets and questionable information reaching HIV-positive individuals, the American and Canadian Dietetic Associations have taken a position, stating that nutrition intervention and education are essential components of complete care for individuals infected with HIV[78] (see Exhibit 4-5).

HUNGER

In November 1989, 23 experts met at the Rockefeller Foundation Conference Center in Bellagio, Italy, to address the problem of world hunger. They produced the Bellagio Declaration.[101] The Declaration identifies methods to reduce world hunger by 50% by the year 2000. Recent projections are that over 100% of the world population could be fed on a basic vegetarian diet of 2,350 kcal/day, but improving the quality of the diet with animal food products would reduce the number of individuals receiving available foodstuff worldwide[102] (see Table 4-4).

Exhibit 4-5   Components of Nutrition Education of HIV-Infected Persons

- Healthful eating principles: what nutrients are important and why, use of vitamin/mineral supplements, frequency of eating
- Healthful eating plan: what to eat and recommended amounts
- Food-safety issues: food storage, food preparation, dining away from home
- Managing nutrition-related symptoms: how to deal with poor appetite, early satiety, nausea/vomiting, diarrhea, food intolerances, mouth sores, swallowing difficulties, and fever
- Alternative feeding methods: use of nutritional supplements, tube feeding, or parenteral nutrition support
- Guidelines for evaluating nutrition information and products: special diet plans, individual vitamin/mineral supplements, or other suggested nutrition practices

Source: Adapted from *AIDS Treatment News-Issues* by J.S. James, pp. 1–75, with permission of the American Dietetic Association, © 1989.

Table 4–4 The Estimated Number of Individuals Supported by the 1992 Global Food Supply

Food Pattern (2,350 kcal/day)	Billions of Individuals	Percent of World Population
Basic: Purely vegetarian cereals, fruits, roots, vegetables	6.3	115
Improved: 15% of kcal from animal products	4.2	77
Complete: 25% of kcal from animal products	3.2	59

Source: Adapted from Uvin P. 1994 The State of World Hunger. *Nutr Rev*. 1994;52(5):151–161.

No single document defines the way to end hunger in the United States and also appeals to multiple contingencies. The 1990 Brown University World Hunger Conference suggested that US organizations concerned with domestic hunger create a "domestic Bellagio." The result was the Medford Declaration to End Hunger in the United States, written during a meeting at Tufts University in Medford, Massachusetts.[103]

Hunger in the United States is serious, but remediable. In the 1970s, the United States mobilized bipartisan support to address hunger.[104] Programs reduced the problem, but hunger returned as a widespread phenomenon. The Medford Declaration targeted 1995 for alleviating hunger. This declaration may have bipartisan support and appeal to the American public; it describes the economic costs and simple unacceptability of domestic hunger and how this problem can be ended. The Medford Declaration may be a seminal document that sets the standard for ending domestic hunger in the United States. It was drafted by a committee of national organizations (e.g., World Hunger Year; Food Research and Action Center; and the Center on Hunger, Poverty and Nutrition Policy at Tufts University). Further, it was reviewed and revised based on comments by foundation presidents, corporate chairpersons, and community leaders.

On April 6, 1992, the Medford Declaration was released to the press, and congressional hearings followed. The declaration brought considerable press and public attention and raised public awareness about hunger in the nation. Congressional hearings have addressed issues and goals raised in the Medford Declaration. Each signature on the declaration has equal prominence and represents a broad spectrum of individuals and organizations.

Estimates are that 5 million US children from birth to 12 years of age are hungry, and 6 million are at risk. Approximately 25 million adults experience hunger. Using medium-range estimates and three methods, projected hunger estimates among Americans are as follows[104,105]:

- epidemiologic model: 28.1 million Americans
- state hunger surveys: 31.6 million Americans
- Breglio survey: 32.4 million Americans

The hunger problem is magnified by the fact that the United States is still considered one of the most desirable countries in which to live. Figure 4–4 profiles hunger data from task force reports, polls, hunger estimates for older adults, harvest estimates, and child hunger surveys from 1984 to 1994.

US Hunger Policies

Policies regarding hunger were first developed in the United States during the Great Depression of the 1930s.[106] Warehouses of surplus food

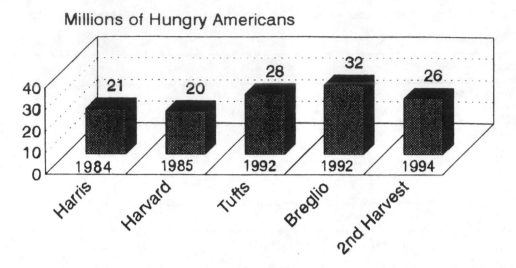

Figure 4-4 A summary of US hunger estimates from various sources from 1984 to 1994. Courtesy of the Center on Hunger, Poverty and Nutrition Policy, Tufts University, Medford, Massachusetts.

were destroyed, while the poor were jobless, standing in breadlines, and unable to buy food. The Federal Emergency Relief Administration distributed surplus farm products as food relief and assisted farmers, as well as the poor.[107] Policies regarding farm prices and production in 1933, food distribution in 1935, and a school lunch program using donated surplus commodities in 1936, all established "hunger-based" policies in the United States. A food stamp concept was tested between 1939 and 1943, and in 1946 the National School Lunch Act converted food aid to cash subsidies. Overall, the decade of the 1930s witnessed the use of surplus agricultural products as the basis of food distribution rather than feeding the poor.[106,108]

The United States prospered from 1950 to 1960, and hunger was thought to be impossible until 1961. In that year President John F. Kennedy initiated a pilot food stamp program in "poverty" areas. The program became nationally available in 1964, and was followed in 1966 with the School Breakfast Program.

Hunger was not identified as a major issue until 1968, when "Hunger USA" and a television documentary, "Hunger in America," evoked national attention.[109] The Senate Select Committee on Nutrition and Human Needs introduced legisla-

tion to expand food assistance.[110] In 1969, President Richard M. Nixon convened the first White House Conference on Food, Nutrition, and Health to establish a national forum and policy direction.[111]

During the 1970s, the purchasing power of families and individuals at the poverty level increased via cash subsidies and vouchers. The Special Supplemental Food Program for Women, Infants and Children (WIC) and nutrition programs for the elderly evolved. Federal food assistance increased from $1.2 billion to $8.3 billion between 1969 and 1977.[110] A second "Hunger in America" report not only acknowledged the continued presence of hunger, but clarified how difficult hunger was to capture and to mediate.[106,112]

During the 1980s, the states and the private sector became more accountable for welfare programs. A "new poor" was identified, consisting of children, unskilled and unemployed youths, and families with limited security and limited incomes.[106] Reports documented an increasing demand for food assistance across most states and various high-risk groups.[113] The Food Research and Action Center in Washington, DC, compiled 250 reports of hunger studies from 1970 to 1991.[113]

By defining hunger in economic terms, the Physician Task Force on Hunger in America identified 12 million children and 8 million adults in 1985 whose income fell below the poverty line or whose food stamp benefits were inadequate.[106,114] Over 40 million US citizens received food assistance to the tune of $21 billion in the 1989 USDA budget alone.[115-118]

Most policy makers are skeptical of data on hunger; they view malnutrition, the extreme of hunger, as a rare occurrence and find it difficult to link malnutrition with hunger. Many believe hunger data are "soft," anecdotal, and unconfirmed. There are a number of real methodological concerns about data on hunger: (1) Many surveys underrepresent the homeless, migrants, and ethnic minorities at risk for hunger and malnutrition.[119] (2) Advocates who lack social survey skills, rather than trained researchers, conduct many of the surveys and construct the methods. Generalizability of the data is limited due to inadequate reliability and validity. The issue of generalizability is paramount to any survey. (3) The link between hunger and a defined disease outcome is hard to document (e.g., the onset of hypertension after inadequate balance of nutrients for several years leading to weight gain, then obesity, then elevated blood pressure, hence hypertension). No easily defined chain reaction exists showing that hunger leads to abnormal biochemical measures, which lead to poor health status, which leads to disease.[106] (4) Ways to suc-

---

Info Line

The Community Childhood Hunger Identification Project (CCHIP) is a rigorous, comprehensive study of childhood hunger in the United States. The purpose of CCHIP is to identify food insufficiency resulting from limited resources. The most recent report, based on interviews with 5,023 low-income households, reports that approximately 13.6 million US children less than 12 years old (29% of all US children in this age group) live in families that have coped with hunger or the risk of hunger at least once during the 12 months prior to the interview.

CCHIP uses seven key survey questions about aspects of hunger occurring because a household lacks resources to procure an adequate amount of food:

1. Does your household ever run out of money to buy food to make a meal?
2. Do you ever rely on a limited number of foods to feed members of your household because you are running out of money to buy food for a meal?
3. Do you or adult members of your household ever eat less than you feel you should because there is not enough money for food?
4. Do you or adult members of your household ever cut the size of meals or skip meals because there is not enough money for food?
5. Do your children ever eat less that you feel they should because there is not enough money for food?
6. Do your children ever say they are hungry because there is not enough food in the house?
7. Do any of your children ever go to bed hungry because there is not enough money to buy food?

Families are classified as "hungry" if they give yes responses to five or more of these questions. Families are considered "at risk of hunger" if they give a yes response to one to four questions. Families are considered "not hungry" if they do not answer any of the seven questions with a yes response.

For more information and a copy of the Executive Summary of the Community Childhood Hunger Identification Project, contact the Food Research and Action Center, 1875 Connecticut Avenue NW, #540, Washington, DC 20009, 202-986-2200 or fax 202-986-2525.

cessfully bring individuals and families out of the vicious poverty and hunger cycle have not been documented. (5) Measuring the extent of hunger is very difficult. The result of acute hunger is not as far-reaching as chronic hunger, which promotes undernutrition and disease. It is difficult to judge who is the "most hungry" or who has the "greatest need." Special concerns relate to persons who are homeless.[120]

Homelessness affects from 250,000 to 2.2 million people in the United States.[121] Socioeconomic and health factors increase the homeless person's nutritional risk. Relevant demographic characteristics of persons who are homeless include family status, age, education, duration of homelessness, income sources, household size, race, sex, social network, and veteran status.[121]

Research on homeless and housed poor children find that eating patterns of homeless children tend to be unbalanced, with a heavy reliance on fast food, and plagued by periods of deprivation. Obesity and iron deficiency in children six months to two years old are common.[122]

Health problems of homeless adults include, among others: dental problems, cardiovascular disease, anemia, hypertension, and alcoholism.[123] Dietary records of 55 urban homeless persons indicated high intakes of fat, cholesterol, and sodium.[124] Anthropometric measures indicated low levels of lean body mass and increased levels of body fat. Nutritional deficiencies commonly found in the homeless include protein-calorie malnutrition and deficiencies of B vitamins, vitamin C, zinc, calcium, thiamin, vitamin B_6, folic acid, and iron.[120]

Measuring clinical or biochemical indices of malnutrition in cross-sectional surveys is expensive. The result has been a cadre of surrogate indicators such as food insecurity, low income, or unemployment.[106] Use of multiple indicators is proposed as a means of increasing the reliability of the measures.[125]

Nestle and Guttmacher[126] reviewed hunger studies authorized by eleven states between 1984 and 1988.[127-137] These studies employed various methods to estimate hunger and food insecurity in the samples, and they commonly used subjective data from questionnaires or interviews.[127-137]

Hunger and food insecurity were frequently reported, as was the need for increased food assistance amid inadequate federal, state, and private resources.[127-137] High-risk subgroups were women, children, and older adults.[127,129-131,133,134,136,137] Many were members of minority groups.[127-129,131,137] Causal factors ranged from poverty and the high costs of housing, to inadequate welfare and food assistance benefits.[126] A summary of Nestle and Guttmacher's findings is presented in Exhibit 4–6.

These studies identified strategies to resolve the hunger problem, and many of the studies' recommendations overlap. They include increasing the federal contribution to state food and welfare assistance programs and enhancing client access to welfare benefits,[127-134,136,137] increasing employment opportunities,[127,130-132,136] higher wages,[137] on-the-job training, accessibility of low-cost housing,[127,131,137] and income redistribution.[137]

Food assistance is currently needed by a large portion of the low-income, minority, single-head-of-household, and older adult US population. Current entitlement programs do not appear sufficient. Table 4–5 outlines the eligibility criteria for food and nutrition assistance programs.[138]

Exhibit 4–6 Observations from US Accumulated Hunger Studies

- Food insufficiency is a chronic US problem.
- Food insufficiency does not reflect food shortages.
- People with lack of access to resources are at greatest risk of hunger.
- The federal poverty level is an inappropriate index of hunger.
- The US social welfare system does not insulate individuals and families from repetitive economic insults.
- Voluntary activities and private charity cannot cure the hunger problem.
- Hunger, poverty, unemployment, and the costs of housing and basic needs are interrelated.

Source: Adapted from Nestle M, Guttmacher S. Hunger in the United States: Rationale, methods, and policy implications of state hunger surveys. *Nutrition Reviews*. 1992;24:18s–22s.

Table 4–5 Eligibility Criteria for Food Assistance Programs

Federal Poverty Income Guideline[a] (%)	Food and Nutrition Assistance Programs[b]
100	Special Supplemental Food Program for Women, Infants and Children, School Breakfast Program (free), School Lunch Program (free), Summer Food Service Program for Children, Food Stamp Program (net income), Temporary Emergency Food Assistance Program, Expanded Food and Nutrition Education Program, Head Start, Commodity Supplemental Food Program
125	All above, plus Food Stamp Program (gross income)
130	Same as above
150–185	All above, but reduced price (not free) School Breakfast Program, reduced price (not free) School Lunch Program
No income standard	Congregate and Home-Delivered Meal Programs for the Elderly

[a]Federal poverty income guidelines are published each year in the *Federal Register* by the US Department of Health and Human Services.
[b]Households at or below poverty level may be eligible. Factors other than income may be considered. The Child Care Food Program guidelines are specific to the sponsor and not listed.

Source: Adapted from *Community Food Resources for Families: An Eligibility Guide* by C. Grandon, Massachusetts Department of Public Health, Office of Nutrition, Boston, Massachusetts, January 1988.

Community nutrition professionals can use information about these programs (e.g., benefits, eligibility, education given, and participation) as demographic or eating behavior data for program planning and implementation. The data can serve as baseline data or sequential variables to monitor individuals and groups.

Today, the attack on hunger in the United States reflects policies of the 1930s and integrates hunger with employment status, poverty, and wages.[139,140] As we enter the 21st century, the hunger problem continues, and its resolution has eluded the US political scene. Empowering low-income groups by training them for jobs and expanding the job market may be a proactive approach toward reducing hunger, as well as a step in the right direction toward reducing health risks and health care costs. Table 4–6 identifies the levels of participation and costs of major food assistance programs.[141]

The US food assistance programs are designed to improve the nutrition and health status of target recipients/beneficiaries by improving their access to food. The second aim of these programs is to support agriculture and ultimately to reduce food insecurity in many US households.[142]

Dimensions of Food Assistance Programs

Three dimensions are identified to explore the impact of food assistance programs on nutrition status, health status, and quality of life for low-income populations: economic, sociopolitical, and nutrition dimensions.

The Economic Dimension

This generally addresses the effects of actions and programs on recipients, society, and delivery costs.[142] Short-term outcomes tend to focus on changes in food intake and immediate indicators of nutritional status (e.g., weight gain in pregnancy, growth in children, and hemoglobin level). Knowledge change denotes short-term outcome. Unless participants are followed in a longitudinal manner, actual impact is difficult to assess.

Medicaid cost savings for newborns was an outcome measure for the cost-benefit evaluation of the WIC program.[143] Noticeable improvements were seen in birth outcomes, with healthier babies and less medical care. Medical care costs were less when women participated in WIC, and program costs were less than medical care costs for

Table 4–6 US Food Assistance Program Participation and Cost, 1989 and 1993

Program	Established	Participation 1989	Participation 1993	Cost (Millions of Dollars)[a] 1989	Cost (Millions of Dollars)[a] 1993–1994
Food Distribution on Indian Reservations	1935	145,777/mo	115,000/mo	52.0	81.6
Child Nutrition					
National School Lunch Program	1946	24.10m/day	25m/day	3,005.0	4,300.0
School Breakfast Program	1966	3.56m/day	5.4m/day	512.0	980.4
Special Milk Program	1954	18.30m pts/mo	NA	19.0	20.3
Food Stamps	1964	18.77m/mo	27m/mo	11,682.0	27,000.0
Food Distribution					
Nutrition Program for Elderly (congregate dining and home-delivered meals)	1965	911,300 meals/day	924,000 meals/day	35.2	150.0
Supplemental Food					
Commodity Supplemental Food	1967	271,146/mo	379,000/mo	144.8	104.5
Women, Infants and Children (WIC)	1972	4.40m	6.5m	1,910.0	3,200.0
Child Care Food Program (including summer)	1968	1.28m	2.0m	745.0[b]	1,500[c]
Temporary Emergency Food Assistance Program	1981	219.0	—	—	120.0
Food Banks and Emergency Feeding	as needed	as needed	as needed	40.0	40.0

[a]Excludes administrative costs, except for WIC.
[b]Includes the summer food service programs for children.
[c]Includes Adult Care Food Program.
Note: m = million; pts = pints; mo = month; NA = not available.

Source: Data from Matsumoto, M., Recent Trends in Domestic Food Programs, *National Food Review*, Vol. 13, No. 2, pp. 31–33, 1990; and from U.S. Department of Agriculture Nutrition Program Facts, Food and Consumer Service, October 1994.

these high-risk women. The cost-benefit precipitates strong national support for the WIC program.[142,143]

Intermediate outcomes of food assistance programs include behaviors, attitudes, and preferences. Eating patterns, food handling procedures, child care alternatives, and medical services all affect nutrition and health status.[142]

Long-term outcomes are reflected in an adequate food and nutrient intake, positive mental and physical development of infants and youths, increased productivity of adults and seniors, and job security of adults.[142]

The Sociopolitical Dimension

This challenges food and nutrition policy makers to improve individual and household food in-

security by distributing resources to meet immediate as well as chronic needs. In addition, two values must be considered: (1) access to food is a basic right; and (2) individuals have the right to free choice.[142]

The concepts of hunger and food insecurity include four components[144]:

1. sufficiency
2. suitability and nutritional adequacy
3. anxiety, lack of choice, or feeling of deprivation
4. acceptability of receiving food[144]

Effective intervention programs must enhance the household's capacity to achieve household goals. Food assistance programs may influence consumer behavior but still allow independent food choice (e.g., food stamps). Or, on the other hand, programs may target specific nutrient deficiencies and package foods accordingly (e.g., WIC coupons).

"Cashing out" of food stamps has been tested in Washington State; San Diego, California; and several counties in Alabama. It substitutes a cash transfer for food stamps. A credit card format has also been tested. Recipients are given a plastic card and personal identification number to use at the checkout counter. A debit is made to the recipient's food account, which is similar to a bank account. These alternatives promote choice and lower administrative costs more than cash payments would. Concern remains, however, about the nutrient quality of products actually purchased and the proportion of the purchase spent on nonfood purchases.[145]

The Nutrition Dimension

This addresses dietary factors that influence morbidity and premature mortality among poorly nourished individuals. Malnourished children are more vulnerable to lead and environmental toxins, increased infectious diseases, school absenteeism, and a muted intellectual achievement. Malnutrition can promote reduced productivity and impaired socialization of young and middle-aged adults. Frail older adults may experience a reduced mobility, impaired digestion and absorption, and an increased risk of malnutrition.[142]

There is no question that hunger exists in the United States. Its presence should motivate the nation to tackle a problem within its borders. From a global perspective, a complex, holistic approach to hunger has been proposed for the world by the International Conference on Nutrition. This perspective is applicable to the United States:

> . . . Food security and nutritional well-being arising from food consumed by households is determined by at least five interrelated factors:

- availability of food through market and other channels,
- ability of households to acquire whatever food the market and other sources have to offer, which is a function of household income levels and flow and the resource base for subsistence farming,
- desire to buy specific foods available in the market or to grow them for home consumption, which is related to food habits, intrahousehold income control, and nutritional knowledge,
- mode of food preparation and to whom the food is fed, which is influenced by income control, time constraints, food habits, and nutritional knowledge, and
- health status of individuals, which is governed by the nutritional status of the individual, nutritional knowledge, health and sanitary conditions at the household and community levels, and caretaking, among others.[146]

VEGETARIANISM

Vegetarians frequently experience lower mortality rates from chronic degenerative diseases than nonvegetarians.[147,148] Diet and other lifestyle patterns of vegetarians are health promoting (e.g., maintaining desirable weight, having regular physical activity, not smoking, not drinking alcohol, and not using illicit drugs).

The vegetarian diet is generally composed of fruits, vegetables, legumes, grains, seeds, and nuts. Eggs, dairy products, or both may be included. Vegetarian diets can vary considerably, depending on the extent to which animal products are avoided.[149]

Total serum cholesterol and low-density lipoprotein cholesterol levels are usually lower among vegetarians. The levels of high-density lipoprotein cholesterol and triglyceride reflect the type of vegetarian diet.[150,151] Low-fat, low-cholesterol, vegetarian diets may decrease apoproteins A, B, and E. Platelet composition and platelet function are altered, and plasma viscosity may decrease. Reversal of severe coronary artery disease has been shown without the use of lipid-lowering drugs.

A vegetarian diet with less than 10% of its energy from fat, smoking cessation, stress management, and moderate exercise have shown a combined effect on reducing artery stenosis.[150] Vegetarians experience hypertension and non–insulin-dependent diabetes mellitus less often than nonvegetarians.[152]

A recent study of 55 Chinese Buddhist vegetarians and 59 nonvegetarian Chinese medical students show major benefits of the Buddhist vegetarian diet which contained 58% to 63% of energy from carbohydrate and 25% to 30% fat. Benefits in lower blood cholesterol were noted, a lower ratio of apolipoprotein A-I to B, and reductions in glucose and uric acid. No positive effect was noted for most hemostatic factors.[153]

One group of vegetarians of particular interest is the Seventh-Day Adventist vegetarians. They have lower rates of mortality from colon cancer than the general population.[154] Their eating pattern promotes high amounts of fiber, less fat and saturated fat, reduced cholesterol and caffeine, and large amounts of fruits and vegetables.

Lactovegetarians consume abundant amounts of calcium. The vegan eating pattern may produce physiologic changes that retard colon cancer.[155] Less meat and animal protein has been associated with decreased colon cancer. A vegetarian eating pattern may lower lung cancer rates, decrease risk for breast cancer, and lower body weight.[156-158]

Because vegetarians have a relatively high intake of complex carbohydrates and fiber, their carbohydrate metabolism may be improved, yielding lower basal blood glucose levels.[159]

A Health-Promoting Eating Pattern

Plant proteins can provide sufficient amounts of the essential and nonessential amino acids if protein sources are varied and an individual eats sufficient calories. Guidelines to assist vegetarians with meal planning are outlined in Exhibit 4-7. Whole grains, legumes, vegetables, seeds, and nuts are excellent sources of essential

Exhibit 4-7 Guidelines To Assist Vegetarians with Meal Planning

Emphasize a variety of foods to meet energy needs:

- Limit low-nutrient-dense foods, such as sweets and fatty foods.
- Choose whole or unrefined grain products and use fortified or enriched cereal products.
- Use a variety of fruits and vegetables.
- Eat a good food source of vitamin C.
- Use low-fat or nonfat milk or dairy products.
- Limit egg intake to 3 to 4 yolks per week.
- Have a reliable source of vitamin B_{12} (fortified commercial breakfast cereals, fortified soy beverages, or a cyanocobalamin supplement).
- Take vitamin D supplement if exposure to sunlight is limited.
- Give vegetarian and nonvegetarian infants who are solely breastfed past four to six months of age a supplement of iron and vitamin D if exposure to sunlight is limited.

Source: Adapted from Position of the ADA: Vegetarian Diets, *Journal of the American Dietetic Association*, Vol. 11, pp. 1317-1319, with permission of the American Dietetic Association, © 1993.

and nonessential amino acids. Soy protein is equivalent to proteins of animal origin.[160]

Most vegetarian diets meet or exceed the Recommended Dietary Allowances for protein.[161] A lower protein intake may improve calcium retention in vegetarians and enhance kidney function in individuals with prior kidney damage. Lower protein intake often leads to lower fat intake.[149]

Plant carbohydrates are rich sources of dietary fiber, which may prevent and/or treat certain diseases such as diverticulosis and colon cancer. In a vegetarian eating pattern, adequate iron intake reflects the amount of dietary iron consumed and absorbed. Inhibitors and enhancers affect nonheme iron absorption. Vegetarians are not at an increased risk of iron deficiency if they consume abundant amounts of ascorbic acid, which enhances nonheme iron absorption. Vegetarians in developing countries consume food staples low in iron. They have fewer sources of ascorbic acid and drink more tea containing tannin. This counters iron absorption and promotes iron deficiency.

Vitamin B_{12} is found in all animal products including milk and milk products. Bacteria produce vitamin B_{12} in the human gut. The site of vitamin B_{12} production is beyond the ileum, where B_{12} is absorbed in the intestine.[149,162] Lack of intrinsic factor in the stomach is the most common cause of vitamin B_{12} deficiency. Atrophic gastritis and the resulting bacterial overgrowth in the upper gut may also contribute to vitamin B_{12} deficiency, especially in older adults.

Plants do not contain vitamin B_{12}. In developing countries, vegans ingest vitamin B_{12} from foods contaminated with organisms that produce the vitamin (e.g., unwashed fruits or vegetables). In Western societies, sanitation is better and the vitamin B_{12} deficiency among vegans may be greater. Cyanocobalamin, the active form of vitamin B_{12}, is available from vitamin supplements or fortified foods such as commercial breakfast cereals, soy beverages, and some brands of nutritional yeast.[149]

Calcium deficiency among vegetarians is rare.[161] Calcium from low-oxalate vegetable greens, such as kale, has been shown to be absorbed as well as or better than calcium from cow's milk.[163]

Zinc is necessary for proper growth and development. Vegetarians in Western countries generally consume adequate amounts of grains, nuts, and legumes and have adequate zinc intake.[149,164]

Infants, children, and adolescents who follow or are fed a vegetarian eating pattern need a reliable source of both vitamin B_{12} and vitamin D.[165,166] If exposure to sunlight is limited, vitamin D supplementation may be required. Vegan diets tend to be high in complex carbohydrate and fiber, creating a feeling of fullness. Daily food intake should be abundant to meet energy needs in infancy and during weaning. Premature infants or infants who are solely breastfed past four to six months of age need a vitamin D supplement if exposure to sunlight is limited. In addition, infants should be given iron from four to six months of age.[167] Vegetarians need iron and folic acid

supplements during pregnancy. In addition, a regular source of vitamin B_{12} is recommended during pregnancy and lactation.[167,168]

HEALTHY PEOPLE 2000 ACTIONS

Many of the *Healthy People 2000* objectives are directed toward improving access to health care, nutrition education, and health education for minorities and other high-risk groups. These specific objectives are integrated within the chapters of this book that deal with the specific disease or disorder (e.g., cancer, cardiovascular disease, and hypertension). Community nutrition professionals have important roles in all aspects of health care delivery, medical nutrition therapy, and general nutrition education of minorities, high-risk groups, and healthy subgroups such as vegetarians.

REFERENCES

1. Loden M, Rosener JB. *Workforce America!* Business One Irwin: 1990.

2. California Department of Health Services. *Health Promotion Section, Multiethnic Health Promotion Task Force Reports.* Sacramento, Calif: California Department of Health Services; 1991.

3. Bronner, Y. Cultural sensitivity and nutrition counseling. *Top Clin Nutr.* 1994;9(2):13–19.

4. Wright PA, Hatamiya F, Kane-Williams E. Cultural competence: Applications to designing materials to prevent alcohol, tobacco, and other drug problems. Presented at the Third Annual National Conference on Social Marketing. Public Health: A New Strategy in Health Promotion; May 1993; Clearwater Beach, Fla.

5. US Department of Commerce, *Statistical Abstracts of the United States.* 112th ed. Washington, DC: US Government Printing Office; 1992.

6. Orlandi MA, Weston R, Epstein LG. *Cultural Competence for Evaluators: A Guide for Alcohol and Other Drug Abuse Prevention Practitioners Working with Ethnic/Racial Communities.* Rockville, Md: US Department of Health and Human Services, Public Health Service, Alcohol, Drug Abuse, and Mental Health Administration, Office of Substance Abuse Prevention; 1992.

7. Bryant CA, Courtney A, Markesbery BA, et al. *The Cultural Feast: An Introduction to Food and Society.* St. Paul, Minn: West Publishing Co; 1985.

8. Kittler-Goyan P, Sucher KP. *Food and Culture*. New York, NY: Van Nostrand Reinhold; 1989.

9. Randall-David E. *Strategies for Working with Culturally Diverse Communities and Clients*. Washington, DC: Association for the Care of Children's Health; 1989.

10. US Department of Agriculture. *Cross Cultural Counseling. A Guide for Nutrition and Health Counselors*. Washington, DC: US Government Printing Office; 1986.

11. Riordan J, Auerbach KA. *Breastfeeding and Human Lactation*. Boston, Mass: Jones and Bartlett Publications, Inc; 1993.

12. Campinha-Bacote J. *The Process of Cultural Competence. A Culturally Competent Model of Care*. Wyoming, Ohio: Transcultural CARE Associates; 1991.

13. Gardenswartz L, Rowe A. What's your diversity quotient? *Working World*. August 31, 1992.

14. US Department of Agriculture. *Cross-Cultural Counseling: A Guide for Nutrition and Health Counselors*. Washington, DC: US Department of Agriculture; 1986.

15. Berlin EA, Fowkes WC Jr. A teaching framework for cross-cultural health care: Application in family practice. *West J Med*. 1983;139:934.

16. *The Fact Is, Reaching Hispanic/Latino Audiences Requires Cultural Sensitivity*. Rockville, Md: National Clearinghouse for Alcohol and Drug Information; September 1990. Publication 20852.

17. Sue DW and Sue D. *Counseling the Culturally Difficult: Theory and Practice*. 2nd Ed. New York, NY: John Wiley & Sons, Inc; 1990.

18. Bronner Y, Burke C, Joubert B. African-American soul foodways and nutrition counseling. *Top Clin Nutr*. 1994;9(2):20–27.

19. Watkins EL, Johnson AE, ed. *Removing Cultural and Ethnic Barriers to Health Care. Proceedings of a National Conference*. Chapel Hill, NC. Washington, DC: US Department of Health, Education, and Welfare, Bureau of Community Health Services, Office of Maternal and Child Health; 1985.

20. Orlandi MA, Weston R, Epstein LG. *Cultural Competence of Evaluators: A Guide for Alcohol and Other Drug Abuse Prevention Practitioners Working with Ethnic/Racial Communities*. Rockville, Md: US Department of Health and Human Services, Public Health Service, Alcohol, Drug Abuse, and Mental Health Administration, Office of Substance Abuse Prevention; 1992.

21. Gittler JB. *Understanding Minority Groups*. New York, NY: John Wiley & Sons, Inc; 1964.

22. Bryant CA, Courtney A, Markesbery BA, et al. *The Cultural Feast: An Introduction to Food, Society, and Change*. St. Paul, Minn: West Publishing Co; 1985.

23. Bennett L. *Before the Mayflower: A History of the Negro in America, 1619–1964*. Baltimore, Md: Penguin; 1966.

24. *Nutrition and Your Health: Dietary Guidelines for Americans*. 3rd ed. Washington, DC: US Dept of Agriculture and US Dept of Health and Human Services; 1990.

25. Block G, Rosenberger WF, Patterson BH. Calories, fat, and cholesterol: Intake patterns in the US population by race, sex, and age. *Am J Public Health*. 1988;78:1150–1155.

26. Lanza E, Jones DY, Block G, et al. Dietary fiber intake in the US population. *Am J Clin Nutr*. 1987;46:790–797.

27. Kerr GR, Amante P, Decker M, et al. Ethnic patterns of salt purchase in Houston, Texas. *Am J Epidemiol*. 1982;115:906–916.

28. Kittler PG, Sucher K. *Food and Culture in America*. New York, NY: Van Nostrand Reinhold; 1989.

29. Bass MA, Wakefield LM. Nutrient intake and food patterns of Indians on Standing Rock Reservation. *J Am Diet Assoc*. 1974;64:36–41.

30. Wolfe WS, Sanjur D. Contemporary diet and body weight of Navajo women receiving food assistance: An ethnographic and nutrition investigation. *J Am Diet Assoc*. 1988;88:822–827.

31. Jackson MY. Nutrition in American Indian health: Past, present, and future. *J Am Diet Assoc*. 1986;86:1561–1565.

32. Storey M, Bass MA, Wakefield LM. Food preferences of Cherokee teenagers in Cherokee, North Carolina. *Ecology of Food and Nutr*. 1986;19:51–59.

33. Chau PP, Lee HS, Tseng R, et al. *Dietary Habits, Health Beliefs, and Health-Related Food Practices among Chinese Elderly: A Pilot Study*. San Jose, Calif: San Jose State University; 1987. Master's project.

34. Leonard AR, Jang VL, Foester S, et al. *Dietary Practices, Ethnicity and Hypertension: Preliminary Results of the 1979 California Hypertensive Survey*. Sacramento, Calif: California Department of Health Services; 1981.

35. Reischauer EO. *Japan: The Story of a Nation*. New York, NY: Alfred A Knopf, Inc; 1974.

36. Tong A. Food habits of Vietnamese immigrants. *Family Economic Review*. 1979;2:28–30.

37. Davis JM, Goldenring J, McChesney M, et al. Pregnancy outcome of Indochinese refugees, Santa Clara County, California. *Am J Public Health*. 1982;72:742–743.

38. Osborne JE, Rogers DE. AIDS Frontline Healthcare Conference Summary. Washington, DC: Health, Education Resources Foundation; 1989.

39. Life Sciences Research Office. *Nutrition and HIV Infection: A Review and Evaluation*. Federation for Experimental Biology American Societies. Bethesda, Md: November 1990.

40. Centers for Disease Control and Prevention. HIV classifications. CDC: Altanta, Ga; 1992.

41. Falloon J, Eddy J, Roper M, et al. AIDS in the pediatric population. In: DeVita VT, Hellman S, Rosenberg SA, eds. *AIDS: Eitology, Diagnosis, Treatment, and Prevention.* 2nd ed. New York, NY: JB Lippincott Co; 1988: 339–351.

42. Goedert JJ, Blattner WA. The epidemiology and natural history of human immunodeficiency virus. In: DeVita VT, Hellman S, Rosenberg SA, eds. *AIDS: Eitology, Diagnosis, Treatment, and Prevention.* 2nd ed. New York, NY: JB Lippincott Co; 1988:33–60.

43. Kotler DP, Wang J, Pierson RN. Body composition in patients with the acquired immunodeficiency syndrome. *Am J Clin Nutr.* 1985;42:1255–1265.

44. Chandra RK. Nutrition, immunity, and infection: Present knowledge and future directions. *Lancet.* 1983; 1:688–691.

45. Krause MV, Mahan LK. *Food, Nutrition, and Diet Therapy.* 7th ed. Philadelphia, Pa: WB Saunders; 1984.

46. Herbert V, Fong W, Gulle V, et al. Low holotrans-cobal-amin II is the earliest serum market for subnormal vitamin B_{12} (cobalamin) absorption in patients with AIDS. *Am J Hematol.* 1990;34:132–139.

47. Brin M. Drugs and environmental chemicals in relation to vitamin needs. In: Hathcock JN, Coon J, eds. *Nutrition and Drug Interrelations.* New York, NY: Academic Press; 1978.

48. Kotler DP, Wang J, Pierson RN. Body composition studies in patients with the acquired immunodeficiency syndrome. *Am J Clin Nutr.* 1985;42:1255–1265.

49. Grunfeld C, Feingold RR. Metabolic disturbances and wasting in the acquired immunodeficiency syndrome. *Seminars in Medicine of the Beth Israel Hospital* (Boston, Mass). 1992;327:329–337.

50. Chlebowski RT, Grosvenor MB, Bernhard NH, et al. Nutritional status, gastrointestinal dysfunction, and survival in patients with AIDS. *Am J Gastroenterol.* 1989;84: 1288–1293.

51. Brozek J, Wells S, Keys A. Medical aspects of semistarvation in Leningrad siege (1941–1942). *Am Rev Soviet Med.* 1946;4:70–86.

52. Fliederbaum J. Clinical aspects of hunger disease in adults. In: Winick M, ed. *Hunger Disease: Studies by the Jewish Physicians in the Warsaw Ghetto.* Osnos M, trans. New York, NY: John Wiley & Sons, Inc; 1979:11–43.

53. Keys A, Brozek J, Henschel A, et al. *The Biology of Human Starvation.* Minneapolis, Minn: University of Minnesota Press; 1950.

54. Cahill GF Jr. Starvation in man. *N Engl J Med.* 1970;282:668–675.

55. Grunfeld C, Kotler DP, Hamadeh R, et al. Hypertriglyceridemia in the acquired immunodeficiency syndrome. *Am J Med.* 1989;86:27–31.

56. Kotler DP, Tierney AR, Brenner SK, et al. Preservation of short-term energy balance in clinically stable patients with AIDS. *Am J Clin Nutr.* 1990;51:7–13.

57. Hommes MJ, Romijn JA, Godfried MH, et al. Increased resting energy expenditure in human immunodeficiency virus-infected men. *Metabolism.* 1990;39:1186–1190.

58. Grunfeld C, Pang M, Shimizu L, et al. Resting energy expenditure, caloric intake, and short-term weight change in human immunodeficiency virus infection and the acquired immunodeficiency syndrome. *Am J Clin Nutr.* 1992;55: 455–460.

59. Brennan MF. Uncomplicated starvation versus cancer cachexia. *Cancer Res.* 1977;37:2359–2364.

60. Grunfeld C, Feingold RR. The metabolic effects of tumor necrosis factor and other cytokines. *Biotherapy.* 1991;3:143–158.

61. Rosenberg ZF, Fauci AS. Immunopathogenic mechanisms in HIV infections. *Ann NY Acad Sci.* 1988;546: 164–174.

62. Patton JS, Shepard HM, Wilking H, et al. Interferons and tumor necrosis factors have similar catabolic effects on 3T3-L1 cells. *Proc Natl Acad Sci USA.* 1986;83: 8313–8317.

63. Beutler BA, Cerami A. Recombinant interleukin 1 suppresses lipoprotein lipase activity in 3T3-L1 cells. *J Immunol.* 1985;135:3969–3971.

64. Keay S, Grossberg SE. Interferon inhibits the conversion of 3T3-L1 mouse fibroblasts into adipocytes. *Proc Natl Acad Sci USA.* 1980;77:4099–4103.

65. Beutler B, Cerami A. Cachectic: More than a tumor necrosis factor. *N Engl J Med.* 1987;316:379–385.

66. Patton JS, Peters PM, McCabe J, et al. Development of partial tolerance to the gastrointestinal effects of high dose of recombinant tumor necrosis factor-alpha in rodents. *J Clin Invest.* 1987;80:1587–1596.

67. Tracey KJ, Wei H, Manogue KR, et al. Cachectin/tumor necrosis factor induces cachexia, anemia, and inflammation. *J Exp Med.* 1988;167:1211–1227.

68. Socher SH, Friedman A, Martinez D. Recombinant human tumor necrosis factor induces acute reductions in food intake and body weight in mice. *J Exp Med.* 1988;167: 1957–1962.

69. Stovroff MC, Fraker DL, Swedenborg JA, et al. Cachectin/tumor necrosis factor: A possible mediator of cancer anorexia in the rat. *Cancer Res.* 1988;48: 4567–4572.

70. Mullen BJ, Harris RBS, Patton JS, et al. Recombinant tumor necrosis factor-alpha chronically administered in rats: Lack of cachetic effect. *Proc Soc Exp Biol Med.* 1990;193:318–325.

71. Mulligan HD, Tisdale MJ. Lipogenesis in tumor and host tissues in mice bearing colonic adenocarcinomas. *Br J Cancer.* 1991;63:719–722.

72. Bartholeyns J, Freudenberg M, Galanos C. Growing tumors induce hypersensitivity to endotoxin and tumor necrosis factor. *Infect Immun*. 1987;55:2230-2233.

73. Grunfeld C, Pang M, Doerrler W, et al. Lipids, lipoproteins, triglyceride clearance and cytokines in human immunodeficiency virus infection and the acquired immunodeficiency syndrome. *J Clin Endocrinol Metab*. 1992;74: 1045-1052.

74. Sarin PS, Gallo RC, Scheer DI, et al. Effects of a novel compound (AL721) on HTLV-III infectivity in vitro. *N Engl J Med*. 1983;309:445-448.

75. Bennett J. NIH-sponsored clinical trials begin for antiviral drug AL721. *Am J Nurs*. 1988;88:432.

76. Mildvan D, Armstrong D, Antoniskis D, et al. An open label dose-ranging trial of AL721 in PGL and ARC (abstract). In: *Proceedings of the Fifth International Conference on AIDS*. June 4-9, 1989; Montreal, Canada: 403.

77. Snipes W, Person S, Keith A, et al. Butylated hydroxytoluene inactivate lipid-coated viruses. *Science*. 1975;188:64-66i.

78. James JS. *AIDS Treatment News-Issues*. 1989; 1-75.

79. Shlian DM, Goldstone J. Toxicity of butylated hydroxytoluene. *N Engl J Med*. 1986;314:648-649.

80. Langsjoen PH, Vadhanavikit S, Folkers K. Response of patients in classes III and IV of cardiomyopathy to therapy in a blind and crossover trial with coenzyme Q-10. *Proc Natl Acad Sci USA*. 1985;82:4204-4244.

81. Folkers KS, Shizukuishi K, Takemura K, et al. Increase in levels of IgG in serum of patients with coenzyme Q-10. *Res Commun Chem Pathol Pharmacol*. 1982;38:335-338.

82. Berger SM. *Dr. Berger's Immune Power Diet*. New York, NY: Penguin Books; 1985.

83. Dwyer JT, Bye RL, Holt PL, et al. Unproven nutrition therapies for AIDS: What is the evidence? *Nutr Today*. 1988;23:25-33.

84. Badgley L. *Healing AIDS Naturally: Natural Therapies for the Immune System*. San Bruno, Calif: Human Energy Press; 1987.

85. Smith MO. AIDS: Results of Chinese medical treatment show frequent symptom relief and some apparent long-term remissions. *Am J Acupuncture*. 1988;16:105-112.

86. Hunan Medical College. Garlic in cryptococcal meningitis: A preliminary report of 21 cases. *Chin Med J*. 1980;93:123-126.

87. Abdullah T, Kirkpatrick DV, Williams L, et al. Garlic as an antimicrobial and immune modulator in AIDS (abstract). In: *Proceedings of the Fifth International Conference on AIDS*. June 4-9, 1989; Montreal, Canada: 466.

88. Ito M, Nakashima H, Baba M, et al. Inhibitory effect of glycyrrhizin on the in vitro infectivity and cytopathic activity of the human immunodeficiency virus [HIV(HTLV-III/LAV)]. *Antiviral Res*. 1987;7:127-137.

89. Hattori T, Ikematsu S, Koito A, et al. Preliminary evidence for inhibitory effect of glycyrrhizin on HIV replication in patients with AIDS. *Antiviral Res*. 1989;11: 255-262.

90. Ikegami N, Yoshioka K, Akatani K. Clinical evaluation of glycyrrhizin on HIV-infected asymptomatic hemophiliac patients in Japan (abstract). In: *Proceedings of the Fifth International Conference on AIDS*. June 4-9, 1989; Montreal, Canada: 401.

91. Muramoto NB. *Natural Immunity: Insights on Diet and AIDS*. Oroville, Calif: George Ohsawa Macrobiotic Foundation; 1988.

92. Weiner MA. *Maximum Immunity Diet*. New York, NY: Pocket Books; 1986.

93. Olson JA, Vitamin A, retinoids, and carotenoids. In: Shils ME, Young VR, eds. *Modern Nutrition in Health and Disease*. 7th ed. Philadelphia, Pa: Lea & Febiger; 1988: 292-312.

94. Blakeslee JR Jr, Yamamoto N, Hinuma Y. Human T-cell leukemia virus I induction by 5-iodo-2'-deoxyuridine and N-methly-N'-nitro-N-nitrosoguanidine: Inhibition by retinoids, L-ascorbic acid, and DL-tocopherol. *Cancer Res*. 1985;45:3471-3476.

95. Fryburg D, Rubinstein A, Rettura G, et al. Vitamin A (VA): Rational for testing VA as therapy for acquired immunodeficiency diseases (AIDS). *Fed Proc*. 1984;43:606.

96. Watson RR, Yahya MD, Darban HR, et al. Enhanced survival by vitamin A supplementation during a retro-virus infection causing murine AIDS. *Life Sci*. 1988;43(6): xiii-xviii.

97. Cathcart RF, III. Vitamin C in the treatment of acquired immune deficiency syndrome (AIDS). *Med Hypotheses*. 1984;14:423-433.

98. Sergio W. Zinc salts that may be effective against the AIDS virus HIV. *Med Hypotheses*. 1988;26:251-253.

99. Crook WG. *The Yeast Connection: A Medical Breakthrough*. Jackson, Tenn: Professional Books/Future Health, Inc; 1985.

100. American Academy of Allergy and Immunology, Executive Committee. Candidiasis hypersensitivity syndrome (position statement). *J Allergy Clin Immunol*. 1986;78: 271-272.

101. Bellagio Declaration. Rockefeller Foundation Conference center. Bellagio, Italy; 1992.

102. Uvin P. The state of world hunger. *Nutr Rev*. 1994;52:151-161.

103. The Medford declaration to end hunger in the United States. *Nutr Rev*. 1992;50:240-242. Editorial.

104. Goodwin MY. Can the poor afford to eat? In: Wright HS, Sims LS, eds. *Community Nutrition: People, Policies and Programs*. Boston, Mass: Jones and Bartlett; 1981.

105. Center on Hunger, Poverty and Nutrition Policy. *Summary of US Hunger Estimates*. Medford, Mass: Tufts University School of Nutrition; 1994.

106. Nestle M, Guttmacher S. Hunger in the United States: Rationale, methods, and policy implications of state hunger surveys. *Nutr Rev.* 1992;24:18s-22s.

107. Poppendieck J. *Breadlines Knee-Deep in Wheat: Food Assistance in the Great Depression.* New Brunswick, NJ: Rutgers University Press; 1986.

108. Kerr NA. The evolution of USDA surplus disposal programs. *Natl Food Rev.* 1988;11(3):25-30.

109. Citizens Board of Inquiry into Hunger and Malnutrition in the United States. *Hunger USA.* Boston, Mass: Beacon Press; 1968.

110. US Senate Select Committee on Nutrition and Human Needs. *Final Report.* Washington, DC: US Government Printing Office; December 1977.

111. White House Conference on Food, Nutrition, and Health. *Final Report: December 24, 1969.* Washington, DC: US Government Printing Office; 1970.

112. Kotz N. *Hunger in America: The Federal Response.* New York, NY: Field Foundation; 1979.

113. Food Research and Action Center. *Hunger Survey Index.* Washington, DC: Food Research and Action Center; 1993.

114. Physician Task Force on Hunger in America. *Hunger in America: The Growing Epidemic.* Middletown, Conn: Wesleyan University Press, 1985, 1986, 1988.

115. *President's Task Force on Food Assistance Report.* Washington, DC: The White House; January 18, 1984.

116. Matsumoto M. Recent trends in domestic food programs. *Natl Food Rev.* 1989;12(4):34-36.

117. *Hunger Counties: Methodological Review of a Report by the Physician Task Force on Hunger.* Washington, DC: US General Accounting Office; March 1986. GAO/PEMD-86-7BR.

118. US House of Representatives, Select Committee on Hunger. *Food Security in the United States.* Washington, DC: US Government Printing Office; 1990.

119. Nestle M. National nutrition monitoring policy: The continuing need for legislative intervention. *J Nutr Ed.* 1990;22:141-144.

120. Strasser JA, Damrosh S, Gaines J. Nutrition and the homeless person. *J Community Health Nurs.* 1991; 8:65-73.

121. Wiecha JL, Dwyer JT, Dunn-Strohecker M. Nutrition and health services needs among the homeless. *Public Health Rep.* 1991;106:364-374.

122. Acker PJ, Fierman AH, Dreyer BP. An assessment of parameters of health care and nutrition in homeless children. *Am J Dis Child.* 1987;141:388.

123. Breakey WR, Fischer PJ, Kramer M, et al. Health and mental health problems of homeless men and women in Baltimore. *JAMA.* 1989;262:1352-1357.

124. Luder E, Boey E, Buchalter B, et al. Assessment of nutritional status of urban homeless adults. *Public Health Rep.* 1989;104:451-457.

125. Anderson SA, ed. Core indicators of nutritional state for difficult-to-sample populations. *J Nutr.* 1990;120(suppl): 1559-1600.

126. Nestle M, Guttmacher S. Hunger in the United States: Rationale, methods, and policy implications of state hunger surveys. *Nutr Rev.* 1992;24:18s-22s.

127. *Hunger in Florida: A Report to the Legislature.* Tallahassee, Fla: Department of Health and Rehabilitative Services and the Florida Task Force on Hunger; April 1, 1986.

128. *Results of the Iowa Food and Hunger Survey.* Des Moines, Iowa: Iowa Department of Human Services and the Governor's Advisory Committee on Commodity Food and Shelter Programs; March 1984.

129. State of Maryland, Governor's Task Force on Food and Nutrition. Interim report, November 1984; final report, executive summary, November 1985.

130. Michigan Department of Public Health. *A Right to Food: Food Assistance—The Need and Response.* Proceedings and recommendations of the Food and Nutrition Advisory Commission Hearings; Lansing, Michigan; May 1984.

131. New Jersey Commission on Hunger. *Hunger: Report and Recommendations.* Trenton, NJ: 1986.

132. Ohio Senate Hunger Task Force. Final report, 1984.

133. The Interim Study Committee on Hunger and Nutrition in South Carolina. *Accounting for Hunger: Hunger and Nutrition in South Carolina.* Columbia, SC: September 1986.

134. Senate Interim Committee on Hunger and Malnutrition. *Faces of Hunger in the Shadow of Plenty: 1984 Report and Recommendations.* Austin, Texas: November 30, 1984.

135. Utahns Against Hunger and Utah Department of Health. *Utah Nutrition Monitoring Project: Study of Low Income Households, Utah 1985.* Salt Lake City, Utah: May 1986.

136. Governor's Task Force on Hunger. *Hunger in Vermont.* June 1986.

137. Governor's Task Force on Hunger. *Hunger in Washington State.* October 1988.

138. Kaufman M. *Nutrition in Public Health—A Handbook for Developing Programs and Services.* Gaithersburg, Md: Aspen Publishers, Inc; 1990:570.

139. Ellwood DE. *Poor Support: Poverty in the American Family.* New York, NY: Basic Books; 1988.

140. Domestic Policy Council Low Income Opportunity Working Group. *Up from Dependency: A New National Public Assistance Strategy.* Washington, DC: The White House; December 1986.

141. Matsumoto M. Recent trends in domestic food programs. *Natl Food Rev.* 1990;13(2):31-33.

142. Splett PL. *Food Assistance Programs: Economic, Sociopolitical, and Nutrition Dimensions*. Chicago, Ill: ADA Research agenda conference proceedings. 1993:127–142.

143. Mathematica Policy Research, Inc. *The Savings in Medicaid Costs for Newborns and Their Mothers from Prenatal Participation in the WIC Program*. Volume I. Washington, DC: US Department of Agriculture, Food and Nutrition Service; 1990.

144. Radimer KL, Olson CM, Green JC, et al. Understanding hunger and developing indicators to assess it in women and children. *J Nutr Ed*. 1992;24(suppl):36S–44S.

145. Blanciforti L. Food stamp program effects in Puerto Rico. *Natl Food Rev*. 1983;23:27–29.

146. Food and Agriculture Organization of the United Nations. *The State of Food and Agriculture 1992*. Rome, Italy: Food and Agriculture Organization of the United Nations, 1992.

147. Burr ML, Butland BK. Heart disease in British vegetarians. *Am J Clin Nutr*. 1988;48:830–832.

148. Fraser GE. Determinants of ischemic heart disease in Seventh-Day Adventists: A review. *Am J Clin Nutr*. 1988;48:833–836.

149. American Dietetic Association. Position of the ADA: Vegetarian diets. *J Am Diet Assoc*. 1993;11:1317–1319.

150. Ornish D, Brown S, Scherwitz L, et al. Can lifestyle changes reverse coronary heart disease? *Lancet*. 1990;336:129–133.

151. Kestin M, Rouse I, Correll R, et al. Cardiovascular disease risk factors in free-living men: Comparison of two prudent diets, one based on lactoovevegetarianism and the other allowing lean meat. *Am J Clin Nutr*. 1989;50: 280–287.

152. Beilin LJ, Rouse IL, Armstrong BK, et al. Vegetarian diet and blood pressure levels: Incidental or causal association? *Am J Clin Nutr*. 1988;48:806–810.

153. Pan W-H., Chin C-J, Sheu C-T, Lee M-H. Hemostatic factors and blood lipids in young Buddhist vegetarians and omnivores. *Am J Clin Nutr*. 1993;58:354–359.

154. Philips R, Snowdon D. Association of meat and coffee use with cancers of the large bowel, breast, and prostate among Seventh-Day Adventists: Preliminary results. *Cancer Res*. 1983;45(suppl):2403–2408.

155. Turjiman N, Goodman GT, Jaeger B, et al. Diet, nutrition intake and metabolism in populations at high and low risk for colon cancer: Metabolism of bile acids. *Am J Clin Nutr*. 1984;4:937.

156. Colditz G, Stampfer M, Willett W. Diet and lung cancer: A review of the epidemiological evidence in humans. *Arch Intern Med*. 1987;147:157.

157. Chen J, Campbell TC, Li J, et al. *Diet, Life-Style and Mortality in China. A Study of the Characteristics of 65 Counties*. New York, NY: Cornell University Press; 1990.

158. Began JC, Brown PT. Nutritional status of "new" vegetarians. *J Am Diet Assoc*. 1980;76:151–155.

159. Nieman DC, Underwood BC, Sherman KM, et al. Dietary status of Seventh-Day Adventist vegetarian and non-vegetarian elderly women. *J Am Diet Assoc*. 1989;89: 1763–1769.

160. Young VR. Soy protein in relation to human protein and amino acid nutrition. *J Am Diet Assoc*. 1991;91: 828–835.

161. Food and Nutrition Board. *Recommended Dietary Allowances*. 10th ed. Washington, DC: National Academy Press; 1989.

162. Herbert V. Vitamin B-12: Plant sources, requirements, assay. In: Mutch PB, Johnston PK, eds. First International Congress on Vegetarian Nutrition. *Am J Clin Nutr*. 1988;48:452.

163. Heaney R, Weaver C. Calcium absorption from kale. *Am J Clin Nutr*. 1990;51:656.

164. Hambige K, Casey C, Krebs N. Zinc. In: Mertz W, ed. *Trace Elements in Human and Animal Nutrition*, II. 5th ed. Orlando, Fla: Academic Press; 1986.

165. Sabate J, Lindsted K, Harris R, et al. Attained height of lactoovovegetarian children and adolescents. *Eur J Clin Nutr*. 1991;45:51–58.

166. O'Connell J, Dibley M, Sierra J, et al. Growth of vegetarian children: The Farm study. *Pediatrics*. 1989;84: 475–480.

167. Food and Nutrition Board, Institute of Medicine. *Nutrition During Lactation*. Washington, DC: National Academy Press; 1991.

168. Food and Nutrition Board, Institute of Medicine. *Nutrition During Pregnancy*. Washington, DC: National Academy Press; 1991.

Appendix 4–A

Rapid Assessment Tool: Food and Culture

Discuss with client. Check yes or no.

Question	Yes	No
Do you have problems purchasing foods that you want?	___	
Do you prepare foods like Grandma at least three times per week?	___	___
Do you eat fast food more than three times per week?	___	___
Do you eat more than three meals per day?	___	___
Do you eat more than one snack a day?	___	___
Do you prepare most of your meals at home?	___	___
Do you eat a special way for religious reasons?	___	___
Are you on a special diet?	___	___
Do you believe that what you eat can make you healthier?	___	___
What is your favorite traditional food?	___	___
Do you eat favorite traditional foods?	___	___
Do you eat favorite traditional foods daily?	___	___
Do you believe children should eat foods different than adults?	___	___
Do you use convenience foods daily?	___	___
Do you avoid any food because it makes you sick?	___	___
Are there certain foods that you don't eat?	___	___
Do you eat only certain foods on holidays?	___	___

Source: Adapted from Bronner Y. Cultural Sensitivity and Nutrition Counseling. *Top Clin Nutr*. 1994;9(2):13–19.

Appendix 4–B

Nutrition Education and Health Care Counseling Sheets for Native American Indians and Alaska Native People

Source: National Institutes of Health, National Heart, Lung, and Blood Institute, and Indian Health Service, U.S. Department of Health and Human Services.

American Indian and Alaska Native People
Keepers of Wisdom
To Strengthen the Hearts

Keep the harmony within you—check your blood pressure!

Strength, wisdom, and good health are American Indian birthrights. Our elders taught us many healthy ways that were practiced for many generations. Over time, some healthy traditions have been traded for unhealthy ways that increase the chances of getting some diseases.

Heart disease is the leading cause of death for American Indians and Alaska Natives today. We can do something to prevent heart disease. Knowing your blood pressure can help you prevent heart disease.

High blood pressure has no signs or symptoms. You can have it and not even know it. High blood pressure can cause heart disease, kidney disease, and stroke. Your chance of having high blood pressure is much less if you watch your weight, stay active, use less salt in your food, and cut back on alcohol.

If you have high blood pressure, here are some useful tips:

- Take extra weight off by eating less and being physically active.

- Use less salt in your food. Add taste by using spices like paprika, pepper, lemon, and others. Avoid using salt at the table.

- Drink less beer, wine, and liquor.

- Take your medicine as your doctor tells you.

Have your blood pressure checked at least once a year.

Go to your doctor or local health clinic to find out more about high blood pressure.

> ## Know Your Blood Pressure
> ### 140/90 or Greater is High

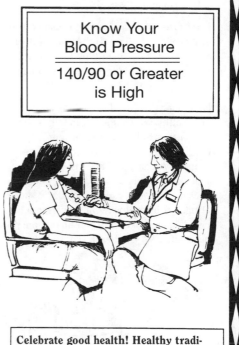

Celebrate good health! Healthy traditions prepare the hearts of tomorrow. Share this wisdom with your family and others.

National Institutes of Health
National Heart, Lung, and Blood Institute
Bethesda, Maryland

Indian Health Service
U.S. Department of Health and Human Services
Washington, D.C.

American Indian and Alaska Native People

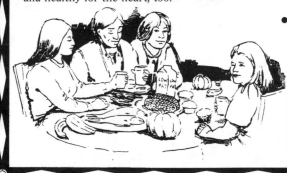

Keepers of Wisdom
To Strengthen the Hearts

Treat your heart to a healthy celebration!

Strength, wisdom and good health are American Indian birthrights. Our elders taught us many healthy ways that were practiced for many generations. Over time, some healthy traditions have been traded for unhealthy ways that increase the chances of getting some diseases.

Heart disease is the leading cause of death for American Indians and Alaska Natives today. We can do something to prevent heart disease. Heathy eating is one way to help your heart stay healthy.

Native foods and traditional ways can help us stay healthy. Native foods can still be found in many places today. We can also grow traditional plants such as beans, corn, pumpkin, squash, and melons. Berries, nuts, plants, fish, caribou, deer, rabbit, duck, and other native foods can be included in healthy eating. Traditional ways of preparing food like drying, baking, stewing, and boiling are good and healthy for the heart, too.

Today, many American Indian families choose foods that are high in fat, sugar, and salt. We also eat more than we used to. Many of today's eating habits can lead to disease.

Here are tips for making healthy food choices:

- Choose fish, fowl, deer, and caribou.
- Eat lean cuts of beef, pork, and mutton.
- Trim the fat from fresh meat. Take off the skin of chicken and other fowl, too!
- Remove fat from canned meat.
- Eat rice, corn, oats, and beans. Use brown rice and whole wheat flour.
- Eat salads and sandwiches with little or no dressing.
- Eat fruits and vegetables.
- Drink low-fat or skim milk and choose low-fat cheese.
- Bake, boil, broil, steam, or roast! Fry foods less often, and use vegetable oil instead of lard or shortening.
- Drain the liquid from canned vegetables and the syrup from canned fruits.

Let us treat our family to healthy eating every day!

> **Celebrate good health! Healthy traditions prepare the hearts of tomorrow. Share this wisdom with your family and others.**

National Institutes of Health
National Heart, Lung, and Blood Institute
Bethesda, Maryland

Indian Health Service
U.S. Department of Health and Human Services
Washington, D.C.

American Indian and Alaska Native People

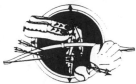

Keepers of Wisdom
To Strengthen the Hearts

Give your heart a workout!

Strength, wisdom, and good health are American Indian birthrights. Our elders taught us many healthy ways that were practiced for many generations. Over time, some healthy traditions have been traded for unhealthy ways that increase the chances of getting some diseases.

Heart disease is the leading cause of death for American Indians and Alaska Natives today. We can do something to prevent heart disease. Being active is one way to keep a healthy heart.

Being active has always been part of our daily life. We hunt animals, play games, dance, run, swim, and ride bikes. Let us keep these healthy ways. At work or at home—give your heart a workout!

Brisk walking can give your heart a workout. It is good for both the young and old. Take a brisk walk for at least 20 minutes three times a week, alone or with your family. Start slowly and build up as you go along by walking longer and farther. Walking is an easy way to stay active.

Staying active is one of the best things we can do for our hearts. Being active is good because:

- It helps take off extra weight
- It helps lower high blood pressure and high blood sugar.

- It is relaxing.
- It gives the body more energy.
- It builds heart and lung strength.

Enjoy being active—it's part of our healthy traditions!

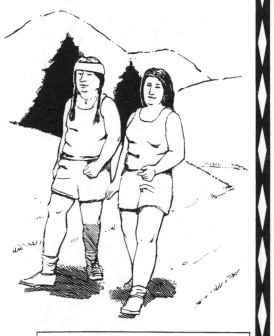

> **Celebrate good health! Healthy traditions prepare the hearts of tomorrow. Share this wisdom with your family and others.**

National Institutes of Health
National Heart, Lung, and Blood Institute
Bethesda, Maryland

Indian Health Service
U.S. Department of Health and Human Services
Washington, D.C.

American Indian and Alaska Native People

Keepers of Wisdom
To Strengthen the Hearts

Help your heart!

Strength, wisdom and good health are American Indian birthrights. Our elders taught us many healthy ways that were practiced for many generations. Over time, some healthy traditions have been traded for unhealthy ways that increase the chances of getting some diseases.

Heart disease is the leading cause of death for American Indians and Alaska Natives today. We can do something to prevent heart disease. One way to keep healthy is not to misuse tobacco.

Tobacco honors life
Tobacco has always been part of our culture. It is used to show respect and honor, and to seek protection on our daily travels. As a gift of the earth, tobacco should not be abused.

Harmful effects of tobacco
Chewing, dipping, and cigarette smoking are not the traditional ways to use tobacco. These ways can lead to heart attacks, cancer, and emphysema. If you chew or dip tobacco, your sense of taste and smell is reduced. If you smoke, your loved ones and you are likely to have more colds and coughs. The smoke from cigarettes can hurt the lungs and hearts of smokers and the people around them. So, if no one in your family smokes, all of you will be less likely to get sick.

So, if you are not smoking cigarettes, chewing, or dipping tobacco, don't start. If you

are–**QUIT**! Go to your local clinic for tips on how to quit smoking, chewing, or dipping tobacco.

Quitting smoking, dipping, or chewing tobacco is the best thing you can do for your family and yourself.

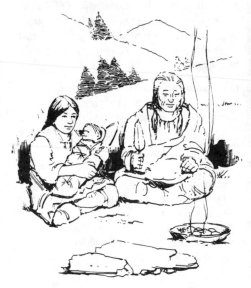

Celebrate good health! Healthy traditions prepare the heart of tomorrow. Share this wisdom with your family and others.

National Institutes of Health
National Heart, Lung, and Blood Institute
Bethesda, Maryland

Indian Health Service
U.S. Department of Health and Human Services
Washington, D.C.

Appendix 4–C

1993 Revision of Adult and Adolescent Case Definitions for AIDS for Surveillance Purposes

For national reporting, a case of AIDS is defined as an illness characterized by one or more of the following "indicator" conditions, depending on the status of laboratory evidence and HIV infection identified below.

I. Without Laboratory Evidence Regarding HIV Infection

If laboratory tests for HIV were not performed or gave inconclusive results and the patient had no other cause of immunodeficiency listed in Section I.A below, then any disease listed in Section I.B indicates AIDS if it was diagnosed by a definitive method.

A. Causes of immunodeficiency that disqualify diseases as indicators of AIDS in the absence of laboratory evidence for HIV infection

1. high-dose or long-term systemic corticosteroid therapy or other immunosuppressive/cytotoxic therapy $\leq$ 3 months before the onset of the indicator disease

2. any of the following diseases diagnosed $\leq$ 3 months after diagnosis of the indicator disease: Hodgkin's disease, non-Hodgkin's lymphoma (other than primary brain lymphoma), lymphocytic leukemia, multiple myeloma, any other cancer of lymphoreticular or histiocytic tissue, or angioimmunoblastic lymphadenopathy

3. a genetic (congenital) immunodeficiency syndrome or an acquired immunodeficiency syndrome atypical of HIV infection, such as one involving hypogammaglobulinemia

B. Indicator disease diagnosed definitively

1. candidiasis of the esophagus, trachea, bronchi, or lungs

2. cryptococcosis, extrapulmonary

3. cryptosporidiosis with diarrhea persisting > 1 month

4. cytomegalovirus disease of an organ other than liver, spleen, or lymph nodes in a patient > 1 month of age

5. herpes simplex virus infection causing a mucocutaneous ulcer that persists longer than 1 month; or bronchitis, pneumonitis, or esophagitis for any duration affecting a patient > 1 month of age

6. Kaposi's sarcoma affecting a patient < 60 years of age

7. lymphoma of the brain (primary) affecting a patient < 60 years of age

Source: Reprinted from HIV Classifications, Centers for Disease Control and Prevention, Atlanta, Georgia, 1992.

8. mycobacterium avium complex or *M. kansaslii* disease, disseminated (at a site other than or in addition to lungs, skin, or cervical or hilar lymph nodes)
9. *Pneumocystis carinii* pneumonia
10. progressive multifocal leukoencephalopathy
11. toxoplasmosis of the brain affecting a patient > 1 month of age

II. With Laboratory Evidence for HIV Infection
A. Indicator conditions diagnosed definitively
1. CD4 T-lymphocyte count < 200 cells/uI, or CD4 T-lymphocyte percent < 14
2. recurrent pneumonia, more than 1 episode in a 1-year period
3. cervical cancer, invasive
4. coccidioidomycosis, disseminated (at a site other than or in addition to lungs or cervical or hilar lymph nodes)
5. IIIV encephalopathy (also called "HIV dementia," "AIDS dementia," or "subacute encephalitis due to HIV")
6. histoplasmosis, disseminated (at a site other than or in addition to lungs or cervical or hilar lymph nodes)
7. isosporiasis with diarrhea persisting > 1 month
8. Kaposi's sarcoma at any age
9. lymphoma of the brain (primary) at any age
10. other non-Hodgkin's lymphoma of B-cell or unknown immunologic phenotype and the following histologic types:
    a. small noncleaved lymphoma (either Burkitt or non-Burkitt type)
    b. immunoblastic sarcoma (equivalent to any of the following, although not necessarily all in combination: immunoblastic lymphoma, large-cell lymphoma, diffuse histiocytic lymphoma, diffuse undifferentiated lymphoma, or high-grade lymphoma)

11. any mycobacterial disease caused by mycobacteria other than *M. tuberculosis*, disseminated (at a site other or in addition to lungs, skin, or cervical or hilar lymph nodes)
12. disease caused by *M. tuberculosis*, pulmonary or extrapulmonary
13. salmonella (nontyphoid) septicemia, recurrent
14. HIV wasting syndrome (emaciation, "slim disease")

B. Indicator diseases diagnosed presumptively
Note: Given the seriousness of diseases indicative of AIDS, it is generally important to diagnose them definitively, especially when therapy that would be used may have serious side effects or when definitive diagnosis is needed for eligibility for antiretroviral therapy. Nonetheless, in some situations, a patient's condition will not permit the performance of definitive tests. In other situations, accepted clinical practice may be to diagnose presumptively based on the presence of characteristic clinical and laboratory abnormalities.
1. recurrent pneumonia, more than 1 episode in a 1-year period
2. candidiasis of the esophagus
3. cytomegalovirus retinitis with loss of vision
4. Kaposi's sarcoma
5. *M. tuberculosis*, pulmonary
6. mycobacterial disease (acid-fast bacilli with species not identified by culture), disseminated (involving at least one site other than or in addition to lungs, skin, or cervical or hilar lymph nodes)
7. *Pneumocystis carinii* pneumonia
8. toxoplasmosis of the brain affecting a patient > 1 month of age

III. With Laboratory Evidence Against HIV Infection
With laboratory test results negative for HIV infection, a diagnosis of AIDS for surveillance purposes is ruled out unless:

A. All the other causes of immunodeficiency listed in Section I.A are excluded; and

B. The patient has had either:
   1. *Pneumocystis carinii* pneumonia diagnosed by a definitive method; or

2. a. any of the other diseases indicative of AIDS listed above in Section I.B diagnosed by a definitive method; and

   b. a T-helper/inducer (CD4) lymphocyte count < 400/mm^3.

Appendix 4-D

An Abbreviated Case Study with an AIDS Patient

Rationale

By reversing the malnutrition that often accompanies HIV disease, a patient may experience an improved level of functioning in activities of daily living, clinical well-being, and long-term survival. Screening for the risk of malnutrition is an important step in early intervention to prevent wasting of lean body mass. Identification of risk factors and indicators for malnutrition by a registered dietitian (RD) is preferred. If risk factors are observed or if malnutrition is suspected, a full assessment is needed.

The main goal of medical nutritional therapy is the maintenance of appropriate weight. Often this is best accomplished by encouraging small, frequent, nutrient-dense meals consumed throughout the day, e.g., three meals plus three snacks, which could include liquid supplements. Emphasis is placed on high-calorie/high-protein foods to offset the metabolic loss.

Consultation

A 36-year-old, Caucasian male, 6 feet tall, and 136 lbs. had contracted the HIV virus through homosexual relations. Past medical history revealed shingles at age 3, a bone tumor at age 10, but otherwise good health until June of 1992. At that time, the patient was admitted to the hospital with a high fever, nausea, and vomiting, which had resulted in a 10–15 lb. weight loss in two weeks. Laboratory data revealed that the patient was HIV positive. He was started on a variety of medications including antivirals and antifungals.

Following this initial episode of illness, the patient was regularly seen by a medical team, including an RD, on an outpatient basis. His health stabilized despite the following medical problems: disseminated chryptosporidium, herpes zoster, herpes simplex II virus, thrombocytopenia, and conjunctivitis. Nutritional problems included nausea, vomiting, diarrhea, early satiety, and insufficient dietary intake with sporadic use of liquid supplements and snacks between meals. Weight loss ranged between 28% to 70% below his usual body weight of 195 lbs., and he reported use of potentially harmful alternative remedies, such as the consumption of raw meat and a fermented mushroom tea known as Kombucha.

At the patient's seventh visit, his weight had stabilized at 136 lbs. His appetite was much improved and he did not complain of nausea, vomiting, or diarrhea. The following recommendations had been discussed previously and he was following them fairly well:

Courtesy of Tracy Lundy, MS, California State University, Long Beach.

If this symptom . . .	then this treatment . . .
Nausea	Eat small, frequent meals. Avoid high fat foods. Try cold foods or those with little aroma. Dry crackers may help settle the stomach.
Vomiting	Try to replace the loss of calories and fluid through the diet. Ask your doctor to prescribe an antiemetic.
Diarrhea	Try to replace the loss of calories and fluid through the diet. Avoid high-fat foods as they may be contributing to the problem.

Patient reported that he had stopped consuming raw meat, however, he was still eating sushi and drinking Kombucha tea despite several past warnings of their potential harm. The patient appeared to have a good understanding of the rationale behind good nutrition. His energy needs were estimated to be 2,800–3,200 kcal/day (35–40 kcal/kg IBW) with 97–122 grams of protein/day (1.2–1.5 gm/kg IBW). A 24-hour dietary recall suggested he was consuming three meals per day and had begun snacking. He was meeting his energy needs for weight maintenance. The nutritional goals for this patient were to maintain good dietary intake and to avoid further weight loss.

5

Nutrition Policy, Health Care Reform, and Population-Based Change

Learning Objectives

- Describe why nutrition care and nutrition services fit within a basic health/medical benefit package.
- Define the major components of a nutrition policy.
- Identify the committees of the US House of Representatives and the US Senate that consider food, nutrition, and health issues.
- Define and give examples of US entitlement programs.
- Explain how to identify state and national legislators.
- Define managed health care and the new health care vocabulary.
- Identify community-based programs that strengthen local resources and return nutrition back to individuals and their community.

High Definition Nutrition

Capitation—a risk-adjusted fixed monthly or annual payment to a community health network to cover all services provided. The priority and focus is on wellness. This is the opposite of the fee-for-service payment system, which requires payment for each service provided.

Clinical pathway—a course of treatment for a specific diagnosis that considers all elements of care, regardless of the effect on patient outcomes.

Critical pathway—a treatment regimen established by a consensus of clinicians. The pathway includes only essential components shown to affect patient outcomes.

Entitlement programs—programs funded directly by Congress for which persons qualify because of certain income or other eligibility requirements. Food stamps and most other food assistance programs are entitlement programs.

Global budgeting—an across-the-board limit on the total public and private health care spending by the federal government. Limits would likely be imposed on states and regions of states.

Health alliance—a group effort by employers and the unemployed to purchase the highest quality of health service for the most economical price from community health networks.

Health maintenance organization (HMO)—a health plan based on relationships between participants and primary care physicians, offering individuals defined benefits monthly or annually with a fee, copayment, or deductible.

Managed care—a system where the care of individuals is carefully planned and monitored. Primary care physicians are assigned, and referrals require preauthorization.

Managed competition—a system by which community health networks compete with one another and provide care based on quality and satisfaction of service by enrollees.

158

Nutrition policy—"a concerted set of actions, often initiated by government, to safeguard the health of the whole population through the provision of safe and healthy food" (World Health Organization, 1989).

Outcome-based monitoring—a statistical approach to measurement, analysis, and reporting of patient recovery rates using categories of illness and injury.

Physician hospital organization (PHO)—a cooperative relationship between hospitals and physicians to form integrated organizations to contract jointly with an employer, managed care plan, insurer, or governmental entity for health services.

Policy making—a dynamic, evolutionary response of individuals or groups to situations and circumstances to improve the public environment, which remains tempered by budget realities.

Preferred provider organization (PPO)—an organizational structure that develops and coordinates contracts among providers and enrollees who purchase service.

Primary care—the first contact made with the health care system resulting in routine medical or preventive care in a physician's office or an ambulatory-care setting.

Tertiary Care—specialized, long-term health services, such as burn treatment, organ transplants, and other highly advanced technical procedures, occurring in a specialty care health facility.

Universal access—health care and insurance available to every American.

Vertical integration—a process to organize all services needed by a specific group with the intent to provide a full continuum of care.

HEALTH CARE REFORM

Health care and welfare reform are the most exciting and far-reaching initiatives influencing community nutrition today. President William Clinton's initial proposal for health care was presented to the nation on Wednesday, September 22, 1993. It included several pathbreaking nutrition components:

- The proposal specifically said local health plans may cover health education and training, and it mentioned nutrition counseling as an example of what that might be.
- Home health coverage for infusion therapy, which is the administration of drugs or nutrients through a tube or intravenously for those unable to swallow or digest, would be covered for the first time.
- The President requested increased funding for the National Institutes of Health (NIH) for research into disease prevention and how nutrition plays a major role.

On Wednesday, October 27, 1993, President Clinton presented the administration's Health Security Act to Congress. The debate began and continues with the printing of this book. The American Dietetic Association (ADA) recommends that the basic health care package should specifically include medical nutrition therapy. This is a tremendous opportunity to recognize nutrition as part of therapy and to cover costs of treatment for some of the most devastating and long-term medical conditions and disease.[1]

Medical conditions such as cancer, acquired immune deficiency syndrome (AIDS), kidney disease, heart disease, high-risk pregnancy, and diabetes can be positively affected by including nutrition therapy in their course of treatment. Medical nutrition therapy, which relies on the science of nutrition, is practiced by highly trained registered dietitians (RDs) who work on a medical team with physicians and other health professionals. It was rare for an insurance policy to cover nutrition therapy in 1995. Patients who would not pay for the services of a dietitian out of their own pockets much more frequently ended up hospitalized and in surgery than patients who could pay for RD services.

Data collected casually by nutrition professionals show that for every dollar spent on nutrition therapy, between $3.25 and $600 in later medical costs is saved, depending upon the severity of the condition. Multiplied by the estimated 17 million patients in the medical system who could benefit from nutrition therapy, the potential benefit for the economy and the cost of health care is enormous.

Several organizations share the same views on including nutrition in health care reform.[2,3] The Coalition for Nutrition Services in Health Care Reform has endorsed a position statement as outlined in Exhibit 5-1. Member organizations of this coalition include the following: American Dietetic Association, Association of State and Territorial Health Officials, American Public Health Association, Center for Science in the Public Interest, American Society for Clinical Nutrition, The Oley Foundation, American Society for Parenteral and Enteral Nutrition, National Association of WIC Directors, Association of the Faculties of Graduate Programs in Public Health Nutrition, and the Society for Nutrition Education.[3]

Questions about Nutrition and Health Care Reform

The debate about nutrition and health care reform has raised many questions. The ADA has

---

Exhibit 5-1 Position Statement of the Coalition for Nutrition Services in Health Care Reform

Preventive, therapeutic, and rehabilitative nutrition services comprise an essential, though often under-appreciated, component of health care. Appropriate nutrition is important to all stages of the life cycle—from prenatal care and infancy to long-term care of the elderly; from developing healthy eating practices and cholesterol screening to high-tech interventions requiring specialized nutrition support services.

It is the position of the Coalition for Nutrition Services in Health Care Reform that:

- Quality health and nutrition services must be available, accessible, and affordable to all Americans.
- Quality nutrition services are essential to meeting the preventive, therapeutic, and rehabilitative health care needs of all segments of the population.

- Any basic benefits plan must include the following nutrition services: screening, assessment, counseling, and treatment for individuals receiving primary care, acute care, outpatient services, home care, and long-term care.
- Quality nutrition services must be reimbursable and provided by qualified professionals.
- Nutrition intervention and education programs that promote health and prevent disease are fundamental to health care reform and must be funded.
- Nutrition services should be coordinated with supplemental food programs and other food assistance programs and be delivered in a variety of settings that are both traditional and innovative.

"If you are among the two out of three Americans who do not smoke or drink excessively, your choice of diet can influence your long-term health prospects more than any other action you might take." (*Surgeon General's Report on Nutrition and Health*. Washington, DC: US Department of Health and Human Services) Public Health Service Publication 88-50210); 1988.

Nutrition programs that promote health and prevent disease must foster personal and community responsibility for healthy behaviors and lifestyles, and be delivered in primary care, public health, and community settings. To maximize the benefit, these nutrition programs must meet the needs of the vulnerable and frequently underserved segments of our population, assure access to a nutritious diet, be culturally appropriate, and be included in preventive care, maternal and child health care, and in health care services for older Americans.

Nutrition services that prevent or ameliorate malnutrition can avert chronic illness or the need for expensive hospital care. For persons suffering from serious illness, specialized nutrition support services such as enteral (tube) and parenteral (intravenous) feeding can save lives as well as promote healing and reduce the length of hospitalization.

A quality health care system must be available, accessible, and affordable; contain mechanisms for monitoring and evaluating the public's health; assure that providers of nutrition care programs and services are qualified and have advanced training or education in nutrition; use clinical and applied research to improve health care practice; and maintain a comprehensive federal, state, and local public health infrastructure to protect the community's health.

Source: Adapted from Position Statement, Coalition for Nutrition Services in Health Care Reform, 1993.

responded to several general questions posed about nutrition's role in health care.[1]

Question: How can people pay for new services, like nutrition assessment and therapies, when they can't even afford the services that insurance and the government currently cover?

Answer: Nutrition services can reduce spending for health care by reducing the need for hospitalization among those with acute and chronic illnesses that have a nutrition component. The issue really is: How can we afford not to cover nutrition services? Exhibit 5-2 gives examples of health care cost savings when nutritional intervention is delivered.[4] The examples also identify useful indicators that could be assessed if systematic, quality data were collected in a prospective manner.

Question: Won't managed care plans simply provide nutrition services since they are cost effective?

Answer: Nutrition services must be available to all patients whose health places them at risk of malnutrition. The lack of reimbursement for nutrition services in our current system has meant that providers learn to practice without these vital services, even when they know that they would

---

Exhibit 5-2 Examples of Health Care Cost Savings by Providing Preventive Nutrition Care

Example 1

Site:	Private Practice, Arcadia, California
Patient/Diagnosis:	80-year-old female with elevated blood glucose, obesity, and knee replacement surgery
RD Intervention:	Medical nutrition assessment and therapy, four visits; patient instructed on 1200-calorie (50% carbohydrate, 20% protein, 30% fat) balanced meal plan
Health Outcome:	25.3 lb weight loss, blood glucose within normal range, avoided hypoglycemic medication
Resources Saved:	Avoided hypoglycemic medication for diabetes
Intervention Cost:	$169.00
Intervention Benefit:	$887.00—cost of medication for five years

Example 2

Site:	County Health Clinic, Riverside, California
Patient/Diagnosis:	63-year-old male with hypercholesterolemia and obesity
RD Intervention:	Medical nutrition assessment and therapy, three visits; instructed patient on 1400-calorie, 30% fat meal plan and low-fat food preparation methods
Health Outcome:	11 lb weight loss; increased exercise; blood cholesterol and low-density lipoprotein (LDL) levels reduced by 19% and 24%, respectively
Resources Saved:	Cost of lipid-lowering medication
Intervention Cost:	$194.40
Intervention Benefit:	$451.00 annually, $2,256.00 over five years

Example 3

Site:	Medical Center, Fresno, California
Patient/Diagnosis:	82-year-old female with dehydration, malnutrition
RD Intervention:	Specialized medical nutrition assessment and therapy during hospitalization; ensure adequate nutrition and hydration with nasogastric tube feeding
Health Outcome:	Patient discharged on nasogastric tube feeding
Resources Saved:	Hospital admission for malnutrition
Intervention Cost:	$33.00
Intervention Benefit:	$700.00—cost of 1-day hospital stay

Source: Adapted from Cost of Services with permission of the California Dietetic Association, © 1994.

be very beneficial to their patients. Managed-care plans currently cover more nutrition services than fee-for-service plans, but these services are not universally available. Fee-for-service plans may extend to nutrition services that make medical treatment more effective and less costly.

Question: Every provider wants to be covered. Why should the plan cover RDs and not others?

Answer: Nutrition assessment and therapies reduce hospital stays,the need for drug therapies, and dialysis; enhance effectiveness of treatments such as chemotherapy; and help people recover from disease faster. Coverage of nutrition services in general results in better outcomes and more efficient use of all provider services.

Question: Registered dietitians aren't well known in the community. Are they really part of the medical treatment team?

Answer: Yes. RDs provide services to clients who are referred by physicians for nutrition services. Many RDs have a private practice, giving group education and one-to-one counseling. RDs collaborate with nurses and other professionals to include a nutrition component in each patient's plan of care. For example, practice guidelines for the care of diabetic and end-stage renal disease patients explicitly call for nutritional assessments, monitoring, and education for routine, effective care.

Question: Why can't physicians provide nutrition therapy?

Answer: Physicians receive extensive training in health and medicine, but their training does not provide the in-depth knowledge of nutrition science and human health. For example, physicians are not trained to provide physical therapy and need physical therapists to provide the physical therapy they prescribe. Dietitians are among the community nutrition professionals who have the vital, in-depth scientific knowledge for medical nutrition therapy.

Question: How are RDs trained and what are their qualifications?

Answer: Registered dietitians (RDs) are highly trained in the science of nutrition and its application to human health. RDs, at a minimum, have a bachelor's degree in nutrition science, have

passed a national registration exam, and serve an internship with a minimum of 900 hours. Over 40% of RDs exceed these minimum qualifications and have completed master's or doctoral degrees.

Question: How do RDs affect patient outcomes?

Answer: Nutrition therapies are designed to establish a balance of nutrient intake that may offset any malabsorption or varied nutritional needs due to the illness. Once appropriate nutrient levels are achieved, the healing process works more effectively. The body can expend its energy on healing rather than dealing with malnutrition (e.g., malnourished HIV-positive individuals who have impaired immune systems are far more susceptible to secondary infections).

Question: Aren't nutrition services just fancy terms for weight-loss clinics and products?

Answer: No. Nutrition assessment and therapies are part of the medical treatment protocols for many diseases and conditions that have nutritional components. Weight-loss programs can be important to the public health in general, but they do not include the breadth of nutrition services that should comprise the medical insurance system.

Question: Shouldn't people do this on their own? How is eating a legitimate part of the health care system?

Answer: For people who have conditions or diseases with a nutritional component, "eating right" is not enough. People who have diabetes, are pregnant, or have renal disease must pay very careful attention to their intake of sugar, protein, fats, calories, and electrolytes. For many, no matter how well they balance their diet, consultation with an expert in the science of nutrition is essential to determine the nutrition therapy most appropriate to their disease.

Question: Why should Congress specify this level of benefit coverage? What organization/ agency should define specific benefits?

Answer: Congress should specify a comprehensive benefit package that includes a broad range of preventive, acute, therapeutic, and rehabilitative services including nutrition services. The establishment of a board that could provide detailed study and rules regarding specific benefit issues may be necessary. Given the historic neglect shown to nutrition services, nutrition professionals would prefer to see Congress specify nutrition services among those that would be covered.

Key Provisions of the Health Security Act

In November 1993, several key provisions were identified in President Clinton's Health Security Act:

- Medical nutrition therapy would be covered if medically appropriate.
- Clinical preventive services specifically included nutrition counseling.
- Nutrition counseling was singled out as an example of health education and training that health plans were allowed to cover.
- Home infusion therapy is covered. It is the administration of drugs or nutrients through a tube or intravenously for those unable to swallow or digest.
- The Special Supplemental Food Program for Women, Infants and Children (WIC) would be fully funded by 1996.
- Public health nutrition was identified as a core public health function with state grant funding available.
- School health education programs that include nutritional health were to be developed.
- Health services research initiatives would focus on promoting health and preventing diseases including breast cancer, heart disease, and stroke—all of which would have a clear nutrition component.

AGENDA OF 104TH CONGRESS

The agenda for the 104th Congress emphasizes the House Republicans' "Contract with America." Reform of the nation's health care system remains a priority, but it will probably be accomplished through smaller, incremental bills rather than one comprehensive proposal.

The newly elected Speaker of the House, Newt Gingrich, Republican from Georgia, promised to bring legislation to the House floor within 100 days. The 104th Congress is more conservative and is expected to push for spending cuts and a reduction in the budget deficit.

Democrats and Republicans are open to possible health care legislation, but passage of items with a broad consensus is unlikely. Health care reform will likely focus on areas of broad agreement (e.g., insurance reform, malpractice reform, and incentives for businesses to promote a healthier lifestyle through their health insurance plans).

Congress is focusing on amendments to the Medicare and Medicaid programs, aimed at reducing the costs of the programs to the federal government. Policy advisors are working on a new health care proposal. The plan is expected to be in the form of key principles, rather than specific legislative language.

An additional concern surfaced in early 1995. Political discussions have been held to consider merging funds for nutrition programs into a single block grant to each state at reduced funding levels. This proposal would cut costs of federal programs. However, it would also reduce food assistance to segments of the population at nutritional risk, require that at-risk populations compete for scarce resources, jeopardize science-based nutrition standards in food assistance programs, and result in a cap on benefits so they cannot be adjusted when the need is greatest.

Not only would fewer funds be available to provide needed benefits, but states could choose to discontinue current programs and/or abandon national science-based nutrition standards. Segments of the population would be left at an increased nutritional risk—especially the very young or very old, and those with physical disabilities, certain medical conditions, and inconsistent incomes. Block grants could negate years of efforts to establish effective programs targeted at high-risk groups. The debate continues as this book goes to press. The Senate Agriculture, Nutrition and Forestry Committee passed a bill that retains both food stamps and child nutrition programs as federal entitlements, although it reduces budget authority for nutrition programs by $19.1

billion over five years, including $16.5 billion in food stamps and $2.4 billion in child nutrition programs. This is a partial departure from the House bill (H.R. 4), which would merge funds for child nutrition programs into block grants. Changes made in child nutrition in the Senate bill include:

- Additional payments for lunches to schools with high participation of free and reduced-price lunches would be terminated.
- Reimbursement policies for breakfasts served to nonpoor children conform with those for lunches.
- Payments under the Summer Food Service Program for Children are limited.
- School Breakfast Startup Grants are abolished.
- Funding for the Nutrition Education and Training Program is reduced to $7 million annually.
- The Child and Adult Care Food Program is targeted to lower-income families.
- The Commodity Distribution Program, the Commodity Supplemental Food Programs, the Emergency Food Assistance Program, the Soup Kitchens Program, and the National Commodity Processing Program are all reauthorized as federal programs through 2000.

The Senate Agriculture Committee bill will be proposed as an amendment to the Senate Finance Committee welfare reform legislation when it is considered on the floor of the Senate. The Finance Committee bill would abolish the Aid to Families with Dependent Children program, replacing it with a "Temporary Family Assistance Grant" or a block grant.

The Senate welfare reform effort has reportedly hit a major snag, because of a major disagreement regarding the formula for dividing federal welfare block grants among the states. Both the House welfare reform bill and the Senate Finance Committee version would freeze block grants for five years at the level that each state received in 1994 for the programs the grants would replace. This formula has raised major concerns among senators from states experiencing increasing population and swelling welfare rolls. On the other hand, senators from states that have flat or decreasing populations are disturbed at the suggestion that their state's piece of the welfare funding pie should be reduced. The debate will continue until a workable plan emerges.

MANAGED HEALTH CARE—THE NEW PARADIGM

Delivering health care in an organized and integrated system is called managed health care. Its goals are as follows[5]:

- to improve the clinical quality of medical services
- to improve the social and client service component of health care
- to reduce costs of delivering quality health care

Managed care is an organized approach to buying and receiving the correct service for a specific health need. Physician hospital organizations (PHOs), health maintenance organizations (HMOs), and preferred provider organizations (PPOs) are types of managed care. The new paradigm is presented simply as $Q/C = V$, where Q = quality service, C = cost, and V = value. In managed care, clients are assigned to one primary physician who refers clients as he or she deems necessary. In this way the single physician manages the care via critical and clinical pathways, and the client pays a fixed monthly payment. Organizations charge the same price for a doctor's visit (e.g., capitation of $40.00). Clients can evaluate different managed-care programs by comparing the type of service provided when the cost is the same. This would be considered the "quality" of care. Higher quality care when the cost is the same results in higher value.

Health care reform in the United States will likely include this new paradigm and use an outcome-based system to monitor patient service. Nutrition care may become a standard component of the preventive approach. It may not only tilt the balance in favor of higher quality service but be a component of health service for which all individuals have universal access.

PUBLIC POLICY

Policy is a framework to make decisions and guide actions that aid the public good.[6,7] Public policies exert significant impact on societal behavior; they are developed when science, economics, social, and political situations evoke government response and direction to meet a need or solve a problem.[6]

In the United States, the legislative branch or Congress has the responsibility of creating policy by passing laws. The executive branch, directed by the elected President, executes all legislation. The judicial branch or court system interprets the laws and settles legal disputes. These three branches formulate, implement, and interpret US laws, respectively (see Table 5–1).

The Congress passes laws that initiate, modify, authorize, and appropriate funds for all programs and services administered by the federal government. Between 10,000 and 15,000 bills are introduced annually. Committees or subcommittees review, conduct hearings, amend, and "kill" or recommend a bill for full congressional action.[6]

Food, nutrition, and health issues are considered by the US Senate in the Agriculture, Nutrition and Forestry Committee and the Labor and Human Resources Committee. In the US House of Representatives, the Agriculture Committee, the Education and Labor Committee, and the

---

Table 5–1 Federal Structures To Initiate, Implement, and Influence Nutrition Policy

Policy Element	Congressional Committees (Legislative Branch)		Administrative Regulatory Agencies (Executive Branch)	External Structures
	House	Senate		
Providing adequate food at reasonable cost	• Agriculture	• Agriculture, Nutrition and Forestry	• USDA	American Farm Bureau Federation, National Farmers Union, Farm Credit Council, National Grange, NCA, Responsible Industry for a Sound Environment, Sierra Club
Ensuring quality, safety, and wholesomeness of food supply	• Agriculture • Energy and Commerce • Science, Space and Technology	• Agriculture, Nutrition and Forestry • Labor and Human Resources	• USDA: Food Safety and Inspection Service, Animal and Plant Health Inspection Service • DHHS: FDA • EPA: Office of Pesticides and Toxic Substances	Public Voice for Food and Health Policy, CSPI, National Food Processors Association, Grocery Manufacturers of America, Food Marketing Institute, Americans for Safe Food

continues

Table 5–1 continued

Policy Element	Congressional Committees (Legislative Branch)		Administrative Regulatory Agencies (Executive Branch)	External Structures
	House	Senate		
Ensuring food access and availability	• Agriculture • Education and Labor	• Agriculture, Nutrition and Forestry • Labor and Human Resources	• USDA: Food and Nutrition Service • DHHS: Administration on Aging	Food Action Resource Center, Children's Defense Fund, Community Nutrition Institute, Center for Budget and Policy Priorities, Bread for the World, American School Food Service Association, National Association of WIC Directors, etc.
Providing research-based information and education programs	• Education and Labor • Agriculture • Energy and Commerce	• Agriculture, Nutrition and Forestry • Labor and Human Resources	• USDA: Cooperative Extension Service, Food and Nutrition Service, Human Nutrition Information Service, FNIC, FSIS • DHHS: FDA • NIH: National Heart, Lung, and Blood Institute, National Cancer Institute	Society for Nutrition Education, American Dietetic Association, National Association of Extension Home Economists, National Exchange for Food Labeling Education
Supporting an optimal science/ research base for food and nutrition	• Agriculture • Science, Space and Technology • Energy and Commerce	• Agriculture, Nutrition and Forestry • Government Affairs • Labor and Human Resources	• USDA: Agriculture Research Service, Cooperative State Research Service, Human Nutrition Information Service • DHHS: NIH, National Center for Health Statistics, FDA	FASEB, American Institute of Nutrition/ASCN, National Association of State Universities and Land Grant Colleges, NAS, Food and Nutrition Board

continues

Table 5–1 continued

Policy Element	Congressional Committees (Legislative Branch)		Administrative Regulatory Agencies (Executive Branch)	External Structures
	House	Senate		
Improving access to nutrition services and integrating them with medical services	• Energy and Commerce • Ways and Means	• Labor and Human Resources • Finance	• DHHS: Health Care Financing Administration, Public Health Service, NIH	American Dietetic Association, American Public Health Association, American Medical Association, American Nurses Association

Note: Authorizing committees for the 103rd Congress are identified. All non-entitlement programs are reviewed by the House and Senate Appropriations Committees.

Key:
ASCN = American Society of Clinical Nutrition
CSPI = Center for Science in the Public Interest
DHHS = US Department of Health and Human Services
EPA = Environmental Protection Agency
FASEB = Federation of American Societies for Experimental Biology
FDA = Food and Drug Administration
FNIC = Food and Nutrition Information Center
NAS = National Academy of Sciences
NCA = National Cattleman's Association
NIH = National Institutes of Health
USDA = US Department of Agriculture

Source: Adapted from Sims, L.S., and Smith, J.S., 1993 Public Policy in Nutrition: A Framework for Action, *Nutrition Today*, March/April 1993, pp. 10–20, with permission of Williams & Wilkins, © 1993.

Energy and Commerce Committee are primarily responsible for nutrition issues.[6]

Federal programs are either entitlement or non-entitlement programs. *Non-entitlement programs* compete for funds through the congressional appropriation process and establish eligibility requirements for recipients. The Special Supplemental Food Program for Women, Infants and Children (WIC) and the National School Lunch Program (NSLP) are examples. *Entitlement programs* guarantee eligible individuals the program benefits. Each year the federal budget may reduce or increase allotments for either type of program. Nutrition policy issues and the level of importance placed on certain programs influence the funded amount. Individuals and organizations can testify at congressional hearings and

make recommendations to modify specific programs[8] (see Exhibit 5–3 and Figure 5–1).

In the United States, nutrition policy issues are represented at the federal level primarily by the US Department of Agriculture (USDA) and the US Department of Health and Human Services (DHHS). USDA ensures the availability of a sufficient, wholesome, and nutritious supply of food and provides information to allow individuals to select a healthful diet. DHHS directs its efforts toward food and health and how dietary excesses and imbalances increase an individual or group's risk for chronic diseases.

Regulatory agencies of the executive branch place restrictions and guidelines on general laws they implement. Regulations may include eligibility criteria, the target audience, amount and

Exhibit 5-3 Washington Watch—Congress Moves Forward on Reauthorization of the Child Nutrition Programs

On May 4, [1994] the Elementary, Secondary and Vocational Education Subcommittee of the House Education Subcommittee of the House Education and Labor Committee voted unanimously to report a substitute H.R. 8, the Healthy Meals for Healthy Children Act of 1994.

On May 18, the full House Education and Labor Committee reported out H.R. 8 with a comprehensive amendment offered by Chair Dale Kildee (D-Mich.) and several important amendments offered by Rep. George Miller (D-Calif.). Sara Parks, 1994 President of the ADA, submitted a letter to USDA in support of their actions. The legislation would among other items:

- Authorize a pilot program for universal school lunch and breakfast
- Allow schools to use 10 percent of their commodity entitlement to obtain fresh fruits and vegetables through a commodity letter of credit if the school so elects
- Reauthorize the National Food Service Management Institute at such sums as may be necessary
- Reauthorize the Nutrition Education and Training Program at such sums as may be necessary
- Require the Secretary of Agriculture to consolidate the National School Lunch and School Breakfast Programs into one comprehensive program without affecting the current reimbursement rates for school lunch and breakfast
- Establish a compromise on the whole milk provision
- Permanently authorize the School Breakfast Start-up Program.

A provision requires the US Department of Agriculture (USDA) to enter into a negotiated rulemaking process before proposed regulations changing the nutrition requirements of the program are published. If enacted by Congress, this provision would require USDA to obtain the advice and recommendations of school foodservice administrators, parents, teachers, public interest organizations, doctors and industry representatives, among others, prior to rulemaking. It also would require USDA to follow the procedures detailed in the Negotiated Rulemaking Act of 1990.

Under the Negotiated Rulemaking Act of 1990, USDA would be required to convene a negotiated rulemaking committee of up to 25 people. The committee must be balanced and represent those parties with an interest in the rulemaking. USDA would provide a description of the subject matter and the scope of the rule to be developed and the issues to be considered. The Secretary would then be required to publish a summary of the negotiated rulemaking committee's recommendations in the *Federal Register*, together with whatever proposed regulations USDA would seek. While new to child nutrition, the Negotiated Rulemaking Act has been used before on other education programs.

It appears that the House and Senate Budget Committee will authorize approximately $150 million in new spending for child nutrition over five years. It is not enough money to allow Congress to consider many of the child nutrition provisions introduced. For example, the provision that would eliminate the reduced-price school lunch and breakfast program in elementary schools would cost approximately $160 million per year and therefore could not be considered under the current budget resolution.

Source: Reprinted from Matz, M., School Food Service and Nutrition, *American School Food Service Journal*, Vol. 48, No. 7, pp. 82–83, with permission of the American School Food Service Association, © 1994.

type of benefits, and qualifications for service providers. The "final rules" are as powerful as the original law.[6]

REGULATORY PUBLICATIONS

The *Federal Register* publishes the proposed rules and notices. The final rules that guide the operation of federal programs appear in the *Code of Federal Regulations* (CFR). This document is revised and published annually. Technical reports or position papers focus on specific subject matter. For example, *Dietary Guidelines for Americans* is a statement of the Federal government's dietary guidance policy.[9]

Info Line

For up-to-the-minute information on child nutrition legislation and policy issues, call the American School Food Service Association Legislative Hotline at (800) 877-1788 and the American Dietetic Association Washington Hotline at (800) 877-0877.

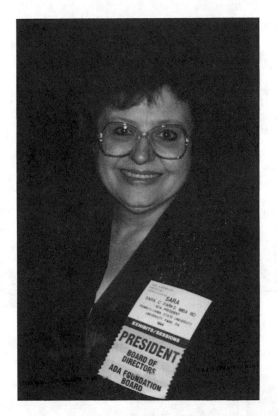

Figure 5-1 Sara Parks, M.B.A., R.D., President of the American Dietetic Association, praised USDA's action to update the school feeding programs by improving nutrient standards and decreasing administrative paperwork.

FORMULATING NUTRITION POLICY

Two major considerations when formulating nutrition policy are (1) providing wholesome food at an affordable cost and (2) recognizing the potential health outcomes resulting from nutrition policy.[10] Nutrition influences health, and it involves individual choice and the social environment. Nutrition is susceptible to modification through social policy changes.[11] No single comprehensive nutrition policy exists in the United States.[12] Instead, a mosaic of separate but related health, social, and food-related programs exist. Each program establishes its own objectives and expected outcomes. The cost-effectiveness of each program is evaluated independently from the others and at various stages of delivery (e.g., after 1 year vs. 2 years of participation). The effect of program participation on nutritional or health

status may not be reported if adequate and well-defined assessments are not designed and implemented. If Congress mandates evaluation within the legislation, evaluation occurs.

Figure 5-2 illustrates the process and factors innate to nutrition policy. *Input* involves issues (e.g., agricultural issues including distribution and marketing) that affect the quantity and quality of available food. *Process* represents events and situations that affect use of the food supply. Food consumption and selections affect the food production. *Output* refers to range outcomes (e.g., individual health or sustainable food environments).[13]

Agricultural policy initiates a nutrition policy process because it influences the quantity and quality of the food supply and the costs of foods presented in the grocery store to the consumer. Health, medical, and environmental policies influence consumer food intake patterns. Health promotion and disease prevention include nutrition as an essential component of any chronic disease prevention policy.[11]

Science policy influences funding priorities for research and new food product development. Approximately $385 million was spent for nutrition research and training in 1988; 78% was used by DHHS, 18% by USDA, and 2% by the Human Nutrition Research and Information Management (HNRIM) system.

Socioeconomic policy affects food costs and food assistance programs when it establishes eligibility criteria. Educational policy affects nutrition education programs and the capability of consumers, youths, and adults to make educated food choices.[12]

Some federal food assistance programs are designed to help economically disadvantaged individuals and families, while other programs are available to any individual. The general types of food assistance programs are family nutrition, child nutrition, supplemental food, and food distribution. In 1992 over $22 million was funded for the Food Stamp Program, which served about 25 million individuals.[6]

Five child nutrition programs exist:

1. National School Lunch Program (NSLP), which is the largest and the oldest

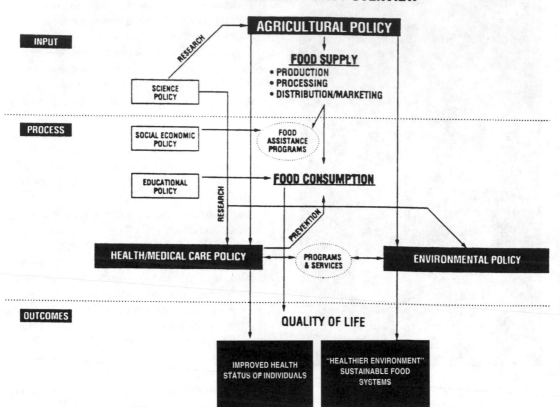

Figure 5-2 The components of nutrition policy. *Source*: Reprinted from McNutt, K., Integrating Nutrition and Environmental Objectives, *Nutrition Today*, Vol. 25, No. 6, pp. 40–41, with permission of Williams & Wilkins, © 1990.

2. School Breakfast Program (SBP)
3. Child and Adult Care Food Program
4. Special Milk Program
5. Summer Food Service Program

The Special Supplemental Food Program for Women, Infants and Children (WIC) provides coupons for a monthly supply of nutritious foods for low-income women and children, nutrition education, health screening, and referral. WIC is generally regarded as one of the most effective of the nutrition programs (see Chapter 7). Several food distribution programs link surplus commodities obtained through farm price supports with people in need (e.g., the Temporary Emergency Food Assistance Program [TEFAP] and the Nutrition Program for the Elderly).[6]

POLICY ELEMENTS IN NUTRITION

There are a limited number of policy options that are considered under the rubric of nutrition. Exhibit 5–4 lists the more common elements of a nutrition policy. Various institutions and groups must be actively involved in the policy formation process because they affect the orientation of the final policy.[6]

Policy Element 1: Provide an Adequate Food Supply at Reasonable Cost

Food production issues are under the jurisdiction of the Agriculture Committee in the House of Representatives and the Agriculture, Nutrition

Exhibit 5-4 The Elements of a Nutrition Policy

- Provide an adequate food supply at reasonable cost to consumers.
- Ensure the quality, safety, and wholesomeness of the food supply.
- Ensure food access and availability to those lacking resources or the ability to obtain sufficient foods.
- Provide research-based information and educational programs to encourage the public to make informed food choices.
- Support an adequate science/research base in food and nutrition.
- Improve access to and integration of nutrition services into preventive health care and medical services.

Source: Adapted from Sims, L.S., and Smith, J.S., 1993 Public Policy in Nutrition: A Framework for Action, *Nutrition Today*, March/April 1993, pp. 10–20, with permission of Williams & Wilkins, © 1993.

and Forestry Committee in the Senate. Implementation rests with USDA in the executive branch. Various farm, environmental, and consumer groups influence this element.

Policy Element 2: Ensure the Quality, Safety, and Wholesomeness of the Food Supply

The Agriculture Committee and the Energy and Commerce Committee in the House, and the Agriculture, Nutrition and Forestry Committee and Labor and Human Resources Committee in the Senate are responsible for food safety and quality. The Science Committee and Space and Technology Committee in the House oversee food enrichment and fortification issues. USDA oversees meat and poultry products. The Food and Drug Administration (FDA) in DHHS and the Office of Pesticides and Toxic Substances in the Environmental Protection Agency (EPA) collaborate on issues of food safety and quality. Public Voice for Food and Health Policy and trade associations like the National Food Processors Association, Grocery Manufacturers of America, and the Food Marketing Institute all influence this element.

Policy Element 3: Ensure Food Access and Availability to Those Lacking Economic Resources or the Ability To Obtain Sufficient Food

The Education and Labor Committee and Agriculture Committee in the House, and the Committee on Agriculture, Nutrition and Forestry in the Senate oversee issues of domestic hunger and food assistance programs. The Food and Nutrition Service of USDA implements almost all programs. Elderly Feeding Programs are under the Senate Committee on Labor and Human Resources and administered by the Agency on Aging in DHHS. Advocacy groups—such as the Food Action Research Center, the Children's Defense Fund, and the Community Nutrition Institute—and associations such as the American School Food Service Association direct their actions toward access and availability. Appendix 5-A includes the actual testimony given by a member of the American Dietetic Association in support of Child Nutrition Reauthorization.[14]

Policy Element 4: Provide Research-Based Information and Educational Programs To Encourage the Public To Make Informed Food Choices

The congressional committee that is assigned to oversee an educational program depends on the agency conducting the program. Educational programs are administered by the Cooperative Extension Service, and dietary guidance programs are directed by the Human Nutrition Information Service. Both programs are run by USDA. Educational initiatives of DHHS are under the Education and Labor Committee in the House, and the Labor and Human Resources Committee in the Senate. These two committees oversee labeling programs (e.g., the Nutrition Labeling and Education Act, which is administered by FDA). Meat and poultry labeling initiatives are in committees that oversee USDA programs. Advocacy groups include professional associations, such as the Society for Nutrition Education and the American Dietetic Association. The American Association of Family and Consumer Sciences and the National Association of Extension Home Economists have also been strong advocates for nutrition education and training programs. The National Exchange for Food Labeling Education convenes trade associations and professional and voluntary health associations to promote nutrition education for the public.

Policy Element 5: Support an Adequate Science/Research Base in Food and Nutrition

Research and nutrition monitoring programs are under the direction of the Agriculture Committee; the Science, Space and Technology Committee; and the Energy and Commerce Committee in the House of Representatives. Governmental Affairs; Agriculture, Nutrition and Forestry; and Labor and Human Resources oversee these activities in the Senate. The nutrition research/ monitoring activities of the Agricultural Research Service, the Cooperative State Research Service, and the Human Nutrition Information Service are under the executive branch. In DHHS, these responsibilities are mainly assigned to the National Institutes of Health (NIH) and the National Center for Health Statistics (NCHS). The Centers for Disease Control and Prevention (CDC) oversee NCHS activities. Trade associations and professional groups such as the National Association of State Universities and Land Grant Colleges closely monitor the areas targeted for research, since their staff and faculty may apply for government research initiatives and funding.

Policy Element 6: Improve Access to and Integration of Nutrition Services into Preventive Health Care and Medical Services

Health care delivery and health care reform have been a top priority for legislators since 1994. This focus illustrates the formation of a new health care paradigm directed toward prevention. The Education and Labor Committee in the House, and the Labor and Human Resources Committee in the Senate oversee this area. The

Health Care Financing Administration in DHHS, and the Public Health Service (PHS) are posed to respond to health care issues.

In response to the new paradigm, the American Dietetic Association has mounted an effort to include medical nutritional services in the basic benefit package of the pending health care reform legislation. The American Medical Association, the American Public Health Association, the American Nurses Association, and the American Dental Association likewise represent their constituents in the health care debate.

ELEMENTS OF CHANGE

Primary, secondary, and tertiary prevention are interventions to change health risk, morbidity, and mortality, respectively. Community nutrition can be positioned in the health care delivery system to improve the health and well-being of US citizens by providing primary, secondary, and tertiary prevention programs.

Health care agencies and organizations are constantly functioning in a changing environment to meet the challenge of a changing health care delivery system. In order to adapt, it is necessary that they initiate several internal activities[15]:

- *Build a sense of urgency*: People tend not to change without discomfort or anxiety. Discomfort with the way something is done creates a sense of urgency that can empower people to accept a new approach to a problem.
- *Create a clear tomorrow*: Create a sense of urgency by showing people what benefits could be possible if a newly defined approach to health care is instituted (e.g., primary prevention efforts directed toward food gatekeepers).
- *Show the way*: Present a clear vision, and then encourage individuals to learn and to practice activities that support the vision. Develop an energizing, inspiring vision that invites individuals in the organization to act. Identify why employees and clients should support the vision. Take the time to lead by giving examples at every opportunity.

- *Create tomorrow*: Select a strategic planning model to achieve goals.
  - Lead from strength.
  - Do what's familiar.
  - Stay a little bit ahead.
- *Remember that vision makes the difference*: Vision is the difference between short-term moves to improve the bottom line and long-term change. Vision translates strategies on paper into a way of life. Vision empowers people and paints a picture of direction. Recommendations include the following:
  - Focus the vision on strategic advantages.
  - Think about how an organization adds value to others.
  - Make the vision clear, so it can be used to make decisions.

    Employees should be able to ask, "Does my action support the vision?" and the vision statement should answer the question.
- *Set the pace with actions*. Demonstrate the vision in action to empower managers and employees. Ensure that managers know that the vision represents what the organization leaders think, feel, and understand. Emphasize the need to change. Use urgency to motivate. Generate specific, concrete actions that support the vision. Emphasize short-term actions to demonstrate immediate change.
- *Expect change or forget it*. Establish quantifiable goals that are short-term and realistic. Review goals continuously to empower and to reinforce individuals. Small successes can build large achievements.

NONLEGISLATIVE PROGRAMS AND APPROACHES

Health care delivery takes many different forms, and government policy can mold the process. In community nutrition, nutrition education and general awareness may be the goal, or primary prevention efforts may be focused on a specific high-risk target group such as physically inactive youth. Secondary prevention may take the form of recruiting free-living individuals with elevated risk factors into a special treatment or study. Tertiary prevention might focus on interventions for individuals with diabetes or hypertension to lower their risk for further complications. Several examples of these different approaches follow. They include an urban farmer's market that brings produce from various agricultural regions to inner-city children and adults, primary prevention efforts for adolescents via planning and intervention grants to community-based organizations, and an international strategy to coordinate prevention and control activities worldwide.

Community Awareness—The Reading Terminal Farmers' Market Trust

The Reading Terminal Farmers' Market Trust is a charitable organization founded in 1991 to promote better nutrition in low-income communities in Philadelphia. The Trust is a core member of a large collaborative program, the Regional Infrastructure for Sustaining Agriculture. The mission of the Trust is to promote the benefits of fresh foods, cultivate links between regional farmers and urban markets, and establish a nutritious food distribution system for low-income residents.[16]

Several situations motivated the Trust to establish programs:

- In Philadelphia, 25% of Reading Terminal Market coupons issued to WIC clients are not redeemed because of the inability of recipients to reach designated markets.
- Local residents are not able to provide input about urban renewal and community programs in their own areas.
- Job training opportunities are limited, unless new programs begin in low-income areas.

The Trust sponsors several programs:

- The Reading Terminal Community Farmers' Market Program, which brings fresh, nutritious foods to low-income communities in Philadelphia. Ten neighborhood markets with high-quality fruits and vegetables at low-cost are each open one-half day a week (see Figure 5–3).

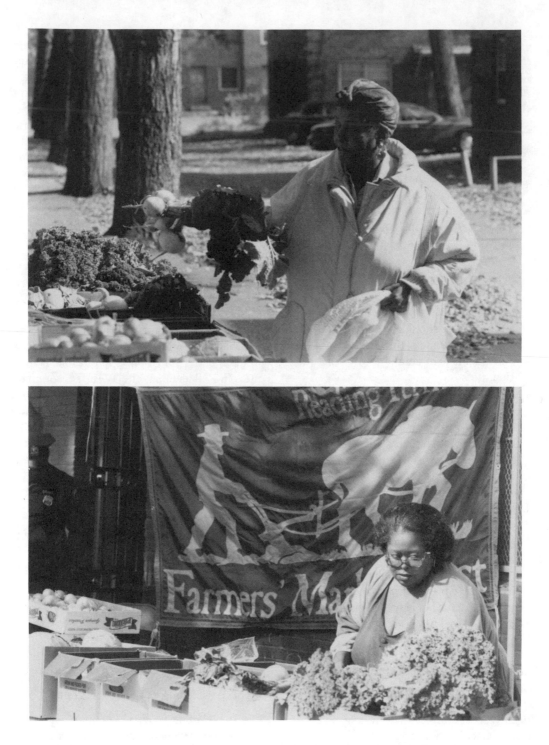

Figure 5-3 The Reading Terminal Community Farmers' Market Program, Philadelphia, Pennsylvania, unites regional agriculture with local access to fresh produce. Courtesy of Mona Sutnick, The Reading Terminal Farmers' Market Trust, Philadelphia, Pennsylvania.

- A food learning network, which teaches low-income school children about healthy foods by visiting the Reading Terminal Market in downtown Philadelphia; tasting fresh fruits, vegetables, and whole-grain breads; and learning how and where the foods are grown (see Figure 5–4).
- The Regional Infrastructure for Sustaining Agriculture, a three-year project that was funded by the Kellogg Foundation to promote adoption of sustainable agriculture in southeast Pennsylvania. Producer-only farmers' markets and a contract program to link low-income consumers with area farmers for fresh foods are components of the project.

Primary Prevention—California Adolescent Nutrition and Fitness Program

The California Adolescent Nutrition and Fitness Program (CANFit) targets California low-income youth by providing significant resources for nutrition education intervention. This initiative is the first of its kind to fund nutrition and fitness outreach to 10-to-14-year-old African-American, Latino, Asian, and American Indian youths[17] (see Chapter 8). Funding is from the settlement of a class action suit.

In 1994, eight planning grants and four intervention grants totaling $265,000 were funded by the CANFit Administrative Board. Planning grants focus on assessing nutritional and fitness needs of youth, developing specific action plans, and identifying the infrastructure to implement the action plans. Intervention grants implement specific programs within community-based organizations among high-risk youth. The grants reflect youth-driven programs, capacity-building activities for the member organizations, and process and impact evaluations.

To further its mission to seed nutrition and fitness programs for youth in California, in its first year CANFit awarded seven $1,000 scholarships for minority college students majoring in nutrition or physical education at California colleges and universities. Recipients submitted competitive essays entitled, "The Three Most Important Nutrition or Fitness Challenges Facing California's Adolescents . . . and Here's What I Would Do." The CANFit program is administered by an administrative board composed of volunteers who are professionals in education, business, medicine, law, and nutrition.

Primary Prevention of Global Proportions— the INTERHEALTH Nutrition Initiative

The World Health Organization's Division of Noncommunicable Diseases (WHO-NCD) initiated a global program for health in 1986 to prevent and control the common risk factors for chronic diseases throughout the world.[18] The noncommunicable diseases include cardiovascular diseases, cancer, diabetes, and osteoporosis. Strategies acceptable by participating countries emphasize total community involvement, health promotion activities, behavioral interventions, and prevention and control activities implemented through existing primary health care systems and community structures.[19,20]

The INTERHEALTH Nutrition Initiative seeks to coordinate prevention and control activities simultaneously for multiple diseases.[19] This approach supports comprehensive population-based screening, developing standardized protocols, and teaching healthy lifestyle behaviors to reduce noncommunicable disease risk factors at the population level. Countries implementing activities to various degrees include Tanzania, Mauritius, Chile, Cuba, United States, Cyprus, Finland, Malta, Lithuania, Russia, Thailand, Sri Lanka, China, Australia, and Japan.

The multicountry activities range from baseline screening to monitoring change in population disease rates and risk factor levels, and from public health policy and nutrition policy development to population-based nutrition interventions focused on chronic diseases.[19] This multicountry approach to common health problems is a global acknowledgment of the ability to prevent and to control noncommunicable disease risk factors. Nutrition intervention is recognized as a viable approach to reduce risk. Future activities at a global perspective may strengthen dietary change activities within each country.[21] Dietary assessment methods being used to collect baseline and

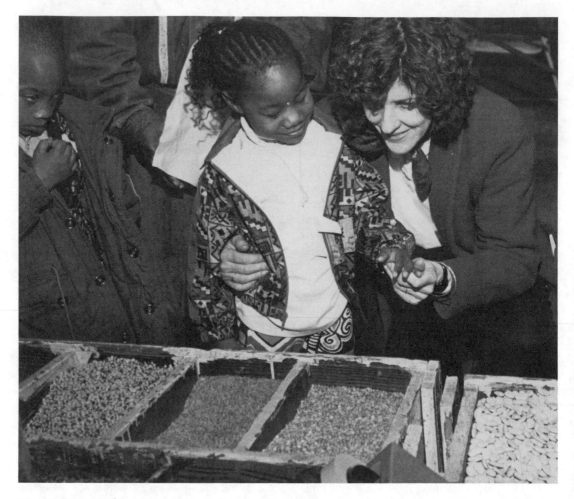

Figure 5–4 Low-income children are taught agriculture in Pennsylvania by on-site visits to the Reading Terminal Market. Courtesy of Mona Sutnick, The Reading Terminal Farmers' Market Trust, Philadelphia, Pennsylvania.

follow-up survey data for the various countries are outlined in Table 5–2. The goal is to standardize the dietary assessment method so food and nutrient intake can be monitored as dietary modification programs are implemented.[21]

Secondary Prevention—Long-Term Adherence to Lipid-Lowering Eating Patterns

One hundred and twenty participants, aged 18 to 70 years, with a fasting plasma cholesterol greater than 5.17 mmol/L (200 mg/dL) were recruited by newspaper advertisement for a three-month prospective intervention using a low-fat, low-cholesterol, Step 1 diet.[22,23] After four weeks, one group was randomly assigned to consume one iodine-enriched egg per day hypothesized to lower blood lipids. A registered dietitian (RD) gave individual counseling at the onset and twice during the first five weeks. Biweekly reinforcement with a nurse practitioner occurred through Week 12. Eating behavior instruction included reading food labels, calculating fat and

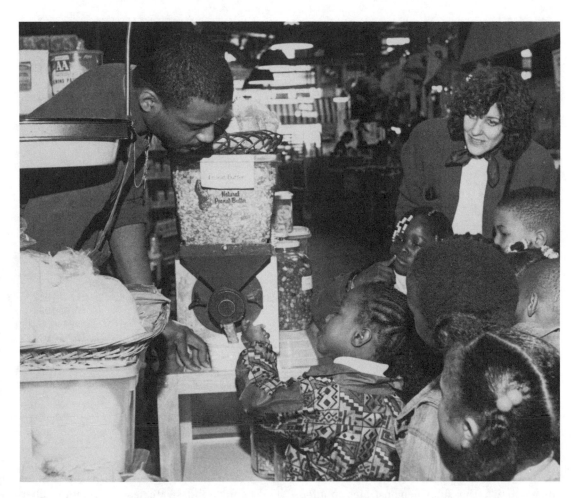

Figure 5-4 continued

cholesterol content, and recording three-day dietary food records weekly. No energy restriction occurred. Fasting blood lipid and lipoprotein levels were analyzed at entry (Week 0), baseline (Weeks 3 and 4), and at the completion of the trial (Weeks 8, 10, and 12). After the initial 12-week trial (N = 105), participants completed a six-month dietary adherence and lipoprotein profile.

Lipid level changes from entry to baseline were plasma total cholesterol 12% to 13% and low-density lipoprotein (LDL) cholesterol 9% to 12.6% for both groups. At the final measure, total cholesterol and LDL levels for the control group had risen from baseline. For the group, there were significantly greater increases of 7.2% and 9.2%, $p<0.01$, respectively, in total cholesterol and LDL levels after ingesting the egg each day while on the diet. More than two-thirds of the participants believed they followed the dietary recommendations successfully during the 12-week study; 30% reported maintaining the diet during follow-up. Those who did not maintain the diet had greater increases in total cholesterol levels.

Table 5–2 Dietary Assessment Methods and Nutrition Monitoring Activities, INTERHEALTH Countries

		Year of Survey	
Site	Method	Baseline	Follow-Up
Australia	Food frequency questionnaire	1985	
China			
(Beijin and Tianjin)	3 days of dietary recall with weighted salt use	1989	1991
Cuba	24-hour recall and food habit questionnaire	1990	
Cyprus	24-hour recall	1989	
Finland	3-day food records, food habit questionnaire	1972	1982
			1991
Japan	24-hour recall	1975–1977	
Lithuania	24-hour recall and food habit questionnaire	1983	1986
			1991
Malta	Food frequency and household budget survey	1984	1989–1990
Mauritius	24-hour recall, diet habit survey, food frequency		
	questionnaire, household inventory	1987	1992
Russia	24-hour recall and food frequency	1986	1990–1991
USA—Florida	Food frequency, food habit questionnaire	1992	
USA—California	24-hour recall and food intake questionnaire	1978–1980	1980–1982
			1982–1984
			1984–1986
			1988–1990
USA—Texas	Food frequency	1985–1987	1991
			1994–1995
Tanzania	Food frequency and food habit survey	1992	

Source: Adapted from Posner BM, Quatromoni PA, Franz M. Nutrition Policies and Interventions for Chronic Disease Risk Reduction in International Settings: The INTERHEALTH Nutrition Initiative. *Nutr Rev*. 1994;52(5):179–187.

Besides evaluating the effect of adding an iodine-rich egg, this study demonstrates an intervention devoid of either a physician-patient relationship, a continuous RD contact for medical nutrition therapy, or a health-risk level. Participants were fairly healthy volunteers, motivation and health beliefs were not measured, and participants did not receive feedback from their physician regarding their blood lipid response. No commitment was made to long-term adherence or a six-month follow-up.

Nonadherence in secondary prevention is common.[22] It often occurs when the regimen is complex, long, dependent on lifestyle alteration, inconvenient, or expensive.[24] Individuals are usually successful achieving modest reductions in lipoprotein levels with short-term dietary changes.

Theories and strategies to promote adherence address the way individuals perceive their illness and treatment and how effective their efforts will be.[24-28] Students are referred to Meichenbaum and Turk's *Facilitating Treatment Adherence: A Practitioner's Guidebook*.[29] General recommendations to increase adherence to group and individual nutrition counseling include the following[30]:

- Keep the messages brief, specific, and clear.
- Prioritize the medical nutrition therapy into small, sequential stages.
- Orient participants to behaviors not just knowledge.

- Tailor recommendations.
- Reward short-term accomplishments.
- Encourage a support system with community nutrition professionals and/or behavior therapists.
- Verify understanding and acceptance of the therapy.
- Conduct frequent booster sessions.
- Keep consistent contact via postcards and preappointment telephone calls.

Info Line

APHIS	Animal and Plant Health Inspection Service (USDA)
ARS	Agricultural Research Service (USDA)
CSRS	Cooperative State Research Service (USDA)
FMI	Food Marketing Institute
FNB	Food and Nutrition Board of Institute of Medicine/ National Academy of Sciences
FSIS	Food Safety and Inspection Service (USDA)
GMA	Grocery Manufacturers of America
NAEHE	National Association of Extension Home Economists
NASULGC	National Association of State Universities and Land Grant Colleges
NAWD	National Association of WIC Directors
NFPA	National Food Processors Association
RISE	Responsible Industry for a Sound Environment

Exhibit 5-5   Model Nutrition Objective for Improved Health Status

By 19____, the prevalence of nutrition-related growth and developmental anomalies and/or risk factor(s), namely (risk factor*) among (target group) will be reduced from _____ to _____.

By 19____, the incidence/prevalence/morbidity/ mortality associated with nutrition-related chronic disease (abnormal exercise stress test, angina, coronary bypass surgery, cancers, hypertension, strokes, diabetes, osteoporosis, dental problems, malnutrition) will be reduced from _____ to _____ among (target group).

*Low birth weight, delayed growth, underweight, iron deficiency, fetal alcohol syndrome, inappropriate infant feeding practices, inadequate pregnancy weight gain, dental caries, eating disorders, inborn errors of metabolism (specific conditions), and "children with special needs" conditions (specify).

Source: Adapted from *Model State Nutrition Objectives*, The Association of State and Territorial Public Health Nutrition Directors, 1988.

HEALTHY PEOPLE 2000 ACTIONS

Community nutrition professionals are closely linked to nutrition policy, health care reform, and population-based change in the United States. Improving the overall health status of the US public is the intended outcome of these three broad movements. Specific nutrition objectives can be established by community nutrition professionals to support the effort.

Exhibits 5-5 through 5-7 provide a framework for developing nutrition objectives to improve health status and services.

Exhibit 5-6 Model Nutrition Objectives for Improved Services/Protection

By 19__, the State Health Agency (in cooperation with other officials, professionals, voluntary agencies, organizations, and industry) will establish dietary guidance recommendations for the general public and (target population) and promote the availability, accessibility, and consumption of a nutritionally adequate and prudent diet in (restaurants, food markets, schools, media, work sites, and institutions).

By 19___, _____ percent of restaurants, _____ percent of secondary school districts will provide/include nutrition education as part of required comprehensive school health education; and _____ percent of school food service programs will comply with established state or federal recommendations for implementation of the Dietary Guidelines.

By 19___, _____ percent of restaurants, _____ percent of work site cafeterias, and _____ percent of food markets exceeding _____ size will participate in point-of-purchase nutrition education and promotion programs.

By 19___, the state will be protected by an operational system of inspection, surveillance, reporting, investigation, intervention, enforcement, follow up, and training for protection against hazardous chemical or biological contamination of food.

By 19___, the state will have a (mass media, training, professional seminar) program to educate the public on the issues of normal nutrition, diet and disease, food safety, and nutrition fraud.

By 19___, ___ percent of (well-child care; prenatal visits; screenings for coronary heart disease or cancer risk factors; medical management of diabetes, hypertension, elevated cholesterol; preventive care of the elderly) contacts should include some element of nutrition screening, assessment, counseling, or education provided by the health professionals in (publicly funded programs, private medical care, health fairs, etc.).

Source: Adapted from *Model State Nutrition Objectives*, The Association of State and Territorial Public Health Nutrition Directors, 1988.

Exhibit 5-7 Model Nutrition Objectives for Improved Surveillance and Evaluation

By 19__, the State Health Agency will have a nutrition monitoring system that will assess and report on any or all of the following:

- nutritional status of various population groups
- food intake patterns
- quantity, quality, and distribution of the food supply including the adequacy of public and private food assistance
- availability and quality of nutrition services and staff
- nutrition education needs

By 19__, the State Health Agency will establish and implement a quality assurance mechanism for monitoring, evaluating, and auditing current activities to measure progress; identify factors that interfere with program effectiveness; and determine the need for continuation or modification of operations and compliance with nutrition standards.

By 19__, the State Health Agency will have a systematic, comprehensive nutrition program plan.

By 19__, the State Health Agency will establish standards for the following:

- nutritional status of the population
- dietary intake of the population
- public and professional nutrition education
- delivery of nutrition services (e.g., nutrition screening, assessment, referral, intervention, and follow up)
- nutrition personnel qualifications and performance

By 19__, mechanisms will be established to finance and/or recover costs for public health nutrition program/services utilizing (federal funds, state and local funds, fee-for-service, third-party reimbursements, grants, contracts, donations, in-kind contributions).

Source: Adapted from *Model State Nutrition Objectives*, The Association of State and Territorial Public Health Nutrition Directors, 1988.

REFERENCES

1. American Dietetic Association. *Health Care Reform Statement*. Chicago, Ill: American Dietetic Association; 1994.

2. *Surgeon General's Report on Nutrition and Health*. Washington, DC: US Department of Health and Human Services; 1988. Public Health Service publication 88-50210.

3. Coalition for Nutrition Services in Health Care Reform. Position statement. Washington, DC, 1993.

4. California Dietetic Association. Cost of services. Playa del Rey, Calif; 1994.

5. Smith JS. Arthur D. Little, Inc; 1993.

6. Sims LS. Public policy in nutrition: A framework for action. *Nutr Today*. 1993;28(2): 10–20.

7. Chapman N. Consensus and coalitions—key to nutrition policy development. *Nutr Today.* 1987;22(5):22–29.

8. Matz M. School food service and nutrition. *American School Food Service Journal.* 1994;48(7):82–83.

9. US Department of Agriculture/US Department of Health and Human Services. *Nutrition and Your Health: Dietary Guidelines for Americans.* 2nd ed. Washington, DC: US Government Printing Office; 1985. Publication HG-232.

10. World Health Organization. Developing a Nutrition Policy Statement. Helsing, Switzerland; 1989.

11. Spasoff RA. The role of nutrition in healthy public policy. *Rapport.* 1989;4:6–7.

12. Sims LS. Nutrition policy through the Reagan Era: Feast or famine? Presented at Pew/Cornell Lecture Series on Food and Nutrition Policy; 1988; Ithaca, NY.

13. McNutt K. Integrating nutrition and environmental objectives. *Nutr Today.* 1990;25(6):40–41.

14. Johnson R. American Dietetic Association. Child nutrition reauthorization. Testimony given before the Senate Agriculture, Nutrition and Forestry Committee. 1994.

15. Belasco JA. Teaching the elephant to dance. In: *Executive Book Summaries.* Bristol, Vt: Soundview Publishers; 1990:1–8.

16. Sutnick M. Personal communication. Philadelphia, Pa: The Reading Terminal Farmers' Market Trust; 1994.

17. CANFit. Berkeley, Calif; 1994.

18. Litrak J, Ruiz L, Restrepo HE, et al. The growing burden of noncommunicable diseases: A challenge for the countries of the Americas. *Bull Pan Am Health Organ.* 1987;21:156–169.

19. Posner BM, Quatromoni PA, Franz M. Nutrition policies and interventions for chronic disease risk reduction in international settings: The INTERHEALTH Nutrition Initiative. *Nutr Rev.* 1994;52:179–187.

20. Epstein FH, Holland WW. Prevention of chronic diseases in the community—one-disease versus multiple-disease strategies. *Int J Epidemiol.* 1983;12:135–137.

21. Posner BM, Franz M, Quatromoni P, and the INTERHEALTH Steering Committee. Nutrition and the global risk for chronic disease: The INTERHEALTH Nutrition Initiative. *Nutr Rev.* 1994;52:201–207.

22. Henkin Y, Garber DW, Osterlund LC, et al. Saturated fats, cholesterol, and the dietary compliance. *Arch Intern Med.* 1992;152:1167–1174.

23. Garber DW, Henkin Y, Osterlund LC, et al. Plasma lipoproteins in hyperlipidemic subjects eating iodine-enriched eggs. *J Am Coll Nutr.* 1992;11:294–303.

24. Eraker SA, Kirscht JP, Becker MH. Understanding and improving patient compliance. *Ann Intern Med.* 1984;100:258–268.

25. Rosenstock IM. Understanding and enhancing patient compliance with diabetic regimens. *Diab Care.* 1985;8:610–616.

26. Green LW. How physicians can improve patients' participation and maintenance in self-care. *West J Med.* 1987;147:346–349.

27. Raab C, Tillotson JL. *Heart to Heart: A Manual on Nutrition Counseling for Reduction of Cardiovascular Disease Risk Factors.* Washington, DC: US Department of Health and Human Services; 1983. NIH publication 83-1528.

28. American Heart Association. *Dietary Treatment of Hypercholesterolemia: A Handbook for Counselors.* Dallas, Tex: American Heart Association; 1988.

29. Meichenbaum D, Turk D. *Facilitating Treatment Adherence: A Practitioner's Guidebook.* New York, NY: Plenum Press; 1987.

30. Kushner RF. Long-term compliance with a lipid lowering diet. *Nutr Rev.* 1993;51(1):16–23.

Appendix 5-A

Testimony of The American Dietetic Association on Child Nutrition Reauthorization, Senate Agriculture, Nutrition and Forestry Committee, May 16, 1994, given by Dr. Rachel Johnson, R.D.

ADA applauds Senator Leahy and this Committee for its strong support and interest in making our nation's child nutrition programs the best they can be. ADA believes that S. 1614, the "Better Nutrition and Health for Children Act," is a step in the right direction as it will benefit our nation's most valuable resource, children.

Dietitians and nutritionists who work with these child nutrition programs know that these programs improve the dietary intake and nutritional health of the nation's children. In addition, studies by the General Accounting Office (GAO), USDA, and others have verified the enormous success of these programs. ADA believes however, that changes could be made to improve these programs and build upon their past successes. For example, children must be provided with learning opportunities to make food choices that can play an important role in their health later in life. The eating habits developed in childhood can last a lifetime, making nutrition education an important component in children's lives.

There are several key issues that must be addressed with legislative action if these programs are to provide leadership in further improving the health and well being of children:

- improved nutritional quality using the principles of balance, variety, and moderation
- increased nutrition education and training
- increased access to the child nutrition programs
- reduced paperwork

First of all, the child nutrition program meals should be required to meet the Dietary Guidelines for Americans, including those for fat and saturated fat. ADA believes that meals served to children should meet a weekly average of 30 percent of total calories from fat and 10 percent of total calories from saturated fat. In addition, emphasis should be put on increasing the amount of fruits, vegetables, fiber, and grain products and on building healthful meals to include moderate amounts of sodium and sugar. . . .

Second, nutrition education and training, geared to making healthier food choices, should be a component of all child nutrition programs. Nutrition education helps the public understand the relationship between what they eat and their future health. Food consumption choices are usually shaped early in life, and schools should be a

Source: Reprinted with permission from Johnson R. American Dietetic Association. Child Nutrition Reauthorization. Testimony given before the Senate Agriculture, Nutrition and Forestry Committee. 1994.

primary source for nutrition education from kindergarten onward.

For nutrition education to be truly successful, school administrators and teachers must work with nutrition professionals to jointly implement classroom-lunchroom programs. Innovative school nutrition education programs demonstrate that students increase consumption of healthful school meals when nutrition taught in the classroom is coordinated with what is served in the lunchroom. Children are not born with good eating habits; they are learned. It has been documented that without nutrition education, student participation rates drop when school meals are abruptly improved. If participation rates drop, this provides a wide open door for competitive foods.

Third, access to each of the programs should be enhanced so that all children who need these services can benefit from them.

Last of all, paperwork must be reduced in order for school feeding programs to further improve the health and nutritional status of the nation's children. Food service personnel could then focus more efforts on improving the nutritional quality of meals rather than complying with a heavy administrative paperwork burden.

ADA has developed specific recommendations that both Congress and USDA could implement to enhance the effectiveness, efficiency, and nutritional quality of the child nutrition programs. ADA's recommendations include:

1. Schools should be allowed to adopt nutrient-based menu planning or a modified USDA meal pattern for meals offered. This would allow schools to plan their menus based on the nutrient content of the meal rather than the current meal pattern method which hampers creative menu planning. . . . ADA supports the change to allow low-fat yogurt as a substitute for eggs, meat, peanut butter, or other meat alternatives.
2. Nutrition education must be expanded. The federal government must make efforts to coordinate the food offered in the lunchroom to the education in the classroom in order to help our nation's children and adolescents develop healthful eating patterns.

3. The whole milk requirement for schools should be repealed. This would allow schools to choose the type(s) of milk appropriate for their students and facilitate efforts to meet the Dietary Guidelines. Eliminating the whole milk mandate is one of the ways Congress can give child nutrition programs the flexibility they need to implement positive changes in school meal patterns.
4. Legal authority should be provided to ensure that foods competing with the child nutrition programs promote the nutritional goals of the Dietary Guidelines. Research shows that the noon-time meals children select from vending machines, snack bars, and ala carte programs are inferior in nutrient content to school lunches. In general, these meals are high in fat, saturated fat, and cholesterol, and *lack* the amount of essential vitamins and minerals contained in school meals. The sale of competitive foods in snack bars, school stores, and banks of vending machines competes with school meals for students' appetites, time, and money. Availability of competitive foods poses three major problems: (1) it diverts income essential to the financial well-being of the school meal program, (2) it encourages the consumption of partial meals, and (3) it fosters the erroneous idea that school meals are only for needy children. Competitive foods create an environment that often is not consistent with sound principles of nutrition education taught in school classrooms and cafeterias.
5. Paperwork must be reduced for all child nutrition programs. School nutrition directors and child care program directors need relief from their burden of paperwork. This will allow them time to concentrate on improving the dietary quality of meals and providing nutrition education.
6. Direct USDA to modify specifications for commodities and to purchase commodities that help schools meet Dietary Guidelines.

In summary, ADA applauds the efforts of Congress to make improvements in the child nutrition programs. It is critical for children to learn good lifelong eating habits. Children are one of the most vulnerable segments of society. They depend on their families and communities to provide a nurturing environment that will enable them to become healthy and productive adults. The improvements that Senator Leahy has proposed for the nation's child nutrition programs will provide America's children with the healthy start they need. We appreciate the opportunity to share our views and stand ready as child nutrition experts to help the Committee with its work on this important issue.

Part II

Primary Prevention of Disease

6

Food-Borne Illness

Learning Objectives

- Contrast infectious disease with noninfectious disease.
- Define the progressive sequence that occurs in a food-borne illness.
- Enumerate the basic food service sanitation procedures, including the steps in the hazard analysis and critical control points (HACCP) system.
- List the major bacteria causing food-borne illnesses.
- Define the role of pesticides in food production.
- List the components of an emergency survival kit.

High Definition Nutrition

Endemic a persistent but low to average disease expression.

Epidemic outbreak—occurrence exceeds the expectation.

Food hazard—a source of danger that is contained within an edible food. Microbial food poisoning or allergic reactions create an immediate effect.

Food risk—an indicator of the probability and severity of harm to human health after expo-

sure to a food hazard. Scientists determine food risk when they identify a hazard; determine the relationship between the dose, amount, or potential for the hazard; and determine the dose or exposure.

Food safety—an estimate of acceptable risk from consuming foods containing potential hazard. A substance in food is considered safe if the risks are estimated as acceptable.

Hyperendemic—persistently high occurrence.

Infectivity—the proportion or ratio of exposed persons who become infected to those who do not become infected.

Pandemic—an epidemic that occurs in several countries or continents.

Pathogenicity—the proportion or ratio of infected persons who develop clinical disease in relation to those exposed.

Sporadic—an irregular occurrence.

Virulence—the proportion of persons with clinical disease who experience morbidity and/or mortality.

INFECTIOUS AND NONINFECTIOUS DISEASES

Community nutrition professionals are generally employed in jobs that address chronic disease rather than infectious disease. The 1990s

187

is witnessing an increasing number of food-borne illnesses, disasters, and deaths from both types of disease. Identifying the cause of a food-borne illness and employing procedures to eliminate the cause have given community nutrition professionals opportunities to apply their skills to food production, provide inservice education for employees and the public, and inspect food facilities. Preparing for and managing disasters such as earthquakes and floods means adequate food supplies must be kept safe and sanitary. This chapter addresses the infectious disease process, food-borne illness, pesticides, sanitation procedures, and preparing for community emergencies.

In infectious disease, health outcomes are influenced by exposure to a causal factor. Some individuals are infectious, yet have no subclinical disease. They are called *carriers*, because they are incubating a disease or infection. The reservoir for an agent is the habitat in which the agent exists. Reservoirs may be humans, animals, or the environment. The reservoir could be the transmission source by which an agent moves to a host. *Clostridium botulinum* exists in the soil, but the medium for infection is often improperly canned food containing the *C. botulinum* spores. Humans and animals are common reservoirs for infectious disease. An infection transfer model begins with disease transmission that occurs when the agent leaves a reservoir or host through a portal of exit and is transferred to another host via a portal of entry. This process is called the *chain of infection*.[1,2]

In contrast, in the noninfectious disease process or chronic disease progression, coinhabitants in one environment (e.g., a family living in one house) may follow similar unhealthy eating and exercise patterns. These individuals are unaware of their risk and are simply blind targets. Does this situation create an invisible chain of disease progression? Does the parent or guardian become the *initiator* of a habit and the environment a *promotor*, with the child an unknowing or passive *recipient*?

Asymptomatic individuals remain at risk. They lack knowledge of their own risk. These individuals are undiagnosed and therefore unable to receive or to attempt intervention to forestall the disease progression. The environment is a major agent for disease progression. The magnitude of influence can range from minimal (if genetics has a large influence), to maximum (if genetics has little influence). In chronic disease development the environment becomes the home, neighborhood, norms, and policies that influence the knowledge, attitudes, and practices of individuals and communities.

PORTAL OF EXIT AND ENTRY

Portal of exit is the path or route an agent takes to leave its source host. Generally the exit corresponds to the site by which the agent creates exposure to others.

When an agent leaves its natural reservoir, it can enter a susceptible host directly, indirectly, mechanically, or biologically. *Direct transmission* is an immediate transfer to a susceptible host usually by direct contact. *Indirect transmission* requires an intermediary. *Mechanical transmission* describes the process by which an agent does not grow or alter its form but is physically placed in the vector. *Biologic transmission* refers to the transfer of an agent to a host followed by an agent modifying its form.[2]

Indirect vehicles (e.g., food, fomites such as plates, forks, and cups) can transmit agents. A dented can of food is an inviting receptacle for *C. botulinum*, which produces the fatal botulism toxin.

Agents enter susceptible hosts through a portal of entry. For example, a fecal-oral transmission involves an intestinal agent that lives in and is excreted by a host's gastrointestinal tract. Later the agent enters the intestinal tract of a new host through another vehicle (e.g., food, water, or an eating utensil).[2]

A susceptible *host* becomes the final stage for infection transfer. Genetic factors, immunity, and nutritional status influence the individual's susceptibility. *Herd immunity* describes the condition of a group when its characteristics slow or limit the dissemination of the disease. Disease can occur at different levels of intensity.[2] Epidemics occur under several conditions as follows:

- an adequate number of agents and hosts exist simultaneously
- an agent moves with ease within a group of susceptible hosts
- virulence of an agent has increased
- an agent has entered a new, receptive environment
- new transfer methods have occurred
- host susceptibility or entry has changed

BACTERIA AND FOOD-BORNE ILLNESS

Bacteria cause 90 percent of the cases of food-borne illness, and symptoms are variable (see Appendix 6–A). Foods containing either a poison or toxin produced by bacteria, chemicals, or viruses can produce a food-borne illness.[2-5] Bacteria are often transferred by infected food handlers, but unsanitary equipment or storage procedures can create the problem (see Exhibit 6–1). Bacteria and toxins contaminate foods through a chain of factors. The sequence is:

food → bacteria → employee → moisture → temperature → time

The Centers for Disease Control and Prevention (CDC) estimates that about six million cases of illness and 9,000 deaths are related to food-borne disease annually in the United States.[3] In California, 324 outbreaks with almost 10,000 illnesses were reported from 1983 to 1992. The agent and transmission mode are illustrated in Figure 6–1.

Factors

Food

Different bacteria have different food needs. Bacteria that cause illness prefer nonacidic foods, such as milk, eggs, meat, poultry, and fish because bacteria thrive best in them. Since most vegetables are slightly acidic, bacteria within them multiply slowly. Fruits, made acidic by adding vinegar or lemon juice, are not good media for bacterial growth. Surprisingly, baked potatoes, refried beans, and cooked rice can be potentially

Exhibit 6–1 Practices That Promote Bacteria Transfer

- improper holding temperatures
- inadequate cooking procedures
- poor personal hygiene practices
- unsanitary equipment
- contaminated food supplies

hazardous when kept barely warm during a long serving period (see Exhibit 6–2).

Bacteria

Many bacteria are beneficial to humans because they assist with the production of cheese, yogurt, buttermilk, and sauerkraut. The majority of bacteria are neither beneficial nor harmful to humans. There are harmful bacteria, however, including salmonella, campylobacter, *Clostridium perfringens, Staphylococcus aureus, Escherichia coli*, and *Clostridium botulinum.*

Handling Procedures

Food service workers control the amount of time and temperature of food during preparation. If proper handling procedures are not followed, then food held for two hours even at ideal temperatures may initiate a food-borne illness. Inservice education of employees and quality controls are essential. Hair nets, caps, chef hats, or painters' caps must be worn in all food preparation and service areas. Clothes, uniforms, and aprons must be clean and free from odors. Employees should brush off their shoulders and clothing after combing or brushing their hair when in restrooms. Hands and fingernails must be kept clean, and dangling jewelry and nail polish should not be allowed.

Smoke-free environments are essential near food storage, preparation, and service. "No smoking" signs must be posted in all food preparation, storage, service, and cleanup areas. Hands must be washed after eating, smoking, blowing one's nose, sneezing, or coughing. Signs about washing hands after using the toilet facilities must be posted in all restrooms.

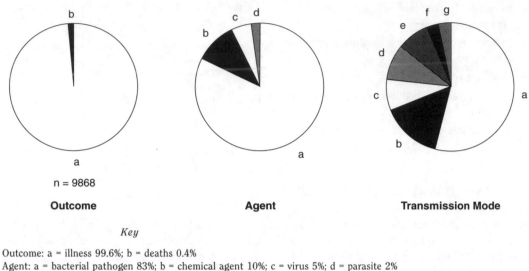

Outcome   **Agent**   **Transmission Mode**

n = 9868

Key

Outcome: a = illness 99.6%; b = deaths 0.4%
Agent: a = bacterial pathogen 83%; b = chemical agent 10%; c = virus 5%; d = parasite 2%
Transmission Mode: a = improper storage or handling temperature 54%;
                    b = poor personal hygiene 15%;
                    c = other mishandling 8%;
                    d = unsafe sources 9%;
                    e = contaminated equipment = 8%;
                    f = inadequate cooling 4%; g = other, unknown 2%

Figure 6-1 A profile of food-borne illness outbreaks, California, 1983–1992 (*N* = 324 reported outbreaks, with 9,868 cases of illness). *Source:* Bruhn C. Safety and Quality of Foods in California. White paper. California Nutrition Council Symposium–Future directions for nutrition policy in California. December 13, 1994. Sacramento, CA.

Exhibit 6-2 High-Risk Foods for Bacterial Growth

- milk and milk products
- eggs
- meat
- poultry
- fish or shellfish
- mayonnaise-based meat and vegetable salads
- baked potatoes
- cooked rice
- refried beans

Food handlers must be free from infections and communicable diseases. All cuts on hands must be covered with a bandage and plastic glove and reported to supervisors.

Inspections of food service facilities are usually conducted by trained staff in the local environmental health agency. Inspection criteria are generally detailed in the state's uniform retail food facilities law.

Moisture

Water or liquid is necessary for bacterial growth. Therefore, milk, water, and juice are viable sources.

Temperature

Temperatures from 45 to 140°F promote bacterial growth with fastest growth between 72 and 98°F. Some bacteria thrive at 113°F or higher and can initiate spoilage in canned foods stored in hot areas. Other bacteria that thrive in cool places can spoil foods stored for extended periods in the refrigerator. A refrigerator checklist can be used to evaluate proper storage procedures (see Exhibit 6-3). Freezing food slows multiplication of bacteria but does not destroy them. During thawing, bacteria start to multiply at about 45°F. Two safety zones that kill and retard the growth of bacteria are 165°F and higher or 40°F and below, respectively.

Exhibit 6-3 Refrigerator Checklist To Evaluate Proper Storage

- Is the refrigerator temperature 40°F or below? Yes___ No___
  If your answer is no, then record the temperature of the refrigerator and report it to your supervisor.
  _____

- Are the foods placed in the proper section? Yes___ No___
  If no, explain _____
  _____
  _____

- Are foods stored in the correct type of containers? Yes___ No___
  If no, explain _____
  _____
  _____

- Are the foods that give off odors separated from those that absorb odors? Yes___ No___
  If no, explain _____
  _____
  _____

- Is the refrigerator overcrowded? Yes___ No___
- Are foods in the refrigerator labeled and dated? Yes___ No___
  If no, explain _____
  _____
  _____

- Are similar foods stored in the same general area? Yes___ No___
  If no, explain _____
  _____
  _____

- Are older foods brought to the front so that they will be used first? Yes___ No___

Hazardous foods must be rapidly cooled to an internal temperature of 40°F or below and checked with a food thermometer. Large quantities of hazardous foods should be placed in shallow pans, stirred frequently, and cooled rapidly. When transporting hazardous foods, refrigerating them ahead of time to 35°F and holding them at 40°F or below is essential.

The golden rule is: Keep hot food hot (140°F or hotter) and cold food cold (40°F or colder).

Time

At favorable temperatures, bacteria double about every 20 minutes. Contaminated foods already begin with thousands of bacteria. See Exhibit 6-4 for a checklist to prevent bacteria growth.

FOOD SERVICE SANITATION PROCEDURES

Certain procedures are recommended for maintaining sanitary food service conditions and eliminating food-borne illnesses.[6]

Exhibit 6-4 Checklist To Prevent Bacteria Growth

- Follow correct hand-washing procedures.
- Keep foods protected.
- Maintain correct refrigerator and freezer storage procedures.
- Thaw foods properly.
- Cook foods adequately.
- Cool foods quickly.
- Maintain correct temperatures during holding and transporting.
- Keep infectious workers away from food.

Protection from Food Safety Hazards

Food must be protected from potential contamination when stored, prepared, displayed, served, or transported. Dust, insects, rodents, unclean equipment and utensils, unnecessary handling, coughs and sneezes, flooding, drainage, and overhead leakage or overhead drippage from condensation are all potential sources of contamination.

Refrigerator Storage Practices

Refrigerators need visible internal thermometers to monitor temperature regularly. A temperature of 40°F or lower is safe. The preferred refrigerator storage procedures for specific foods are listed in Table 6–1. Food containers should be:

- covered to protect the food from contamination
- arranged for ease of cleaning and air circulation
- stored six inches or more above the floor in walk-in refrigerators

Freezer Storage Practices

Frozen foods should be frozen at 0°F or below. A thermometer should be kept in freezers, and foods should be arranged to allow air to circulate. Proper packaging can prevent freezer burn and protect foods. Potentially hazardous foods must be thawed in refrigerators below 40°F, under clean running water of 70°F or below, or in a microwave—and cooked immediately.

Dry Storage Practices

Dry storerooms should be monitored to protect the food from insects, rodents, high temperatures, and high humidity. A range of 55 to 70°F discourages bacterial action and food deterioration.

Hot Storage Practices

Potentially hazardous foods must have an internal temperature of 140°F or above during service or transportation.

Table 6–1 Guidelines for Refrigerating Specific Foods

Food	Procedure
Butter	Wrap butter to prevent absorption of odors and to protect it from exposure to light and air, which hastens rancidity. Remove soiled shipping container.
Cheese	Wrap cheese lightly to prevent drying out. Do not freeze, because freezing breaks the grain and causes cheese to crumble (or shred cheese and then freeze it).
Dairy products and eggs	Refrigerate milk, cheese, butter, and eggs immediately. Store dairy products and eggs away from strong-flavored foods. Cross-stack egg crates for air circulation.
Fresh fruits and vegetables	Refrigerate fresh fruits and vegetables immediately to preserve color, flavor, texture, and nutritive value. Leave paper wrappings on fruits to prevent spoilage and moisture loss. Store fruits and vegetables so cold air can circulate. Examine produce for freshness before storing. Use very ripe items immediately.
Meats, fish, and poultry	Refrigerate fresh meats, fish, and poultry immediately. For most items, remove outer paper wrapping and cover lightly.
Cooked foods	Use clean, covered containers that promote quick cooling. Quick cool (within two hours) hot foods to refrigeration temperature to avoid food poisoning. Keep precooked foods refrigerated until serving (e.g., cream- or custard-filled pastries, puddings, salads, sandwiches, cold meats). Use foods within two to three days, preferably within 24 hours. Discard cooked foods if they have been removed from refrigeration and reheated for serving more than two times.

Food Preparation and Service Procedures

Food should be touched rarely by human hands. Disposable plastic gloves are essential. Clean and sanitary utensils and preparation surfaces are essential to prevent cross-contamination from other foods. Raw fruits or vegetables should be thoroughly washed with clean, running water before being cooked or served. Poultry, poultry stuffing, stuffed meats, and stuffing containing meat must be cooked to 165°F or higher. Pork and any food containing pork must be cooked to at least 165°F. Rare roast beef must be cooked to an internal temperature of at least 130°F. Food served to a customer but not eaten should be discarded.

Food Transportation Practices

To prevent contamination during transportation (e.g., transfer to a school or congregate feeding site), food and food utensils must be covered, completely wrapped, or packaged. Hot foods must be 165°F or higher before they are placed in transport carts or containers, and cold foods must be at a temperature of 35°F. Written records should be kept for a year of food temperatures before transport, upon arrival, and prior to service.

HIGH-RISK GROUPS FOR FOOD-BORNE ILLNESS

Several groups are considered at high risk if they eat contaminated seafood. This includes individuals with liver disease, diabetes mellitus, immune disorders, and gastrointestinal disorders (see Exhibit 6–5). Children, older adults, individuals receiving chemotherapy or radiation treatment, and individuals suffering from a debilitating disease (e.g., diabetes) are at high risk for severe illness if they acquire a food-borne illness.[7,8]

CONTROL PROCEDURES

In a report from the Centers for Disease Control and Prevention (CDC), 97% of food-borne ill-

Exhibit 6–5 FDA Warning and High-Risk Groups

The Food and Drug Administration (FDA) warns that patients with diabetes are at serious risk of *Vibrio* infection from eating raw shellfish. While this infection is not a threat to most healthy patients, certain susceptible patients can be exposed to the infection by eating raw or undercooked molluscan shellfish (oysters, mussels, clams, and whole scallops). The population groups that are particularly vulnerable to severe illness or even death if they ingest contaminated seafood are those with liver disease, diabetes mellitus, immune disorders, and gastrointestinal disorders.

The high-risk season for raw shellfish consumption begins in April, when warmer water encourages the growth of the bacteria *Vibrio vulnificus*. The symptoms of the infection include fever, chills, nausea, vomiting, and abdominal pain. The bacteria are killed when shellfish are thoroughly cooked.

More information is available in a series of four brochures entitled "Get Hooked on Seafood Safety." For a free copy, write to: FDA, Seafood Brochures, HFI-40, 5600 Fishers Lane, Rockville, MD 20857. Indicate which brochure you want: diabetes mellitus, gastrointestinal disorders, immune disorders, or liver disease.

Source: American Diabetes Association. *Professional Section Newsletter.* Summer 1993.

nesses that occurred from 1983 to 1987 were preventable if individuals had used improved food-handling practices.[3] A copy of the form developed by CDC to investigate food-borne outbreaks is given in Exhibit 6–6.

The most common food-borne pathogens remain the same, decade after decade, and the ways they can be controlled rarely change. The problems are the lack of basic knowledge by consumers and food handlers, and the lack of personal commitment to acceptable, safe procedures. For all foods, individuals should check the dates on the packages and not violate the "keep refrigerated," "sell by," and "use by" dates. Some specific guides for reducing exposure to or proliferation of common bacteria that cause food-borne illness follow.

Campylobacter jejuni

This microorganism is commonly found in raw foods of animal origin.[9] Wash hands and utensils

Exhibit 6-6 Form for Investigating Outbreak of Food-Borne Illness

1. Where did the outbreak occur?

State _____

City or Town _____   County _____

2. Date of outbreak: (Date of onset 1st case)

_____

MO/DA/YR

3. Indicate actual (a) or estimated (e) numbers:

Persons exposed _____

Persons ill _____

Hospitalized _____

Fatal case _____

4. History of Exposed Persons:

No. histories obtained _____

No. persons with symptoms ____

Nausea _____

Diarrhea _____

5. Incubation period (hours):

Shortest _____ Longest _____

Approx. for majority _____

6. Duration of illness (hours) _____

Shortest _____ Longest _____

Approx. for majority _____

7. Food - Specific attack rates:

Food Items Served	Number of persons who ATE specified food _____				Number who did NOT eat specified food _____			
	Ill	Not	Total	Percent Ill	Ill	Not	Total	Percent Ill

8. Vehicle responsible (food item incriminated by epidemiological evidence): _____

9. Manner in which incriminated food was marketed: (Mark all Applicable)

	Yes	No			Yes	No
(a) Food Industry			(c) Not Wrapped......		Y	N
Raw........	Y	N	Ordinary Wrapping.		Y	N
Processed	Y	N	Canned....................		Y	N
Home Produced			Canned - Vacuum Sealed		Y	N
Raw.........	Y	N	Other (specify)........		Y	N
Processed	Y	N				
(b) Vending Machine	Y	N	(d) Room Temperature		Y	N
			Refrigerator.............		Y	N
			Frozen....................		Y	N
			Heated....................		Y	N

10. Place of Preparation of Contaminated Item:

Restaurant	1
Delicate	2
Cafeteria	3
Private Home	4
Caterer	5
Institution:	
School	6
Church	7
Camp	8
Other, specify	9

11. Place where eaten:

Restaurant	1
Delicate	2
Cafeteria	3
Private Home	4
Picnic	5
Institution:	
School	6
Church	7
Camp	8
Other, specify	9

If a commerical product, indicate brand name and lot number _____

Source: Reprinted with permission of the Centers for Disease Control and Prevention. US Department of Health and Human Services. Public Health Service. Atlanta, Georgia 30333.

that contact raw meats prior to using the utensils with cooked foods. Use warm, soapy water. Cook ground meats (e.g., beef, pork, veal, and lamb) to an internal temperature of 160°F, and cook ground poultry to 165°F. Reheat leftovers to 160°F. Don't drink unpasteurized milk or other dairy products, don't drink untreated water, and don't eat raw or undercooked foods from animals. Do not allow dogs and pets in restaurants or other food preparation environments.

Clostridium perfringens

This microorganism contributed to major food-borne outbreaks recorded from 1978 to 1987.[3] Instruct employees to divide leftover roasts, turkey, stuffing, soups, stews, and casseroles into two-inch-deep portions before cooling or freezing. Reheat to 160°F. Wash all soil off vegetables.

Escherichia coli

This microorganism has appeared as a major public health problem for North America.[3] Instruct food service staff to cook all ground meats to a uniform internal temperature of at least 160°F, ground poultry to 165°F, and nonground meat cuts to 145°F. Reheat foods to 160°F. Avoid unprocessed fruit and vegetable juices and unpasteurized milk and milk products.

Salmonella

This was one of the most common microorganisms to cause food-borne illness recorded from 1978 to 1987.[3] Instruct employees to thaw poultry and meat in the refrigerator or microwave and cook them immediately after thawing. Avoid cross-contamination of raw and cooked foods, utensils, and work surfaces. Never eat unpasteurized, raw, or undercooked animal products. Cook ground meats to an internal temperature of 160°F, ground poultry to 165°F, and nonground meat to 145°F. Keep cold foods at 40°F. Reheat leftovers to 160°F. Buy eggs from refrigerated cases.

NEW FOOD-BORNE PATHOGENS

We are experiencing an era of new food-borne pathogens (see Table 6–2). Much of this is the result of environmental and societal changes, especially lifestyle. For example, the organic and natural food industry quotes 1990 sales at over $4 billion—a 7.4% increase from the previous year (even though these products cost 20 to 25% more than conventional items).[5,10] The demand for natural foods, minimally processed foods, novel or innovative food processes, and changes in agricultural practices and distribution are some of the factors behind this new order of food-borne pathogens.

Table 6–2 Food-Borne Pathogens for the 21st Century

Pathogen Status	Type
Previously unrecognized	*Salmonella enteritidis* *Vibrio vulnificus* Norwalk virus *Escherichia coli* 0157:H7
Not previously recognized as agents of food-borne disease	*Yersinia enterocolitica* *Listeria monocytogenes* *Campylobacter jejuni*
Recognized as an agent of food-borne disease, now able to grow in unique situations	*Clostridium botulinum* Conventional botulism Infant botulism

Source: Adapted from Matthews ME, Theis M. Relationship Between the Environment, the Food Supply and the Practice of Dietetics. Research Agenda Conference. *J Am Diet Assoc.* 1993.

Info Line

USDA Meat and Poultry Hotline
Monday–Friday, 10 AM–4 PM (Eastern Time)
(800) 535-4555

Centers for Disease Control and
    Prevention
Foodborne Illness Line
24-hour recorded information:
    (404) 332-4597
In Washington, DC, area, call
    (202) 720-3333

National Live Stock and Meat Board
Consumer Information Department
444 North Michigan Avenue
Chicago, Illinois 60611
Monday–Friday, 9:30 AM to 5:30 PM
    (Eastern Time)
(312) 467-5520

County Extension Home Economists
(Look in phone book under: county
    government, Cooperative Extension
    Service, or a state university)

Food and Drug Administration, Rockville,
    MD
Call (301) 443-3170, or check phone
    book under federal government listing
    for regional offices in major cities

PREPARING FOR COMMUNITY EMERGENCIES

A community emergency is an unforeseen combination of circumstances that call for immediate action, such as an earthquake, flood, hurricane, or tornado. Such a definition can encompass a wide array of circumstances, even in the area of food and nutrition. The first rule is for households to always keep a supply of familiar, easy-to-prepare, nonperishable basic foods on hand, replacing each item as it is eaten.

Water is an absolute necessity for life, and in times of emergency it may be the scarcest re-source. A 72-hour supply (three gallons per family member) is needed for food preparation and personal cleansing. In an emergency, immediately shut off the water and use the uncontaminated supply in the toilet tank and water heater. Use discarded water to flush commodes. If one suspects that the water supply is contaminated, purify by boiling, or by using 16 drops of household bleach per gallon or 24 drops of iodine per gallon, until water appears clear. Purification tablets may also be used and can be purchased at local sporting goods stores.[11]

Authorities recommend that at least a three-day supply of food for each family member be available in the event of an emergency. Ideally, these foods should be stored separately, apart from the cupboard basics. A nutrition survival plan should include the following[11]:

- the "Top 10 Staples" (see Exhibit 6–7)
- infant food needs
- pet food (for the family friend)
- barbecue and briquettes (outdoors only)
- comfort foods, such as instant coffee, cocoa, nuts, raisins, instant pudding

Minimum quantities should be planned per family member for a three-day period:

- milk: four 12-oz cans low-fat, evaporated milk

Exhibit 6–7 The Top 10 Long-Lasting, Nutritious, and Inexpensive Staples for Emergency Use

- pasta, rice, and canned or instant potatoes
- all-purpose biscuit mix
- canned fruits, vegetables, and juices
- peanut butter
- canned meats, chicken, and fish
- powdered and canned milk
- canned stew or other main dishes
- canned or dried beans (all types)
- quick-cooking or enriched dry cereals
- canned or dried soups

Source: California Dietetic Association. *Nutrition Survival Plan: A Food Guide for Emergencies, Big and Small.* 1990.

- fruits and vegetables: five 15-oz cans, assorted
- protein: three 6-oz cans of meat, or three 1-cup servings of beans
- cereals, pastas: 9 cups or 72 crackers

Storage and maintenance tips include:

- Store foods in a dry, cool area, below 70°F.
- Containers should be water resistant and dated.
- Store in basement or garage.
- Rotate foods into normal eating patterns every three to six months to maintain freshness.

HACCP IN FOOD SERVICE

HACCP, pronounced "haysap," is an acronym for hazard analysis and critical control points. This is a term for a food safety system for food service directors to prevent contamination of the food served to clients.[12]

HACCP was created in 1965 by Pillsbury Company. Pillsbury was selected by the National Aeronautics and Space Administration to provide food for US astronauts during extended space missions. The food had to be virtually 100% free of contamination. Pillsbury devised a prevention-oriented system of quality control by starting at the very beginning of food preparation. This HACCP system is applied in all steps of the preparation process. It starts with the selection of vendors and ends when the meal is eaten.

Community nutrition professionals are generally not involved in the inspection or remediation process, but it might be wise to rethink the situation. A merger between community nutrition professionals, who plan and oversee food production, and environmental specialists, who inspect and monitor food production facilities, seems practical.

The *HA* in HACCP stands for *hazard analysis*, which is the identification of any potentially hazardous ingredient or food preparation method. The *CCP* in HACCP stands for *critical control point*, which is any food preparation step where loss of control could result in an unacceptable health risk (see Exhibit 6-8).

Exhibit 6-8 Steps in the HACCP System

1. Assess hazards.
2. Determine critical points.
3. Establish limits.
4. Develop monitoring plan.
5. Devise corrective action.
6. Organize recordkeeping.
7. Verify reliability of system.

Source: HACCP: Making the System Work, *Food Engineering*, August 1988:7;70–80.

Food Service Standards and Regulations

Regulations and standards for food service sanitation and safety are enforced at the local, state, and federal levels. Local environmental health departments manage these tasks. Standards require that appropriate safeguards against contamination exist. HACCP principles can be integrated into existing regulations and standards using *HACCP Principles for Food Production*.[13]

Food service employees are trained in food safety precautions to maintain acceptable standards and can be taught HACCP principles during ongoing inservice sessions. *Applied Foodservice Sanitation*, a resource for directors, covers HACCP guidelines and employee sanitation training.[6]

Food manufacturers can analyze their products for microbes before they are distributed to the general public. Table 6-3 lists common bacteria that can cause food-borne illness.[14] The importance of preparing a safe product for clients is clear because there is no opportunity for second chances in a food service setting. Food-borne illness can have devastating consequences.

Developing a HACCP System

Not all products require extensive methods for quality control. Individually packaged prepared food products, such as crackers, muffins, chips, and cookies, have a low potential for food-borne illness.

The important first step is to identify and to evaluate any food products or preparation pro-

Table 6–3 Major Microbes in Food

Microbe	Where Found	How To Control
Salmonella	Poultry, meat, eggs	Cook thoroughly.
S. aureus	High-protein foods, foods kept at room temperature for prolonged periods	Keep hot foods hot and cold foods cold.
C. perfringens	Beef and poultry, leftover foods	Cook thoroughly. Chill rapidly and reheat leftovers thoroughly.
C. jejuni	Meat, poultry, fish	Cook thoroughly.
C. botulinum	Home-canned foods and tightly wrapped cooked potatoes, meatloaf, meat pies, stews	Use commercially canned foods. Chill rapidly and reheat leftovers thoroughly.

cedures that have potential for causing food-borne illness. For example, the potential hazards in serving canned peaches would be far less than the potential hazards for preparing ground beef for tacos. Ground beef has a high potential for bacterial contamination and goes through several critical steps in its preparation—storing, thawing, cooking, and holding. Canned peaches are free from bacterial contamination and do not require many handling steps by the food service workers.

Ground beef for tacos is used as an example to illustrate the steps of the HACCP system:

- *Step 1:* Assess hazards associated with growing and harvesting raw materials and ingredients, processing, manufacturing, distributing, marketing, preparing, and consuming the food. Each food item served by the food service organization would undergo this assessment. The hazard associated with ground beef is the potential for bacterial contamination.
- *Step 2:* Determine critical control points required to control the identified hazards. The critical control points for ground beef preparation are those steps when hazardous microorganisms need to be controlled or destroyed. Vendor selection is important to ensure that the raw product is processed and handled according to US Department of

Agriculture protocol. Storing, defrosting, cooking, holding, and possibly chilling and reheating are all critical steps for control of bacterial contamination.

- *Step 3:* Establish the critical limits that must be met at each identified critical control point. Each critical control point in food preparation must have specific limits, such as time and temperature. For example, ground beef should be kept frozen in a freezer no higher than 0°F. The meat should be defrosted in such a way as to keep its temperature below 45°F, and it should be held at a temperature of greater than 140°F. Raw ground beef should be kept separate from cooked or prepared foods at all times.
- *Step 4:* Develop procedures to monitor critical control points. A monitoring schedule must be established. The temperature of the freezer in which the ground beef is stored is probably already monitored in an organization. Continuous monitoring of critical control points is important because of the possibility for food contamination if these limits are not met (e.g., freezer temperature greater than 0°F).
- *Step 5:* Devise corrective action to be taken when there is a deviation identified by monitoring a critical control point. The limit for the critical control point of cooking ground

beef is that the beef must be cooked to 165°F. If the supervisor sees an area of beef that is not fully cooked and still pink, then this likely occurred because the cook failed to stir the ground beef thoroughly while cooking. A corrective action would be to stir the ground beef immediately to attain even heating. Long-term correction of this problem would be to add this step of frequent stirring to the list of critical limits.

- *Step 6:* Organize effective recordkeeping systems to document the HACCP plan. This step is important because the food service director may keep and use these records for continuous improvement of the organization. These records may also be made available to regulatory agencies to show compliance to specific standards.
- *Step 7:* Verify that the HACCP system is working correctly. This step is carried out by retracing the flow of ground beef during its path to reach the consumers. Reports of food poisoning should be reviewed and recorded. Controls and procedures can be reviewed periodically. Adjustments can be made to improve the food preparation process.

Food safety, along with sensory quality and client acceptance, has always been a top priority among food service operations. Over the years, food service systems in the United States have done a good job preventing food contamination. However, an immaculate and sanitary kitchen will not suffice for preventing food contamination. HACCP is an approach to ensure that food safety is integrated into the whole food path from purchase to service.

FOUR PRIORITY AREAS FOR REDUCING FOOD-BORNE DISEASE

Doyle outlined four priority areas for reducing food-borne disease.[15] These are:

1. *Emphasize risk analysis, management, and communications.* Since many foods carry an inherent risk because of the occurrence of microbial pathogens, foods could be regulated on the basis of risk. Information systems can identify foods most often associated with illnesses, identify minimum infectious dose of harmful microorganisms, determine the survival and growth characteristics of food pathogens, and determine which pathogens may or may not be tolerable in certain foods.
2. *Develop innovative approaches to produce pathogen-free foods from animals.* Innovative yet practical approaches to reduce external contamination of foods during slaughter and processing are needed to reduce the conveyance of pathogens by animals.
3. *Conduct research to support the implementation of effective HACCP programs.* Current areas needing further research are procedures to detect and to isolate pathogens in the facilities where food is processed. Procedures currently take one to four days to isolate pathogens. Tests that require minutes or hours would allow processors to respond with quick, corrective action when pathogens are detected. Steps can be applied at critical points to destroy pathogens. Innovative, practical methods are needed in food-processing plants.
4. *Develop innovative approaches to educate consumers and food preparers about proper food-handling practices.* Improper handling of foods by consumers at home and by employees in commercial food preparation has increased the incidence of salmonellosis. New approaches are needed to educate consumers and food preparers about proper food preparation and storage techniques and to clarify the risks of food-borne illness from eating raw or undercooked foods of animal origin.

Info Line

The routine measures that can be used to control further food-borne outbreaks are as follows:

1. Collect appropriate specimens for laboratory analysis, and then destroy remaining foods to prevent their consumption.
2. Prevent a recurrent event by
   a. Educating food handlers in proper food preparation and storage techniques; stress the importance of time-temperature associations.
   b. Acquiring necessary equipment for properly cooking, cooling, serving, and storing foods.
   c. When applicable, eliminating sources of contaminated food.
3. Implement basic principles in prevention of the pathogen, such as for *C. perfringens*:
   a. Cook all foods to minimum internal temperature of 165°F.

b. Serve immediately or hold at >140°F.
c. Discard any leftovers, or immediately chill and hold food at <40°F in shallow pans.
d. Reheat all leftovers and hold at proper temperatures.

The rationale for "working up" an outbreak is as follows:

1. To identify factors associated with the outbreak occurrence and to institute the necessary measures to prevent future recurrences.
2. To document that a premeditated and deliberate act of poisoning was not involved.
3. To demonstrate that public health officials can react promptly to a problem and identify causative factors using epidemiologic methods.

Source: Reproduced with permission of Paige R, Cole G, Timmrock T. *Basic Epidemiologic Methods and Biostatistics.* Boston, MA: Jones and Bartlett Publishers; 1993.

PESTICIDES IN FOODS

To combat damage to crops by insects, pesticides were introduced. Americans are as concerned about exposing their families to pesticides as they are about food-borne illnesses. Foods are not the only source of pesticides in the environment. Pets, home gardens, parks, and specialty gardens can all embody pesticides and residues. However, home and private application of pesticides are not monitored by the Food and Drug Administration (FDA) to the degree that growers are regulated. Reports from recent federal and state monitoring indicate no detectable residues in 90% or more of food test samples. When residues are detected, however, they are only a fraction of the FDA tolerance level.[16]

The FDA's total diet study is performed annually and gives a very accurate comparison of pesticide exposure estimates using health criteria.[17] The procedure involves purchasing foods at retail outlets and in "table-ready" form. Analysis reveals that infants and children are exposed to pesticide residues at less than 1% of the allowable level based on long-term animal toxicology studies.

Important information that frames the discussion about pesticides includes the fact that different quantities of different pesticides produce a toxic effect on humans. A child's exposure to pesticides is greater than an adult's, because children tend to eat a narrower range of foods, consume more processed foods, and ingest more food per kilogram of body weight. The exposure of children to pesticides varies by geographic region.[16]

The Environmental Working Group's 1994 report, *Washed, Peeled, Contaminated: Pesticide*

Residues in Ready-to-Eat Fruits and Vegetables,[18] has voiced selective concern for pesticide exposure to children. The report recommends an increase in the availability and promotion of certified organic foods.[19] Reviewers of the report make the following points[18]:

- Dose makes the poison. It is the amount of pesticide residue–not merely its presence or absence–that determines harm.
- The report did not include a risk assessment to calculate estimates of infant and child exposures to pesticides.
- The wording of the report implies that washing and peeling do not eliminate residues, which is incorrect.
- It is important to differentiate between *reduction* and *elimination* of pesticide residues.

A well-publicized scare involved daminozide (tradename Alar) in 1989. Daminozide is a plant growth regulator that has been used on apples and other fruits. The Natural Resources Defense Council released a report, "Intolerable Risk: Pesticides in our Children's Food." After the hysteria from the report and an apple boycott, factual information emerged. This included acknowledging that no human cancers had ever been linked to Alar and that no well-designed clinical trials had ever been conducted on Alar to warrant a ban on its use. Later, in a well-controlled study with mice, a dose more than 250,000 times the highest amount thought consumable by children was used. No tumors were noted in the mice.[20]

Info Line

The Food and Drug Administration publishes an annual pesticide program report, "Residue Monitoring," in the *Journal of AOAC International.*

Exhibit 6–9 *Healthy People 2000* Objectives Targeting Foodborne Outbreaks

12.1   Reduce infections caused by key foodborne pathogens to incidences of no more than:

Disease (per 100,000)	1987 Baseline	2000 Target
Salmonella species	18	16
Campylobacter jejuni	50	25
Escherichia coli 0157:H7	8	4
Listeria monocytogenes	0.7	0.5

12.2   Reduce outbreaks of infections due to Salmonella enteritidis to fewer than 25 outbreaks yearly. (Baseline: 77 outbreaks in 1989.)

12.3   Increase to at least 75% the proportion of households in which principal food preparers routinely refrain from leaving perishable food out of the refrigerator for over 2 hours and wash cutting boards and utensils with soap after contact with raw meat and poultry. (Baseline: For refrigeration of perishable foods, 70%; for washing cutting boards with soap, 66%; and for washing utensils with soap, 55%, in 1988.)

12.4   Extend to at least 70% the proportion of states and territories that have implemented model food codes for institutional food operations and to at least 70% the proportion that have adopted the new uniform food protection code ("Unicode") that sets recommended standards for regulation of all food operations. (Baseline: For institutional food operations currently using FDA's recommended model codes, 20%; for the Unicode, 0%, in 1990.)

Source: Reprinted with permission from *Healthy People 2000: National Health Promotion and Disease Prevention Objectives.* Washington, DC: US Department of Health and Human Services; 1991. DHHS (PHS) Publication 91-50212.

Info Line

Common Consumer Questions and Appropriate Answers

Q: My child is in day care five days each week. How can I help protect him from food-borne illness when I'm not there?

A: Make sure that the people who manage the day care center practice appropriate sanitation and food handling techniques. Ask the providers to teach children to wash hands with warm, soapy water before and after going to the bathroom. It's critical for child care providers and parents to remember to wash hands thoroughly after every diaper check and change. Spread of disease does not require ingestion of food or beverage.

Q: When preparing food at home, should I use a plastic or wood cutting board?

A: Though the advice for years has been to use plastic cutting surfaces instead of wood, there is discussion as to whether wooden surfaces may actually be better at preventing bacterial growth than plastic surfaces, which seem to harbor them. Whether you choose wood or plastic, use separate boards for raw and cooked foods, and make sure to clean and sanitize after each use. To sanitize cutting boards, wash with warm, soapy water, and then wash again with a solution of two to three teaspoons of household bleach in one quart of warm water. Rinse with plain, hot water.

Q: My kids love to eat raw cookie dough when I bake cookies. Is this safe?

A: If your cookie dough contains raw eggs, there is a risk involved. Other foods to think twice about are traditional Caesar salad (the dressing is made with raw eggs) or anything made with homemade mayonnaise or soft poached eggs. If you make homemade mayonnaise, ice cream, or other recipes requiring eggs that will not be cooked, use pasteurized eggs. Commercially prepared dressing, mayonnaise, commercially prepared cookie dough, and "cookie dough" ice cream, all use pasteurized eggs.

Q: What causes mold? If a food has mold on it, is it unsafe to eat?

A: Mold is a result of spoilage. If there is mold on hard cheese, cut off the mold to a depth of one inch, and it should be fine to eat. Other foods with mold on them should be thrown out.

Q: What should I do if I suspect I have a food-borne illness?

A: First, if possible, preserve the suspected food, marking it with a warning label to make sure no one else eats it. Second, call or see a medical professional. If the suspected food was served at a large gathering or in a public place (such as a restaurant, a sidewalk vendor, or an employee cafeteria), or if the food is a commercial product or was prepared by a grocery store, contact your local health department to report the incident. If vomiting or diarrhea are symptoms, drink lots of fluids to prevent dehydration. Physicians and laboratories have a responsibility to contact the health department for some diagnoses of food-borne illness. However, most food-borne illness is not diagnosed; symptoms are treated to alleviate discomfort. If food is the suspected source of illness, be sure to advise a physician. (Reproduced with permission of the National Livestock and Meat Board, Consumer Pamphlet.[22])

Pesticides have two major functions: to regulate plant growth and to prevent crop damage caused by insects, weeds, and plant disease. Herbicides are the most common pesticides and are used to control weeds. Insecticides and fungicides control insects and plant disease. As a result of the concern over pesticides in foods and the cost of pesticides, new ways have been developed to produce crops and to replace the exclusive use of pesticides. One approach is the use of compounds that are highly specific to certain pests and that require only a small

Exhibit 6-10 Model Nutrition Objectives for Reduced Risk Factors

By 19__, the following contaminants will not be present in the state food supply above toxic/hazardous levels as defined by state or federal agencies.

- Agricultural: pesticides, fertilizers, growth regulators
- Drugs: antibiotics, steroids/hormones, growth regulators
- Environmental: organics, inorganics/heavy metals
- Food additives: preservatives, colors, flavors, sweeteners, stabilizers
- Industrial: organics, inorganics/heavy metals, radioactives
- Microbial: bacteria, molds, fungi, virus, protozoa, and related toxins
- Naturally occurring toxins: carcinogens, mutagens, neurotoxins

Source: Reprinted with permission from *Healthy People 2000: National Health Promotion and Disease Prevention Objectives.* Washington, DC. US Department of Health and Human Services; 1991. DHHS (PHS) Publication 91-50212.

Exhibit 6-11 Model Nutrition Objectives for Increased Public and Professional Awareness

By 19__, there will be an ongoing interdisciplinary information program for public health and food industry professionals on food safety, labeling, health claims, nutrition fraud, and the reporting of food-borne illness.

Source: Kaufman M. *Nutrition in Public Health—A Handbook for Developing Programs and Services.* Gaithersburg, Md: Aspen Publishers, Inc; 1990:570.

dosage. A new agricultural approach called integrated pest management (IPM) seeks alternatives that produce the least impact on the environment.[16]

IPM techniques have been used by the state of Washington apple growers to control mites, moths, and apple scab. To control mites, miticides are replaced with predator mites. The codling moth is controlled by the use of pheromone, a natural sex-attractant odor that traps moths by disrupting mating patterns. To control apple scab, a fungal disease that attacks leaves and fruit, farmers use a moisture timetable and spray at the peak of potential attack.[21]

HEALTHY PEOPLE 2000 ACTIONS

Specific HP2K objectives target food-borne outbreaks and actions that can be taken in the home as well as in institutional food service settings (see Exhibit 6-9). Model nutrition objectives for community nutrition professionals are given in Exhibits 6-10 and 6-11.[23]

REFERENCES

1. Centers for Disease Control and Prevention. *Principles of Epidemiology: An Introduction to Applied Epidemiology and Biostatistics.* Atlanta, Ga: Centers for Disease Control and Prevention; 1992.

2. Page R, Cole G, Timmrock T. *Basic Epidemiologic Methods and Biostatistics.* Boston, Mass: Jones and Bartlett Publishers; 1993.

3. Centers for Disease Control and Prevention. Foodborne disease outbreaks, 5-year summary: 1983-1987. In: CDC Surveillance Summaries. *MMWR.* 1990;39(SS-1):15-57.

4. Matthews ME, Theis M. Relationship between the environment, the food supply and the practice of dietetics. Research Agenda Conference. *J Am Diet Assoc.* 1993.

5. Expert Panel on Food Safety and Nutrition. Government regulation of food safety: Interaction of scientific and societal forces. *Food Technol.* 1992;46(1):73-80.

6. National Restaurant Association. The Education Foundation. *Applied Foodservice Sanitation.* 4th ed. New York, NY: John Wiley & Sons, Inc; 1992.

7. American Diabetes Association and the Diabetes Care and Education Practice Group of the American Dietetic Association. *Maximizing the Role of Nutrition in Diabetes Management.* Alexandria, Va: American Diabetes Association; 1994.

8. American Diabetes Association. *Professional Section Newsletter,* June, 1993.

9. Ryser ET, Marth EH. "New" food-borne pathogens of public health significance. *J Am Diet Assoc.* 1989;89:948-956.

10. "Green consumers" boost organic sales over $1 billion. *Magic Mill Newsletter of Food, Health and Environmental Issues.* 1992;2(1):1.

11. California Dietetic Association. *Nutrition Survival Plan: A Food Guide for Emergencies, Big and Small*. Playa del Rey, Calif:California Dietetic Association; 1990.

12. HACCP: Making the system work. *Food Engineering*. August 1988;7:70–80.

13. National Advisory Committee for Microbiological Criteria for Foods. *HACCP Principles for Food Production*. Washington, DC: US Department of Agriculture, Food Safety and Inspection Service; 1989.

14. *Bacteria That Cause Foodborne Illness*. Washington, DC: US Department of Agriculture, Food Safety and Inspection Service; December 1990. FSIS-40.

15. Dolye MP. Reducing foodborne disease—what are the priorities. *Nutr Rev*. 1993:51;346–347.

16. Committee on Pesticides in the Diets of Infants and Children. *Pesticides in the Diets of Infants and Children*. Washington, DC: National Academy Press; 1993.

17. Yess NJ, FDA monitoring program. Residues in foods. 1990. *J Assoc Anal Chem*. 1991;74:121a–141a.

18. Winter CK. *Washed, Peeled, Contaminated: Pesticide Residues in Ready-to-Eat Fruits and Vegetables*: A Critical Review. Position Paper. University of California, Davis. 1994.

19. Expert Panel on Food Safety and Nutrition. Organically grown foods. *Food Technol*. 1990;44(12):123–130.

20. Smith K. *Alar Three Years Later: Science Unmasks a Hypothetical Health Scare*. New York, NY: American Council on Science and Health; 1992.

21. Washington Apple Commission. *Apple Production Information*. Wenatchee, Wash: Washington Apple Commission; 1992.

22. National Livestock and Meat Board. *Safety—Preventing Foodborne Illness*. Consumer Pamphlet. Chicago, Illinois.

23. Kaufman M. *Nutrition in Public Health—A Handbook for Developing Programs and Services*. Gaithersburg, Md: Aspen Publishers, Inc; 1990:570.

Appendix 6–A

Food-Borne Illnesses: Agents, Symptoms, and Incubation Periods

Agent	Average Incubation/ Range (Hours)	Common Symptoms	Pathophysiology	Food Sources
Short incubation period with vomiting and little or no fever				
Staphylococcus aureus	2–4/1–6	N,C,V; D,F may be present	Preformed enterotoxin	Sliced/chopped ham and meats, custards, cream fillings
Bacillus cereus	2–4/1–6	N,V,D	Preformed enterotoxin	Fried rice
Heavy metals (cadmium, copper, tin, zinc)	5–15 minutes/ 1–60 minutes	N,V,C,D		Foods and beverages contaminated by metal
Moderate to long incubation period, with diarrhea and usually with fever				
Clostridium perfringens	12/8–16	C,D (V,F rare)	Enterotoxin formed in vivo	Meat, poultry
Salmonella (nontyphoid)	12–36/6–72	D,C,F,V,H septicemia or enteric fever	Tissue invasion	Poultry, eggs, raw milk, meat or cross-contamination
Vibrio parahaemolyticus	12/2–48	C,D,N,V,F,H,B	Tissue enterotoxin	Seafood
Moderate to long incubation period, with diarrhea and fever				
Escherichia enterotoxigenic	16–48	D,C	Enterotoxin	Uncooked vegetables, salads, water, cheese
Escherichia coli enteroinvasive	16–48	C,D,F,H	Tissue invasion	Same
E. coli enterohemorrhagic (E. coli 0157:H7) 48–96	B,C,D,H,F	infrequent Cytotoxin	Beef, raw milk,	water
Bacillus cereus	8–16	C,D	Enterotoxin	Custards, cereals puddings, sauces, meat loaf

Source: Adapted from Page R, Cole G, Timmrock T. *Basic Epidemiologic Methods and Biostatistics.* Boston, MA: Jones and Bartlett Publishers; 1993.

Agent	Average Incubation/ Range (Hours)	Common Symptoms	Pathophysiology	Food Sources
Shigella	24–48	C,F,D,B,H,N,V	Tissue invasion	Foods contaminated by infected food handler; usually not food borne
Yersinia enterocolitica	3–5 days	F,D,C,V,H	Tissue invasion enterotoxin	Pork products, food contaminated by infected human or animal
Vibrio cholerae 01	24–72	D,V	Enterotoxin formed in vivo	Shellfish, water, or foods contaminated by infected person or obtained from contaminated environment
Vibrio cholerae non-01	16–72	D,V	Enterotoxin formed with tissue invasion	Shellfish
Campylobacter jejuni	3–5 days	C,D,B,F	Unknown	Raw milk, poultry, water
Parvovirus-like agents (Norwalk, Hawaii, Colorado, cockle agents)	16–48	N,V,C,D	Unknown	Shellfish, water
Rotavirus	16–48	N,V,C,D	Unknown	Food-borne transmission not well documented
Clostridium botulinum	12–72	V,D; descending paralysis	Preformed toxin	Improperly canned or preserved foods that provide anaerobic conditions
Diagnosed from intake of certain foods				
Poisonous mushrooms	Variable	Variable		Wild mushrooms
Other poisonous plants	Variable	Variable		Wild plants
Scombroid fish poisoning	5 minutes–1 hour	N,C,D,H, flushing, urticaria	Histamine	Mishandled fish (tuna)
Ciguatera poisoning	1–6	D,N,V, paresthesias, reversal of temperature sensation	Ciguatoxin	Large ocean fish (barracuda, snapper)

Common symptom codes: B=bloody stools, C=cramps, D=diarrhea, F=fever, H=headache, N=nausea, V=vomiting

7

Healthy Eating in Early Life— Infants and Preschoolers

Learning Objectives

- Describe the development of a healthy eating pattern for children.
- List the factors influencing normal growth and development of young children.
- Identify the nutrition programs available for all infants and preschoolers and low-income children in particular.
- Enumerate the major nutrition issues in early life.
- Identify the roles and responsibilities of caregivers including community nutrition professionals in providing a safe and healthy eating and playing environment for infants and preschoolers.

High Definition Nutrition

Atherogenic—description of an eating pattern that promotes heart disease.

Day care center—a facility licensed by a sponsor to keep more than 12 infants or children and responsible for their safety, well-being, and food.

Day care home—a personal residence licensed by a sponsor to keep 12 or fewer infants or children and responsible for their safety, well-being, and food.

Kid culture—commonalities among day care centers and home facilities regarding foods served to children (e.g., spaghetti, fish sticks, hot dogs, potato chips, and cookies) that may be extremely popular but nutrient poor.

Salutogenic—health-promoting quality of food or eating pattern.

INTRODUCTION

The nutritional health of a child depends on the foods ingested and how the body uses them. Excess weight predisposes children to high blood cholesterol and sets them on a track for chronic disease.[1] At the other extreme, underweight and malnourished children present a different mosaic of nutritional problems, many of which begin during infancy and the preschool years.

The most common problems among Massachusetts Head Start children were excess weight (13%), short stature (13%), and iron deficiency anemia (12%). About 20% of physically or developmentally disabled children had short stature compared with 15% of the Asian children. Acute undernutrition was not prevalent. Excess weight among Hispanic, African-American, and white children was 17%, 13%, and 11%, respectively.[2]

Migrant children are a special group of children suspected of receiving inadequate nutrition prior to school entrance. These children experience poor housing with limited cooking facilities. They are victims of a lack of prenatal care, because their mothers have inadequate money for nutritious foods. Migrant children exist at a poverty level that has negative effects on their health and school potential.[3]

Infants and preschoolers are fun to watch, to teach, and to love. Their vitality, exuberance, and innocence capture the eye of parents, relatives, and caregivers. The nutritional needs of young children are as important as their emotional and social needs. Children who do not grow according to a standard growth chart or who remain either listless or overactive at school may not be receiving their nutrient needs on a daily basis. These nutrient needs may have escaped the living environment of the child when still a fetus.

Adult concerns for preschoolers' health should begin at conception or even before. The foundation for healthy infants and preschoolers remains an adult task. For each cohort born in the United States annually, attention must be paid not only to how well but also to how poorly the nutrient needs of young children are met.

Current scientific research links cognitive development of infants and children to nutrition.[4] The Center on Hunger, Poverty and Nutrition Policy at Tufts University School of Nutrition summarized the research findings[5]:

- Undernutrition, along with environmental factors associated with poverty, can permanently retard physical growth, brain development, and cognitive functioning.
- The longer a child's nutritional, emotional, and education needs go unmet, the greater the livelihood of cognitive impairments.
- Iron deficiency anemia, affecting nearly 25% of low-income children in the United States, is associated with impaired cognitive development.
- Low-income children who attend school hungry perform significantly below their non-hungry, low-income peers on standardized test scores.

- There exists a strong association between family income and the growth and cognitive development of children.
- Improved nutrition and environmental conditions can modify the effects of early undernutrition.
- Iron repletion therapy can reduce some of the effects of anemia on learning, attention, and memory.
- Supplemental feeding programs can help to offset threats to children's capacity to learn and perform in school that result from inadequate nutrient intake.
- Once undernutrition occurs, its long-term effects may be reduced or eliminated by a combination of adequate food intake and environmental support—both at home and at school.

US infant mortality rates (IMRs) have declined by almost two-thirds since 1970. However, IMRs for African-American and Native American infants remain at 18 and 13 per 1,000 live births compared to 10 per 1,000 live births for the total population (see Figure 7–1, and see Chapter 9 for prenatal nutrition). The Special Supplemental Program for Women, Infants and Children (WIC) reaches high-risk pregnant mothers, infants, and children to change the direction of their health (see Appendix 7–A).

WIC has been shown to dramatically reduce infant mortality by 25% to 66% among Medicaid beneficiaries who are WIC participants, compared to non-WIC Medicaid beneficiaries. The incidence of low-birth-weight babies can be lowered by 3.3%, and preterm births can be reduced by 3.5% (see Chapter 9).

THE FIRST FOOD FOR NEWBORNS

Milk remains the first choice, and breast milk remains the best choice to feed a newborn. The reasons are as follows[6]:

- Breastfeeding protects from disease and infections. There is less illness and hospitalization of breastfed babies than bottle-fed

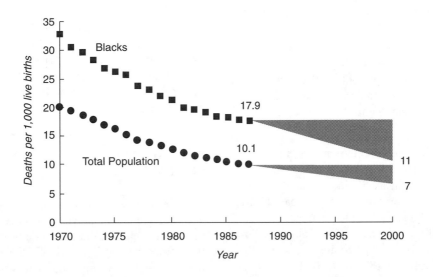

Figure 7-1 US infant mortality rates. *Source:* Reprinted with permission from *Healthy People 2000: National Health Promotion and Disease Prevention Objectives*. Washington, DC: US Department of Health and Human Services; 1991. DHHS (PHS) Publication 91-50212.

babies. Breast milk contains many immunological factors that protect babies.

- Breast milk is less allergenic. Breast milk rarely causes allergic reactions in babies, whereas cow's milk formula may create these problems.

- Breastfeeding improves learning. Breastfeeding has a positive effect on learning, memory, and other brain functions of young children.

- Breastfeeding reduces cancer risk. Cancer of the breast, ovaries, and cervix are less common among women who have breastfed an infant.

- Breastfeeding improves the mother's shape. Breastfeeding allows a woman to lose weight after pregnancy and reduces uterine bleeding. Milk production requires an additional 300 to 600 calories daily, which is partially obtained from the fat stores accumulated during pregnancy.

- Breastfeeding reduces overfeeding. A mother becomes more sensitive to her baby's satiety cues and does not simply empty a bottle.

- Breastfeeding promotes bonding. Having skin contact, smelling the mother, and hearing the mother's heartbeat all contribute to the baby's bond to mother. Mother feels special because she is providing baby's food.

- Breastfeeding provides optimal nutrient content. The protein, fat, mineral, vitamin, and calorie content of breast milk is superior to any other form of milk. It is made by humans for humans, and its nutrient content changes as the baby's needs change.

- Breastfeeding is convenient. When baby is hungry, the milk is always there. Milk is at the right temperature and clean, with no bottles to heat and no formula to prepare.

- Breastfeeding is economical. It is less expensive to breastfeed than to formula feed. Breast pumps are not a requirement.

- Breast milk is digestible. It is made by humans for humans, is easy to digest, and creates less constipation and diarrhea.

- Breastfeeding is natural. It is the natural extension of a pregnancy; 95% of all women can be successful with encouragement, support, and basic information.

- Breastfeeding is safe. It is bacteriologically safe and always fresh.
- Breastfeeding promotes infant bone formation. The breastfed infant has good jaw and tooth development.

Even with the benefits of breastfeeding known, cow's milk is commonly used for infants early in life. The role of cow's milk or cow's milk-based formula in food allergy remains unclear, but it is generally thought that increased intestinal permeability early in life contributes significantly to the development of food allergies. Cow's milk protein is the most common food allergy in childhood, affecting 0.4 to 7.5% of infants.[7] The effect of limiting foods with cow's milk proteins to reduce the incidence of allergy is not known.[8,9] Milk, both bottle and breast, is implicated in 20% of colicky infants who persistently cry and are sleepless and irritable during the first three to four months of life.[10] Breast milk is contraindicated when women are HIV positive, drug abusers, or required to take multiple or powerful drugs.

A recurring question is whether breastfed infants have a slower growth rate after the second or third month compared with bottle-fed infants. In the DARLING Study (Davis Area Research on Lactation, Infant Nutrition and Growth), researchers observed 46 breastfed and 41 formula-fed infants, 2,500 to 5,000 g at birth, who were given no solid food before four months. At three-month intervals of observation, formula-fed infants drank a signficiantly higher total energy and protein intake. No difference was noted in weight, length, lean body mass, or fat mass during the first three months of life, but the breastfed infants had a slower weight gain from three to nine months. From three to twelve months, the breast-fed infants consistently showed a positive correlation between total energy ingested and lean body mass gain. Fat mass deposition was more apparent for the formula-fed infants. A higher incidence of illness from six to nine months occurred for infants having higher protein intakes.[11]

General recommendations for infants and young children less than two years old are that fat not be restricted.[12] Breast milk and commercial infant formula contain 50% of energy as fat. Risks associated with low-fat diets appear to outweigh the theoretical risk associated with a high-fat intake. Lower-fat milk is a good source of protein, calcium, and vitamin D for older children.

SHAPING FOOD PATTERNS IN YOUNG CHILDREN

Eating behaviors and food choices are formed early in life. Primary prevention efforts to reduce the onset of chronic disease might be improved if the factors shaping food patterns early in life were understood. Parents influence food-related behaviors, but several factors interact to shape food choices. These factors include but are not limited to nutrition attitudes and knowledge of parents and child care providers, economic and social status of the family, birth order of the child, and number of siblings. Peers, media and advertising, access to the health care system, and the source of food (ranging from the home, to day care, to fast-food restaurants) all shape children's food choices.

A conceptual model to identify the determinants of eating behavior and the outcome of actual nutrient intakes is given in Table 7-1. This model suggests that actual nutrient intake is the end result of a progressive sequence of actions. The actions begin with a stimulus, which may be physiological or environmental. The stimulus creates a response—the child's eating behavior. The behavior causes food to be ingested, which is the first stage of response. The second stage of response is the resulting nutrient intake.

This model relates to the theory of reasoned action, which has been successful in predicting intent to perform health behaviors including eating in a fast-food restaurant.[13] *Reasoned action* postulates that one's behavior is predictable and based on the individual's intention to perform that behavior. *Intention* is a function of attitude about the behavior and the perception that one has about the way significant others would feel if one performs the behavior.

Four elements are inherent to the definition of the behavior: specified action, target for the

Table 7–1 Conceptual Model To Identify Determinants of Eating Behavior of Children

Stimulus (Determinants)	*Response* (Behaviors[a])	*Result* (Nutrients)
Parents	Fat avoidance or excess	Fat
School	Salt use or limit	Saturated fatty acids
Siblings	Snacks eaten or limited	Sodium
Environment	Meals eaten or missed	Energy
Physiology	Sugar use or amount	

[a]An abbreviated list of possible behaviors for demonstration purposes.

action, context in which the behavior occurs, and time frame for the action. For example, fat avoidance is the specified action; it is reflected in the target for action as total fat intake or the percentage of energy from fat. The context for the behavior might be the home-prepared meals or eating out. The time frame for action might be the one-half hour around mealtime.

Factors that have been evaluated for their influence on the eating pattern of young children are texture, taste, familiarity of food, preferences of the child compared with those of parents and other significant adults, and interaction patterns of parents and children around food. The child's willingness to eat is affected by the sensory appeal of the food, immediate hunger and nutritional status, the child's prior experience with food (both good and bad), and the child's personal beliefs and feelings about food.

Preference for a sweet taste is expressed early in life but appears modifiable.[14] Beauchamp et al demonstrated that to maintain a newborn's level of preference for sugar water, sweetened water must be repeatedly offered to the infant.[15] With no exposure during the newborn period, the relative acceptance of the sweetened water decreases.

Dislike of bitter tastes appears early in life, and an infant's reaction to salty tastes tends to be indifference.[14] The preference for a salt taste begins at about four months of age, as different foods are entered into the newborn's eating repertoire. Young children and infants prefer a salty taste; in fact, studies have shown that preschoolers favor higher levels of salt compared to adults.[16]

For preschool children, sweetness and familiarity enhance choice; familiarity is less impor-

tant to older children.[17] Preference rankings of preschool children are highly correlated with consumption,[18] yet their preferences are strongly influenced by their peers. Fear of new foods decreases with exposure to the food. Food preferences of young children are influenced by parents and child care staff, but not unequivocally.[18]

Burt and Hertzler observed that both mother and father can equally influence a child's food preferences, if weight is given to the father's preferences specifically at mealtime.[19] Birch reported that adults from the same ethnic group as the child, but not related to the child, influence the child's food preferences as much as the parents.[20] When parents are involved in nutrition education, the eating patterns of their children are more nutritious than when the parents are not included.[21]

Evaluations of mother-child choices generally show a stronger influence of what the mother chooses rather than what the father chooses. As a child advances through the preschool years, the parental and child food choices become more similar and stronger than when the child was younger, for example, age 2. Food choices of younger children also mirror those of the child's siblings.[22]

EATING BEHAVIOR OF CHILDREN

Interactions

Eating interactions form a continuum influenced by parental attitudes, values, interests, and beliefs and the child's cognitive, physical, and emotional maturity. Parent-child interactions determine children's acceptance of healthy and not-so-healthy foods and attitudes toward eating. Parents are often anxious and may pressure children to eat. In response, children often assume control of the eating environment. Battles may intensify, and a child's nutrient intake may suffer. Disordered eating including excessive weight, obesity, and failure to thrive may occur.

Parent-child eating interaction is complex and reciprocal. Each response to an action can cause future behaviors, both healthy and unhealthy. Eating behavior becomes both the cause and the effect of other behaviors. Because of the dependence of children on parents and caregivers for food, this section will address the role of adult-child interactions on food intake and nutrient intake. Community nutrition professionals may learn new ways to approach old problems.

Parent-child interactions can be initiated by the child and influence the child, as seen by the cries of a hungry infant stimulating the parent or guardian to respond with food. Eating behaviors increase, stay the same, or decrease, depending on the consequence that follows initial eating. In fact, the consequences can reinforce or punish.[23] Determining what is reinforcing rather than punishing depends on the outcome or preceding event.

Reinforcers can be either positive or negative. Positive reinforcement—such as a smile, food, or money—can create a positive environment. Negative reinforcement, such as silence, often removes or ends a behavior. All reinforcers increase the behavior that follows. However, positive reinforcement adds pleasure, and a negative reinforcement removes something. Shouting is a punisher that adds reinforcement to a child who eats something that she or he should not eat.

Peterson[24] suggests considering interaction in terms of A (antecedent events), B (behavior), and C (consequences). For example, a father takes his four-year-old son to a baseball game. The boy asks for candy and cries when the father refuses to buy it. The child cries and kicks the seat in front of him, and the father ends up buying the candy. In buying the candy, the father reinforced the kicking and the crying, but the father received negative reinforcement because the kicking stopped after he gave candy. By giving candy, he stopped something annoying to him. Both father and son were reinforced for their behaviors (i.e., the son was positively reinforced for kicking; the father was negatively reinforced, because the kicking stopped when he gave in). The tendency would be for each person to repeat their behavior. Table 7–2 classifies the behaviors and consequences of a similar situation—a negative reinforcement for a parent and a positive reinforcement for a child.[25]

Parents and caregivers often become trapped and unable to see their own ineffectiveness in directing their children's eating behavior. Mealtimes can create difficult, volatile eating interactions. Affection, praise, and touch often create secondary reinforcement when they are paired with a positive eating event. Money can become a reinforcer, and food is often used as a reinforcer for various other behaviors such as physical activity.[25]

Assessing the antecedent behaviors of eating is pivotal for community nutrition professionals to understand why children eat certain foods or

Table 7–2 Negative Reinforcement for Parent and Positive Reinforcement for Child

A (Mother)	B (Child)	C (Mother)
1. Pours milk into glass	2. Starts crying 4. Cries 6. Stops crying and drinks soda	3. "Drink your milk." 5. Removes milk and gives child soda

Source: Adapted from Pipes PC. Management of mealtime behavior. In *Nutrition in Infancy and Childhood.* 4th ed. Times Mirror. Boston, MA. p. 405.

persist with certain behaviors. Assessment is essential if effective behavioral change is needed for primary prevention and health promotion. Adults can review the foods that are reinforcers, help children learn appropriate behaviors, and then use the foods with other reinforcers—such as affection and praise—until the child understands how the two behaviors reinforce one another. Then the food can be removed as the reward but the secondary reinforcer retained. A circular interaction that reinforces a child's control of eating and a possible solution is given in Table 7–3.[25]

Selections

Young children learn to differentiate food from nonfood substances and place items into edible and inedible categories. Very young children show a high to moderate level of acceptance of all categories of food and nonfood items, but the acceptance of dangerous, disgusting, or unacceptable substances (e.g., ketchup on mashed potatoes) decreases with age.[26]

Energy regulation appears keener for children than adults. When given a high-calorie instead of a low-calorie snack before lunch, 95% of the children and 60% of adults ate less lunch.[27] Food contingencies, for example, "eat this and you can do this," can discourage rather than encourage food consumption among preschoolers, and variety increases intake.[28,29]

When asked to group foods, children group foods based on commonalities, such as sweet foods or foods served at breakfast, but not based on nutritional value.[30] Categories tend to match the cognitive level of children (e.g., food recognition is based on sensory perceptions or differentiating animal versus plant sources).[31]

For decades, the basic four food groups have been a common grouping to teach children about food selection. However, not all children know and use the food groups correctly. In one study, all children identified a "sweets" group; one-half put foods in a fruit, vegetable, or beverage group;

Table 7–3 Circular Interaction To Reinforce a Child's Control of Eating Environment and Solution

A (Mother)	B (Child)	C (Mother)
Interaction in which child controls eating		
1. Presents applesauce to toddler in highchair	2. Cries and whines, points to the refrigerator	3. "What do you want?"
	4. Cries, points to cupboard	5. "Do you want a cracker?"
	6. Cries, points to cupboard and refrigerator	7. "What do you want? Here is some cereal."
	8. Cries, points to refrigerator	9. "No, you can't have ice cream."
	10. Screams	11. "OK, here is some ice cream."
	12. Stops crying	
Solution **Interaction in which parent controls eating**		
1. Presents applesauce to toddler in highchair	2. Cries, points to cupboard	3. Leaves room (can see child but child can't see her)
	4. Slowly stops crying, starts eating applesauce	5. Returns and says "My, what a big boy!"
	6. Child laughs and keeps on eating	

Source: Adapted from Pipes PC. Management of mealtime behavior. In *Nutrition in Infancy and Childhood*. 4th ed. Times Mirror. Boston, MA. p.405.

one-fourth identified a dairy group; and one-fifth identified a breads and cereals category.[30] The US Department of Agriculture (USDA) Food Guide Pyramid is the current visual aid for grouping foods and the focus of games, mobiles, and refrigerator magnets.[32] It replaces the basic four food groups.

Other Factors

The extent to which nutrition knowledge is used in family and child care menu planning may relate to a child's self-esteem, problem-solving skills, and family organization.[33] Older children, by virtue of their age, appear to influence the mother's food selection more than younger siblings, irrespective of the mother's nutrition knowledge.[34] Day care providers who report limited nutrition knowledge still value the role they play in influencing eating patterns of children.[35] Further, family role modeling and reinforcement may set the stage for strong interactive environmental conditioning.[36] Differences have been observed between thin parents and their thin children, compared with heavy parents and their children. Birch[37] observed more interaction and positive reinforcement for thin children and their mothers compared to their heavier counterparts.[36]

Food rewards can influence food preferences of children.[38] Nonfood rewards such as stickers, sports equipment, amusement tickets, and sports cards are preferred incentives in behavior modification. Reinforcement procedures of cueing have been used to redirect snack choices, but once the cues are removed, prior habits return.[39] Satter views the parent or caregiver as the individual who is responsible for what is offered to the child. The child is responsible for the amount of food eaten.[40,41]

Role of Media

The role of mass media has increased proportionately to the amount of time children are in contact with the media. Young children are mesmerized by television before they can speak, and the preschooler cannot differentiate between commercials and actual programs.[42,43] There ap-

pears to be an inverse association between income and the amount of time children spend watching television.[44] The specific television segments that influence children are advertisements. On the average, children watch three hours of advertisements per week and 19,000 to 22,000 commercials over a year.[45] Advertisements categorize foods by first establishing their enjoyability and pleasure in terms of sweetness and richness. Children's repeated exposure to messages that do not build positive images about crisp, fresh vegetables or the bone-building capacity of milk and dairy products has motivated national healthy eating campaigns directed toward children, such as the "5-A-Day" campaign.[46]

Since preschool children may spend over 26 hours a week watching television, physical activity may be displaced by sedentary activities. Six-to-16 year olds still average 25 hours of television watching per week.[47] Understanding and trusting commercials has been explored among children; it appears that older children recognize commercials as sales pitches and not educational, and they even tend to distrust the information.[43]

An overriding concern of health professionals and educators has been the long-term impact of television commercials and messages on the health of all children, including preschoolers. When television can influence what a family purchases and which snacks are provided to children, and confuses the role of food with other outcomes—smoking, sexual appeal, and popularity—then the real message about healthy eating has been lost. The more television children watch, the greater the tendency for weight gain. This can be considered from two perspectives. First, fewer calories are expended when sitting, and one is more likely to eat while watching television. Second, seeing thin, active children eat gooey chocolate and high-fat foods on television is interpreted as an acceptable habit that does not cause excess body weight.

ATHEROGENIC VERSUS SALUTOGENIC EATING PATTERNS

Data from the 1987–1988 Nationwide Food Consumption Survey indicated that children 1 to 19 years old averaged 35 to 36% of their total calories from fat. Saturated fat was 14% of their intake, polyunsaturated fat was 6%, and monounsaturated fat was 13 to 14%; dietary cholesterol levels were 193 to 296 mg.[48] This eating pattern has predisposed children to a health-risk behavior resulting in excess weight and high blood cholesterol levels. At least 25% of American children exceed the acceptable 170 mg% serum cholesterol level.[48]

However, fat-avoiding behaviors have been observed in a cross-sectional sample of Mexican-American preschoolers and their parents.[49] Significantly higher fat-avoiding scores were noted for Anglo-American preschoolers (N = 143) than Mexican-American preschoolers (N = 198) (maximum score = 7.0, sum score = 4.85 compared to 4.35, $p < 0.0001$).[50]

The eating patterns of young children two to five years of age reflect intraindividual and interindividual variability. To evaluate the influence of food choices on actual health risk,

nutrient intake can be compared with a standard. A conceptual guide that characterizes the salutogenic (health-promoting) quality of food versus the atherogenic (heart-disease-promoting) quality of an eating pattern is outlined in Table 7–4.

Standards used as cutoff points reflect consensus recommendations of such organizations as the American Heart Association, the American Cancer Society, and the National Cholesterol Education Program. Achieving the standards means achieving a healthy eating pattern. If young children can be taught to make wise food choices and if their parents and other adults plan and prepare healthy meals and snacks, then a primary prevention effort can unfold. If the salutogenic approach (i.e., health-promotion) is consistent, then over time the eating pattern will promote positive health of the child. If the usual eating pattern is atherogenic, then the risk factors for chronic disease may appear early in the life of a child.

Table 7–4 Conceptual Model for Describing Eating Pattern of Children and Its Relation to Health Risk versus Health Promotion

Component	Salutogenic[a]	Standard	Atherogenic[a]
Total fat	25–29% kcal	30%	>30%
Saturated fat	8–9% kcal	10%	>10%
Polyunsaturated fat	8–9% kcal	10%	<8%
Monounsatured fat	12–14% kcal	10–12%	<10%
Carbohydrate	55–60% kcal	53–55%	<53%
Starch	30–40% kcal	28–30%	<28%
Cholesterol	100–150 mg/kcal	140–150 mg/kcal	>150 mg/kcal
Sodium (1–3y)	<975 mg	325–975 mg	>975 mg
(4–6y)	<1350 mg	450–1350 mg	>1350 mg
Potassium (1–3y)	>1650 mg	550–1650 mg	<1650 mg
(4–6y)	>2325 mg	775–2325 mg	<2325 mg
Fiber	>10 g	10–20 g	<5 g
CSI[b]	<37	35–37	>37
FAS[c]	>3.5	3.5	<3.5

(Health Risk: − ←——————————————→ +)

[a]Both accepted (American Heart Association and National Cholesterol Education Panel) and author-hypothesized values
[b]Cholesterol saturated fat index
[c]Fat/cholesterol avoidance scale

FACTORS IN CHILDHOOD THAT PREDISPOSE TO ADULT DISEASE

Obesity

Obesity among 6-to-11-year-old US children has increased by 54% since 1970, compared with a 39% increase among 12-to-17 year olds.[51] Excessive energy intake from sugar and fat or simply eating too many calories and not expending excess calories leads to excess adiposity.[51] Fitness for preschoolers involves regular physical activities such as those identified by the President's Council on Physical Fitness and Sports (see Appendix 7–B).

A recent 20-year longitudinal study reported that 41% of children defined as fat at one year of age maintained their fat into early childhood, preadolescence, and adulthood 21 years later.[52] Heights, weights, and triceps skinfold measures for boys and girls from six months to five years old, collected in the Health and Nutrition Examination Survey and the Hispanic Health and Nutrition Examination Survey are given separately for boys and girls and then by ethnic group in Appendix 7–C.

Obese infants at six months of age are at an increased risk of being obese adults, and tracking of obesity is more pronounced for children at or above the 95th percentile for age-specific measures.[53] A higher percentage of Hispanic children are obese compared to their white and African-American peers.[54] Obesity increases the risk of hypertension, high serum cholesterol, adult-onset diabetes mellitus, and certain cancers.[55,56] Hispanic subgroups in the United States demonstrate a two-to-four times higher risk for developing non-insulin-dependent diabetes mellitus primarily linked to body weight.[57] High sodium intake and excess body weight promote high blood pressure.[58]

The correlation between a child's body fat and his or her responsiveness to caloric-dense cues was observed for 77 preschoolers, two to four years old. Children at higher levels of body fat were not able to regulate energy intake as well as children at lower levels. More parental control over intake lessened the child's ability to self-regulate ($r = -0.67$, $p < 0.0001$).[59]

High Blood Pressure and Hyperlipidemia

Blood pressure and serum total cholesterol are indicators of a child's health status. Direct relationships are reported between incidence of coronary heart disease (CHD) and both the average level of adult serum total cholesterol ($r = 0.80$) and the amount of saturated fat in the diet ($r = 0.84$).[60] Serum total cholesterol and blood pressure have been shown to track or remain in a set position for some children relative to their peers.[61] Determining a child's dietary intakes, serum total cholesterol, and blood pressure levels establishes a baseline to forecast and to track associations and future risk.

The Pediatric Nutrition Surveillance System provides the opportunity to explore the tracking question. Using serum total cholesterol data of a multiethnic group of preschoolers from low-income families in Arizona, an initial level was compared with a follow-up level about 13 months later ($N = 1169$).[62] The correlation of the two measures was $r = 0.54$ and did not vary by ethnicity, sex, relative weight, or changes in weight. Association increased when the age was higher at the initial measure. The correlation of $r = 0.64$ for four year olds and their follow-up measure was identical to that observed by the Bogalusa Heart Study.[63]

Of the children, 34% or five times the number expected had an initial and follow-up cholesterol level equal to or greater than 200 mg/dL. This contrasts with 25% who had their subsequent measure at less than 170 mg/dL. Although intravariability exists, multiple measures portray the cholesterol and subsequent risk beginning in childhood.[62]

Eating pattern models that integrate both the nutrient intakes and the behaviors of preschoolers are needed to explore the combined role of eating patterns on the chronic disease process early in life. How well these eating patterns and blood levels persist or whether new practices can be taught that become habits remain areas of interest and research.

NUTRITION GUIDELINES FOR PRESCHOOL CHILDREN

General nutrition guidelines for children have evolved over the years. For proper growth and development, all young children need an array of nutrients on a daily basis. The Recommended Dietary Allowances (RDAs) are the standards used to evaluate the sufficiency of a child's total daily food intake.[63] RDAs are set for energy, protein, 10 vitamins, and seven minerals. Minimum requirements are set for sodium, chloride, and potassium (see Chapter 2 for a listing of the RDAs for infants and young children).

The USDA bases the meal planning guide for child care, day care, summer foods programs, and home meals on the assumption that children should consume one-third of the RDAs for lunch and about one-fourth of the RDAs for breakfast.[64]

To reduce heart disease, the current recommendation is to lower fat and saturated fat consumption. Current dietary recommendations call for energy reduction and a concomitant replacement of dietary fat with complex carbohydrate.[65,66] The revised *Dietary Guidelines for Americans*[66] apply to healthy individuals two years and older and address the progression of chronic diseases (e.g., CHD and hypertension). General goals include "Choose a diet low in fat, saturated fat, and cholesterol" and "Use salt and sodium only in moderation." Specific goals include the following:

- total fat 30% or less
- saturated fat <10%
- fewer animal sources of fat
- less salt and sodium in cooking, at the table, and when planning meals.

NUTRITION GUIDELINES FOR TODDLERS AND INFANTS

Specific statements are made in the Pediatric Panel Report of the National Cholesterol Education Panel (NCEP) regarding healthy food choices for toddlers and infants.[65] Toddlers two and three years of age are in a transition period during which they gradually adopt the eating patterns of the rest of the family. The RDAs for zinc, iron, and calcium are high for young children,[67] and preschoolers generally do not meet the RDAs for iron and zinc.[68] Foods that provide these nutrients are lean meat for iron and zinc, and low-fat dairy products for calcium. Fortified or enriched bread and cereal products, beans, and peas supply iron.

The NCEP excludes newborns to two years of age from dietary fat recommendations. These infants require energy-rich foods and a higher percentage of calories from fat than older children. The American Academy of Pediatrics, the American Heart Association, the National Institutes of Health Consensus Development Conference on Lowering Blood Cholesterol, and the NCEP all recommend that fat and cholesterol should not be restricted during infancy.[69-72]

Breast milk is recommended as the main source of nutrients from birth to six months of age, with infant formula substituted when breastfeeding is not possible. Breast milk and infant formula have a caloric density of about 0.7 kcal/mL and 50% of energy from fat to sustain growth and meet the small volume held by the stomach. After four to six months of age, pureed and mashed table foods, which provide fewer calories from fat than breast milk or formula, can be added gradually to replace some milk or formula. Fatty acid content of breast milk fat is partially influenced by a women's eating pattern and by her body fat stores. In fact, a low saturated fat or total fat eating pattern has limited effect on a woman's breast milk.[73,74]

The NCEP does not recommend feeding skim milk to infants because it provides a very high solute load per calorie from mineral salts and protein. This requires extra water for excretion in the urine and may lead to serious dehydration of the infant.

The NCEP's recommended eating pattern for toddlers does not require major changes from what young children currently eat. Preschool children have lower energy and nutrient needs per kilogram of body weight compared to toddlers, but protein and other nutrient needs are higher. Reduction in saturated fatty acids and total fat from the dairy and meat groups are recommended. A wide variety of foods from all food groups; regular, scheduled meal times; and low-fat snacks at midmorning, midafternoon, and bedtime are advised since toddlers have a limited capacity for food at one sitting.

These recommendations form the basis of primary prevention efforts early in life. They are supported by the *Healthy People 2000* health objectives for the year 2000,[75] the recommendations of the National High Blood Pressure Control Program,[76] and by the following:

- studies that report, for example, an average decrease among adults of 1% to 10% in plasma cholesterol from a higher intake of fiber-rich fruits, vegetables, grains, and legumes[77]

- the integration of nutrition education into preschool education for children and parents to encourage healthy behaviors (e.g., the "Fun Kit" with puppets, music cassettes, and stickers[78])

- documentation that positive mealtime behavior of child care providers (e.g., eating alongside children and giving positive comments about food) is associated with structured activities such as cooking and baking, tasting new foods, artwork, and storytelling[79]

Info Line

Although food labels for infants less than two years old look like labels on adult foods, there are differences:

- Food labels for infants do not list calories from fat, saturated fat, or cholesterol, but they do show total fat content.
- Serving sizes for infant foods are based on average amounts usually eaten at one time.
- Daily values are listed only for protein, vitamins, and minerals; they do not include fat, cholesterol, sodium, potassium, carbohydrate, or fiber.

Source: Adapted from National Center for Nutrition and Dietetics. *Nutrition Fact Sheet. Food Labels for Infants under Two Years.* 1994. page 1.

ROLE OF CAREGIVERS

In 1992, 24,361 child care centers and 161,533 day care homes were participating in the USDA Child and Adult Care Food Program. This program involved approximately 1.9 million children who ate at least one meal on the premises.[80]

Much of the protection and health promotion of children rests with caregivers. Today's parenting lifestyle often includes assigning responsibility of infants or preschoolers to caregivers for the majority of the waking hours. Caregivers are responsible for encouraging healthful behavior patterns including exercise, sleep, and play and for practicing healthful food preparation, sanitation, and safety procedures. The latter are necessary to reduce the potential of foodborne illness (see Chapter 6).

Most communicable illnesses are transferred from one child to another in group settings via coughing; sneezing; and improperly sanitized eating utensils, toys, and toilets. Simple handwashing procedures and proper toileting and handling of colds and diarrhea can reduce the spread of illness.[81]

Meeting the nutrient need of infants and children in group care settings requires attention to the following[81-83]:

- *A variety of foods:* Presenting different foods promotes awareness and generates interest.
- *Interesting shapes, colors, and temperatures:* Children enjoy crisp, finger-size foods that are easy to chew and handle. Cool and warm foods are preferred to hot and very cold foods, since a child's mouth is sensitive to temperatures. Foods that can cause choking include tough or stringy meat, grapes, nuts, small pieces of hard raw vegetables and fruits, miniature hot dogs, popcorn, and small pieces of fried foods. Single foods rather than mixed foods or casseroles are preferred. Individually wrapped servings teach self-service and dexterity.
- *Appropriate servings:* Preschoolers can meet the RDAs for their age group by eating small servings rather than adult servings (1 tablespoon per year of age).
- *Ethnic variety and awareness:* Table manners and common foods of preschoolers vary by ethnic group. For example, Japanese often wash their faces and hands with a wet towel at the table before the meal and use a

low table for eating; Asians often drink soup directly from the bowl; Europeans may cut fruit and some sandwiches with a knife and fork. Children may be used to certain foods with their meals. For example, tortillas are common with Mexican Americans, sliced bread with Anglo Americans, and biscuits or cornbread with African Americans. Activities that develop an awareness of the richness of many cultures include the following[84]:

1. activities that build on the shared experiences of all people, not on the emphasis of difference
2. programs that reach outside the immediate child care environment
3. projects that use racial, cultural, and socioeconomic backgrounds of the children in care
4. planned curricula with incidental teaching opportunities giving a multicultural perspective

- *Frequent feedings:* Preschoolers' small stomachs, small appetites, and short attention spans demand an eating approach that provides nutrient-dense foods in small and frequent feeding times. Snacks of fruit, dairy products, or cereal should be served two hours from meals.

- *Family-style meal service:* Providing bulk quantities of each food allows teaching staff to serve small portions of single foods first and then to promote second helpings. This encourages capacity building among the children, for example, acquiring the capacity to eat a variety of foods rather than focusing on any one favorite food.

- *Avoidance of certain foods:* Foods to avoid include foods that are hard to control, chew, or swallow such as whole nuts and grapes, raw carrots, and hard candies. Remove obvious hazards such as fruit pits and fish bones (except canned salmon, which has bones that can be mashed into the meat). Quarter breads and sandwiches.

- *Elimination of conflict around food:* Conflicts about food and preoccupation with eating can lead to negative attitudes and behaviors about food. Realistic and positive expectations by parents and food service

staff about food are essential if eating is to be a primary prevention training ground for children and if children are to establish positive eating behaviors early in life.

NUTRITION STANDARDS FOR CHILD CARE PROGRAMS

Caring for Our Children—National Health and Safety Performance Standards: Guidelines for Out-of-Home Child Care Programs[85] is a joint publication of the American Academy of Pediatrics and American Public Health Association. It provides a consensus of direction regarding how to provide quality care for children in child care programs. A written plan for the food and nutrition services is a key standard; a comprehensive plan written under the direction of a nutrition specialist is preferred. Three guiding principles set the tone of the nutrition section of the standards[85]:

1. Food should help to meet the child's daily nutritional needs and reflect individual and cultural differences. Foods should provide an opportunity for learning, and activities should complement and supplement those of the home and the community. The facility can assist the child and family to understand the association between nutrition and health and various ways to meet the nutritional needs.
2. A nutrition specialist or food service expert is a vital member of the facility's planning team to ensure the implementation of an efficient and cost-effective food service.
3. To prevent food-borne illness, proper equipment and food handling are essential.

The American Dietetic Association (ADA) has published a position paper entitled "Nutrition Standards for Child Care Programs."[86] The standards cited by ADA reflect those of the following groups:

- US Department of Health and Human Services (DHHS) as established for the Head Start Program
- USDA for the Child and Adult Care Food Program

- American Public Health Association for home child care
- American Academy of Pediatrics for home child care
- Society for Nutrition Education for child care facilities

The ADA recommendations include the following:

- *Meal plans:* One-third of the RDAs should be met if the child is present four to seven hours per day; one-half to two-thirds of the RDAs should be met for a child present eight or more hours per day. Meals and snacks with a variety of nutritious foods should comprise the foods offered. Attention should be given to cultural food patterns, appetizing colors and textures, and appropriate portions.
- *Preparation and food service:* Salt, fat, and sugar should be kept to a minimum. Fruits, vegetables, and whole-grain foods should be promoted. Preparation that promotes nutrient retention is essential.
- *Nutrition consultation and guidance:* Registered dietitians (RDs) knowledgeable of the child care environment and the nutrient needs of infants and preschoolers should be employed to review and guide a quality program.
- *Nutrition education and training:* Education for children, parents, and caregivers should be routine. Parents can serve as instructors and facilitators.
- *Physical and emotional environment:* A positive, enjoyable interaction among children and adults is preferred.
- *Compliance with local and state regulations:* All tasks to ensure wholesomeness of foods and the sanitation and safety of the facility should be followed.

HEALTHY MENU PLANNING IN CHILD AND FAMILY DAY CARE CENTERS

In one study, researchers reviewed child care facility menus in 10 states and found that the menus were not consistently nutritionally adequate. The variety of foods is often limited, servings of cruciferous fruits and vegetables are rare, and fat content is high.[87]

To evaluate the menu planning process, Briley et al used a mailed survey to 300 child care centers located across six US states in different geographic regions.[87] Menu planners ($N = 153$) were described and included the following: 98% were female, 46% were older than 45 years of age, 80% were full-time employees, 72% were at current site more than 5 years, and 36% were program directors. The study reported 40% of the menu planners also served as cook at the center, 66% received training in food service, 58% received training on the job, 41% completed college-based training, and 33% used home study courses.[87]

Another study identified factors that influenced menu planning in three child care centers in Texas. Each center was comprised of children from different ethnic groups, but the findings across centers were similar. The most influential menu factors were the food program requirements, staff perceptions of children's food preferences, the background of the food program, and the fee for the child care service. The conclusions of the study were as follows[88]:

- Menu improvement is needed.
- Training for center or home care staff should be sensitive to ethnic composition of the center's client base.
- Staff's nutrition knowledge has an indirect influence on menu quality.
- Program requirements and monitoring activities need revision.

In California, the California Department of Education, Child Nutrition and Food Distribution Division has developed a healthy meal pattern planning guide, called "The New SHAPE Meal Pattern"[89] for child care food programs that feed children from 1 to 12 years of age (see Table 7–5).

For infants, meal planning centers around breast milk or formula for the first four to six months of age. Solid foods are introduced between four and six months. Portions listed are the minimum amount needed to ensure achieve-

Table 7–5 The New SHAPE Meal Pattern for California Child Care Food Programs, 1994

Meal and Meal Components	Age	
	1 to 3 years	3 to 6 years
Breakfast		
Milk, fluid	½ C	½ C
Vegetable, fruit, or full-strength juice	¼ C	½ C
Bread/bread alternates (whole grain or enriched)	2 servings total[a]	4 servings total[a]
• Bread	½ slice	½ slice
• Or cornbread, rolls, muffins, biscuits	½ serving	½ serving
• Or cold dry cereal (volume or weight, whichever is less)	¼ C or ⅓ oz	⅓ C or ½ oz
• Or cooked cereal, pasta, noodle products, or cereal grains	¼ C	¼ C
Lunch/Supper		
Milk, fluid	½ C	½ C
Vegetable and/or fruit (two or more kinds)	¼ C total	¾ C total
Bread/bread alternates (whole grain or enriched)	2 servings total[a]	2 servings total[a]
• Bread	½ slice	½ slice
• Or cornbread, rolls, muffins, biscuits	½ serving	½ serving
• Or cold dry cereal (volume or weight whichever is less)	¼ C or ⅓ oz	⅓ C or ½ oz
• Or cooked cereal, pasta, noodle products, or cereal grains	¼ C	¼ C
Meat/meat alternates[b,c]		
• Lean meat, fish, or poultry (edible portion as served)	1 oz	1½ oz
• Or cheese, cottage cheese	1 oz	1½ oz
• Or egg	1 egg	1 egg
• Or cooked dry beans or peas[b]	¼ C	⅜ C
• Or peanut butter, soy nut butter, or other nut or seed butters	2 T	3 T
• Or peanuts, soy nuts, tree nuts, seeds	½ oz[c]	¾ oz[c]
• Or an equivalent quantity of any combination of the above meat/meat alternates		
AM or PM Supplement (Snack)—Select 2 of these 4 components:		
Milk, fluid[d]	½ C	½ C
Vegetable, fruit, or full-strength juice[d]	½ C	½ C
Bread/bread alternates (whole grain or enriched)	2 servings total[a]	2 servings total[a]
• Bread	½ slice	½ slice
• Or cornbread, rolls, muffins, biscuits	½ serving	½ serving
• Or cold dry cereal (volume or weight, whichever is less)	¼ C or ⅓ oz	⅓ C or ½ oz
• Or cooked cereal, pasta, noodle products, or cereal grains	¼ C	¼ C
Meat/meat alternates[b,c]		
• Lean meat, fish or poultry (edible portion as served)	½ oz	½ oz
• Or cheese or cottage cheese	½ oz	½ oz
• Or egg	½ egg	½ egg
• Or cooked dry beans or peas[b]	⅛ C	⅛ C
• Or peanut butter, soy nut butter, or other nut or seed butters	1 T	1 T
• Or peanuts, soy nuts, tree nuts, seeds· or yogurt	½ oz[c]	½ oz[c]
• Or an equivalent amount of any combination of the above meat/meat alternates	¼ C	¼ C

[a]Any combination of bread/bread alternates may be served, as long as the required number of servings is met.

[b]In the same meal service, dried beans or dried peas may be used as a meat alternate or as a vegetable; however, such use does not satisfy the requirement for both components.

[c]No more than 50% of the requirement shall be met with nuts or seeds. Nuts or seeds shall be combined with another meat/meat alternate to fulfill the requirement. For the purpose of determining combinations, 1 oz of nuts or seeds is equal to 1 oz of cooked lean meat, poultry, or fish.

[d]Juice may not be served when milk is served as the only other component.

continues

Table 7–5 continued

Note: General selection guides:

Milk:
- Use breast milk or iron-fortified formula for children under one year of age.
- Use whole milk for children one to two years of age.
- Emphasize use of 2% low-fat milk for children two years and older.

Fruits/Vegetables:
- Must offer raw fruits or vegetable at least once a day.
- Serve vitamin A and vitamin C rich foods daily.

Bread/bread alternates:
- One-half of all bread/bread alternates served must be a minimum of 25% whole grain (with recommended levels of 33% or more whole grain) or list whole grain as first ingredient.

Meat/meat alternate:
- Emphasize lean and lower-sodium choices.
- At least ⅛ cup beans per week must be served as replacement for ½ ounce meat/meat alternate.

Source: Adapted from California Department of Education. Child Nutrition and Food Distribution Division. *The New Shape Meal Pattern*. Sacramento, CA. 1994.

---

ment of the RDAs. The meal planning guide uses whole milk for children from one to two years of age and emphasizes 2% low-fat milk for children two years and older. A raw fruit or vegetable must be offered at least once a day, and foods rich in vitamin A and vitamin C must be served daily. One-half of all bread/bread alternates served must be from 25% to 33% whole grain, or list whole grain as the first ingredient. Emphasis must be placed on lean and lower-sodium choices. At least one-eighth cup of beans must replace one-half ounce of meat or meat alternate each week.

While several changes would have to be made to incorporate these guidelines into child care food programs outside of California, an overriding goal is to lower the fat intake of young children. This message motivates menu planning in many programs throughout the United States due to the recommendations of the National Cholesterol Education Panel (NCEP) Report on Blood Cholesterol Levels in Children and Adolescents.[65]

The extent of limiting fat in preschool menus depends on the age of the child and the primary prevention population approach to be used. Some skeptics have asked if 30% to 35% of energy from fat can provide adequate calories for two-to-six-year-old preschoolers. To lower fat and still meet the recommendations for all nutrients including fat, each meal and snack must provide variety and adequate amounts of fruits, vegetables, grains, breads, cereals, and legumes each day.

Low-fat dairy products and moderate portions of lean meats and poultry must be served.[90] While targeting a lower fat content means lowering the fat in food, menu planners must address the smaller appetites of preschoolers and control the salt and sugar content of the foods planned. A transition phase may be warranted to lower the fat, salt, and sugar content while maintaining taste and visual appeal.[91]

Zimmerman et al used computer modeling to determine menu planning components to reduce fat but retain two-thirds of the RDAs for young children.[92] The following techniques were applied: medium-fat meats (MMt) replaced high-fat ones; lean meats (LMt) replaced higher-fat ones; lean meats were used with three high-fat meats a week (LMt-mod); skim milk (Skim) replaced whole milk and 2% milk; fat-modified products (FMP) were used; low-fat preparation techniques (PrP) were used; and extraneous sources of fat (EF) were removed.

For children two and three years old, single strategies of LMt, LMt-mod, Skim, FMP, EF, and a combined strategy of MMt + PrP achieved the goal of less than 30% ± 1% of calories from fat, and reduced energy intake by 54 to 107 kcal. Only strategies Skim and MMt + PrP also met the criteria of providing at least 67% of the RDAs for one-to-three year olds. Zinc and Vitamin D were low. Menus were made isocaloric or the same by adding carbohydrates. Then strategies LMt,

FMP, and LMt-mod also achieved both goals. All techniques led to a decrease in saturated fatty acids and monounsaturated fatty acids. Only the isocaloric strategy Skim approached the recommended ratio of saturated to monounsaturated to polyunsaturated fatty acids.

For children four and five years old, strategies LMt, LMt-mod, Skim, FMP, EF, and MMt + PrP achieved the goal of less than 30% ± 1% of calories from fat, met at least 67% of the RDAs, and reduced energy intake by 58 to 131 kcal. When strategies LMt and Skim were made isocaloric, saturated fatty acids and monounsaturated fatty acids fell at or below 10% ± 1% of total calories.

Several strategies can be used to lower total fat in the menu for preschoolers. Planners must recognize and alter saturated and monounsaturated fatty acids sources. Menus must be isocaloric, if variety is to be achieved, but nutrient-rich to ensure micronutrient adequacy.[92]

Info Line

Children's Choices is a unique, culturally sensitive cookbook for family day care providers. It contains more than 100 recipes for breakfast, lunch/supper, snacks, and party/special occasions, with a minimum of two preparation and tasting tests per recipe. A four-week menu cycle incorporates many of the recipes that meet the Child Care Food Program requirements. Recipes are analyzed for key nutrients and projected for eight preschool and eight school-age portions. Symbols designate if the recipe is microwavable, quick and easy, vegetarian, prepared ahead of time, party/special occasion, or a "kids can help" dish.

Children's Choices was developed under the direction of the California Department of Education, Nutrition and Food Distribution Education Section.[93] For more information, contact: California State Department of Education, Nutrition and Food Distribution Division, PO Box 944272, Sacramento, CA 94244.

ROLE AND STATUS OF CHILD CARE EMPLOYEES

The major responsibility of staff in child care centers and family child care homes is to protect young children from any hazards in the eating environment and to provide enjoyable and nutritious foods. Specific information needed by all employees includes the following[94]:

- basic concepts of nutrition, including nutrition issues in the child care setting
- interpretation and application of nutrition information and resources
- likes and dislikes, cultural beliefs and practices, and the food acceptability of preschoolers
- procurement and production techniques with attention to specifications, labels, storage, cost, nutrient retention, and standardized production

One avenue to disseminate the information is continuing education activities that enrich the skills of employees. Management can provide these activities with hands-on learning experiences, discussions, simulations, and problem-solving exercises. Often, connecting the daily activities of the center or home to a state or national initiative (e.g., "5 A Day") increases staff commitment and gives direction. Integrating parents into program planning with staff and providing incentives for staff participation in continuing education strengthen the chances that employees will buy into the activities.

What is a typical child care facility? In 1993, a statewide survey of child care centers was conducted in California.[95] A mass mailing of 707 questionnaires was sent to agencies that sponsored a Child Care Food Program (CCFP). These respondents were called *sponsors*. A 20% random sample (*N* = 23) of the 114 agencies that only sponsor day care homes was identified. Day care homes are actual residences in which an individual takes care of children as a daytime job. This random sample of agencies received the sponsor questionnaire and a questionnaire for day care home providers.

Completed questionnaires were returned by 445 CCFP sponsors out of 707 agencies, for a 63% response rate; 16 agencies or 70% of the random sample returned questionnaires regarding day care homes. These are high response rates for mailed questionnaires. Of the CCFP sponsors, 40% represented urban areas; 16% represented rural areas; 25% served both rural and urban areas; and 13% served the suburban areas of California. Of the respondents, 34% served metropolitan areas with more than 250,000 people; 15% served towns with less than 25,000 people.

The title of the respondents included director, coordinator, administrator, nutrition coordinator, and program director. Of the respondents, 47% had served in their current position between one and five years; 39% were 41 to 50 years of age, and 30% were 31 to 40 years of age; 39% had either a B.A. or B.S. degree, and 28% held Master's degrees. Only 4% of the respondents were registered dietitians. There was an almost equal percentage of agency directors who earned either $15,000 to $24,999 (27%) or $25,000 to $34,999 (28%); 19% earned above $35,000 a year.

Agencies provided various incentives for their director or supervisor to gain professional training. Paid time for training was provided for 59% of the directors/supervisors, whereas only 3% had received a single salary increase and 1% a single promotion after additional training. Of the respondents, 9% had both pay increases and promotion when they participated in continuing education and training, but 26% reported receiving no incentive (neither paid time for training, salary increase or promotion) for continuing education.

Of the sponsors, 54% managed some developmentally disabled children. Due to the multiethnic population in California, 59% of nutrition staff members were bilingual. Of the sponsors, 19% employed a nutrition education specialist.

Average daily participation at child care centers varied (i.e., 63% had fewer than 200 children, 15% kept 200 to 799 children, and 7% cared for more than 800 children). The number of centers sponsored by a single sponsor across the state ranged from 1 to over 20; 68% sponsored one to five centers, 17% sponsored 6 to 10 centers, 4% sponsored 11 to 20, and 6% sponsored more than 20 day care centers. Agencies reported sponsoring from 1 to 1,500 individual home child care providers.

Sponsors were asked how well prepared they felt on topics related to their job. Over 40% of the sponsors felt very well prepared on the topics of food sanitation, interpersonal skills, organization management, healthy menu planning, personnel management, and arranging pleasant mealtimes. They reported not at all prepared for special feeding concerns (53%), infant feeding (31%), recycling waste (28%), cultural foods (23%), and disaster planning (19%).

Of the sponsors, 18% had a regular quarterly or annual training schedule for their staff members that commonly used demonstrations, handouts, and video tapes. On-the-job training was continuous. Demonstrations, handouts, group discussions, and on-the-job training were common for home care providers.

Menu and food service system characteristics included 54% of sponsors preparing meals on-site, 13% subcontracting, and 13% using bulk preparation at a central kitchen. Of the sponsors, 37% followed a menu planning system consistently.

Breakfast and lunch were commonly served at centers and homes. About one-half of centers and homes served dinner. Snacks were also popular at both types of facilities.[95]

TECHNIQUES TO ASSESS FOOD LIKES OF PRESCHOOLERS

A common procedure in child care facilities is to regulate a child's food intake to reduce food waste and to control overeating. A 29-day study assessed self-selected feeding of 20 preschool children who were three years old and 20 who were four years old. Preschoolers could select and eat as much as they wanted. Using a 2×2 factorial design, a significant interaction of class and feeding method was noted. Four year olds increased their intake more than three year olds; but no significant difference was noted in plate waste, whether self-selection or portion-control was used. A significant difference was noted in plate waste by age: younger children wasted more than older children.[96] Based on this study, child care providers should review their menu planning and portion-control procedures.

It has been the norm to use adult food preferences when planning meals and snacks for children.[97] Some researchers report that young children are not reliable respondents; others have observed that children can report preferences better than their parents.[98,99] Three-year-old children have been found to be reliable and consistent when reporting their likes and dislikes about food.[100] Several techniques that have been useful to day care center staff are as follows:

- *A facial hedonic scale:* This has shown consistency by having children rate preferences for a sample of food by circling the face that reflects how they feel about a food.[101]
- *A ranking scale:* With this method, preschoolers are presented with a group of foods, asked to taste them, and then asked to identify the ones they like the best. The preferred item can be removed and the procedure repeated to establish a list of preferred foods.[97]
- *Plate waste method:* This technique is used when a standard portion is served to a child. The amount remaining is subtracted from the standard portion to determine how much was eaten.
- *Informal tasting with sample bites:* By using this method, children can sample foods at a classroom learning center in science or health and associate what they eat with their health.[97]

Info Line

A "kid culture" or "child care culture" may exist in day care centers and home facilities. Common menu items served across a group of child care facilities in Texas included spaghetti, fish sticks, hot dogs, potato chips, and cookies, which may be extremely popular but are nutrient poor.[88,102]

SUMMER FOOD SERVICE PROGRAM

The summer can often create a time of deficit food intake for children. Organizations may sponsor a Summer Food Service Program (SFSP), but sponsorship is limited to the following[103]:

- public and private nonprofit school food authorities, residential summer camps, and colleges and universities that participate in the summer programs for youth
- private, nonprofit organizations that meet specific criteria defined in SFSP regulations
- local, county, municipal, state, or federal government units.

Both private, nonprofit organizations and governmental units must have direct operational control over each site under their sponsorship. This means that they will be responsible for (1) managing site staff, including such areas as hiring, conditions of employment, and termination; and (2) exercising management control over SFSP operations at sites during the period of program participation.[103]

Potential sponsors must demonstrate that they have the necessary financial and administrative capability to meet SFSP objectives and to comply with program regulations. They must also accept final financial and administrative responsibility for all sites under their auspices. Approved sponsors must operate the program according to the federal and state regulations. Management responsibilities cannot be delegated below the sponsor level. The quality of the meal service, the conduct of site personnel, and the adequacy of recordkeeping reflect the sponsor's performance, which is subject to audit by the administering agency, by the USDA Office of the Inspector General, and by the General Accounting Office.

Sponsors may operate the SFSP at one or more sites (i.e., the physical locations where program meals are served to children). Regular sites and sites primarily for homeless children may be approved to serve up to two meals daily, either lunch and breakfast or lunch and a snack. Sites serving primarily migrant children and camps may be approved to serve up to four meals per day—breakfast, snack, lunch, or supper.[103]

Sponsors must demonstrate that their proposed open sites are located in areas in which poor economic conditions exist. Two methods to demonstrate this are use of school data and use of census tract data.

Sponsors of sites where meals are served only to an enrolled group of children must document eligibility based on statements of the household size and income, food stamp numbers, or Aid to Families with Dependent Children (AFDC) case numbers of children enrolled at each site. Sponsors must demonstrate that at least 50% of the enrolled children have been individually determined eligible for free or reduced-price school meals.[103]

Sponsors may either prepare their own meals, obtain meals from a school food service authority, or obtain meals from a food service management company. Meals must meet meal pattern requirements as outlined in Appendix 7–D. Sponsors must comply with the following rules[103]:

- Serve the same meal to all children.
- Ensure that children eat all meals on-site. Site personnel must be sure to supervise all children on the site while they are eating meals. Only meals that children eat on-site are eligible for reimbursement.
- Serve meals during the times of meal service posted and approved by the administering agency.
- Ensure that all children at the site receive one meal before any child is served a second meal.
- Ensure that there is a three-hour interval between meals. When nonresidential camp sites and sites serving primarily migrant children serve lunch and supper with no afternoon snack between the two meals, a four-hour interval must occur between lunch and supper.
- Except at feeding sites for homeless children, ensure that the meal service period is no more than two hours for lunch and supper and no more than one hour for all other meals, including snacks.

- Adhere to local health and sanitation regulations.
- Arrange for delivery and adequate storage of meals if not prepared at the site.

In a Summer Food Service Program, several job positions are essential to conduct an effective and efficient program. These include the director, the bookkeeper, site monitors, and the site supervisor. The responsibilities of these positions are listed in Appendix 7–E.

SPECIAL NUTRITION-RELATED CONCERNS

Several of the special nutrition concerns during gestation, infancy, and childhood are discussed briefly below.

Fetal Alcohol Syndrome

Data from the last decade show that several kinds of birth defects and mental retardation may result from ingestion of alcohol by pregnant women. This condition is known as fetal alcohol syndrome. Fetal alcohol syndrome is considered the third leading cause of birth defects and mental retardation among newborns. These harmful effects on fetal development occur in the first few weeks or months of prenatal development, which is when much of the nervous system is being formed. The level of alcohol in the fetus's blood may be 10 times greater than the blood alcohol content of the mother. A few drinks during pregnancy can endanger normal fetal development.[104]

Neural Tube Defects

In 1960 researchers discovered that folic acid deficiency causes birth defects in animals. A deficiency of folic acid during pregnancy paired with a family history of birth defects appears to increase the risk of neural tube defects in humans. Studies have shown that women with no previous history of children with neural tube defects can reduce their risk by 60% to 75% by taking a supplement of 0.4 mg to 0.8 mg of folic acid each day.[105]

Often, defect of the neural tube occurs in an embryo before a woman is aware that she is pregnant. Incidence in the United States is 1 to 2 infants per 1,000 live births. The average daily intake of folic acid for women is 0.2 mg. The Food and Drug Administration has recently proposed fortification of foods to ensure an adequate intake among childbearing women (i.e., 140 micrograms per 100 grams or 3.5 ounces of bread, rolls, buns, corn grits, cornmeal, rice, noodles, and farina). Good sources of folic acid include leafy green vegetables, citrus fruits, beans, and fortified breakfast cereals.

There are two types of neural tube defects: anencephaly, which means that a baby does not develop a brain, and spina bifida, which is a defect of the spinal column. An infant with anencephaly dies soon after birth. In an infant with spina bifida, the bones of the spinal column may surround the spinal cord but do not fuse correctly within the first month after conception. As a result, the cord or spinal fluid bulge in the lower back. Paralysis and incontinence occur. The severity of the condition ranges from a mild, often undiagnosed form to spina bifida aperta, which creates a sac called a meningocele on the infant's back. Symptoms range from hydrocephalus, to foot and knee deformities that require braces, to obesity due to limited ability to move.[105]

Phenylketonuria

Phenylketonuria (PKU) is a metabolic disorder characterized by a deficiency of phenylalanine hydroxylase. Hyperphenylalaninemia occurs when phenylalanine is not metabolized to tyrosine. A screening test, the Guthrie bacterial inhibition assay, is performed on blood from the heel of newborns within 28 days of life. Undiagnosed PKU infants without diet alteration (i.e., a low-phenylalanine diet, primarily Lofenalac formula) are severely mentally retarded and function with an IQ of about 40. Diagnosed and treated infants have a normal range of functioning and intelligence.[106]

Iron Deficiency Anemia

A significant decline in the prevalence of iron deficiency anemia has been observed among healthy children from 1969 to 1986, with credit given to improved prenatal and infant care among recipients of the Special Supplemental Food Program for Women, Infants and Children (WIC) (see Chapter 9). Iron deficiency (less than 3.5 mg%) remains the most common nutrient deficiency among US children six months to three years of age.[107]

Lead Poisoning

Lead exposure has now become the most common environmental disease of childhood.[108] A strong relationship between blood lead level, hematocrit, and age has been noted. The higher the blood lead level, the greater the probability of iron-deficiency anemia; a toxic level is from 10 to 25 micrograms/dL.[109] Lead affects nutrition by displacing essential divalent cations (e.g., iron, zinc, and calcium) in several metabolic functions; thereby, lead toxicity is associated with deficiencies of iron, zinc, and calcium.[110] Since the body absorbs lead more efficiently during times of growth, children and infants are susceptible to toxicity.

Even at low levels, lead can affect the central nervous system, hearing, blood pressure, and physical growth. Initial signs of lead poisoning include diarrhea, irritability, and lethargy. The long-term effects of exposure include lower IQ scores, poorer speech and language performance, impaired attention, and an increased risk of attention deficit disorder and hyperactivity.

In one study, 55% of African-American children living in poverty had blood lead levels greater than 10 micrograms/dL. The blood lead levels of 579 children, aged one to five, who lived near a lead smelter ranged from 11 to 164 micrograms/dL. The younger children with higher blood lead levels had a higher probability of anemia.[110]

Hyperactivity

Many dietary links to hyperactivity are presented as testimonials, parental reports, and case studies. Feingold's alarming statement in 1975 regarding food additives made many parents fearful of food additives, but clinical trials have not supported the allegations.[111] Only preschool children who had extremely high levels of food dyes or who were allergic to food dyes were observed to have adverse effects from diet.[112-114]

Sugar and aspartame have been reported to produce behavioral problems including hyperactivity among young children. A double-blind, controlled trial involving 25 normal three-to-five year olds and 23 "sugar sensitive" six-to-ten year olds was conducted by Wolraich and colleagues.[115] Three consecutive three-week modified diets were followed by the children and their families: (1) a diet with about 5,600 mg of sucrose per kg and no artificial sweeteners; (2) a diet low in sucrose with 38 g aspartame/kg; and (3) a diet low in sucrose but containing 12 mg saccharin as a placebo sweetener. None of the test foods had additives, artificial food coloring, or preservatives.

School-age children were given about 4,500 mg of sucrose/kg, 32 mg of aspartame per kg, and 9.9 mg saccharin per kg. The results showed that for 39 different behavioral and cognitive variables measured during the three diets, only preschool parents reported significantly better cognition during the sucrose diet versus the aspartame and saccharin diets and that a decreased pegboard performance occurred when the sucrose diet was followed. No significant differences were noted for the school-age children, and no adverse reaction occurred when children followed the sucrose or aspartame diets.[115] Overall, sugar, saccharin, and aspartame do not appear to affect behavior and cognitive functioning of young children.

RECAP OF COMMUNITY NUTRITION SERVICES—A PUBLIC HEALTH PERSPECTIVE

Since the 1920s, the United States has supported public health programs for infants and children. Title V of the Social Security Act of 1935 confirmed a state and federal collaboration to address the needs of this cohort. During the last 20 to 30 years, the US Congress has responded with appropriations for programs including the Special Supplemental Food Program for Women, Infants, and Children (WIC)[112-115]; the Food Stamp Program; Maternal and Child Health Services Block Grant Programs; the Preventive Health Services Block Grant Programs; the Medicaid Early Periodic Screening, Diagnosis and Treatment Program; and programs in the Indian Health Service.

WIC has been a highly funded program, primarily because evaluation has been conducted and positive results are visible.[116] For example:

- WIC lowers the rate of anemia among participating children ages six months to five years. The data show an average decrease in the anemia rate of more than 16% for each year from 1980 to 1992.[117]
- WIC significantly improves children's diets, particularly when it comes to vitamins and nutrients including iron, vitamin C, thiamin, protein, niacin, and vitamin B_6.[118]
- Four-and-five year olds who participate in WIC in early childhood have better vocabularies and digit memory scores than comparable children who do not participate in WIC.[118]
- WIC participants have higher rates of immunization against childhood diseases.[118]

Approximately 15,000 community nutrition professionals, commonly referred to as public health nutritionists, function at the local, state, and federal level to assess the needs of infants and children, to develop and direct programs, and to evaluate the impact of WIC and other programs.[119]

HEALTHY PEOPLE 2000 ACTIONS

Currently in the United States, public programs combine with the newer wave of community-based primary prevention activities of schools, universities, professional organizations, hospitals, clinics, and private industry to provide services and interventions for young children. The collaborative and complementary efforts of these groups are needed to address immediate health and nu-

Exhibit 7-1 *Healthy People 2000* Objectives for Infants and Preschoolers

---

2.4   Reduce growth retardation among low-income children aged 5 and younger to less than 10%. (Baseline: Up to 16% among low-income children in 1988, depending on age and race/ethnicity.)

Special Population Targets

Prevalence of Short Stature		1988 Baseline	2000 Target
2.4a	Low-income black children <age 1	15%	10%
2.4b	Low-income Hispanic children <age 1	13%	10%
2.4c	Low-income Hispanic children aged 1	16%	10%
2.4d	Low-income Asian/Pacific Islander children aged 1	14%	10%
2.4e	Low-income Asian Pacific Islander children aged 2-4	16%	10%

Note: Growth retardation is defined as height-for-age below the fifth percentile of children in the National Center for Health Statistics' reference population.

2.10   Reduce iron deficiency to less than 3% among children aged 1 through 4 and among women of childbearing age. (Baseline: 9% for children age 1 through 2, 4% for children age 3 through 4, and 5% for women aged 20 through 44 in 1976–80.)

Special Population Targets

Iron Deficiency Prevalence		1976–80 Baseline	2000 Target
2.10a	Low-income children aged 1-2	21%	10%
2.10b	Low-income children aged 3-4	10%	5%
Anemia Prevalence		*1983–85 Baseline*	*2000 Target*
2.10d	Alaska Native children aged 1-5	22-28%	10%

Note: Iron deficiency is defined as having abnormal results for two or more of the following tests: mean corpuscular volume, erythrocyte protoporphyrin, and transferrin saturation. Anemia is used as an index of iron deficiency. Anemia among Alaska Native children was defined as hemoglobin <11 gm/dL or hematocrit <34%. For pregnant women in the third trimester, anemia was defined according to CDC criteria. The above prevalences of iron deficiency and anemia may be due to inadequate dietary iron intakes or to inflammatory conditions and infections. For anemia, genetics may also be a factor.

2.11   Increase to at least 75% the proportion of mothers who breastfeed their babies in the early postpartum period, and to at least 50% the proportion who continue breastfeeding until their babies are 5 to 6 months old. (Baseline: 54% at discharge from birth site and 21% at 5 to 6 months in 1988.)

Special Population Targets

Mothers Breastfeeding Their Babies: during Early Postpartum Period		1988 Baseline	2000 Target
2.11a	Low-income mothers	32%	75%
2.11b	Black mothers	25%	75%
2.11c	Hispanic mothers	51%	75%
2.11d	American Indian/Alaska Native mothers	47%	75%
At Age 5–6 Months			
2.11a	Low-income mothers	9%	50%
2.11b	Black mothers	8%	50%
2.11c	Hispanic mothers	16%	50%
2.11d	American Indian/Alaska Native mothers	28%	50%

continues

Exhibit 7–1 continued

2.12 and 13.11   Increase to at least 75% the proportion of parents and caregivers who use feeding practices that prevent baby bottle tooth decay. (Baseline data available in 1991.)

Special Population Targets

Appropriate Feeding Practices		Baseline	2000 Target
2.12a and 13.11a	Parents and caregivers with less than high school education	–	65%
2.12b and 13.11b	American Indian/Alaska Native parents and caregivers	–	65%

14.1   Reduce the infant mortality rate to no more than 7 per 1,000 live births. (Baseline: 10.1 per 1,000 live births in 1987.)

Special Population Targets

Infant Mortality per 1,000 Live Births	1987 Baseline	2000 Target
14.1a Blacks	17.9	11
14.1b American Indians/Alaska Natives	12.5	8.5
14.1c Puerto Ricans	12.9	8

14.5   Reduce low birth weight to an incidence of no more than 5% of live births and very low birth weight to no more than 1% of live births. (Baseline: 6.9% and 1.2%, respectively, in 1987.)

Special Population Targets

Low Birth Weight	1987 Baseline	2000 Target
14.5a Blacks	12.7%	9%

Very Low Birth Weight	1987 Baseline	2000 Target
Blacks	2.7%	2%

Note: Low birth weight is weight at birth of less than 2,500 grams; very low birth weight is weight at birth of less than 1,500 grams.

20.8   Reduce infectious diarrhea by at least 25% among children in licensed child care centers and children in programs that provide an Individualized Education Program (IEP) or Individualized Health Plan (IHP). (Baseline data available in 1992.)

Source: Reprinted with permission from *Healthy People 2000: National Health Promotion and Disease Prevention Objectives.* Washington, DC: US Department of Health and Human Services; 1991. DHHS (PHS) Publication 91-50212.

trition needs, as well as long-term goals for a healthier population of children in the United States.

Eating behaviors and nutrient intakes early in life set the stage for lifelong habits. HP2K objectives include ensuring healthy body weight from birth to the preschool age (see Exhibit 7–1). Breastfeeding, iron deficiency anemia, and diarrhea are nutrition-related topics.[75] The meal and snack pattern and its blend with appropriate physical activity set the agenda for preschool and day care facilities. Community nutrition professionals have a visible role and responsibility to work with children, parents, teachers, administrators, and caregivers who work with preschool and day care facilities to achieve these HP2K objectives.

REFERENCES

1. Berenson G. Causation of cardiovascular risk factors. In: *Children—Perspectives on Cardiovascular Risk in Early Life*. New York, NY: Raven Press; 1986:408.

2. Wiecha JL, Grandon CA, Fisher-Miller P, et al. *Nutrition Counts: Massachusetts Nutrition Surveillance System, FY90 Annual Report*. Boston, Mass: Department of Public Health; 1991. ERIC Document Reproduction Service No. ED 338; 423.

3. Good ME. *A Needs Assessment: The Health Status of Migrant Children as They Enter Kindergarten*. San Jose, Calif: San Jose State University; 1990. ERIC Document Reproduction Service No. ED 338; 460.

4. Nutrition Cognition Initiative. 1994.

5. Center on Hunger, Poverty and Nutrition Policy. *The Link between Nutrition and Cognitive Development in Children*. Medford, Mass: Tufts University School of Nutrition; 1994:16.

6. County of Riverside Health Services Agency. *"Best Feeding" Lactation Counselors' Manual*. 2nd ed. Riverside, Calif: Department of Public Health Nutrition Services Branch; 1994.

7. American Academy of Pediatrics, Committee on Nutrition. The use of whole cow's milk in infancy. *Pediatrics*. 1992;89:1105–1109.

8. Kramer MS. Does breast-feeding help protect against atopic disease? Biology, methodology, and a golden jubilee of controversy. *J Pediatr*. 1988;112:181–190.

9. American Academy of Pediatrics, Committee on Nutrition. Hypoallergenic infant formulas. *Pediatrics*. 1989;83:1068–1069.

10. Clyne PS, Kulczycki A. Human breast milk contains bovine IgG. Relationship to infant colic? *Pediatrics*. 1991;87:439–444.

11. Heinig MJ, Nommsen LA, Peerson JM, et al. Energy and protein intakes of breast-fed and formula-fed infants during the first year of life and their association with growth velocity: The Darling study. *Am J Clin Nutr*. 1993;58: 152–161.

12. American Academy of Pediatrics. Committee on Nutrition. Statement of cholesterol. *Pediatrics*. 1992;90:469–473.

13. Ajzen I, Fishbein M. *Understanding Attitudes and Predicting Social Behavior*. Englewood Cliffs, NJ: Prentice Hall; 1980:250.

14. Lawless H. Sensory development in children: Research in taste and olfaction. *J Am Diet Assoc*. 1985;85:577.

15. Beauchamp GK, Cowart BJ. Congenital and experimental factors in the development of human flavor preferences. *Appetite*. 1985;6:357.

16. Cowart BJ, Beauchamp GK. The importance of sensory context in young children's acceptance of salty tastes. *Child Dev*. 1986;57:1034.

17. Birch LL. Dimensions of preschool children's food preferences. *J Nutr Ed*. 1979;11:77.

18. Birch LL. Preschool children' food preferences and consumption patterns. *J Nutr Ed*. 1979;11:189–192.

19. Burt JV, Hertzler AA. Parental influence on the child's food preference. *J Nutr Ed*. 1978;10:127.

20. Birch LL. The relationship between children's food preferences and those of their parents. *J Nutr Ed*. 1980;12:14.

21. Kirks BA, Hughes C. Long-term behavioral effects of parent involvement in nutrition education. *J Nutr Ed*. 1986;18:203.

22. Pliner P, Pelchant ML. Similarities in food preferences between children and their siblings and parents. *Appetite*. 1986;7:333.

23. Cooper JO, Heron TE, Heward WL. *Applied Behavior Analysis*. Columbus, Ohio: Charles E. Merrill Publishing Co; 1987.

24. Peterson LW. Operant approach to observation and recording. *Nurs Outlook*. 1967;15:28.

25. Pipes PC. *Nutrition in Infancy and Childhood*. 4th ed. Boston, Mass: Times Mirror/Mosby College Publishing; 1989:405.

26. Rozin P, Hammer L, Osler H, Horowitz T, Marmora Y. The child's conception of food: Differentiation of categories of rejected substances in the 16 months to 5 year age range. *Appetite*. 1986;7:141.

27. Birch LL, Deysher M. Conditional and unconditioned caloric compensation: Evidence for self-regulation of food intake in young children. *Learning and Motivation*. 1985;16:341.

28. Birch LL, Marlin DW, Rotter J. Eating as the 'means' activity in a contingency: Effects on young children's food preferences. *Child Dev.* 1984;55:431.

29. Rolls BJ. Experimental analysis of the effects of variety in a meal on human feeding. *Am J Clin Nutr.* 1985;42:932.

30. Michela JL, Contento IR. Spontaneous classification of foods by elementary school-aged children. *Health Ed Q.* 1984;11:57.

31. Bybee RW, Sund RB. *Piaget for Educators.* 2nd ed. Columbus, Ohio: Charles E. Merrill Publishing Co; 1982.

32. Food and Nutrition Service. *Food Guide Pyramid.* Washington, DC: US Dept. of Agriculture; 1992.

33. Swanson-Rudd J. Nutrition orientations of working mothers in the North Central region. *J Nutr Ed.* 1982;14:132.

34. Phillips DE, Bass MA, Yetley E. Use of food and nutrition knowledge by mothers of preschool children. *J Nutr Ed.* 1978;10:73.

35. Gillis DEG, Sabry JH. Daycare teachers: Nutrition knowledge, opinions, and use of food. *J Nutr Ed.* 1980;12:200.

36. Hertzler AA. Obesity—impact on the family. *J Am Diet Assoc.* 1981;79:525.

37. Birch LL. Mother-child interaction patterns and the degree of fatness in children. *J Nutr Ed.* 1981;12:17.

38. Birch LL, Zimmerman SI, Hind H. The influence of social-affective context on the formation of children's food preferences. *J Nutr Ed.* 1981;13:115.

39. Stark LJ, Collins FL, Osnes PG, Stokes TF. Using reinforcement and cueing to increase healthy snack food choices in preschoolers. *J Appl Behav Anal.* 1986;19:367.

40. Satter EM. The feeding relationship. *J Am Diet Assoc.* 1986;86:352.

41. Satter E. *Child of Mine.* Palo Alto, Calif: Bull Publishing Co; 1991.

42. Somers AR. Violence, television, and the health of American youth. *N Engl J Med.* 1976;294:811.

43. Blatt J, Spencer L, Ward S. A cognitive developmental study of children's reactions to television advertising. In: Rubinstein EA, Comstock GA, Murray JP, eds. *Television and Social Behavior, Vol 4: Television in Day to Day Life: Patterns of Use.* Washington, DC: US Government Printing Office; 1972.

44. Reid LN, Bearden WO, Teel JE. Family income, TV viewing, and children's cereal ratings. *Journalism Q.* 1980;57:327.

45. Choate R. Statement presented before the House Subcommittee on Communications of the Committee on Interstate and Foreign Commerce, US House of Representatives. Washington, DC: US Government Printing Office; 1975.

46. California Department of Health and Human Services. *5 a Day for Health.* Sacramento, Calif: California Department of Health and Human Services; 1992.

47. *Television, 1976,* North Brook, Ill: A.C. Nielson Co; 1976.

48. Wotecki CE. Nutrition in childhood and adolescence—Parts 1 and 2. *Contemporary Nutr.* 1992;17(2):1-2.

49. Knapp JA, Hazuda HP, Haffner SM, et al. A saturated fat/cholesterol avoidance scale: Sex and ethnic differences in a biethnic population. *J Am Diet Assoc.* 1988;88:172-177.

50. Frank GC, Zive M, Nelson J, et al. Fat and cholesterol avoidance among Mexican American and Anglo preschool children and parents. *J Am Diet Assoc.* 1991;91:954-961.

51. Gortmaker SL, Dietz WH, Sobol AM, et al. Increasing pediatric obesity in the US. *Am J Dis Children.* 1987;141:535-540.

52. Rolland-Cachera MF, Deheeger M, Avons P, et al. Tracking adiposity patterns from 1 month to adulthood. *Ann Hum Biol.* 1987;14:219-222.

53. Charney E, Goodman HC, McBride M, et al. Childhood antecedents of adult obesity: Do chubby infants become obese adults? *N Engl J Med.* 1976;295:6-9.

54. Owen JA, Frankle RT. *Nutrition in the Community.* St. Louis, Mo: Times Mirror-Mosby College Publishing; 1986:427.

55. Gutin B, Basch C, Shea S, et al. Blood pressure, fitness, and fatness in 5- and 6-year-old children. *JAMA.* 1990;264:1123-1127.

56. US Department of Health and Human Services. *Surgeon General's Report on Nutrition and Health.* Washington, DC: US Government Printing Office; 1988. Publication no. 88-50210.

57. Center for Disease Control and Prevention. Prevalence of overweight for Hispanics—United States, 1982-1984. *JAMA.* 1990;263:631.

58. Heinbach JT. Sodium, hypertension and the American public: Second tracking survey. *Public Health Rep.* 1985;100:371.

59. Johnson SL, Birch LL. Parents and children's adiposity and eating styles. *Pediatrics.* 1994;94:1-9.

60. Keys A. Coronary heart disease in seven countries. *Circulation.* 1970;41:1-211.

61. Webber LS, Cresanta JL, Voors AW, et al. Tracking of cardiovascular disease risk factor variables in school-age children. *J Chronic Dis.* 1983;36:647-660.

62. Freedman DS, Byers T, Sell K, et al. Tracking of serum cholesterol levels in multiracial sample of preschool children. *Pediatrics.* 1992;90:80-85.

63. Frerichs RR, Weber LS, Voors AW, et al. Cardiovascular disease risk factor variables in children at two successive years: The Bogalusa Heart Study. *J Chronic Dis.* 1979;32:251-262.

64. US Department of Agriculture. *Food Buying Guide for Child Nutrition Programs.* Washington, DC: US Government Printing Office; 1981. Program aid 1331.

65. National Cholesterol Education Panel. *Report of Cholesterol Levels of Children*. Bethesda, Md: National Cholesterol Education Panel; April 8, 1991.

66. US Department of Health and Human Services. *Nutrition and Your Health: Dietary Guidelines for Americans*. Washington, DC: US Government Printing Office; 1989.

67. National Research Council, Commission on Life Sciences, Food and Nutrition Board. *Recommended Dietary Allowances*. 10th ed. Washington, DC: National Academy Press; 1989.

68. Human Nutrition Information Service. *Nationwide Food Consumption Survey: Continuing Survey of Food Intakes by Individuals, Women 19–50 Years and Their Children 1–5 Years, 4 Days, 1986*. Hyattsville, Md: US Department of Agriculture; 1988. CSFII report no. 86-3.

69. National Cholesterol Education Program. *Report of the Expert Panel on Population Strategies for Blood Cholesterol Reduction*. Bethesda, Md: US Department of Health and Human Services, Public Health Services, National Institutes of Health, National Heart, Lung, and Blood Institute; November 1990. NIH pub. no. 90-3046.

70. Weidman W, Kwiterovich P Jr, Jesse MJ, et al. Diet in the healthy child. Task Force Committee of the Cardiovascular Disease in the Young Council of the American Heart Association. *Circulation*. 1983;67:1411A–1414A.

71. Consensus conference. Lowering blood cholesterol to prevent heart disease. *JAMA*. 1985;253:2080–2086.

72. American Academy of Pediatrics Committee on Nutrition. Prudent life-style for children: Dietary fat and cholesterol. *Pediatrics*. 1986;78:521–525.

73. Jensen RG, Ferris AM, Lammi-Keefe CJ, et al. Hypocholesterolemic human milk. *J Pediatr Gastroenterol and Nutr*. 1990;10:148–150.

74. Insull W Jr, Hirsch J, James T, et al. The fatty acids of human milk. II. Alterations produced by manipulation of caloric balance and exchange of dietary fats. *J Clin Invest*. 1959;38:443–450.

75. *Healthy People 2000: National Health Promotion and Disease Prevention Objectives*. Washington, DC: US Department of Health and Human Services; 1990. DHHS (PHS) publication 91-50212.

76. National Heart, Lung and Blood Institute. National High Blood Pressure Control Program. Bethesda, Md. 1994.

77. Connor WE, Connor SL. The dietary prevention and treatment of coronary heart disease. In: Connor WE, Bristow JD, eds. *Coronary Heart Disease: Prevention, Complications and Treatment*. Philadelphia, Pa: JB Lippincott Co; 1985.

78. Portland Unified School District. *"Fun Kit" Preschool Curriculum*. Portland, Ore: Portland School Food Service Department; 1992.

79. Clough CB, Forbes RL. Child care providers' backgrounds, nutrition competence, and provision of food and nutrition-related experiences. *American Dietetic Association Annual Meeting Abstracts Supplement*. 1992;92(9): A-96.

80. Willer B, Hofferth SL, Kisker EE, et al. *The Demand and Supply of Child Care in 1990*. Washington, DC: National Association for the Education of Young Children; 1991.

81. Duyff RL, Giarratano SC, Zurich MF. *Nutrition, Health and Safety for Preschool Children*. New York, NY: Glencoe-McGraw-Hill; 1994:238, 210–211.

82. Fredericks D. Safe and easy to eat meals. *Poppy Seeds*. Summer 1991:6.

83. Fredericks D. The eating challenge. *Poppy Seeds*. Spring 1993:15.

84. Fredericks D. Nutrition, food, fun and cultural awareness. *Poppy Seeds*. Fall 1990:8.

85. American Public Health Association and American Academy of Pediatrics. *Caring for Our Children—National Health and Safety Performance Standards*. Ann Arbor, Mich: Edward Brothers; 1992.

86. American Dietetic Association. Position of the American Dietetic Association: Nutrition standards for child care programs. *American Dietetic Association Annual Meeting Abstracts Supplement*. 1992;92(9):A-75.

87. Briley ME, Coyle E, Roberts-Gray C, Sparkman A. Nutrition knowledge and attitudes and menu planning skills of family day-home providers. *J Am Diet Assoc*. 1989;89:694–695.

88. Briley ME, Roberts-Gray C, Simpson D. Identification of factors that influence the menu at child care centers: A grounded theory approach. *J Am Diet Assoc*. 1994;94: 276–281.

89. Child Nutrition and Food Distribution Division. *The New Shape Meal Pattern*. Sacramento, Calif: California Department of Education; 1994.

90. Fredericks D. Cutting the fat . . . Proceed with caution! *Poppy Seeds*. Fall 1994:8.

91. Fredericks D. Nutritious meals using children's choices. *Poppy Seeds*. Winter 1994:6–7.

92. Zimmerman SA, Kris-Etherton P, Sigman MJ. Nutrient adequacy and effectiveness of dietary fat reduction techniques for preschool children. *American Dietetic Association Annual Meeting Abstracts Supplement*. 1992;92(9): A-112.

93. California Department of Education. *Child Nutrition and Food Distribution. Children's Choices*. Sacramento, Calif: California Department of Education; 1994.

94. Fredericks D. Staff development to fuel excellence. *Poppy Seeds*. Summer 1994:28.

95. Frank GC, Adsen MA. *Final Termination Report of the Statewide Survey of Child Care Food Program Sponsors*. Long Beach, Calif: California State University Long Beach, Child Nutrition Program Management Center; 1993:1–144.

96. Branen L, Fletcher J. Effects of restrictive and self-selected feeding on preschool children's food intake and waste at snacktime. *J Nutr Ed*. 1994;26:273–277.

97. Fredericks D. Measuring consumer acceptance. *Poppy Seeds*. Fall 1991:20–21.

98. Bryan MS, Lowenberg ME. The father's influence on young children's food preferences. *J Am Diet Assoc*. 1958;34:30–35.

99. Glaser A. Nursery school can influence food acceptance. *J Home Econ*. 1964;56:680–683.

100. Birch LL. Dimensions of preschool children's food preferences. *J Nutr Ed*. 1979;11:77–80.

101. Phillips BK, Kolasa KK. Vegetable preferences of preschoolers in day care. *J Nutr Ed*. 1980;12:192–195.

102. Briley ME, Simpson D, Roberts-Gray C. *Factors that Influence the Menu at the Child Care Center*. Austin, Tex: Texas Nutrition Education and Training Program; August 1992.

103. US Department of Agriculture, Food and Nutrition Service. *Summer Food Service Program for Children. Sponsor's Handbook*. Washington, DC: US Department of Agriculture; 1991. FNS-206.

104. Edlin G, Golanty E. *Health and Wellness: A Holistic Approach*. 4th ed. Boston, Mass: Jones and Bartlett Publishers; 1992:285–294.

105. Williams RD. FDA proposes folic acid fortification. *FDA Consumer*. 1994;11–14.

106. Mahan LK, Arlin MT. *Krause's Food Nutrition and Diet Therapy*. 8th ed. Philadelphia, Pa: WB Saunders Company; 1992:704.

107. Johnson AA. Iron deficiency: Pediatric epidemiology. In *Functional Significance of Iron Deficiency*. Annual Nutrition Workshop Series, Volume III, ed. C. Enwonuw. Nashville, Tenn: Meharry Medical College; 1990:57–65.

108. Needleman H. Lead exposure: The commonest environmental disease of childhood. *Bulletin of National Center for Clinical Infant Programs*. 1991;11:1–6.

109. Schwartz J, Landrigan PJ, Baker EL, et al. Lead-induced anemia: Dose-response relationships and evidence for a threshold. *Am J Public Health*. 1990;80:165–168.

110. Whitney EN, Rolfes SR. *Understanding Nutrition*. 6th ed. St Paul, Minn: West Publishing; 1993.

111. Feingold BF. Hyperkinesis and learning disabilities linked to artificial food flavors and colors. *Am J Nurs*. 1975;75:797–803.

112. Harley JP, Ray RS, Tomasi L, et al. Hyperkinesis and food additives: Testing the Feingold hypothesis. *Pediatrics*. 1978;61:818–828.

113. Swanson JM, Kinsbourne M. Food dyes impair performance of hyperactive children on a laboratory learning test. *Science*. 1980;207:1485–1487.

114. Weiss B, Williams JH, Margen S, et al. Behavioral responses to artificial food colors. *Science*. 1980;207:1487–1489.

115. Wolraich ML, Lindgren SD, Stumbo PJ, et al. Effects of diets high in sucrose or aspartame on the behavior and cognitive performance of children. *N Engl J Med*. 1994;330:301–307.

116. US Department of Agriculture, Food and Nutrition Service. *The Savings in Medicaid Costs for Newborns and Their Mothers from Prenatal Participation in the WIC Program*. Washington, DC: US Department of Agriculture; Oct 1990.

117. Henchy G, Parker L. *WIC Works—Let's Make It Work for Everyone*. Washington, DC: Food Research and Action Center; May 1993.

118. Rush D, Leighton J, Sloan L, et al. Study of infants and children. *Am J Clin Nutr*. 1988;48:484–511.

119. Kaufman M. *Nutrition in Public Health—A Handbook for Developing Programs and Services*. Gaithersburg, Md: Aspen Publishers, Inc; 1990:570.

Appendix 7-A

A Glimpse into the Past—The WIC Program's Humble Beginnings in the 1960s

Physicians from neighborhood clinics began filling the conference room in the Health, Education and Welfare Department (HEW), joining the staff from the Bureau of Women and Children in Public Health Service. I was the only stranger in the meeting, sitting there wondering why I, as the administrator of Consumer and Marketing Service (CMS) at the Department of Agriculture (USDA), had been invited.

The doctors, all young and tired looking, uneasy about being away from their clinics, began to discuss the problem that brought them to Washington that spring day in 1968. Young women were coming into the clinics, they said, often pregnant, complaining of various ailments. The women had various symptoms, the doctors said, but they were not suffering from any diseases. Some brought infants who cried a lot and otherwise were listless. . . . I asked, "Why don't you prescribe food?" realizing why I had been invited to the meeting.

With exasperation, one doctor said, "We don't have the authority to prescribe food." The head of the Bureau, a kindly woman whose name I cannot recall, said "Even if we could authorize food as a prescription, we don't have the funds. It would be too expensive for the service, and it isn't in the budget."

"Is there anything the Department of Agriculture could do?" she asked. They described the kinds of foods, including infant formula, that would be needed. "I don't know. Let me look into it," I said lamely. "We don't have any programs that would fit that problem. I'll get back to you."

"Could we build food commissaries attached to the neighborhood clinics, stock them with the commodities the doctors say they need, and let the doctors or clinic staff prescribe food, with the prescription serving as a voucher the women could use to receive a food package?"

The CMS staff thought the agency had many of the commodities already in stock as surplus, and there was authority and funding to purchase additional food in the market, if the Secretary of Agriculture determined such an action was in the department's interest.

I said, "Get a schematic drawing of a prototype commissary. Check with the Bureau on the commodities they will need, and work out where they should be located for easy access. Get the paperwork ready, and see where the Bureau would want the first units located. Come back in two weeks and let me know where we are." Two months later one summer day, the schematic drawing was brought to my office accompanied

Note: This is an account written by Rodney E. Leonard when he was the administrator of Consumer and Marketing Service at the US Department of Agriculture in 1968.

Source: Reprinted in part from Leonard RE. Recalling WIC Program's humble beginnings in the 1960's. *Consumer Nutrition Institute.* April 22, 1994. pp. 4–7.

by the proud smiles of the commodity division staff.

In Atlanta, Georgia, in the early fall of 1968 the first commissary was dedicated. Herman Talmadge was the Chairman of the Senate Agriculture Committee and the Senator from Georgia. The young doctor who was most vocal in the HEW meeting was from that clinic in Atlanta, and the politics fit the need perfectly. The first Women, Infant and Children (WIC) supplemental food program site was opened.

The Nixon administration began and a muted approach to WIC followed. Dr. David Paige, a physician at the Johns Hopkins School of Medicine, had started a voucher program in the Cherry Hills neighborhood in nearby Baltimore. Using his project as a model we developed legislative language which would authorize the concept as law.

By 1972, we were ready to move and crafted the legislation carefully. The WIC program would be only a two-year demonstration. We knew from the results of Dr. Paige's project that the benefits would be so overwhelming that WIC would easily be continued as a full program. We wrote the language to instruct that USDA shall carry out the demonstration program; in legislative language the word "shall" is a legally binding term that requires the agency to do exactly what the legislation says. Funding would be provided at $20 million a year, directing funds be taken from Section 32 of the statute authorizing the farm programs (obligating one-third of previous year customs receipts to USDA bypassing the Appropriation committee).

Senator Hubert H. Humphrey arranged hearings in the Agriculture Committee, which cast a tie vote on the legislation. Normally a bill cannot be reported to the Senate without an affirmative vote. Humphrey knew that a House committee chair could bring legislation to the floor without first holding a hearing as a matter of personal privilege, and Humphrey asked for help that day. Representative Carl Perkins, Chairman of the House Education and Labor Committee, was a fierce advocate for children and spearheaded the effort. The result was that the House adopted the WIC legislation by unanimous consent.

The Nixon administration inadvertently removed any final obstacle to the WIC program as a permanent feature of the federal nutrition program. Following enactment, USDA refused to carry out the legislative mandate. Food and Nutrition Service was ordered to ignore the law, but the head of Food Research and Action Center (FRAC) stepped in with a lawsuit arguing that the word "shall" removed any discretionary authority the Secretary might believe he possessed. USDA's obstinacy delayed the first year of the two-year demonstration, so the judge ordered USDA to spend the full amount of the funding, or $40 million, in the second year, 1973. Perkins introduced legislation to permanently authorize the WIC program in 1974. The program received overwhelming support and easily passed both the House and the Senate.

None of this would have been possible if Senator Humphrey had not returned to the Senate as the putative leader of the Democratic party, willing to champion the legislation with his considerable energy and political prestige. Nor could WIC have become the program it is today had not Rep. Perkins used his authority as chairman to expand the substantial political capital and risk defeat on a matter of personal privilege. And for all of that, millions of infants, children, and pregnant women are healthier today than would otherwise be possible.

Appendix 7–B

An Abbreviated List of Activities for Preschoolers with and without Adult Assistance

Activities with Adults

- *Over-under-around:* Adult sits on floor, legs apart. Child moves around parent going over legs. Parent forms a bridge. Child goes under and around.

- *Jump the stick:* Parent holds a pole just above the floor and child jumps over.

- *Jumping beans:* Hold the child's hands in yours. Child starts bouncing, then jumping up and down. Stop, rest, and start again.

- *Wheelbarrow:* Child lays face down on the floor. Parent grasps child's ankles and lifts upward. Ask the child to push up with arms until arms are straight. With head up, walk the hands forward. Child's body should not sag.

- *Row, row, row your boat:* Parent sits with legs apart, child sits opposite with legs in the middle. Grasp the child's hands. Child leans back as if "rowing a boat," then pulls to sit upright. Repeat. Sing "Row, row, row your boat."

Activities without Adults

- *Twister:* Child takes a pole and holding it with both hands, steps through the triangle formed by the arms and pole. The child then should be able to step foot-by-foot forward and backward without letting go of the stick.

- *Jump the brook:* Use a towel or mark the sidewalk with the "banks of the brook." Child stands on one side of the brook and attempts to jump the brook without "falling in."

- *Simon says:* Simon says: "Can you touch your toe to your chin?" Select body parts that encourage stretching.

- *Wall push-ups:* Stand about an arm's distance away from a wall with your legs together. Place your hands on the wall just a little wider than your shoulders. Lean forward and touch your nose to the wall and push back to your starting position. Be sure to keep your body in a straight line and your heels on the floor.

- *Toe-walking:* Walk around on your toes.

Source: Adapted from President's Council on Physical Fitness and Sports. Kids in Action: Fitness for Children 2-17.

Appendix 7–C

Anthropometric Measures for Children
Six Months to Five Years of Age

Table 7–C1 Height in Centimeters for Boys and Girls 2–5 Years of Age—Number Examined, Mean, Standard Deviation, and Selected Percentiles, by Sex and Age: United States, 1976–80

| Sex and Age | N | Mean | ± SD | Percentile | | | | | |
				10th	25th	50th	75th	85th	95th
Boys									
2 years	375	91.2	4.3	85.8	88.2	91.3	94.2	95.8	97.6
3 years	418	99.2	4.5	94.3	96.5	98.8	102.0	103.9	107.0
4 years	404	106.0	5.2	99.5	102.5	106.4	109.2	111.0	115.0
5 years	397	112.6	5.4	105.8	109.4	112.6	115.6	118.1	121.2
Girls									
2 years	336	89.7	4.2	84.4	86.7	89.8	92.2	93.6	97.2
3 years	366	97.5	4.8	91.1	94.5	97.6	100.8	102.5	104.5
4 years	396	104.6	5.0	98.2	101.5	104.5	108.2	109.8	112.4
5 years	364	111.6	5.3	105.1	108.1	111.6	115.2	116.5	120.3

Source: Reprinted with permission of National Center for Health Statistics. *Vital and Health Statistics: Anthropometric Data and Prevalence of Overweight for Hispanics 1982–1984.* Series 11: data from the National Health Survey. No. 239. March, 1989. Hyattsville, Md. DHHS Publication No. (PHS) 89-1689.

Table 7–C2 Height in Centimeters for Boys 2–5 Years of Age by Specified Hispanic Origin and Age: Hispanic Health and Nutrition Examination Survey, 1982–84

Hispanic Origin/Age	N	Mean	±SD	Percentile 10th	25th	50th	75th	85th	95th
Mexican-American Boys									
2 years	110	91.5	4.0	86.1	88.9	91.7	93.8	95.6	98.2
3 years	131	98.6	4.8	91.2	95.6	99.5	101.7	103.6	105.5
4 years	118	105.3	4.8	99.3	101.7	104.9	108.7	111.2	113.1
5 years	115	111.9	5.4	105.1	108.5	111.6	115.6	117.6	121.4
Puerto Rican Boys[+]									
2 years	34	93.4	5.3	*	89.1	94.0	96.6	*	*
3 years	38	99.5	4.7	*	95.6	99.0	102.3	104.1	*
4 years	41	107.3	6.2	*	104.5	107.3	110.1	112.1	*
5 years	22	*	*	*	111.8	113.4	116.1	*	*

[+]Cuban data not presented because of insufficient sample size.
* No data available.

Table 7–C3 Height in Centimeters for Girls 2–5 Years of Age by Specified Hispanic Origin and Age: Hispanic Health and Nutrition Examination Survey, 1982–84

Hispanic Origin/Age	N	Mean	±SD	Percentile 10th	25th	50th	75th	85th	95th
Mexican-American Girls									
2 years	116	89.2	3.8	84.5	86.9	89.4	91.9	93.4	94.4
3 years	97	97.9	4.6	90.0	94.2	98.4	101.6	102.3	*
4 years	96	105.1	4.9	98.1	102.2	105.1	108.6	110.1	*
5 years	109	111.7	5.2	104.7	107.9	111.7	115.1	116.4	120.1
Puerto Rican Girls[+]									
2 years	27	88.9	4.1	*	85.8	88.1	91.6	*	*
3 years	40	98.0	3.9	*	95.9	97.6	100.6	101.6	*
4 years	34	106.7	4.7	*	103.4	106.0	110.2	*	*
5 years	30	115.0	4.9	*	111.5	114.3	117.1	*	*

[+]Cuban data not presented because of insufficient sample size.
* No data available.

Table 7–C4 Weight in Kilograms for Boys and Girls 6–11 Months to 5 Years of Age

Sex and Age	N	Mean	±SD	Percentile 10th	25th	50th	75th	85th	95th
Boys									
6–11 months	179	9.4	1.3	7.6	8.6	9.4	10.1	10.7	11.4
1 year	370	11.8	1.9	10.0	10.8	11.7	12.6	13.1	14.4
2 years	375	13.6	1.7	11.6	12.6	13.5	14.5	15.2	16.5
3 years	418	15.7	2.0	13.5	14.4	15.4	16.8	17.4	19.1
4 years	404	17.8	2.5	15.0	16.0	17.6	19.0	19.9	22.2
5 years	397	19.8	3.0	16.8	17.7	19.4	21.3	22.9	25.4
Girls									
6–11 months	177	8.8	1.2	7.3	7.9	8.9	9.4	10.1	10.9
1 year	336	10.8	1.4	9.1	9.9	10.7	11.7	12.4	13.4
2 years	336	13.0	1.5	11.2	12.0	12.7	13.8	14.5	15.9
3 years	366	14.9	2.1	12.3	13.4	14.7	16.1	17.0	18.4
4 years	396	17.0	2.4	14.3	15.2	16.7	18.4	19.3	21.1
5 years	364	19.6	3.3	16.1	17.2	19.0	21.2	22.8	26.6

Table 7–C5 Weight in Kilograms for Girls 6 Months–5 Years of Age by Specified Hispanic Origin and Age: Hispanic Health and Nutrition Examination Survey, 1982–84

| Hispanic Origin/Age | N | Mean | ±SD | Percentile | | | | | |
				10th	25th	50th	75th	85th	95th
Mexican-American Girls									
6–11 months	63	8.9	1.2	7.6	8.0	8.7	9.5	10.3	*
1 year	119	11.0	1.5	9.3	9.8	10.9	12.0	12.7	13.6
2 years	121	13.1	1.7	11.2	12.0	12.9	13.8	14.7	15.7
3 years	97	15.3	2.3	12.8	13.8	15.0	16.8	17.5	*
4 years	96	17.7	2.7	14.9	15.8	17.6	19.1	20.4	*
5 years	109	20.0	4.3	16.3	17.3	18.9	21.3	23.3	27.6
Puerto Rican Girls+									
6–11 months	18	*	*	*	*	9.2	*	*	*
1 year	33	11.2	1.6	*	9.8	11.3	12.3	*	*
2 years	27	13.1	2.0	*	11.9	12.8	14.4	*	*
3 years	40	15.5	3.3	*	13.7	15.1	16.5	17.1	*
4 years	34	18.7	3.6	*	16.1	17.6	20.4	*	*
5 years	30	21.6	2.7	*	19.3	22.4	24.1	*	*

+Cuban data not presented because of insufficient sample size.
* No data available.

Table 7–C6 Weight in Kilograms for Boys 6 Months–5 Years of Age by Specified Hispanic Origin and Age: Hispanic Health and Nutrition Examination Survey, 1982–84

| Hispanic Origin/Age | N | Mean | ±SD | Percentile | | | | | |
				10th	25th	50th	75th	85th	95th
Mexican-American Boys									
6–11 months	57	9.7	1.4	8.1	8.8	9.7	10.3	10.6	*
1 year	105	11.8	1.8	9.8	10.8	11.5	12.5	13.1	15.0
2 years	111	14.0	1.7	11.7	13.0	14.1	15.0	15.5	17.0
3 years	131	15.8	2.3	13.0	14.5	15.4	16.8	17.7	19.9
4 years	118	17.7	2.1	14.9	16.2	17.6	18.9	19.5	21.7
5 years	116	20.0	3.5	16.2	17.9	19.5	21.3	22.8	26.0
Puerto Rican Boys+									
6–11 months	17	*	*	*	*	9.7	*	*	*
1 year	34	11.8	2.0	*	10.6	11.8	12.7	*	*
2 years	35	14.7	2.1	*	13.1	14.8	15.4	16.0	*
3 years	38	15.5	2.0	*	13.9	15.5	16.7	17.4	.*
4 years	41	19.2	4.1	*	16.4	18.3	21.1	22.0	*
5 years	22	*	*	*	19.2	20.2	23.3	*	*

+Cuban data not presented because of insufficient sample size.
* No data available.

Table 7–C7 Triceps Skinfold in Millimeters for Boys and Girls 6–11 Months to 5 Years of Age

Sex and Age	N	Mean	±SD	Percentile					
				10th	25th	50th	75th	85th	95th
Boys									
6–11 months	179	10.4	3.1	7.0	8.0	10.0	12.0	14.0	16.0
1 year	370	10.4	2.7	7.0	8.5	10.0	12.0	13.0	15.5
2 years	375	10.2	2.9	7.0	8.0	10.0	12.0	13.0	15.0
3 years	418	10.0	2.6	7.0	8.0	9.5	11.5	12.5	15.0
4 years	404	9.6	3.0	6.5	7.5	9.0	11.0	12.0	15.0
5 years	397	8.9	2.9	6.0	7.0	8.0	10.5	11.5	14.5
Girls									
6–11 months	177	9.9	2.6	7.0	8.0	10.0	11.5	12.5	14.5
1 year	336	10.6	3.3	7.0	8.0	10.5	12.0	13.5	16.5
2 years	336	10.6	3.0	7.0	8.0	10.5	12.5	13.5	16.0
3 years	366	10.3	2.9	7.0	8.0	10.0	12.0	12.5	16.5
4 years	396	10.4	3.1	6.5	8.0	10.0	12.0	13.0	15.5
5 years	364	10.6	3.2	7.0	8.5	10.5	12.5	14.0	16.0

Table 7–C8 Triceps Skinfold in Millimeters for Girls 6 Months–5 Years of Age by Specified Hispanic Origin and Age: Hispanic Health and Nutrition Examination Survey, 1982–84

Hispanic Origin/Age	N	Mean	±SD	Percentile					
				10th	25th	50th	75th	85th	95th
Mexican-American Girls									
6–11 months	63	10.4	2.5	7.5	9.0	10.5	12.0	12.5	*
1 year	119	9.8	2.5	7.0	8.0	9.5	11.5	12.5	14.0
2 years	118	10.6	2.9	7.0	8.5	10.5	13.0	13.5	16.0
3 years	96	10.5	2.9	7.0	8.5	10.5	12.5	13.0	*
4 years	96	11.0	3.4	7.5	8.0	10.5	13.0	14.5	*
5 years	109	10.6	4.2	7.0	7.5	10.0	12.0	13.5	17.5
Puerto Rican Girls[+]									
6–11 months	15	*	*	*	*	10.5	*	*	*
1 year	31	9.2	2.5	*	7.0	8.0	11.0	*	*
2 years	27	11.3	3.2	*	8.5	10.0	13.5	*	*
3 years	40	10.3	2.5	*	9.0	10.0	12.0	12.5	*
4 years	34	11.2	3.3	*	9.0	11.0	13.0	*	*
5 years	30	11.1	3.7	*	7.5	11.0	13.5	*	*

[+]Cuban data not presented because of insufficient sample size.
* No data available.

Table 7–C9 Triceps Skinfold in Millimeters for Boys 6 Months–5 Years of Age by Specified Hispanic Origin and Age: Hispanic Health and Nutrition Examination Survey, 1982–84

| Hispanic Origin/Age | N | Mean | ±SD | Percentile | | | | | |
				10th	25th	50th	75th	85th	95th
Mexican-American Boys									
6–11 months	57	10.5	2.6	7.5	8.5	10.0	12.0	13.0	*
1 year	104	10.2	3.2	6.5	8.0	10.0	11.5	13.0	16.0
2 years	111	10.2	2.7	6.5	8.0	10.0	12.0	13.0	14.5
3 years	130	10.0	3.1	6.5	7.5	9.5	11.5	13.0	16.0
4 years	118	9.3	2.7	6.0	8.0	9.0	10.5	11.5	14.5
5 years	116	9.3	3.8	5.5	7.0	8.0	10.5	13.0	17.0
Puerto Rican Boys[+]									
6–11 months	17	*	*	*	*	10.0	*	*	*
1 year	32	9.5	2.5	*	8.0	9.0	10.0	*	*
2 years	34	10.5	3.5	*	8.0	9.5	12.0	*	*
3 years	38	8.9	2.2	*	7.5	8.5	10.0	11.5	*
4 years	41	10.6	3.7	*	8.5	9.5	11.0	15.0	*
5 years	22	*	*	*	7.0	9.0	12.0	*	*

[+]Cuban data not presented because of insufficient sample size.
* No data available.

Appendix 7-D

Summer Food Service Program Meal Requirements

Summer Food Service Program meal pattern requirements must be followed for reimbursement. The meal or snack component and minimum serving sizes are outlined below.

Component	Minimum Amount
Breakfast	
Milk	1 C
Fluid milk	(½ pt)
Vegetables and fruits	½ C
Vegetables and/or fruits or full-strength vegetable or fruit juice	
Bread and bread alternates	
Bread (whole-grain or enriched) or	1 slice
Bread alternates (whole-grain or enriched):	1 serving
cornbread, biscuits, rolls, muffins, etc. or	
Cooked pasta or noodle products or cooked cereal grains,	
such as rice, corn grits, or bulgur or	½ C
(Whole grain, enriched, or fortified): cooked cereal or	¾ C or 1 oz (whichever is
cereal grains or cold dry cereal	less)
Meat and meat alternates (optional, serve as often as possible):	
Meat	1 oz
Meat alternate	½ amount listed under lunch or supper
Snack (supplemental food)	
Serve two food items selected from	
any two of the following four components:	
Milk	1 C
Fluid milk	(½ pt)
Meat and meat alternates	
Lean meat or poultry or fish or	1 oz (edible portion as served)
Meat alternates:	
Cheese or	1 oz
Egg or	1 large
Cooked dry beans or peas or	¼ C
Peanut butter or other nut or seed butters or	2 T

Component	Minimum Amount
Nuts and/or seeds or	1 oz
Yogurt (plain, sweetened, or flavored)	4 oz
Vegetables and fruits	
Vegetables and/or fruits or full-strength juice	¾ C
Bread and bread alternates	
Bread (whole-grain or enriched) or	1 slice
Bread alternates (whole-grain or enriched):	
Cornbread, biscuits, rolls, muffins, etc. or	1 serving
Cooked pasta or noodle products or	½ C
Cooked cereal grains, such as rice, corn grits, or bulgur or	½ C
(Whole-grain, enriched, or fortified): cooked cereal or cereal grains or cold dry cereal	¾ C or 1 oz (whichever is less)
Lunch or Supper	
Milk	1 C
Fluid milk	(½ pt)
Meat and meat alternates	
Lean meat or poultry or fish or	2 oz (edible portion as served)
Meat alternates:	
Cheese or	2 oz
Egg or	1 large
Cooked dry beans or peas or	½ C
Peanut butter or other nut or seed butters or	4 T
Nuts and/or seeds	1 ounce = 50%*
Vegetables and fruits	
Vegetables and/or fruits (2 or more selections for a total of ¾ cup) or full-strength juice	¾ C
Bread and bread alternates	
Bread (whole-grain or enriched) or	1 slice
Bread alternates (whole grain or enriched):	
Cornbread, biscuits, rolls, muffins, etc. or	1 serving
Cooked pasta or noodle products or	½ C
Cooked cereal grains, such as rice, corn grits, or bulgur	½ C

*No more than one-half of the requirement shall be met with nuts or seeds. Nuts or seeds shall be combined with another meat/meat alternate to fulfill the requirement.

Key: cup = C, tablespoon = T, ounce = oz

Appendix 7-E

Summer Food Service Program Job Positions

In a Summer Food Service Program, the director is responsible for the overall integrity and quality of the program and in this capacity directs the activities of the other major positions. The bookkeeper is responsible for the fiscal management of the program and processing of food purchases. The monitor oversees the activities at various sites by routine visits during meal service. S/he may be responsible for 15 to 20 sites. At each site, a supervisor administers the day-to-day activities and has direct contact with the children, parents, and staff. Specific tasks are as follows:

DIRECTOR

- providing overall management
- supervising the program
- selecting sites
- submitting applications
- corresponding with administering agency
- coordinating with other agencies
- conducting outreach efforts
- hiring, training, and supervising staff
- arranging for food preparation or delivery
- ensuring that all monitoring requirements are met
- adjusting meal orders

- submitting reimbursement vouchers
- ensuring civil rights compliance
- handling all contracts, bidding, and negotiations with food service management companies

BOOKKEEPER

- maintaining records
  - daily site reports, invoices, and bills
  - food costs
  - labor costs
  - administrative costs
  - other costs
  - program income
- preparing reimbursement vouchers
- preparing payroll
- purchasing office supplies

MONITOR

- checking on-site operations to ensure that site personnel maintain records and program operates according to requirements
- visiting and reviewing all sites within 1–4 weeks of food service operations
- preparing reports of visits and reviews
- revisiting sites as necessary

Source: US Department of Agriculture, Food and Nutrition Service. *Summer Food Service Program for Children. Sponsor's Handbook.* Washington, DC: USDA; 1991. FNS-206.

- suggesting corrective actions for problems encountered
- ensuring that the site takes corrective actions
- conducting on-site training as necessary

SITE SUPERVISOR

- serving meals
- cleaning up after meals

- ensuring safe and sanitary conditions
- receiving and accounting for delivered meals
- ensuring that children eat all meals on-site
- ensuring that only eligible children receive meals
- planning and organizing daily site activities
- making meal arrangements during bad weather

8

Nutrition for School-Age Children

- Identify a healthy eating pattern for children.
- Name the major child nutrition responsibilities of schools, families, and health care professionals.
- Define *comprehensive school health education* and identify how child nutrition fits within the definition.
- Describe preventive efforts directed toward youth, such as Guidelines for Adolescent Preventive Services (GAPS), *Healthy Youth 2000* efforts, and specific community-based initiatives.
- Name the *Healthy People 2000* objectives that are specific for child nutrition.

High Definition Nutrition

Comprehensive school health education—a primary prevention strategy for teaching life skills for disease prevention and health promotion to children and parents, involving a planned, sequential pre-K through 12th grade curriculum that addresses the physical, mental, emotional, and social dimensions of children.

Guidelines for Adolescent Preventive Services—an initiative to address current adolescent morbidity and mortality in the United States. It is a part of the "Healthier Youth 2000 Project" of the American Medical Association

and directed to primary and secondary prevention.

Iron deficiency—the most common nutrient deficiency among US adolescents. It is defined as a hemoglobin level less than 3.5 mg%.

National School Lunch Program—the program for school-age children established by Public Law 79-396 for the purpose of protecting the health and well-being of all US children with nutritious foods.

School Breakfast Program—the program for school-age children established by the Child Nutrition Act of 1966, Public Law 89-642, as a pilot program but extended to all schools in 1975 for the purpose of providing a nutritious breakfast to all US children.

NUTRITION AND SCHOOL-AGE CHILDREN

An overriding concern about school-age children (ages 6 to 18) is the general lack of acceptance of two concepts: (1) eating behavior influences health; and (2) eating behavior in childhood initiates adolescent and adult eating patterns. Parents and other adults who are responsible for the foods served to children must understand and acknowledge the benefits of nutrition for children's long-term health (e.g., prevention of cancer, heart disease, obesity, and osteoporosis). Further, they must integrate facts and recommendations into their meal planning and any formal or informal nutrition education they provide.[1]

Healthy children have better athletic performance, mental prowess, and physical attractiveness than unhealthy children. They have good skin and hair quality and body leanness complemented with a small amount of body fat. Good nutrition contributes to positive feelings and an energetic nature.

Children associate with desirable role models (e.g., athletes and entertainers) and the eating patterns they project. Teachers influence eating patterns via the knowledge they impart and the personal habits they practice, especially among elementary students. Peers emerge as an adolescent's major role model, and peers who practice unhealthy eating habits may serve as negative role models. Overemphasis of lean bodies with no fat may lead students to distorted body perceptions, lack of interpersonal trust, and bizarre weight control methods.

On the other hand, hunger still exists. This is especially true for low income families where children face additional pressures in school due to their high-risk status.

The eating patterns and nutritional well-being of school children are influenced by the multiple environments of their daily living (see Figure 8-1). This means that the home and family, school with teachers and food services, all forms of media, the health care setting, fast food establishments, and peer groups all influence what a child chooses to eat. The effect can be positive or negative on the overall health of the child.[2]

The nutritional well-being of a child depends on the foods ingested and how the body uses them. During the school-age years, growth and development will be a continuous process. Recommended daily nutrient intakes may or may not be achieved with the child's meal and snack choices. The child's eating pattern—both in and outside of school—contributes to overall intake.

GROWTH AND DEVELOPMENT

Growth and development are monitored by two common nutritional indicators, height and weight.

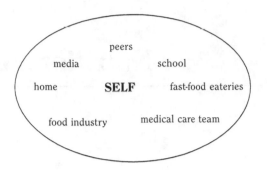

Figure 8-1 Multiple environments of youth that influence daily living and eating behaviors

Many US students today exist at one of the extremes: They are either too heavy or too light for age or height. Children who exceed their recommended weights by 15% are considered *overweight*, and those who exceed recommendations by 20% are considered *obese*. For adolescents, overweight is defined as body mass index equal to or greater than 23.0 for males aged 12 through 14, 24.3 for males aged 15 through 17, 25.8 for males aged 18 through 19, 23.4 for females aged 12 through 14, 24.8 for females aged 15 through 17, and 25.7 for females aged 18 through 19. The values for adolescents are the age- and gender-specific 85th percentile values of the 1976 to 1980 National Health and Nutrition Examination Survey (NHANES II), corrected for sample variation.[3]

Various anthropometric measures for children 6 to 19 years old in US surveys including the Hispanic Health and Nutrition Examination Survey (HHANES) are presented in Appendix 8-A. Excess weight predisposes children to high blood cholesterol and sets them on a track for chronic disease.[4] At the other extreme, underweight and malnourished children present a different mosaic of nutritional problems, many of which begin during infancy and the preschool years.[1]

HHANES 1982 to 1984 found that Mexican-American children were shorter than non-Hispanic whites but had larger anthropometric measurements and greater weight for height than average American children. Hispanic children in all age groups were heavier than non-Hispanic children, and their excess weight represented increased fatness in the trunk. Of these Hispanic children, 23% had an abnormal weight for their age: 19% were overweight and 4% were underweight. Of these Hispanic children, 10% had abnormal hemoglobin and/or hematocrit levels, and this increased to 23% when borderline cases were counted.[1]

ACCESS TO FOOD

The lack of access to food greatly influences the natural growth and development of children. Key findings in a 1991 survey of childhood hunger in the United States were as follows[5]:

- About 5.5 million children under 12 years of age are hungry.
- An additional 6.0 million are at risk of hunger.
- Hungry children were two to three times more likely than children from nonhungry, low-income families to suffer from individual health problems such as unwanted weight loss, fatigue, irritability, headaches, and inability to concentrate in the six months prior to the survey.
- Children with a specific health problem are absent from school almost twice as many days as those not reporting specific health problems.

NUTRIENT RECOMMENDATIONS

To achieve the expected growth and development, children need an array of nutrients on a daily basis. The Recommended Dietary Allowances (RDAs) are the standards used to evaluate the sufficiency of children's total daily food intakes.[6,7] RDAs are set for energy, protein, 10 vitamins, and seven minerals. Minimum requirements are set for sodium, chloride, and potassium.

Children generally consume about one-fourth of their day's energy, fat, and protein intakes at lunch and one-third or more of their calcium and sodium levels.[8,9] The 1987–1988 Nationwide Food Consumption Survey (NFCS) found that 20% of

adolescent boys and 40% of adolescent girls did not drink milk on the day of the survey.[3] Milk is essential for growing children and their major source of calcium.[10] Chan studied 164 healthy white children and found that those who consumed at least 1,000 mg of calcium per day had a higher bone mineral content than children with intakes of less than 1,000 mg.[11] The higher bone mineral content is especially crucial for girls to prevent osteoporosis later in life.

Iron deficiency (less than 3.5 mg%) remains the most common nutrient deficiency among US adolescents. There is an increased demand for iron to compensate for the increased hemoglobin level with growth.[12] National surveys report that adolescent girls 12 to 19 years old have the highest anemia prevalence rates (between 6% and 14%). These adolescents become our mothers of tomorrow.[10]

The meals served at school are under the direction of a child nutrition professional, but the food service budget and the likes and dislikes of the children dictate what foods are offered and how food is prepared. Parents have more control over the eating environment of younger children, but they control fewer food choices as children age and peers gain more influence. Teachers mediate choices not only by what they say informally, but also by the direct nutrition information they present in the classroom.

MEALS PROVIDED BY SCHOOLS

In 1946, Public Law 79-396 created the National School Lunch Act for the purpose of protecting the health and well-being of the nation's children.[13] The act directs students to pay the full price for lunches but allows local school districts to serve lunch without cost or at a reduced cost to any child who is unable to pay the full cost. Schools use surplus commodities when possible in meal planning and do not discriminate against any child who is unable to pay a full price. Some of the meal ticket systems, however, may label children inappropriately.

The Child Nutrition Act of 1966, Public Law 89-642, authorized the School Breakfast Program as a pilot program; the program was extended to all schools in 1975 using grants-in-aid.[14] During the 1970s, legislation improved the quality of meals, emphasized nutrition education, and enlarged coverage of programming. The Omnibus Budget Reconciliation Act of 1981, Public Law 97-35, targeted benefits based on need and improved program management and accountability at the local (school-site) level.

The Food and Nutrition Service (FNS) of the US Department of Agriculture (USDA) implements programs legislated by Congress. FNS establishes regulations, policies, and guidelines about school foods and monitors program performance. In addition, FNS provides program and administrative funds to states via seven regional offices. States generally assign the responsibility for program administration to the state educational agency (e.g., the state department of education), which assists local school districts by establishing fiscal recordkeeping systems and monitoring performance. The individual school is responsible for preparing nutritious meals and serving them to children. A list of federally funded food and nutrition programs is given in Table 8–1.

Table 8–1 Federally Funded Food and Nutrition Programs

Program (Dollars Appropriated by Congress FY 1995)	Provider	Funding/ Agency
National School Lunch Program Provides nutritious low-cost lunch to children enrolled in school ($4.2 billion)	All public schools; voluntary in private schools	A/1
School Breakfast Program Provides nutritious breakfast to children in participating schools or institutions ($1.1 billion)	Voluntary by public and private schools	A/1
Special Milk program Provides milk to school-age children, in child care centers, and in schools or institutions where there is no school lunch program ($18.1 million)	Schools, camps, and child care institutions not participating in other school nutrition programs	A/1
Summer Food Service Program for Children Provides one nutritious meal to children as a substitute for the National School Lunch Program and School Breakfast Program during summer vacation ($254.6 million)	Public and nonprofit private schools; public residential facilities of local, municipal, or county government	A/1–3
Child Care Food Program Provides financial assistance for nutritious food in child care setting ($1.5 billion)	Licensed child care centers or family day care homes; Head Start programs	A/1–3
Head Start Program Provides comprehensive health, educational, nutrition, social, and other services to low-income preschool children and their families	Local Head Start program	8/B
Special Supplemental Food Program for Women, Infants and Children (WIC) Provides supplemental food and nutrition education as an adjunct to health care to low-income pregnant, postpartum, and breastfeeding women and to infants and children at nutritional risk ($3.5 billion)	Health agencies, social services, community action agencies	4/A

continues

Table 8–1 continued

Program (Dollars Appropriated by Congress FY 1995)	Provider	Funding/Agency
Commodity Supplemental Food Program (CSFP)		
Provides commodity foods to low-income women (pregnant, breastfeeding, or postpartum), infants and children to 6 years of age, and the elderly in certain cases	Public and private nonprofit agencies (community health or social service agencies)	4/A, C/6
Food Stamp Program		
Provides low-income households with coupons to increase food purchasing power ($27.7 billion)	Local public assistance or social services offices	5/A
Temporary Emergency Food Assistance Program (TEFAP)		
Provides commodity foods to low-income households through local public or private nonprofit agencies; quarterly distributions by emergency providers ($65 million)	Public and private nonprofit agencies (community action agencies, councils on aging, local health or local school districts)	5/A
Cooperative Extension—Expanded Food and Nutrition Education Program (EFNEP)		
Provides nutrition education to low-income families and individuals	Local cooperative extension office where program is available	9/A
Food Distribution Program on Indian Reservations (FDPIR)		
Operates as a substitute for food stamps for eligible needy families living on or near Indian reservations ($33.2 million)	Local agency	7/A

Key: Funding sources: A = US Department of Agriculture, B = US Department of Health and Human Services, C = Aging Administration.
Administrative agency: 1 = state departments of education, local school districts; 2 = nonprofit, community-based organizations; 3 = for-profit, community-based organizations; 4 = state health agency; 5 = state welfare or social service agency; 6 = state and area aging agencies; 7 = Indian tribal councils; 8 = federal and regional departments of health services; 9 = state and land grant universities.

Source: Adapted from Mildred Kaufman, *Nutrition in Public Health.* Aspen Publishers, Gaithersburg, MD, 1990 Chapter 4: "Reaching Out to Those at Highest Risk" p 72–82.

Schools can serve foods in addition to the requirements at breakfast and lunch at their own discretion. An "offer-versus-serve" parameter (i.e., must offer five items but student can select three) is now extended to all elementary, junior, and senior high students (Public Law 97-35). New FNS regulations allow students to request smaller portions of food items than the amount defined in the five-item pattern.

School districts receive a reimbursement for meals that are served according to USDA menu standards. Milk yields an additional reimbursement. Schools can choose whether to participate in the School Breakfast Program. However, with hunger and high-risk children slipping through the cracks, schools should ensure that their policies allow access for all children to the School Breakfast Program, National School Lunch Program (NSLP), and Summer Food Service Program. The "Contract with America" that is currently being discussed in Congress may alter the accessibility of school meals and their nutrient composition.

In addition to serving food, the mission of school food service has included nutrition education since the 1940s; when a total school program was defined as one in which students learned the relation between food, nutrition, and health. Public Law 91-248 was enacted in 1970 and was the first federal legislation to specify nutrition education provisions authorizing training school food service workers in nutrition. Public Law 95-166 established the Nutrition Education and Training (NET) program; this program gave new impetus not only to teach children the value of a nutritionally balanced diet through positive daily lunchroom experience and classroom reinforcement, but also to train teachers and school food service personnel to implement programs.[15] The NET funding is decentralized, with state departments of education directing the award and evaluation of programs.

Cross-Sectional Surveys

In cross-sectional surveys among a biracial sample of 10- and 15-year-old children in Bogalusa, Louisiana, school lunch analysis reported 22% and 29% of total energy intake from fat and 20% and 29% from carbohydrate, respectively. Sugar intake represented over one-half the total carbohydrate intake. Sodium averaged one-third of the recommended daily range.[16] Parcel et al analyzed school lunch aliquots in a cross-sectional sample of schools in Galveston, Texas, and reported that 39% of the day's total fat intake was from lunch.[17]

The School Nutrition Dietary Assessment Study (SNDA) collected information from a nationally representative sample of 545 schools and 3,350 students attending 1st to 12th grade in those schools. The schools provided information about the food service operation and all meals served during a one-week period between February and May 1992.[18] Approximately 3,350 students in 1st to 12th grade completed a 24-hour recall. Parents assisted students in grades 1 and 2; but students in grades 3 to 12 served as their own respondent. The study compared the dietary components from school and other meals with several standards (see Table 8-2).

SNDA data show that the National School Lunch Program is available to 92% of all students in the United States but only 56% participate. Children whose family income is less than or equal to 130% of the poverty guidelines qualify for free meals, and children whose family income is between 130% and 185% qualify for reduced-price meals. All other children pay full price, but full-price lunches are also federally subsidized.[18]

The average full price for a school lunch in the 1991–1992 school year was $1.14; average prices ranged from $1.11 in elementary schools to approximately $1.22 in middle and high schools. The average price of a reduced-price meal was $0.38. About 39% of school lunches were provided free, 7% were reduced price, and 53% were full price.[18]

Table 8–2 Dietary Standards Used in the School Nutrition Dietary Assessment Study, 1993

Guideline	Standard
National School Lunch Program and School Breakfast Program goals	• One-third of the RDAs for lunch • One-fourth of the RDAs for breakfast
Dietary Guidelines for Americans	• Limit intake of total fat to 30% or less of calories • Limit intake of saturated fat to less than 10% of calories
National Research Council's Diet and Health Recommendations	• Limit daily sodium intake to 2,400 mg or less • Limit daily cholesterol intake to 300 mg or less • Increase daily carbohydrate intake to more than 55% of calories

Source: Adapted from Burghardt J and Devaney B. *The School Nutrition Dietary Assessment Study—Summary of Findings.* October 1993. Mathematica Policy Research, Inc. Alexandria, VA. p. 3.

Approximately 99% of public schools and 83% of all public and private schools participate in the NSLP. Only a small fraction of schools offer neither the NSLP nor a non-USDA lunch program.

In 1993, the school lunch subsidy was $0.1625 per meal for full-price lunches, $1.2950 for reduced-price lunches, and $1.6950 for free lunches. Schools at which at least 40% of the lunches are served free and where costs are greater than the regular rate (severe-need schools) receive additional assistance of $0.02 per lunch. All schools may receive entitlement commodities, valued at $0.14 per lunch in FY 1993.[18]

More than 50% of the schools offer a la carte items in addition to NSLP meals. This is much more common in middle and high schools than elementary schools. Cookies and cakes, beverages, frozen desserts, and snack foods are the most commonly offered a la carte items. Nearly 40% of high schools that participate in the NSLP offer at least one a la carte entree (e.g., pizza, cold cut sandwiches, and hamburgers). The following section summarizes data from the SNDA and highlights the NSLP, the School Breakfast Program, and the overall eating patterns of students.[18]

National School Lunch Program

Who participates? Participation in the NSLP varies with household income, age, gender, and region of the United States. More elementary school students than middle and high school students take part in the program. Generally, more students who are eligible for free and reduced-price meals get NSLP lunches than students who pay full price. More students participate in the program where the full price is comparatively low, and more boys than girls participate.

More students participate in rural than in urban and suburban schools. Students in the Northeast and West participate less than students in the Southeast, Southwest, and Mountain states. If students are allowed to leave school at lunchtime, NSLP participation declines.[18]

NSLP meals in about 50% of schools include a choice of entree daily; 35% of schools have two

or three entrees, and 8% have six or more. High schools and middle schools offer more choices than elementary schools. About half of high schools and 16% of elementary schools have a food bar once a week. Schools must offer whole milk plus one type of low-fat, unflavored milk, and a low-fat chocolate milk is common. About 25% of schools offer four types of milk. Desserts are not required, but 39% of lunch menus offer dessert.

Lunches provide one-third or more of the RDAs for most nutrients. Nutrient intakes that are low in the NSLP meals include iron for 11-to-18-year old females, zinc for 11-to-18-year-old males, and calories and vitamin B_6 for 15-to-18-year-old males. The average percentage of energy from total fat is 38%, with 15% from saturated fat. A meal's average sodium content is 1,479 mg, which is nearly twice the target of 800 mg or less. Cholesterol in meals averages 88 mg.

Only 1% of schools offer lunches that average 30% or less of calories from fat. Only one school in the sample reported having a weekly lunch menu providing an average of less than 10% of calories from saturated fat. Many schools offer at least one low-fat lunch choice; 44% offer at least one full lunch per week that meets the goal of 30% or less of energy from fat. Low-fat lunches have fewer calories than the average lunches, but they contain similar amounts of protein, vitamins, and minerals. Schools whose average NSLP lunches approach 30% fat employ several menu planning, food purchasing, and food preparation practices to lower the fat content.

Schools that provide lunches with less than 32% of energy from fat offer ground-beef entrees less often and poultry and meatless entrees more often. They offer an extra bread item frequently, in addition to the bread or bread alternate included in an entree (e.g., bread plus rice or spaghetti). They offer fewer vegetables with added fat. Schools that provide low-fat lunches offer fruit and fruit juice more often and offer juice in addition to other items. They serve 2% milk less frequently, with 1% or nonfat milk served often. Salad dressing is served less frequently, but low-calorie dressing is served often. Cakes and cookies are served less frequently than low-fat, high-carbohydrate desserts like yogurt, pudding made from skim milk, and gelatin.

It is important to note that the schools that offer low-fat lunches have 6% lower NSLP participation rates than other schools. Participation rates in schools serving lunches that average 32 to 35% of calories from fat resemble participation rates of schools with lunches averaging greater than 35%. Schools can modify fat content of lunches without adversely affecting NSLP participation, but fat content below 32% appears to cause a decline in student participation.[18]

School Breakfast Program (SBP)

The USDA subsidizes school breakfasts with cash reimbursements and commodities if breakfasts achieve one-fourth the RDA. In 1992, reimbursement rates were $0.1875 for full-price breakfasts, $0.6450 for reduced-price breakfasts, and $0.945 for free breakfasts. For severe-need schools, subsidies are $0.8225 for reduced-price breakfasts and $1.1225 for free breakfasts.[18]

The SBP is available to slightly more than 50% of the nation's students, but fewer than 20% participate. Students who are more likely to participate include those certified for free and reduced-price meals, students from low-income families, younger students, male students, African-American students, and students living in rural areas. Average full breakfast price in 1991–1992 was $0.60, and the average reduced price was $0.28. Nearly all SBP breakfasts are provided free or at a reduced price. More than half of all schools participate in the SBP, but rates are higher among elementary and middle schools. Snacks, not breakfast, are especially prevalent in high schools.[18]

In nearly 40% of nonparticipating schools, principals consider joining the program but do not join. They report no need for the program, foresee transportation or scheduling problems, report resource constraints, or have an overall lack of interest or support for the SBP. Many schools serve breakfast after school begins and during the nutrition break, which may increase participation.[18]

About 50% of the breakfasts served do not include a meat or meat alternate; milk options replicate lunch choices. Breakfasts generally contain breads and ready-to-eat cereals, and orange juice or noncitrus juice. SBP breakfasts provide less than one-fourth of the energy RDAs for male students greater than 10 years of age and less than one-fourth of the zinc RDA for all ages of boys and girls. Breakfasts average 31% fat and 14% saturated fat.

Forty-four percent of schools offer SBP breakfasts having less than 30% of calories from fat, but only 4% offer breakfasts with less than 10% from saturated fat. The reason that SBP meals have lower fat than NSLP meals is that a meat or meat alternate is not required at breakfast. More than 50% of the SBP breakfasts do not serve a meat item; those with a meat or meat alternate tend to serve sausage, eggs, or cheese. Cholesterol averages 73 mg, and carbohydrate averages 57%. The average sodium content is 673 mg.

FOODS CONSUMED IN THE HOME AND LEISURE-TIME ENVIRONMENT

The home and leisure-time environment of the child may either complement or contradict nutrition knowledge, attitudes, and behaviors learned in the school environment.[2] Parents serve as important role models. Kirk and Gillespie coined two new roles of parents that affect children's food choices: the "meaning creator" and the "family diplomat."[19] Previously, mothers functioned as nutritionist, economist, and manager-organizer; today, preparation time, individual preferences, and whether the mother works outside the home influence food choices as much as nutrition. Kids seem to mimic the "all or nothing" attitude of their parents. Many identify foods as "good" or "bad." In fact, 73% of 4th to 8th graders surveyed in a national sample worried about fat and cholesterol. About 85% felt they should avoid all high-fat foods, while 77% felt they should never eat high-sugar foods.

About one-half of school-age children eat with their family every day; 89% eat with their family at least 3 to 5 times per week. Students who give themselves the best nutrition rating eat more frequently with their family.[20]

TYPICAL EATING BEHAVIOR

Describing a typical eating behavior and nutrient intake of children and youth is challenging. The USDA 1987–1988 Nationwide Food Consumption Survey (NFCS) profiles the intakes of US children and demonstrates that the fat content remains well above recommended levels (see Table 8–3).[3] Typical eating behavior may be described as follows.

Skipped Meals

Many school-age children skip meals. In a sample of US 4th through 8th graders, more have skipped breakfast (57%) than lunch (41%), followed by dinner (17%).[21] Meal and snack skipping influences dietary adequacy. Of 639 4th and 6th grade students, 9% reported skipping breakfast within the past 24 hours and 5% reported eating nothing the entire morning. The most common reason for missing meals was dislike of particular meals or snacks, lack of time, or forgetting to bring food. Of the respondents, 30% met the recommended number of servings from the four food groups, but 44% did not achieve their recommended fruit and vegetable servings. Students who ate breakfast and had a morning snack were three times more likely to meet all food group recommendations.[22]

Breakfast Habits

Breakfast influences behavior and cholesterol level. The breakfast habits and behavior of younger children (N = 382) in the 3rd and 4th grades revealed that children who ate breakfast exhibited other healthful habits such as brushing teeth and taking vitamin/mineral supplements. Students who skipped breakfast were significantly more tired and hungry when they arrived at school; however, no significant social and emotional behavior problems or concerns were noted.[23]

Resnicow[24] studied the relationship between breakfast habits and plasma cholesterol in school children, 9 to 19 years old. Only 4% reported not eating breakfast regularly, and these children were less likely to believe in the benefits of breakfast. Controlling for age, gender, and body mass index, those who skipped breakfast had significantly higher total cholesterol levels (172 mg%) than breakfast consumers (160 mg%). The ready-to-eat fiber cereal group had lower cholesterol levels than all other breakfast eaters. Those who skipped breakfast reported higher intake of high-fat snacks, and traditional breakfast eaters reported significantly lower intake of high-fiber/low-fat snacks.[24]

Fat-Avoiding Behaviors

Fat-avoiding behaviors can be observed. In a cross-sectional sample of Mexican-American preschoolers and their parents, significantly higher fat-avoiding behaviors were noted for Anglo-American preschoolers (N = 143) than Mexican-American preschoolers (N = 198) (max score = 7.0, sum score = 4.85 versus 4.35, p <0.0001).[25] Preliminary data from 1987–1988 NFCS report that children 1 to 19 years old aver-

Table 8–3 Reported Nutrient Intakes of Youth Compared with Recommended Levels

Dietary Component	NFCS (1987–1988)	Recommended
Saturated fatty acids (% energy)	14	<10
Total fat (% energy)	35–36	Average no more than 30
Polyunsaturated (% energy)	6	Up to 10
Monounsaturated (% energy)	13–14	10–15
Cholesterol (mg/day)	193–296	<300

Source: Adapted from NIH Population Panel Report. p. 27.

age 35% to 36% of their total calories from fat. Saturated fat was 14%, polyunsaturated fat was 6%, monounsaturated fat was 13 to 14%, and dietary cholesterol was 193 to 296 mg.[10] This eating pattern has predisposed children to a health-risk behavior that illustrates itself in excess weight and high blood cholesterol levels. At least 25% of American children and adolescents exceed the acceptable 170 mg% serum cholesterol level.[10]

Fruit and Vegetable Intakes

Fruit and vegetable intakes are low. Murphy et al analyzed food group intake from the 1982–1983 HHANES data set composed of 3,356 Mexican-American children.[26] Fruits and vegetables were consumed less often than the other food groups. Children chose their calories instead from the meat, dairy, and breads/cereals groups.

The low fruit and vegetable intake of children is common and problematic. About 90% of children participating in a National Heart, Lung, and Blood Institute demonstration/education project called "CATCH" state that they eat fresh fruit at home most of the time; about three-fourths of Anglo-American and African-American children appeared sure they could eat fresh fruit instead of a candy bar. However, of 407 Los Angeles Latinos, 3% consume four servings a day, compared with HHANES reporting 5% and 3% of children 6 to 10 and 11 to 15 years eating four a day.[27]

Student Selections

Students are increasingly responsible for making most of their own food selections. This is true especially by the time children reach the 4th grade. Approximately 65% choose their own breakfast, 46% their lunch, and 74% their snacks; whereas 73% report that their mother chooses their dinner. Most students (87%) are responsible for cooking or preparing some of their own meals, with 80% making their own breakfast and 57% involved in buying food for meals or snacks.[21]

Food Allergies

Food allergies are uncommon. If parents think their children's eating habits are unhealthy because they avoid certain foods due to intolerances or hypersensitivities, the avoidance may not be well-founded. Although many individuals think they have a food allergy, true food allergies affect only 0.3 to 7.5% of children and fewer than 1% of adults. Food allergies must be verified by a physician using an immunological procedure.[28] If confirmed, 95% of true allergies are caused by one of four major foods: nuts (43%), eggs (21%), milk (18%), and soy (9%). The remaining 5% are caused by fish and wheat.[29]

Food intolerance is more common and refers to an abnormal physiologic response to a food where the mechanism is unknown or non-immunologic. Hyperactivity is a different condition, distinguished by signs of developmentally inappropriate inattention occurring in 5 to 10% of young school children.[30,31] Food allergies do not cause hyperactivity. However, two dietary excesses that stimulate the nervous system are caffeine and alcohol (see section on alcohol and caffeine later in this chapter).

RDA Achievement

RDA achievement varies. The SNDA study assessed students' dietary intakes over a 24-hour period and the contribution of NSLP and SBP meals to their intakes. Students eat at least three times a day, and more than 50% eat at least five times a day. For students of all ages, 88% eat breakfast, 93% eat lunch, and 99% eat dinner. Two-thirds have an afternoon snack, and 58% eat an evening snack. Only 15% have a morning snack. Total daily food intake averages 111% of the energy RDAs. Adolescent males consume 17% more calories than the RDA, while females consume 4% more. Students from families below the poverty level average 129% of the energy RDA. Except for adolescent females, vitamin and mineral intake for all age and gender subgroups exceeds the RDAs. Calcium intake is relatively low (80% for 15- to-18 year olds and 87% for 11-to-14 year olds).[18]

Overall eating patterns average 34% of calories from fat and 13% from saturated fat. Students from low-income families have higher fat intakes than students from higher-income households. Carbohydrate averages 53% of the calories; sodium averages 4,800 mg, and strikingly high intakes are reported for boys.[18]

NSLP participants waste or discard about 12% of the energy in the food they are served. They are more than twice as likely as NSLP nonparticipants to eat cheese, milk, meat, poultry, fish, and meat mixtures than nonparticipants. The result is that NSLP participants' have a higher percentage of energy from fat and saturated fat.

Students who are nonparticipants in the NSLP consume more sweets and sweet drinks. They purchase food from vending machines, the school store, or a la carte from the cafeteria. Nonparticipants consume about 23% of their energy RDA, and less than 20% of the RDAs for vitamin A, vitamin B_6, calcium, iron, and zinc at lunchtime. Students who brought lunch from home met 31% of their energy RDA, but less than one-third of the vitamin A, vitamin B_6, calcium, and zinc RDAs. Students who ate off campus met 34% of their energy RDA, but one-third of the vitamin A, vitamin B_6, calcium, and zinc RDAs.[18]

Students who brought lunch from home or purchased a non-NSLP lunch at school had fewer calories from fat and more from carbohydrate than students who went off campus for lunch. The sodium and fat content of lunches bought off campus is similar to NSLP lunches.

SBP participants' breakfast intakes average 31% of energy from fat (compared with the *Dietary Guidelines* goal of 30% or less) and 13% from saturated fat (compared with the *Dietary Guidelines* goal of less than 10%). Differences in the breakfast consumption of specific types of foods by SBP participants and nonparticipants are consistent with differences in dietary intakes. Although only one-half of SBP breakfasts include a meat or meat alternate, SBP participants are three times more likely than nonparticipants to consume meat, poultry, fish, or meat mixtures at breakfast. SBP participants are also more likely than nonparticipants to consume milk or milk products at breakfast. The higher proportion of SBP participants consuming foods from these two groups explains their higher breakfast intakes of calories, protein, calcium, fat, and saturated fat.[18]

SBP participation is associated with an increased intake of calories over 24 hours. The difference between the 24-hour intakes of SBP participants and nonparticipants is about the same as the calorie difference in their breakfast intake. The effects of SBP participation on the percentage of calories from fat, saturated fat, and carbohydrate eaten at breakfast disappear over 24 hours. The SBP contributes to higher intakes of protein and calcium, both at breakfast and over 24 hours.[18]

HIGH-RISK BEHAVIORS OF YOUTHS

Risk-Taking Behaviors

The 1987 National Student Health Survey assessed risk-taking behaviors of a national random sample of 11,319 adolescents. Among the participants, 5,859 were 8th graders and 5,560 were 10th graders; 51% were female and 49% were male. All students responded to 11 questions about behaviors related to tobacco, cigarettes, seat belts, illegal drugs, alcohol, exercise, and fried foods. The adolescents were randomly divided into three groups with almost equal age and sex distributions. Each group completed an in-depth questionnaire on two or three risk-taking behaviors.[32]

Data from a subsample of students were analyzed. These students had a high-risk status defined by extreme tobacco, cigarette, seat belt, illegal drug, alcohol, exercise, and fried food eating behaviors. Factor scores were determined for the high-risk students to identify any potential clustering of risk-taking behaviors. Significant clusters were identified.[33]

Cigarette smoking, drug use, and alcohol intake were the major behaviors forming a high-risk cluster for 8th and 10th grade girls. These three behaviors plus chewing tobacco use were the major behaviors forming high-risk behavior for 8th and 10th grade boys. Statistically, 27% to 32% of the variability of the behaviors was explained with these variables.

Each high-risk factor was the outcome variable in a multilinear regression analysis. Significant predictors of the high-risk behavior were identified ($p < 0.05$). Different antecedent behaviors predicted high-risk behavior for girls compared with boys, and for 8th graders compared with 10th graders. Antecedent behaviors that were the major predictors of a high-risk behavior for all 8th graders were mixing alcohol and drugs with swimming and other water sports, using "stay awake" pills, using psychedelic drugs, and believing it is "OK for peers to use drugs." Major predictors for all 10th graders were mixing alcohol and drugs with swimming and other water sports, using marijuana, and believing it is "OK for peers to use drugs."

For 8th grade girls, other significant predictors included swimming unsupervised, riding with a driver on drugs or alcohol, and controlling weight by throwing up. Serious thoughts of suicide, thoughts about getting a handgun, and salty snack behavior were significant predictors for 8th grade boys.

For 10th grade girls, other significant predictors were riding with a driver on drugs or alcohol, having serious thoughts of suicide, using marijuana, and using diet pills to control weight. Riding with a driver on drugs, using alcohol and drugs within the past month, eating fried foods as snacks, and not warming up before exercise were the major predictors for 10th grade boys.[33]

These data emphasize the importance of two major objectives listed in *Healthy People 2000* for adolescents and young adults: (1) "to reduce the proportion of youth using alcohol, marijuana and cocaine in the past month" and (2) to increase "the individuals 10+ who have discussed with their family these topics in the past month: nutrition, alcohol, physical activity, sexual behavior, tobacco, drug and safety issues."[34] The overall intent of the adolescent and young adult health objectives is to reduce the death rate by 15% to no more than 85 per 100,000 for 15-to-24 year olds by the year 2000.[34]

Antecedent behaviors that predict high-risk behaviors were identified in this secondary data analysis of the 1987 National Student Health Survey. These behaviors can form the basis of parent, peer, and classroom discussion and education to improve the health and well-being of our youth.

Alcohol and Caffeine Consumption

Alcohol provides calories and energy, but most adolescents drink it for fun and pleasure. Supplanting nutrient-rich foods with alcohol sets a child in a dangerous nutrition and accident-prone track.[1]

In Michigan, 45% of white and 48% of Native American high school students reported using alcohol; almost one-half of white, Native American, and Hispanic male users reported heavy alcohol use.[35] Prevalence may be higher among dropouts.

The 1990 Youth Risk Behavior Survey of 9th to 12th graders reported that 88% of youths had consumed alcohol during their lives; 59% reported drinking at least once during the past 30 days. Males were more likely than females (62% and 55%, respectively), and 12th graders were more likely than 9th graders to drink. Of the males, 37% had consumed more than five drinks at least once during the past 30 days.[36]

Sarvela et al[37] evaluated drinking habits of rural students in 7th to 12th grades and noted that 39% had ridden in a car with a drinking driver in the past six months and 16% had driven after drinking. There was an increased level of both activities as grade level increased.[37]

Caffeine is a nervous system stimulate and not viewed as a negative dietary component. However, caffeine may be of increasing concern as it lowers calcium absorption and increases heart rate and respiration. Arbeit and colleagues reported that caffeine intake per kilogram of body weight of white children 10 to 15 years old was comparable to adults (2.5 versus 2.6 mg/kg). Caffeine sources for children are carbonated beverages, chocolate candy, chocolate pudding and ice cream, and tea.[38]

Inactivity and Obesity

Obesity has been shown to track from childhood into adulthood.[39,40] It is estimated that 40% of children who are obese at seven years of age carry their obesity into adulthood, and approximately 70 to 80% of adolescents retain their obesity as adults.[41] Two large surveys of physical activity among US youths—the National Children and Youth Fitness Study (NCYFS I) and the Youth Risk Behavior Survey (YRBS)—profiled physical activity in this population.

NCYFS I reported that if one considers an entire year, typical youths participate in about one to two hours of moderate to vigorous physical activity per day. However, about 20 to 30% of students average less than one-half hour a day. The YRBS presented physical activity data showing that about 50% of boys and 75% of girls do not have moderate to vigorous activity three or more times a week.[42-44] Girls are less active than boys, especially for vigorous activities, and both groups have reduced physical activity with aging.

The President's Council on Physical Fitness and Sports reports that boys 6 to 15 years old scored an average of 20 seconds lower in 1985 than in 1980 for six of ten age categories. In 1981 and 1985, boys experienced lower scores on pull-ups than in 1979.[45] Adolescent girls 12 to 17 years had lower scores on the one mile run in 1979 to 1981 than in 1985.

One overarching concern is that physical activity has been shown to be inversely associated with adiposity.[44,46] An inactive lifestyle in youth sets the stage for inactivity in adulthood and the propensity for obesity.[47]

A number of controlled, primary prevention studies show that by increasing physical activity, one can modestly slow the rise in adiposity among obese youths. Increasing physical activity alone is not as effective as coupling activity with dietary changes and behavior modification. Including parents of obese youths in the combined strategy to change physical activity and eating behavior gives the greatest impact on weight loss.[48,49]

Since 1970, the prevalence of obesity among children 6 to 11 years old has increased 54%, and it has increased 39% for 12-to-17 year olds. Thus, a focus on physical activity and food choices is relevant.[41] Hispanic children are among those experiencing as much as a 120% increase in the prevalence of obesity over the past 20 years. The excess intake of high fat and low complex carbohydrate foods amid minimal physical activity is a major, potential culprit for the obesity trend.[41]

The relationship between consumption of high-fat foods, low physical activity, and obesity was studied using a case-control design for a group of school children with a 30% prevalence of obesity. Of the girls, 35% were obese compared with 26% of the boys. The children who consumed high-fat foods but had low physical activity had a 38% increased risk of obesity compared with children consuming low-fat foods and having a high physical activity.[50]

Most cross-sectional data show no significant population increase in the average amount of total calories consumed, but a possible trend toward a lower amount of total fat is noted in the eating patterns of children and the general public.[51] If the trend is real, a concern remains since the percentage of calories from fat still averages more than 35% for boys and girls at all ages.[43,52]

Conditioning and equipping children with skills not only to shift food intakes toward higher fruit and vegetable consumption but also to increase physical activity and reduce television watching is an eating behavior strategy to alter this obesity trend. In a 1991 study by Tucker et al, the amount of television viewing was inversely correlated with amount of exercise in a sample of 4,771 adult females. Women who reported four or more hours of watching television each day had twice the prevalence of obesity compared with females who watched less than one hour daily. Women who watched three to four hours of television had almost twice the prevalence of obesity compared to the group that watched less than one hour.[53]

Are the television-watching patterns similar for children? Children who watch more television than their peers have greater prevalence of obesity and superobesity.[54] During prime-time television programs and commercials, references to food focus on low-nutrient beverages and sweets consumed as snacks. Emphasis is on "good taste" and "fresh and natural" with minimal attention given to foods consistent with healthy guidelines for children.[55] Data from NHANES II and III found an increase in the prevalence of obesity by 2% for each additional hour of television viewing. These findings remained after controlling for prior obesity status, region of the United States, season, population density, ethnicity, and socioeconomic status.[56]

The prevalence of obesity among children of military dependents was observed at two major medical centers.[57] The prevalence was greater among adolescents than among young children. The percentage of very obese children increased from 5.5% in 1978 to 9.0% in both 1986 and 1990. Children of active duty staff were less frequently obese compared with children of retirees (18% versus 24%), irrespective of age and rank of the parent.

Eating Disorders

Approximately 1 million adolescents are affected by anorexia nervosa and bulimia, which are thought to occur from a variety of reasons including pressure to be thin, depression, biological errors, and poor self-concept. As many as 10% of these adolescents may die prematurely as a result of the disorder. Medical and physical signs of disordered eating are listed in Exhibit 8–1; early behavioral identification signs of eating disorders are listed in Exhibit 8–2. The American Psychiatric Association delineates diagnostic criteria for four types of eating disorders.[31]

Anorexia Nervosa

Two subtypes of anorexia nervosa include the *restricting* and the *binge eating/purging* types. In the binge eating/purging type, the person regularly engages in binge eating or purging behavior such as self-induced vomiting or the misuse of laxatives, diuretics, or enemas. In the restricting type, the person does not regularly en-

Exhibit 8–1   Medical and Physical Signs of Disordered Eating

- amenorrhea or irregular menstrual cycles
- abrasions on hand or fingers from purging efforts
- changes in hair, skin, and nails
- blood chemistry irregularities in electrolytes, serum iron, serum glucose, and/or cholesterol levels

Source: Adapted from Sloan R. Developing an Awareness of Eating Disorders: Identifying the High-Risk Client. *On the Cutting Edge.* 1994. 15(6):22.

Exhibit 8–2   Behavioral Identification Signs of Eating Disorders

ANOREXIA NERVOSA

- restriction of food to "safe" foods
- excessive rituals around food and its consumption
- intermittent episodes of binge-eating
- exercise taken to an extreme
- compulsive drive for perfection in various areas of life

BULIMIA NERVOSA

- rigid restriction of food, followed by binges
- binges of high-calorie, sweet, or salty foods
- secretive eating
- leaving for bathroom immediately after meals
- laxative and/or diuretic use, and/or vomiting
- frequent mood swings
- erratic behavior such as kleptomania, gambling, substance abuse, compulsive spending, or self-mutilation

Source: Adapted from Sloan R. Developing an Awareness of Eating Disorders: Identifying the High-Risk Client. *On the Cutting Edge.* 1994. 15(6):22.

gage in these behaviors. Criteria for anorexia nervosa are as follows:

- refusal to maintain body weight at or above a minimal normal weight for age and height (i.e., weight loss leading to maintenance of body weight less than 85% of that expected);

or failure to make expected weight gain during periods of growth, leading to body weight 15% below that expected

- intense fear of gaining weight or becoming fat, even though underweight
- disturbance in the way in which one's body weight or shape is experienced, undue influence of body weight or shape on self-evaluation, or denial of the seriousness of the current low body weight
- amenorrhea in postmenarchal women (i.e., the absence of at least three consecutive menstrual cycles)

Bulimia Nervosa

Two subtypes exist and include the *purging* and the *nonpurging* types. The purging type regularly engages in self-induced vomiting or the misuse of laxatives, diuretics, or enemas. The nonpurging type does not regularly engage in these behaviors, but uses other inappropriate compensatory behaviors, such as fasting or excessive exercise. Criteria for this classification are as follows:

- recurrent episodes of binge eating where a binge includes both of the following:
  1. eating in a discrete period of time, such as two hours, an amount of food that is definitely larger than most people would eat during a similar period of time under similar circumstances
  2. a sense of lack of control over eating during the episode so that the individual cannot stop eating or control what or how much she or he eats
- recurrent inappropriate compensatory behavior in order to prevent weight gain, such as self-induced vomiting; misuse of laxatives, diuretics, or other medications; fasting; or excessive exercise
- occurrence of binge eating and inappropriate compensatory behaviors, on average, at least twice a week for three months
- self-evaluation unduly influenced by body shape and weight

- disturbance does not occur exclusively during episodes of anorexia nervosa

Binge Eating Disorder

This disorder involves recurrent episodes of binge eating and at least three of the following:

- eating much more rapidly than normal
- eating until feeling uncomfortably full
- eating large amounts of food when not feeling physically hungry
- eating alone because of being embarrassed by how much one is eating
- feeling disgusted with oneself, depressed, or very guilty after overeating

Criteria also involves marked distress regarding binge eating, which occurs at least twice a week for six months. Regular use of purging, fasting, and excessive exercise does not occur.

Eating Disorder Not Otherwise Specified

This is a transient behavior and characterized by the following criteria:

- All of the criteria for anorexia nervosa are met except the individual has regular menses.
- All of the criteria for anorexia nervosa are met except that, despite substantial weight loss, the individual's current weight is in the normal range.
- All of the criteria for bulimia nervosa are met except binges occur at a frequency of less than twice a week or for a duration of less than three months.
- An individual of normal body weight regularly engages in inappropriate compensatory behavior after eating small amounts of food (e.g., self-induced vomiting after the consumption of two cookies).
- An individual repeatedly chews and spits out, but does not swallow, large amounts of food.
- Individual meets the criteria for binge eating disorder (recurrent episodes of binge eat-

ing in the absence of the regular use of in-appropriate compensatory behaviors charac-teristic of bulimia nervosa).

More about Eating Disorders

The age of onset for anorexia seems to peak between 14 and 18 years of age.[58] The precise beginnings of anorexia is difficult to discern, as the US population views "dieting" as a hobby. The mean age of onset for bulimia is about 18 years. If the onset of bulimia occurs after 25 years of age, then chemical dependency problems, sui-cide attempts, or depression may be linked.[58] Pre-adolescent and adolescent girls are at high risk for anorexia and bulimia. Youths with insulin-dependent diabetes mellitus are probably more prone to eating disorders than youths with non-insulin-dependent diabetes mellitus.[59]

Eating disorders occur in all population groups, but a culture-bound syndrome may exist.[60] Spe-cific personality and sociocultural factors may predispose certain individuals to the development of eating disorders. Individuals in the middle to upper socioeconomic levels who are high achiev-ers are prone to developing an eating disorder. Situations that promote food restrictions and diet regulating may be antecedents to eating disor-ders.[61] Youths who are involved in extracurricu-lar activities that stress body form (e.g., ballet or gymnastics) or any highly competitive sport are also at risk.[62]

The Youth Risk Behavior Survey[63] of 9th through 12th graders reports that 69% of male students considered themselves at the right body weight and 17% thought they were underweight; females reported 59% and 7%, respectively. Black students considered themselves less overweight than white or Hispanic students. About 44% of the girls reported that they were trying to lose weight, but only 15% of the boys reported this intent. Even 27% of girls who considered them-selves at the right weight reported currently try-ing to lose weight. Their weight loss methods included exercise, skipping meals, taking diet pills, and inducing vomiting—which they reported sig-nificantly more often than boys.

Shisslak implemented a program to educate high school students, staff, and teachers about eating disorders and found more questions about eating disorders answered correctly by partici-pants than by controls.[64] Larson reported that 454 white girls, 14 to 19 years old, who responded that their guardians "always" lectured them about food, had significantly higher scores on the "drive for thinness" and "ineffectiveness" subscales. Students who responded that their guardians were unaware of their problems also had higher scores on the "ineffectiveness" and "interpersonal distrust" subscales.[65]

Info Line

Nightmare Alive
We use our filthy hands
to feed our hungry hearts.
We stuff our mouths
with food we hate
and bury guilt inside.
Our bowls are dirty,
the plates are too.
Why even bother to clean?
It's on to the next
disgusting feast,
it's on to the cookies and cream.
We can't seem to stop
when we're into a binge
and nothing else matters at all.
Our feelings we push down,
our anger we hide.
Our lives seem so out of control.
We next rush upstairs
to rid all this waste
and swear it won't happen again.
We watch as our lives
and our souls go around
as they flush away into the rot.
And before we know it
it happens again.
We stand at the freezer door
impulsively grabbing whatever is there
reaching out for the food we crave
    and the cycle begins
        all over again
            until finally this life must end.

Source: Author is an unidentified youth with bulimia.

In another study, 12% of black, low-income adolescents thought they had an eating disorder. Those who were 14 years or older were more likely to think about vomiting to lose weight. Females identified more emotional concerns about being overweight or the need to lose weight. The "desire to do everything perfectly" was related to eating disorders among middle school students, whereas "feeling ineffective as a person" was related to eating disorders among high school students. Students who had a self-perceived eating disorder were more often above the 50th percentile for weight for height, and they accurately perceived themselves as such.[66]

Desmond et al administered a 22-item questionnaire on weight perceptions to inner-city black and white adolescent students, 12 to 17 years old. Of the respondents, 40% of heavy black females perceived themselves as overweight, compared to 100% of heavy white females; the trend was similar for heavy males. Black males were more likely to believe that emotions affected eating behavior than white males; black females felt that lack of exercise and white females felt that eating habits accounted for their excess weight. Girls obtained their weight control information from television, family, friends, and magazines. Boys used television, family, and athletic coaches for advice.[67]

Important questions about what influences disordered eating behavior and what triggers and perpetuates the condition include the following[68]:

- Do media images control or influence the thinking of youths about their body size? What is the impact of advertising and entertainment media that promote thin bodies on the behavior of young men and women?
- Is there a critical mass of nutrition knowledge that is needed for long-term stability of eating behavior of youths?
- Are specific groups of dieters at greater risk for developing eating disorders?
- Is there an association between physical activity and food restriction in initiating and perpetuating anorexia nervosa?

Community Nutrition Professionals and Eating Disorders

Community nutrition professionals, often registered dietitians, are part of the health care team working with anorexic and bulimic youth. They must recognize and treat these behaviors. Individual and group sessions with clients can focus on nutritional concerns and restoration of normal eating patterns.[69]

Another alternative is employing medical nutrition therapy in a two-phase approach as recommended by the American Dietetic Association.[70] The education phase consists of collecting relevant information; establishing a collaborative relationship; and defining and discussing relevant principles and concepts of food, nutrition, and weight regulation. Other objectives are to present examples of hunger patterns, typical food intake patterns, and the total energy intake of an individual who has recovered from an eating disorder, and to educate the family, thereby decreasing their frustrations while supporting the recovery process. In addition, attention should be given to separating food- and weight-related behaviors from feelings and psychological issues; changing food behaviors in an incremental manner until the food intake pattern is normalized; slowly increasing or decreasing body weight; learning to maintain a weight that is healthful for that individual; and learning to be comfortable in social eating situations.

The success rate of recovery from bulimia nervosa is greater when the individual has:

- positive self-image and body image
- strong relationships with others
- maintenance of an ideal body weight

The outcome is highly variable and ranges from chronic symptoms and relapses to full remission at follow up.[71] Rates of recovery can be as low as 13% at follow up among hospitalized bulimia nervosa patients, to up to one-half, to over two-thirds of patients at follow up.[72-74]

Teen Pregnancy

In 1985, 1,031,000 teenagers became pregnant, and 477,710 teenagers gave birth to an infant. Of those becoming pregnant, 10,000 were less than 15 years of age.[75] In 1991, pregnancy rates were 75 per 1,000 teenagers 15 to 17 years old and 171 per 1,000 girls 18 to 19 years old. In the same year, teen birth rates were the highest for black non-Hispanic girls compared to other ethnic groups.[76] Unless the adolescent's growth at the time she conceives is completed, there will be a greater demand for food energy and nutrients.[77]

Most adolescents who become pregnant after age 16 do not have an increased nutrient need for growth. However, eating patterns of adolescents reflect a high consumption of fast foods, frequent snacking, independence of food choice, dieting, and skipping of meals, with a preoccupation with physical appearance and peer influence. A study of 1,268 adolescents 13 to 19 years of age showed that 69% of the teens had previously dieted; 33% were dieting at the time of the inquiry, and 14% were considered "chronic dieters."[78]

Community nutrition professionals can teach pregnant adolescents skills for healthy eating. These skills might include learning to read food labels, analyzing their own intake and showing the difference between what they eat and what they should eat, and practicing food preparation methods for nutrient-dense foods and snacks they like.

Important research questions that need to be asked on this topic include the following[68]:

- Is there an optimal weight gain for pregnant adolescents at different ages? (see Chapter 9)
- Are the nutrient needs of pregnant adolescents at different ages based on data from pregnant adolescents at different ages?
- What are predisposing cultural factors that can influence the incidence of pregnancy in adolescence?
- Do effective methods exist to teach and to train pregnant adolescents how to modify their eating patterns for the health of their babies and themselves?

CURRENT CHALLENGES AND MAJOR NUTRITION INITIATIVES TO ACHIEVE *HEALTHY YOUTH 2000*

Primary prevention efforts are more effective if children over two years old who are at high risk for chronic disease are identified. Lifestyle changes early in life can affect the course of disease. It is assumed that changes may be more readily achievable at young ages, before lifelong habits are established.

Anatomical data have become available to strengthen the argument for a low-fat eating pattern in youth. No information was available regarding associations between serum lipid or lipoprotein levels and atherosclerosis in youth until data from the Bogalusa Heart study were published. This study reported an association between low-density lipoprotein (LDL) cholesterol concentrations and aortic lesions in 44 deceased adolescents in Bogalusa, Louisiana.[79,80] About the same time, in 1983, a group of pathologists and scientists organized the Pathobiological Determinants of Atherosclerosis in Youth Study. They focused on atherosclerosis among individuals 15 to 34 years old who were victims of violent death. The data involved 390 young men.[81]

Pathologists at central laboratories graded the arteries for atherosclerotic lesions. Serum total lipoprotein cholesterol and thiocyanate concentrations were measured. The percentage of intimal surface having atherosclerotic lesions in both the aorta and the right coronary artery had a positive association with serum very-low-density lipoprotein plus LDL cholesterol concentration. The percentage was negatively associated with serum high-density lipoprotein (HDL) cholesterol concentration.

Smoking was measured indirectly with serum thiocyanate concentration. It was strongly associated with prevalence of raised lesions, especially in the abdominal aorta. Lipoprotein levels did not explain the effect of smoking. Even after adjusting for lipoprotein cholesterol levels and smoking, black children had more extensive total surface involvement of the aorta than white children. These associations clarify the role of serum lipoprotein cholesterol concentrations and smoking on the early stages of atherosclerosis among youths and young adults.[81]

Primary prevention efforts are fueled by the important finding that risk factors for cardiovascular disease tend to remain or track in the same relative rank within a population. Children with high levels of cardiovascular risk are earmarked for adult disease. The concept of tracking yields two major implications: (1) that a relative ranking of an individual with respect to his peers can be maintained, and (2) that the potential exists for identification of risk.

Several studies demonstrated an association of cardiovascular risk factor variables within school-age children as they age. These studies were conducted in Bogalusa, Louisiana, and Muscatine, Iowa[4,82-85] and within young adults in the Naval Aviator Study,[86] the Evans County Study,[87] and the Tecumseh Study.[88]

In the Bogalusa Heart Study, tracking of serum total cholesterol, anthropometric measures, and blood pressure were noted early in the longitudinal observations as follows[84]:

- *Anthropometric measures:* Pearson product moment correlation coefficients for height were the lowest due to changes noted for growth. For weight, coefficients between readings three years apart were 0.82 to 0.91 across all age groups of children (p <0.0001); readings four years apart ranged from 0.70 to 0.85 (p <0.0001). Right triceps skinfolds tracked with correlations from 0.72 to 0.83 for a three-year span and 0.64 to 0.77 for a four-year span.
- *Blood pressure:* The Pearson product moment correlation coefficient for systolic blood pressure for a three-year span was 0.57 and for a four-year span was 0.50 (for both, p <0.0001). Diastolic pressure correlations were 0.40 (p <0.001) and 0.38 (p < 0.0001), respectively.
- *Serum total cholesterol:* For the three- and four-year spans, a 0.64 and 0.61 correlation coefficient were observed (for both, p <0.0001). LDL cholesterol yielded correlation coefficients of 0.70 and 0.67 (for both, p <0.0001).

These tracking data indicate that specific children can be identified who will continue to have abnormal levels of risk factors. Specific primary preventive measures can be taken to meet the needs of individual children.

DIETARY RECOMMENDATIONS FOR CHILDREN OVER TWO YEARS OF AGE

Several objectives in *Healthy People 2000* set the nutrition agenda for school-age children.[34] The Pediatric Panel Report of the National Cholesterol Education Panel (NCEP) underscores these objectives for all children two years and older by recommending maintenance of a healthy body weight and an eating pattern with less than 30% of total energy as fat, 10% as saturated fat, and less than 300 mg of cholesterol per day.[89] This is called the Step 1 eating pattern.

Step 1 Eating Pattern

The preferred eating pattern for all children aged two and above requires a high complex carbohydrate intake to reach the lower fat composition and to achieve adequate calories for growth and development of children.

If children are identified to have an elevated LDL level greater than or equal to 130 mg/dL, then the Step 1 pattern should definitely be followed. If LDL level is not reduced after three to six months, then Step 2 is recommended by NCEP.

Step 2 Eating Pattern

In the Step 2 eating pattern, fat provides 30% or less of total energy intake, saturated fat is lowered to 8 to 9% of total energy, and dietary cholesterol is decreased to less than 150 mg per day. A 5 to 15% reduction in the LDL cholesterol level has been noted with the Step 2 eating pattern. A 23% decrease has been reported when oat bran, psyllium, or lotus bean gum has been added as a supplement to a low-fat eating pattern. Even a 10 to 15% reduction in LDL cholesterol has been noted when psyllium is added to a Step 1 pattern, but the research data are not consistent.

Fiber

A fiber recommendation for all children is needed for a healthy gastrointestinal tract, yet a broad-based recommendation remains speculative at this time. Fiber intake of 10-year-old Bogalusa Heart Study children from 1973 to 1982 averaged 4 to 5 grams. Fiber data from the 1977–1978 NFCS were compared with data from the 1987–1988 Nationwide Food Consumption Survey and showed that the total average dietary fiber intake of all children decreased. Vegetables and fruits were the major source of dietary fiber for children aged two to eleven in the 1977–1978 data. A decade later, bread and cereal were the two major dietary fiber sources. Children who ate breakfast consumed more fiber than children who did not.[9,90]

Wynder et al have suggested a 25/25 standard: 25% of the total energy intake for children as fat and 25 grams of fiber per day.[91] An increase in complex carbohydrate to achieve a fat intake of 30% or less creates a high-fiber eating pattern. In 1994, The American Health Foundation convened child nutrition researchers to explore support for a fiber recommendation for children. Based on the current state of the science, a 0.5 gram per kilogram recommendation appears unrealistic, especially for large 18-year-old boys; the 10 grams per 1,000 kcal creates high intakes for very young children.

A new, age-sensitive formula was proposed to determine children's dietary fiber needs. It is called the "Age of Child Plus 5 Rule" (see Figure 8–2). The formula is proposed to ensure that children from 3 to 18 years grow into their fiber requirements as a natural way of eating, with an annual increase in fiber above their basal needs. An objective of the recommendation is to introduce a consensus of thinking about fiber and encourage all health care groups and professional organizations to use the guide in their programs and materials.[92]

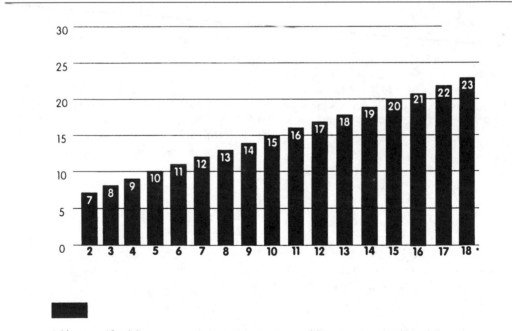

* After age 18 adult recommendations of 20-35 grams of fiber per day should be followed.

Figure 8–2 American Health Foundation recommended fiber intake for children: "Age of Child Plus 5 Rule." *Source:* American Health Foundation, New York, NY. 1994.

General Eating Pattern Guide for Children

To achieve a healthy eating pattern, children and adults who prepare food for children can use USDA's Food Guide Pyramid as the planning blueprint.[93] The pyramid is the visual presentation of the *Dietary Guidelines.*[94] It was presented to the public by Secretary of Agriculture Madigan in April 1992. Fats, oils, and sweets are at the tip, followed by low-fat meats and dairy products. Whole-grain starches, breads, and cereals; fruits; and vegetables form the bottom segments, signifying more servings for a healthier food pattern. The edible fiber content of foods is described in Figure 8–3.

Three general concepts conveyed in the Food Guide Pyramid are: (1) balance foods higher in nutrients with those lower in nutrients, (2) choose a variety of foods each day, and (3) have moderate portions of foods. The Food Guide Pyramid was preceded in 1989 by California's Assembly Bill 2109. This bill mandated the California Department of Education to develop nutrition guidelines for all food and beverages sold on school campuses in California.[95,96] The "Nutrition Guidelines for California School Foods" that resulted represented a three-tiered approach to dietary modification of lunch and breakfast menus. Each level reduces the fat content and increases the fiber content through the increase in whole-grain foods, fruits, and vegetables:

- Tier 1 has the least change with modification primarily in the quality of the food that children receive. For example, this includes serving a fresh fruit rather than a canned one, or serving whole-grain bread rather than plain white bread.
- Tier 2 decreases the quantities of certain foods and replaces them with increased quantities of other foods to maintain the calories children need for energy and growth. For example, butter, gravies, and rich desserts—which all add calories primarily in the form of fat—are served less frequently. Instead, the lower-fat forms of meat, cheese, milk, and desserts are used, and calories are increased by adding servings of bread and bread alternates, fruits, and vegetables.

- Tier 3 has the greatest change. It is the last step for increasing servings of beans, fruits, and vegetables. All high-fat desserts are replaced with fresh fruits; whole-grain breads are served and minimal fat is added in cooking. Reaching this tier achieves the nutrition guidelines for child nutrition programs. Nutrient content reflects 30 to 35% of the total calories as fat and one-third of the RDAs for vitamins and minerals with moderation of sodium and sugar.

The eating pattern identified in California's school nutrition guidelines are based on the *California Daily Food Guide,*[96] currently used by California for all nutrition programs. These guidelines could be used for all snacks and meals planned for children throughout the United States. The *California Daily Food Guide* provides quantitative, life-cycle dietary recommendations with ethnic-, age-, and gender-specific food guides. The importance of these guidelines is the continuity they provide for programs and for the public. If the pattern is followed in childhood, then continuing the pattern into adolescence and adulthood is easier and probable.

CHILD NUTRITION AS A COMPONENT OF COMPREHENSIVE SCHOOL HEALTH

Comprehensive school health education is a primary prevention strategy for teaching disease prevention and health promotion life skills to children, parents, and future parents.[97-99] Comprehensive school health education is based on a planned, sequential pre-K through 12th grade curriculum that addresses the physical, mental, emotional, and social dimensions of children.[100]

Health education has evolved from emphasizing dissemination of knowledge to emphasizing modification of health behavior.[101] Table 8–4 contrasts traditional health education with health instruction that emphasizes health-promoting behaviors. Several theoretical models explain health behavior including the Health Belief Model, Theory of Reasoned Action, Multiattribute Utility Theory, and Social Learning Theory.[102]

Edible Fiber Of Foods
(per serving)

Food	Serving Size	Moderate Fiber (2-4 gm)	High Fiber (5+gm)
Breads	1 slice	Whole wheat, cracked wheat, bran muffin	———
	4	Rye wafers	———
Cereals	1 oz.	Bran Flakes, Raisin Bran, Shredded Wheat, oatmeal	All Bran, Bran Buds, Corn Bran
Vegetable	1/2 cup	Beets, broccoli, brussel sprouts, cabbage, carrots, corn, green beans, green peas	Spinach
	1 med	Baked potato with skin	Corn on the cob
	1/2	Avocado	———
Fruits	1 med	Apple with peel, date, fig, mango, nectarine, orange, pear	———
	1/2 cup	Applesauce (unsweetened), raspberries, blackberries	Cooked prunes
Meat substitutes	1/2 cup	———	Baked beans, black beans, garbanzos, kidney beans, lentils, lima beans, pinto beans
	2 tbsp	Peanut butter	———
	1/4 cup	Peanuts, roasted	———

Figure 8–3 Edible fiber of foods identified by serving size. *Source:* Reprinted with permission of the American Academy of Pediatrics, *AAP: Pediatric Nutrition Handbook*, Nutrition Committee, Chapter 11, Table 13, 1993 edition.

Table 8-4 Traditional Health Education versus Health Instruction in a Health-Promoting School

Traditional Health Education	*Health Instruction in a Health-Promoting School*
Emphasizes knowledge and attitude changes predisposing to behavior change.	Applies multiple theories and models to development and intervention designed to promote health-enhancing behaviors.
Organizes the health instruction program around 10 content areas.	Focuses on 6 priority health behaviors within the 10 content areas.
Views the school health program as instruction, health services, and a healthful school environment.	Expands the program to include health promotion regarding food services, physical education, guidance, worksite, and integration of school and community.
Considers health instruction as the focal intervention strategy.	Replaces the health instruction model with a health promotion model that employs multiple strategies.
Considers health education only in limited classroom terms.	Coordinates health promotion activities with community programs and infuses health content throughout the curriculum.
Promotes coordination of the health education program via a school health advisory council.	Promotes coordination of the school health program within the school through interdisciplinary and interagency teams.
Concentrates on didactic, teacher-led health instruction and acquisition of facts.	Promotes active student participation matching teaching techniques with instruction.
Tends to respond to a series of problems or crises one-by-one.	Includes common skills in the curriculum.
Considers the adoption of health-promoting behaviors a result of health instruction.	Develops caring schools and communities with high expectations for pupil success.
Does not routinely involve parents actively in the school health program.	Considers family support and involvement in health and development of the total school health program as the nucleus of the health-promoting school.

Source: Adapted from Young IM. Encouraging Parental Involvement in School. In Nutbeam D, Haglund B, Farley P, Tellgren P, eds. *Youth Health Promotion: From Theory to Practice in School and Community*. London, England: Forbes Publication Ltd; 1991:218–232.

Critical factors influencing an individual's health behavior include the following[103]:

- knowledge about the disease
- perceived threat of illness
- attitudes about health care
- social interaction
- social norms
- social structure
- accessibility of health services
- demographic factors

Health status and health risk result from multiple factors. Therefore, researchers believe that multiple interventions are needed to effect behavioral, environmental, or social changes.[104-109]

The 10 content areas essential for a comprehensive program are: community health, consumer health, environmental health, family life, growth and development, nutrition, personal health, prevention and control of disease, safety and accident prevention, and substance use and abuse. Common content areas required by state mandates include drug and alcohol abuse prevention (required in 29 states), tobacco use prevention (required in 20 states), and nutrition (required in 19 states).[110,111]

The Public Health Service identified four major factors that contribute to premature illness and death in the general population[112]: heredity (20%), environment (20%), health care delivery system (10%), and unhealthy lifestyle (50%). The Centers for Disease Control and Prevention targeted education for behavior change in six areas as critical to reducing premature illness and death among adolescents: nutrition, physical activity, intentional and unintentional injury, alcohol and other drug use, smoking, and reproductive health.[113] These priority behaviors complement objectives from *Healthy People 2000*, one-third of which focus on children and youths.

Two of the six education goals set by the Centers for Disease Control and Prevention would be difficult to attain without implementation of an effective school health program—readiness for learning; and a safe, disciplined, drug-free, and violence-free environment.

"Child nutrition and food services" is one of the 10 components of comprehensive school health. School cafeterias are a primary prevention arena—a potential learning laboratory for children and campus food sales where demonstration and education studies can be conducted to evaluate menu changes and acceptability to students.[114-116] With national efforts to legislate comprehensive school health programs, support for a comprehensive approach strengthens each component (e.g., child nutrition or physical education and their respective programs). Appendix 8-B outlines strategies to promote 5-A-Day messages in a comprehensive school health program.

Coordination of Food Service with Classroom Education

A relatively newly defined role for community nutrition professionals is nutrition education in schools. Even though nutrition education has been taught for decades in the classroom as part of health, science, and home economics, the 1990s have seen an increase in specific professional positions of school nutrition and child nutrition educators and specialists. Placement of child nutrition specialists on the school campus to coordinate food service activities with classroom instruction strengthens the role of nutrition in health and in comprehensive school health education. Creative approaches to nutrition education in the classroom are needed (see Figure 8-4).

In a survey of 407 4th to 8th grade students, 94% thought that the food they eat can affect their future health. Of the respondents, 99% understood the importance of exercise for good health; 80% could identify three of the four food groups; and 98% recognized the importance of eating plenty of fruits, vegetables, and high-fiber foods.[117]

Simply knowing about fruits, vegetables, and fiber is not enough to make individuals eat more. Because students report that their primary sources of nutrition information are schools (95%), parents (86%), and health professionals (73%), it behooves schools to be actively involved in nutrition education. Surveys support nutrition education as an acceptable method for reducing population risk factors for chronic disease, and nutrition education provides a more inexpensive approach compared to medical and clinical strategies.[118] Roper surveys have identified nutrition at a consistently high level of interest in the United States since the mid 1970s. Almost all individuals from 1976 to 1985 reported that the nutritional value of food (90% reported) and their specific diets (60% reported) were very important to their health.[119]

The "Food for Thought, All About Nutrition and You!" program in the Palm Beach (Florida) School District revealed that 10% of children were either underweight or overweight. Age-appropriate nutrition education activities were placed in the curriculum, and students prepared healthy snacks in the classroom. An increased acceptance of vegetables, skim milk, and other foods that had been used during class were noted by the child nutrition employees in the cafeteria. The majority of teachers, principals, and students wanted to continue the program the following year, and test packets were distributed to other district schools.[120]

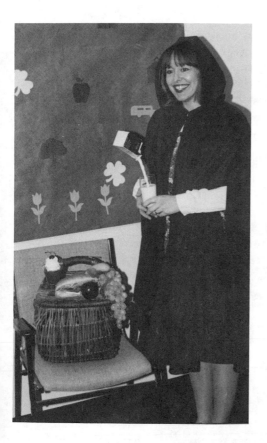

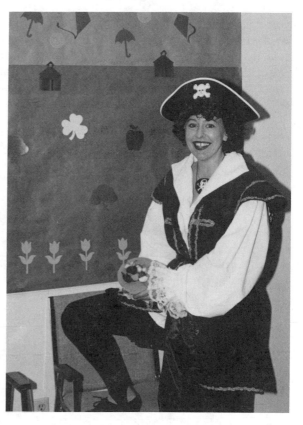

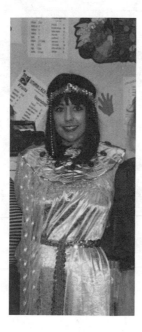

Figure 8-4 Child nutrition specialist, Anna Apoian, R.D., sports costumes to carry nutrition messages to Corona-Norco Unified School District students. She disguises as Patti the Pirate, Phonecia the Egyptian, and Little Red Riding Hood. *Source:* Reprinted with permission of Anna Apoian. Corona-Norco Unified School District. Norco, CA.

It appears that the earlier nutrition education is integrated into the classroom, the more likely students will practice healthy eating behaviors. The "FUN Kit" provides nutrition education for preschoolers with puppets, music cassettes, and stickers.[121] Liang developed nutrition lessons using musical compositions about "my body, my friends" (see Figure 8-5).[122] The International Food Information Council and the National Center for Nutrition and Dietetics have developed classroom posters and materials that present nutrition as fun and something children will want to do. The American Heart Association, the American Cancer Association, and the National Dairy Council are only a few of the many nonprofit groups that have developed numerous curricula for all ages of school children. Each of these organizations has developed nutrition education materials that are generally available at a minimal cost, such as "Changing the Course," "Early Start," and "Heart Works." These organizations support community outreach and training of allied health and education professionals. Working collaboratively with these organizations and volunteers can be advantageous to schools with budget restrictions. Continuing education hours can be accrued for teachers and child nutrition employees. Additionally, complete up-to-date and effective curricula from these organizations can link classroom education with the cafeteria and parents and tap community resources.

Info Line

A 192-page guidebook published in 1995 entitled, "How to Teach Nutrition to Kids," written by Connie L. Evers, MS, RD, is designed for educators, nutrition professionals, parents, and other caregivers. It outlines the tools they need to provide an integrated approach to nutrition for early elementary aged children (6-10 years old). The guidebook combines strategies for the classroom, the cafeteria, and the home environments. It contains nutrition education activities and strategies that have been used with children and endorsed by teachers.

The guidebook is available from 24 Carrot Press, P.O. Box 23546, Tigard, OR 97281-3546. Telephone 503-524-9318. $18.00.

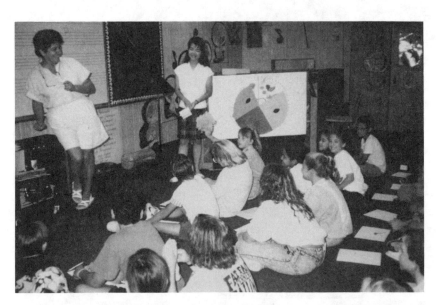

Figure 8-5 A creative, age-sensitive nutrition education curriculum for upper elementary children. *Source:* Reprinted with permission of Liang T. and Frank G. Hello My Friend—What Did You Eat Today? *Journal of Nutrition Education.* 1994;26: 205B–206B.

ACTION PLAN—TARGETING SUCCESS

To create or adapt child nutrition programs to achieve *Healthy People 2000* objectives, any action plan should include the RDAs, the Food Guide Pyramid, and the National Cholesterol Education Panel recommendations. If achieved, these objectives collectively have the potential to reduce eating disorders, promote healthy weight management, and reduce nutrient imbalance. They enhance nutrition education in the classroom and assist students with skills such as making healthy food choices during leisure eating time. In addition, they promote healthy and acceptable meal planning in schools.

The Predisposing, Enabling and Reinforcing or PRECEDE model for school health intervention can serve as a blueprint for developing a nutrition education and food service management action plan. PRECEDE addresses predisposing, enabling, and reinforcing factors in schools[123]:

- *Predisposing factors* are the demographic and population norms often beyond the scope of a program and usually nonmodifiable. However, increasing fruit and vegetable intake to 5-a-day in the population would establish a new, preferred norm.
- *Enabling factors* concern availability and accessibility in the school, such as the cafeteria, vending machines, and campus stores.
- *Reinforcing factors* address attitudes and behaviors of peers, parents, teachers, administrators, and media that either support or discourage behavioral change.

Community nutrition professionals can structure their action plans based upon this framework and reduce unknowns, thereby focusing their energies and budgets on specific modifiable factors. In addition to action plans directed toward comprehensive school health, the health and nutrition plight of many children must be curtailed. Direct health services are essential in some settings to complement meals and education at school.

The 1992–1993 Healthy Start Initiative in California provides immediate care clinics on school grounds for high-risk populations. This approach should be considered for a national mandate. Nutrition services in the form of the School Breakfast Program should be visible and incorporated at the beginning of each Healthy Start program as a direct service. This is a priority when obesity, anorexia nervosa, iron deficiency anemia, lead poisoning, hunger, and nutrient imbalances are prevalent among youths. In addition, each district should work to increase their reimbursement rate by offering nutritious meals and promoting participation of all students in the School Breakfast Program and National School Lunch Program through marketing to the community, school boards, parents, teachers, and students.

As changes are made, action plans must be monitored to identify what works and what does not work. Often community nutrition programs lack sufficient evaluation. Evaluation is crucial if major issues are to be corrected and if successful program components are identified for generalizability to other locations and situations.

Implementation and process evaluation may include questionnaires and observational measures to assess readiness of the students and faculty prior to the program implementation. Outcome evaluation may include questionnaires and observational measures to assess program effects on food consumption and nutrient outcome. Evaluation tools can include instruments for staff, as well as for students. Examples of evaluation tools include:

- *Meal quality assessment instrument:* a checklist that can be used by school nutrition staff to address food preparation and menu planning consistent with dietary guidelines for school children. It might require 15 to 20 minutes of direct observation, marking observations on a scantron form. The assessment tracks qualitative changes in menus.
- *Pre/post test:* 5 to 10 items that can be used at a training class to establish baseline knowledge of employees or teachers.
- *Basic nutrition knowledge questionnaire:* may contain 10 to 25 items directed toward general information students should have

(e.g., ability to identify foods by specific food group, the role of foods in chronic disease prevention, food misconceptions, and nutrition message in the media).

- *Attitudinal questionnaire:* may focus on student likes and dislikes, such as fruits and vegetables or high-fat and protein foods. Scales using facial expressions are helpful when assessing attitudes of younger children.
- *Other:* Behavior can be measured with one- to three-day food records, a specific instrument such as the Fat/Cholesterol Avoidance Scale, or a food frequency questionnaire set up specifically for adolescents.[25]

WHO IS RESPONSIBLE FOR SOUND NUTRITION IN SCHOOLS?

Schools have two major child nutrition responsibilities: (1) to protect the health and well-being of students with wholesome foods, and (2) to provide an enjoyable environment that makes healthful foods accessible to all children. To achieve these responsibilities, coordinating classroom learning with cafeteria decision making and supporting inservice training for child nutrition employees and teachers are paramount.

The key national players are the US Department of Agriculture (USDA) and its Nutrition Education and Training Program, National School Lunch Program, breakfast and commodity programs, the American School Food Service Association,[124] the School Nutrition Services Dietetic Practice Group of the American Dietetic Association, state child nutrition directors, and numerous food manufacturers. These groups and organizations such as the Society of Nutrition Education and the American Public Health Association are likewise responsible for informing legislators of the needs and priorities for effective and efficient school nutrition programs across the United States. As school nutrition is integrated with comprehensive school health, the Centers for Disease Control and Prevention and other national survey and professional organizations gain importance.

On June 8, 1994, new child nutrition program regulations were announced by USDA Secretary of Agriculture, Mike Espy, and the Assistant Secretary for Food and Consumer Services, Ellen Haas. The regulations, entitled "School Meals Initiative for Healthy Children," will take effect by the 1998–1999 school year. After a series of public hearings and roundtables, USDA considered the suggestions and insights of school food service, nutrition, health, medical, and education professionals and the general public. The regulations are set to update the nutrition standards for meal plannings dramatically. Three specific components include the following[125]:

1. "Nutrient Standard Menu Planning" (NuMenuS) to provide a one-week assessment of meals to reflect nutrient content
2. the nutrient composition of commodities, variety among the commodities, and new product development
3. reduction of administrative paperwork for the claims process and the review/certification process

By the 1998–1999 school year, school food service planners and directors must ensure that lunches offered to school children (aged 2 years and older) meet nutrient standards. School districts can use a nutrient-standard computerized menu planning procedure or an assisted nutrient-standard menu planning process available through USDA. Breakfast and lunch must provide ¼ and ⅓ of the RDA for a child as a minimum standard for planning meals and the 1990 Guidelines for Americans must be achieved (i.e., <30% of energy from total fat and <10% of energy from saturated fat).

The American School Food Service Association has led the challenge to postpone implementation because school districts do not have the resources needed to computerize their menus. The association does not believe that the administrative controls have been streamlined sufficiently. USDA plans to launch a nationwide nutrition education campaign aimed at the lunchroom and the classroom to introduce children, food service staff, classroom teachers, and parents to an improved way to plan meals and make improved meal planning a part of their lifestyle.[125]

TARGETING CHANGE IN THE SCHOOL EATING ENVIRONMENT

Specific ways to target change in the eating environment of schools are presented below.[1]

Time Allocation for Meals

Students may have 12 to 25 minutes for lunch. This includes obtaining their meal, finding a place to sit, eating, socializing, and discarding waste. This rushed environment decreases chances for optimal food intake. Children probably need a minimum of 15 to 20 minutes from the time they are seated to eat, talk a little, and experience lunch without rushing.

Meal monitors are employed in some schools as "traffic controllers" and "time keepers." If their efforts are positive and not demeaning for students, a receptive environment occurs. Some schools even present lunch as a pleasant social time with music and citizenship awards for cleanup and manners.

Acceptability of Menus

Student meal acceptance has usually been based on plate waste. To lower plate waste, menu planners have developed potato, salad, and sandwich bars. High school youth advisory groups have been devised by the American School Food Service Association to bring students into the planning, tasting, and decision-making process.[126] Upper elementary students should be given similar choices to build their food decision-making skills.

The multicultural environment found in many schools today requires school foods that are diverse in taste and enhance the cultural pride of the students. To increase acceptability, cultural foods should be incorporated. However, with westernization, the benefits of nutritious foods from different cultures have been lost (e.g., tofu has been deleted from Asian dishes and high-fiber ingredients have been left out of salads and vegetables of the Middle East). Individual student tastes and cultural practices have been shaped by societal norms and food preferences of the West.

Hong et al identified the top five school lunch entrees for 5th and 6th grade students in the ABC Unified School District in Los Angeles County.[127] The 172 students were 30% Hispanic; 30% Asian; 30% Caucasian; and 10% Portuguese, East Indian, and other. A significant correlation was noted between the acceptance and the frequency of eating the routine entrees and acceptance of a new recipe for a tofu (low-fat) Chinese meat bun: nacho beef and cheese, $r = 0.739$; pepperoni pizza, $r = 0.753$; spaghetti, $r = 0.739$; chicken chunks, $r = 0.717$; diced turkey, $r = 0.786$; Chinese meat bun, $r = 0.850$ (for all, $p < 0.001$). When given culturally diverse foods, culturally diverse children select and eat them.

Healthful Content of Menus

Several education/demonstration studies have successfully reduced the fat and saturated fat content of school recipes. The "Go for Health" program focused on influencing the student environment by enhancing physical activity classes and by lowering the fat content of school lunches (saturated fat from 16% to 10%, and total fat from 32% to 19%). Dietary recalls of students indicated that they consumed fewer calories, less total fat, and less sodium than students who were not offered the modified menus.[128]

The "Heart Smart" program developed a complementary approach for cardiovascular health promotion. The school cafeteria and classroom were effective vehicles to translate reduced fat, sodium, and sugar content of menus into acceptance foods.[115,116]

The American School Food Service Association initiative called "Healthy EDGE" (Eating, the Dietary Guidelines and Education) focuses on (1) team building in schools and communities to work together to make the *Dietary Guidelines for Americans* a part of school policy, and (2) activities that will effectively improve the nutritional health of students.[124] This initiative is the impetus for child nutrition employees to practice healthy menu planning for school children.

Trained Food Service Personnel

The American School Food Service Association has a strong commitment to continuing education that addresses sanitation, safety, meal planning, and meal preparation for health promotion in schools. Schools districts should support the food service staff and share expenses in training and upgrading this aspect of the school environment. Often child nutrition employees are at the low end of pay scales; their work may be seen as tertiary to education and physical fitness. This is demeaning and unnecessary: no hunger or malnourished child can think, concentrate, or participate at his or her fullest potential.

In California, Frank and Adsen[129] conducted a statewide census of training needs, querying 547 directors and 1,266 managers. Respondents indicated that "training programs" was the number one factor in influencing their personal career development and retention. "Food Preparation" and "Healthy Menu Planning" were the two courses they felt would be most helpful in their daily work. On-the-job-training was the most common form of training, and respondents preferred either their school site or their district office for training.

To train child nutrition employees in healthy menu planning, "Shaping Healthy Meals for School Children" was developed as a 10-lesson curriculum to be taught in a train-the-trainer format.[130] "Shaping Healthy Meals" uses the California Daily Food Guide (CDFG) and has been approved for continuing education units by the *California School Food Service Association*. The curriculum integrates several worksheets from the American Cancer Society's cafeteria training manual, "Changing the Course" discussed earlier. This is one of several excellent hands-on curricula and model programs that blend multiple materials with the immediate need in schools for

relevant training about low-fat, tasty, and nutritionally adequate foods.

Cafeteria intervention in the form of inservice education training can follow a population-based approach and be given to all participating schools in a district or to multiple districts in a county. Training in most school districts is not but should be formalized in a consistent, sequential manner on a monthly or bimonthly basis. A train-the-trainer format, which identifies employees who are trained and then become trainers for their peers, strengthens the likelihood that school districts will sustain the program.

Food Service Delivery System

The ability of school cafeterias to link with classroom education is often influenced by the skills of child nutrition employees, the type of food service delivery system, and the degree to which the teachers are aware of the food service system.

A *centralized service* is a food service system in which all food is prepared in a central kitchen. Such a service often uses a "cook-chill" process—transporting the food daily to specific school sites, refrigerating, and then heating it before serving it. This system provides an opportunity to train a kitchen staff and influence thousands of meals daily prior to distribution. The major concerns are that foods are often purchased pre-portioned and that cooking equipment is automated in an assembly line. Menu changes must fit into the equipment and production process and the food specifications required of food companies.[1]

The *decentralized service* is a food service system in which all food is prepared on each school campus under the supervision of a site manager. This type of service creates a sense of ownership by the staff, who feel very responsible for their "kids." Training at the site involves identifying the "readiness" of each employee, who may be responsible for only single types of foods (e.g., the baker, the main entree cook, etc.). For this type of service, training is directed toward skill development of the different preparation positions.[1]

For either delivery system, training food service staff in the use of point-of-choice nutrition information is a basic marketing effort. Nutrition information can be placed adjacent to foods to complement classroom education. For example, a label could read, "Tossed salad with flaked tuna, 1½ cups: 144 calories, 241 retinol equivalents (RE) vitamin A, 36 mg vitamin C," or "Hamburger on whole-wheat bun: 266 calories, 41% fat, 362 mg sodium." Point-of-choice nutrition information has been used to guide individuals in making healthy food choices with comparisons and nutrient information.[131-134] Color-coding like a stop light has been effective with children.[128]

Because school menus are increasingly being evaluated by a nutrient standard, computerized databases are being used by employees. Increasing the technical skills of child nutrition employees can be accomplished by integrating the computer training into routine procedures.

Many programs are available, such as Computrition, Inc., DINE Systems, and Nutri-Kids.[135-138] Each system has unique characteristics—ranging from extensive food production, purchasing, and inventory programs on Computrition to evaluation by USDA meal components on NutriKids. NutriKids is a food database designed specifically for child nutrition programs. It contains over 1,100 common ingredients and 200 recipes. The DINE System has over 7,200 foods and produces a printout with an overall menu score based on consensus dietary recommendations (e.g., less than 30% fat and less than 3,300 mg of sodium[136,138]) (see Chapter 9).

High-Risk Youth Programs

Part of the solution to the problem of obesity is school involvement in secondary prevention programs. Schools can develop goals and plans to provide low-fat food choices matched with ample opportunities for continuous physical activities and sports participation. Dedicated school staff and faculty must be identified to champion the cause. Parental involvement in the program should be garnered to build self-esteem, reinforce positive behavior change, and identify depression among youth and their families.

The SHAPEDOWN program is a secondary prevention program for obese adolescents, which has produced significant long-term outcomes. It is transferable to various settings and may provide the foundation for a school-based program.[139]

Partnership with the Community

Developing a partnership with the community is a growing trend for child nutrition directors. A community advisory group of 8 to 12 individuals can consist of a community leader, a local pediatrician or family practice physician, a grocery store owner, a restaurant owner, an American Cancer Society representative, an elementary school teacher, a newspaper/radio or television reporter, a member of the clergy, a health agency representative, a local nutritionist, and/or a popular personality. The advisory group can respond to a program's philosophy, needs, progress, and any changes in format. This group can reinforce and publicize positive efforts occurring in child nutrition programs.

At the same time, child nutrition directors and the nutrition education specialists they employ can serve as nutrition resources for the media and community health efforts. For example, Connie Evers, M.S., R.D., a specialist once employed by the Portland Public Schools, periodically wrote a column focusing on child nutrition in the *Portland Oregonian*. A concern is that only 8% of child nutrition directors employ such a specialist, often due to lack of funds.[129]

Working with USDA and Regional Offices

The USDA and regional offices provide the major direction and impetus for school food programs. The nutritional well-being of children is greatly influenced by USDA's acceptance and integration of national nutrition directives into its own programs. USDA oversees the commodity program that provides surplus foods to schools annually.

The trend has been to provide healthier commodities to schools who need the price break that commodities offer. For example, common commodities in 1970 included American cheese, ground beef with fat not to exceed 30%, fruit packed in heavy syrup, and hydrogenated vegetable fat. These have been replaced with mozzarella cheese, ground beef with fat not to exceed 22%, and soybean salad oil. Today, ground turkey, extra-lean frozen beef patties, and diced chicken appear on the commodity list, along with processed cheese with reduced sodium, sliced peaches in light syrup, and almond butter. Changes are still needed, but improvements in commodities are evident.

USDA has established a National Food Service Management Institute at the University of Mississippi, which was authorized by the Child Nutrition and WIC Reauthorization Act of 1989. The institute aims to "build the future through child nutrition" and designs and conducts activities to improve the operation and quality of child nutrition programs. The institute, which is a national resource center for all child nutrition programs, has three divisions:

1. *Development and Applied Research:* conducts research designed to provide appropriate management tools that ensure cost effectiveness, quality, nutritious food service, and employee performance standards.
2. *Education and Training:* designs and develops competency-based training modules and materials for child nutrition program employees and provides technical assistance.
3. *Technology Transfer:* acts as a clearinghouse and information center for all areas of relevant research and information and collects, evaluates, and disseminates materials.

Info Line

The National Food Service Management Institute is authorized by the US Congress and administered by the US Department of Agriculture. For information write to P.O. Drawer 188, University, MS 38677-0188. Telephone: (601) 232-7658 or 1-800-321-3054.

Participation in Professional Organizations

The American School Food Service Association (ASFSA) and state chapters support a national membership of more than 65,000. ASFSA is the mouthpiece for child nutrition professionals and has active lobbying efforts in Congress. Legislative efforts are directed toward universal feeding and challenging block grants to fund the National School Lunch Program, the School Breakfast Program, and the Summer Food Service Program.

The American Dietetic Association (ADA) and the School Food Services Dietetic Practice Group are major professional organizations of registered dietitians (RDs) employed in school systems. The ADA collaborates with other national organizations to produce nutrition education materials for school-age children. In addition, many food companies employ RDs who manage complete health care lines and specialty lines for schools (e.g., SE Rycoff, Arrow-Sysco, and ConAgra). Child nutrition directors and managers work directly with the food companies to achieve products lower in fat, sodium, and sugar for their menus.

The Association of State School Nutrition Directors and Supervisors meets annually to update programs on USDA guidelines and pending federal legislation affecting school meals, to discuss innovations, and to provide continuing education. These directors oversee all USDA food programs in schools and day care facilities in their respective states.

GUIDELINES FOR ADOLESCENT PREVENTIVE SERVICES

A major area of concern is the current adolescent morbidity and mortality. This toll on young lives creates a health crisis for today's youths. Problems include unplanned pregnancy, sexually transmitted disease including human immunodeficiency virus (HIV), alcohol and drug abuse, and eating disorders.[140] Adolescence is a period of experimentation and risk taking. The resulting behaviors of youths threaten their current health and may have long-term consequences on their adult functioning. In addition, youths should be screened for substance abuse and certain behavioral and biomedical conditions. Vaccinations to protect youths from infectious diseases such as measles and rubella are also an important part of primary care.

The American Medical Association (AMA) has received funding to focus on the adolescent population through the "Healthier Youth 2000 Project." This project is being implemented in conjunction with the AMA National Coalition on Adolescent Health. It includes the publication of a multidisciplinary, modular newsletter, *Target 2000*, and the creation of the National Adolescent Health Promotion Network (NAHPNet). NAHPNet is comprised of several thousand individuals who serve as resources for information on adolescent health and as consultants to community efforts.

The AMA has developed the Guidelines for Adolescent Preventive Services (GAPS), a comprehensive set of recommendations for community organizations that can serve as the potential content of preventive health services. These recommendations address problems common to youths of all ethnic groups (e.g., suicide, unplanned pregnancy, sexually transmitted disease), and they are directed to primary and secondary prevention. Because schools and community organizations have increased health education programs, and primary care physicians and other health care providers including community nutrition professionals are bringing preventive services into their clinical practice, GAPS provides a blueprint for the delivery of services.[130]

Info Line

Healthy Youth 2000 is a part of the "Healthier Youth 2000 Project" of the American Medical Association. The cornerstone of this initiative is *Healthy People 2000: The National Health Promotion and Disease Prevention Objectives*. For further information contact the American Medical Association, Department of Adolescent Health, 515 N State Street, Chicago, IL 60610, 312-464-5570.

The GAPS guidelines emphasize health guidance and prevention of behavioral and emotional disorders. Health guidance includes health education, health counseling, and anticipatory guidance. Because adolescence is a time of experimentation and risk taking, the resulting behaviors may threaten current health or may have long-term consequences. Four types of services are identified: health care delivery, health guidance, screening for specific conditions, and immunizations for the primary prevention of selected infectious disease.[130]

The health conditions addressed in these four services are listed in Exhibit 8–3. Developing healthy eating patterns is the health promotion focus to prevent high blood cholesterol, alcohol abuse, and depression. In addition, a series of annual health visits between the ages of 11 and 21 years are recommended for all youths. Adolescents who have initiated health-risk behaviors can be identified. If they are at early stages of physical or emotional disorders, opportunities for communication and support can be formed. The recommended frequency of specific GAPS preventive services is outlined in Exhibit 8–4. These services can reinforce health promotion messages for adolescents and their parents.

Rapid behavioral changes occur during adolescence. Frequent visits that screen youth for health risk behaviors can provide health guidance and ensure that accurate information is recorded. Because the clients are adolescents, GAPS recommend that all information given by adolescents during the medical visit should remain confidential to build a medical bond and promote future contact.

In 1993, the Public Health Service conducted a cross-sectional review of progress on *Healthy People 2000* objectives related to adolescents and young adults. Sixty objectives target youths, with 11 objectives pertaining to tobacco, alcohol, and other drugs. Some reductions in tobacco and substance abuse have occurred among young people. Progress in meeting objectives for tobacco, alcohol, and other drugs is listed in Table 8–5.

The lack of adequate access to appropriate health services and the selective approach of certain existing programs are barriers to quality

Exhibit 8–3   Health Conditions Addressed in the Guidelines for Adolescent Preventive Services

---

HEALTH PROMOTION

To increase parents' ability to respond to the health needs of their adolescents:
- for healthy psychosexual adjustment

To adjust to puberty and adolescence:
- for safety and injury prevention
- for physical fitness
- for healthy eating patterns

DISEASE PREVENTION

To prevent eating disorders and obesity
To prevent the negative health consequences of sexual behaviors
To prevent hypertension
To prevent hyperlipidemia
To prevent the use of tobacco products
To prevent the use and abuse of alcohol and other drugs
To prevent severe or recurrent depression and suicide
To prevent physical, sexual, and emotional abuse
To prevent learning problems
To prevent infectious diseases

Source: Adapted from American Medical Association. *Guidelines for Adolescent Preventive Services.* Chicago, IL. 1992, page 3.

---

health care for adolescents and young adults. Action items for achieving the objectives for adolescents and young adults from 1995 to 2000 include[141]:

- reevaluating the targets and strategies for sexual activity
- identifying and supporting catalyst agencies to help move strategies from a categorical to a broader life view
- assessing the impact and periodicity for clinical preventive services proposed for adolescents

PRIMARY PREVENTION–CALIFORNIA ADOLESCENT NUTRITION AND FITNESS PROGRAM

The California Adolescent Nutrition and Fitness Program (CANFit) provides $5,000 to $50,000 grants for nutrition education and fitness intervention. This initiative is the first of its kind to fund outreach directly to community-based organizations serving 10-to-14-year-old African-American, Latino, Asian, and American Indian Youths.[142]

Eight planning grants and four intervention grants totaling $265,000 were funded by the CANFit administrative board in 1994. Planning grants focus on assessment of needs, development of specific action plans, and defining the intrastructure to implement those plans. Intervention grants implement specific programs within community-based organizations among high-risk youths. The content of the grants reflect youth-driven programs, capacity-building activities for the member organizations, and process and impact evaluations. A brief description of the CANFit planning and intervention grants funded initially is found in Appendix 8–C.[142]

To further its mission to seed nutrition and fitness programs for the youth in California, CANFit awards about ten $1,000 scholarships annually to minority college students majoring in nutrition or physical education at California colleges and universities. Applicants submit competitive essays entitled, "The Three Most Important Nutrition or Fitness Challenges Facing California's Adolescents . . . and Here's What I Would Do." The CANFit program is administered by an administrative board composed of volunteers who are professionals in education, business, medicine, law, health, education, and nutrition. The program provides a unique model that could be replicated in other states and communities.

NATIONAL INSTITUTES OF HEALTH INTERVENTIONS

Several major intervention studies have been funded by the National Institutes of Health to alter the high-risk status of certain children. Results may have implications for future health policy and medical practice. A brief description of these studies follows.[143]

Dietary Intervention Study in Children

This study was initiated in December 1986 to assess the feasibility, acceptability, efficacy, and

Exhibit 8-4   Recommendations Developed for Guidelines for Adolescent Preventive Services (GAPS)

1. From age 11 to 21, all adolescents should have an annual preventive services visit.
2. Preventive services should be age and developmentally appropriate, and should be sensitive to individual and sociocultural differences.
3. Physicians should establish office policies regarding confidential care for adolescents and how parents will be involved in that care. These policies should be made clear to adolescents and their parents.
4. Parents or other adult caregivers should receive health guidance at least once during their child's early adolescence, once during middle adolescence and, preferably, once during late adolescence.
5. All adolescents should receive health guidance annually to promote a better understanding of their physical growth, psychosocial and psychosexual development, and the importance of becoming actively involved in decisions regarding their health care.
6. All adolescents should receive health guidance annually to promote the reduction of injuries.
7. All adolescents should receive health guidance annually about dietary habits, including the benefits of a healthy eating pattern, and ways to achieve it and safe weight management also.
8. All adolescents should receive health guidance annually about the benefits of exercise and should be encouraged to engage in safe exercise on a regular basis.
9. All adolescents should receive health guidance annually regarding responsible sexual behaviors, including abstinence. Latex condoms to prevent STDs, including HIV infection, and appropriate methods of birth control should be made available, as should instructions on how to use them effectively.
10. All adolescents should receive health guidance annually to promote avoidance of tobacco, alcohol, and other abusable substances, and anabolic steroids.
11. All adolescents should be screened annually for hypertension according to the protocol developed by the National Heart, Lung, and Blood Institute Second Task Force on Blood Pressure Control in Children.
12. Selected adolescents should be screened to determine their risk of developing hyperlipidemia and adult coronary heart disease, following the protocol developed by the Expert Panel on Blood Cholesterol Levels in Children and Adolescents.
13. All adolescents should be screened annually for eating disorders and obesity by determining weight and stature, and asking about body image and dieting patterns.
14. All adolescents should be asked annually about their use of tobacco products including cigarettes and smokeless tobacco.
15. All adolescents should be asked annually about their use of alcohol and other abusable substances, and about their use of over-the-counter or prescription drugs for nonmedical purposes, including anabolic steroids.
16. All adolescents should be asked annually about involvement in sexual behaviors that may result in unintended pregnancy and STDs, including HIV infection.
17. Sexually active adolescents should be screened for STDs.
18. Adolescents at risk of HIV infection should be offered confidential HIV screening with the ELISA and confirmatory test.
19. Female adolescents who are sexually active or any female 18 or older should be screened annually for cervical cancer by use of a Pap test.
20. All adolescents should be asked annually about behaviors or emotions that indicate recurrent or severe depression or risk of suicide.
21. All adolescents should be asked annually about a history of emotional, physical, and sexual abuse.
22. All adolescents should be asked annually about learning or school problems.
23. Adolescents should receive a tuberculin skin test if they have been exposed to active tuberculosis, have lived in a homeless shelter, have been incarcerated, have lived in or come from an area with a high prevalence of tuberculosis, or currently work in a health care setting.
24. All adolescents should receive prophylactic immunizations according to the guidelines established by the federally convened Advisory Committee on Immunization Practices.

Source: Adapted from American Medical Association. *Guidelines for Adolescent Preventive Services.* Chicago, IL. 1992, pages 1–9.

safety of dietary intervention in children and adolescents with elevated low-density lipoprotein (LDL) cholesterol levels. The study population comprises children of both genders with elevated LDL cholesterol levels, ages 8 to 10 at entry, and includes at least 45% girls.

Participants are either in a control or a special-care group and receive intensive dietary intervention. If dietary modification is to become an acceptable public health or primary prevention strategy for children, this study must confirm that dietary modification has no detrimen-

Table 8–5 Progress Report on Health Objectives for Adolescents

Objective		1987 Baseline	1991	1992	Year 2000 Target
3.5	Reduce initiation of smoking by children and youths so no more than 15% are regular smokers by age 20	30%	24%	—	15%
3.5a	Lower socioeconomic status youth	40%	31%	—	18%
3.9	Reduce smokeless tobacco use by males aged 12 through 24				
	Males aged 12–17	6.6%	5.3%	—	4%
	Males aged 18–24	8.9%	9.9%	—	4%
3.9a	American Indian/Alaskan native youths	18–64%	19.7%	—	10%
4.1b	Reduce deaths among youths aged 15–24 caused by alcohol-related motor vehicle crashes	21.5	—	14.1	18.0
4.5	Increase by at least 1 year the average age of first use of:				
	Cigarettes	11.6	—	11.5	12.6
	Alcohol	13.1	—	12.6	14.1
	Marijuana	13.4	—	13.5	14.4
4.6	Reduce substance use in the last month				
	Alcohol: 12–17 yr-olds	25.2%	—	15.7%	12.6%
	18–20 yr-olds	57.9%	—	50.3%	29.0%
	Marijuana: 12–17 yr-olds	6.4%	—	4.0%	3.2%
	18–25 yr-olds	15.5%	—	11.0%	7.8%
	Cocaine: 12–17 yr-olds	1.1%	—	0.3%	0.6%
	18–25 yr-olds	4.5%	—	1.8%	2.3%
4.7	Reduce heavy drinking of alcoholic beverages in past two weeks among:				
	High school seniors	33%	—	27.9%	28%
	College students	41.7%	—	41.4%	32%

Source: Adapted from American Medical Association. *Target 2000*, Fall 1994, page 6.

tal effects on children's growth. At the end of six months of intervention, the percentage of energy from total fat and saturated fat was reduced by 5.1% ($p = 0.004$) and 2.9% ($p < 0.001$).[144] The children will potentially be followed until the year 2000.

NHLBI Growth and Health Study

The National Heart, Lung, and Blood Institute Growth and Health Study began in September 1985 to assess the occurrence of obesity in young women, factors that could predict and correlate with the transition to obesity, and the association of obesity with various risk fac-

tors for heart disease. The study population includes both African-American and white girls, 9 to 10 years old at entry. The group is 51% African American. Dietary and physical activity, socioeconomic status, and lifestyle variables are assessed.

Child and Adolescent Trial of Cardiovascular Health

This trial began in 1987 to measure and to compare the effects of school-based interventions to promote lifelong behavior among elementary school children and adolescents to reduce cardiovascular risk. About 12,000 girls and boys in the third, fourth, and fifth grades, and from all major US ethnic groups are involved. Total serum cholesterol is the primary outcome measure. Interventions include classroom curricula, family-focused dietary modifications, physical activity, and tobacco use.

Coronary Artery Risk Development in Young Adults

This is a prospective observational study focusing on precursors and determinants of risk factors including lifestyle for heart disease. These factors will be studied over time in a population of African-American and white women and men, 18 to 30 years old. The group is 55% women and 52% African American.

Framingham Heart and Offspring Study

This study has been identified as the landmark longitudinal study of risk factors associated with the development of cardiovascular disease. The Framingham Study began in 1948 and provides surveillance of adults in Framingham, Massachusetts. The Framingham Offspring Study began in 1971 with 5,135 participants, of which 3,555 were offspring of the original cohort. Endpoints for both studies are coronary heart disease, stroke, hypertension, congestive heart failure, and peripheral arterial disease.

The most well-known finding from the Framingham Study was that high blood cholesterol, high blood pressure, and cigarette smoking were identified as the three major risk factors for heart disease. In addition, smoking was listed as a significant independent variable contributing to the risk of stroke, and specifically brain infarction. Obesity was identified as a major independent risk factor.

The Framingham Offspring Study reports that offspring have slightly lower blood cholesterol and blood pressure levels than their parents. Children of parents with hypertension have higher blood pressures than other children. Smoking among men has decreased to half that of their fathers, but women smoke more than

their mothers. Heart disease mortality has declined, but the reason remains unclear.

PRESIDENT'S COUNCIL ON PHYSICAL FITNESS AND SPORT

In 1995, US President Bill Clinton appointed a diverse group of 15 physical fitness, sports, health, and community leaders to serve on the President's Council on Physical Fitness and Sport. The current appointees are from the fields of medicine, professional and amateur sports, physical education, and training and advocacy for physically disabled persons. The council supports activities throughout the United States to energize Americans to become more physically active, healthier, and more physically fit.[145]

School-age youths can participate in the President's Council annually via the physical education department at their schools. Planned activities commonly comprise routine evaluation of the fitness level of youths. Standards are set and awards are given for students who meet and/or exceed the criteria for several measures.

HEALTHY PEOPLE 2000 ACTIONS

Nutrition-related objectives are outlined for school-age children in Exhibit 8-5. Obesity and dental caries are major concerns. Alcoholic beverage consumption, high-fat intakes, and low calcium and complex carbohydrate intakes are the focus of specific directives. Community nutrition professionals have a new frontier and opportunity for their services. Attention to adolescent health has gained prominence during the 1990s. Nutrition services need to be integrated and clearly defined to effect positive change in the lives of the newest generation of young adults.

Strategies to achieve nutritionally healthy and fit youths by the year 2000 include embellishing efforts for comprehensive school health education for all children;[146-148] enhancing complementary physical activity and child nutrition programs at schools; assessing the readiness of students and faculties for change before programs are

Exhibit 8-5 *Healthy People 2000* Nutrition Objectives for School-Age Children

2.3   Reduce overweight to a prevalence of no more than 20% among people aged 20 and older and no more than 15% among adolescents aged 12 through 29. (Baseline: 26% for people aged 20 through 74 in 1976–80, 24% for men and 27% for women; 15 percent for adolescents aged 12 through 19 in 1976–80.)

   Note: For people aged 20 and older, overweight is defined as body mass index (BMI) equal to or greater than 27.8 for men and 27.3 for women. BMI is calculated by dividing weight in kilograms by the square of height in meters. The cut points used to define overweight approximate the 120% of desirable body weight definition used in the 1990 objectives.

2.5   To reduce dietary fat intake to an average of 30% of calories or less and average saturated fat intake to less than 10% of calories among people aged 2 and older.

2.6   To increase complex carbohydrate and fiber-containing foods in the diets of adults to 5 or more daily servings for vegetables (including legumes) and fruits, and to 6 or more daily servings for grain products.

2.7   To increase to at least 50% the proportion of overweight people age 12 and older who have adopted sound dietary practices combined with regular physical activity to attain an appropriate body weight.

2.8   Increase calcium intake so at least 50% of youth aged 12 through 24 and 50% of pregnant and lactating women consume three or more servings daily of foods rich in calcium, and at least 50% of people aged 25 and older consume two or more servings daily. (Baseline: 7% of women and 14% of men aged 19 through 24 and 24% of pregnant and lactating women consumed three or more servings, and 15% of women and 23% of men aged 25 through 50 consumed two or more servings in 1985–86.)

2.17   Increase to at least 90% the proportion of school lunch and breakfast services and child care food services with menus that are consistent with the nutrition principles in the *Dietary Guidelines for Americans*. (Baseline data available in 1993.)

2.19   Increase to at least 75% the proportion of the nation's schools that provide nutrition education from preschool through 12th grade, preferably as part of quality school health education. (Baseline data available in 1991.)

4.1b   Reduce deaths among people aged 15 through 24 caused by alcohol-related motor vehicle crashes to no more than 18 per 100,000. (Baseline: 21.5 per 100,000 in 1987.)

4.5   Increase by at least 1 year the average age of first use of cigarettes, alcohol, and marijuana by adolescents aged 12 through 17. (Baseline: Age 11.6 for cigarettes, age 13.1 for alcohol, and age 13.4 for marijuana in 1988.)

4.6   Reduce the proportion of young people who have used alcohol, marijuana, and cocaine in the past month, as follows:

Substance/Age	1988 Baseline	2000 Target
Alcohol/aged 12–17	25.2%	12.6%
Alcohol/aged 18–20	57.9%	29.0%
Marijuana/aged 12–17	6.4%	3.2%
Marijuana/aged 18–25	15.5%	7.8%
Cocaine/aged 12–17	1.1%	0.6%
Cocaine/aged 18–25	4.5%	2.3%

4.7   Reduce the proportion of high school seniors and college students engaging in recent occasions of heavy drinking of alcoholic beverages to no more than 28% of high school seniors and 32% of college students. (Baseline: 33% of high school seniors and 41.7% of college students in 1989.)

   Note: Recent heavy drinking is defined as having 5 or more drinks on one occasion in the previous 2-week period as monitored by self-reports.

4.8   Reduce alcohol consumption by people aged 14 and older to an annual average of no more than 2 gallons of ethanol per person. (Baseline: 2.54 gallons of ethanol in 1987.)

4.9   Increase the proportion of high school seniors who perceive social disapproval associated with the heavy use of alcohol, occasional use of marijuana, and experimentation with cocaine, as follows:

continues

Exhibit 8-5 continued

Behavior	1989 Baseline	2000 Target
Heavy use of alcohol	56.4%	70%
Occasional use of marijuana	71.1%	85%
Trying cocaine once or twice	88.9%	95%

> *Note:* Heavy drinking is defined as having 5 or more drinks once or twice each weekend.

4.10   Increase the proportion of high school seniors who associate risk of physical or psychological harm with the heavy use of alcohol, regular use of marijuana, and experimentation with cocaine, as follows:

Behavior	1989 Baseline	2000 Target
Heavy use of alcohol	44.0%	70%
Regular use of marijuana	77.5%	90%
Trying cocaine once or twice	54.9%	80%

> *Note:* Heavy drinking is defined as having 5 or more drinks once or twice each weekend.

4.11   Reduce to no more than 3% the proportion of male high school seniors who use anabolic steroids. (Baseline: 4.7% in 1989.)

4.13   Provide to children in all school districts and private schools, primary and secondary school educational programs on alcohol and other drugs, preferably as part of quality school health education. (Baseline: 63% provided some instruction, 39% provided counseling, and 23% referred students for clinical assessments in 1987.)

4.16   Increase to 50 the number of states that have enacted and enforce policies, beyond those in existence in 1989, to reduce access to alcoholic beverages by minors.

> *Note:* Policies to reduce access to alcoholic beverages by minors may include those that address restriction of the sale of alcoholic beverages at recreational and entertainment events at which youth make up a majority of participants/consumers, product pricing, penalties and license-revocation for sale of alcoholic beverages to minors, and other approaches designed to discourage and restrict purchase of alcoholic beverages by minors.

4.17   Increase to at least 20 the number of states that have enacted statutes to restrict promotion of alcoholic beverages that is focused principally on young audiences. (Baseline data available in 1992.)

8.4   Increase to at least 75% the proportion of the nation's elementary and secondary schools that provide planned and sequential kindergarten through 12th grade quality school health education. (Baseline data available in 1991.)

8.9   Increase to at least 75% the proportion of people aged 10 and older who have discussed issues related to nutrition, physical activity, sexual behavior, tobacco, alcohol, other drugs, or safety with family members on at least one occasion during the preceding month. (Baseline data available in 1991.)

> *Note:* This objective, which supports family communication on a range of vital personal health issues, will be tracked using the National Health Interview Survey, a continuing, voluntary, national sample survey of adults who report on household characteristics including such items as illnesses, injuries, use of health services, and demographic characteristics.

13.1   Reduce dental caries (cavities) so that the proportion of children with one or more caries (in permanent or primary teeth) is no more than 35% among children aged 6 through 8 and no more than 60% among adolescents aged 15. (Baseline: 53% of children aged 6 through 8 in 1986–87; 78% of adolescents aged 15 in 1986–87.)

continues

Exhibit 8–5 continued

Special Population Targets

Dental Caries Prevalence		1986–87 Baseline	2000 Target
13.1a	Children aged 6–8 whose parents have less than high school education	70%	45%
13.1b	American Indian/Alaska Native children aged 6–8	92%[*] 52%[**]	45%
13.1c	Black children aged 6–8	61%	40%
13.1d	American Indian/Alaska Native adolescents aged 15	93%[**]	70%

[*]In primary teeth in 1983–84.
[**]In permanent teeth in 1983–84.

13.2   Reduce untreated dental caries so that the proportion of children with untreated caries (in permanent or primary teeth) is no more than 20% among children aged 6 through 8 and no more than 15% among adolescents aged 15. (Baseline: 27% of children aged 6–8 in 1986; 23% of adolescents aged 15 in 1986–87.)

Special Population Targets

Untreated Dental Caries among Children		1986–87 Baseline	2000 Target
13.2a	Children aged 6–8 whose parents have less than high school education	43%	30%
13.2b	American Indian/Alaska Native children aged 6–8	64%[*]	35%
13.2c	Black children aged 6–8	38%	25%
13.2d	Hispanic children aged 6–8	36%[**]	25%

[*]1983–84 baseline.
[**]1982–84 baseline.

Note: The number of servings of foods rich in calcium is based on milk and milk products. A serving is considered to be 1 cup of skim milk or its equivalent in calcium (302 mg). The number of servings in this objective will generally provide approximately three-fourths of the 1989 Recommended Dietary Allowance (RDA) of calcium. The RDA is 1200 mg for people age 12 through 24, 800 mg for people age 25 and older, and 1200 mg for pregnant and lactating women.

Source: Reprinted with permission from *Healthy People 2000: National Health Promotion and Disease Prevention Objectives.* Washington, DC: US Department of Health and Human Services; 1991. DHHS (PHS) publication 91-50212.

planned and implemented; developing youth-driven programs; and incorporating the family, the various living and eating environments of adolescents, and the community.[149]

The National Commission on the Role of the School and the Community in Improving Adolescent Health has called the nation to action to address the problems of youth. In *CODE BLUE:* *Uniting for Healthier Youth*, the commission states that the situation is an emergency and that life-threatening events are occurring in the lives of US youths. These events threaten the very survival and healthy functioning of adolescents, the future of the children birthed by adolescents, and the viability and competitiveness of the American work force in general. All sectors of society are involved, and their dedication is needed to redirect the future of this generation.[149]

REFERENCES

1. Frank GC. Nutrition issues. In: *The Comprehensive School Health Challenge*. Santa Cruz, Calif: ETR Assoc; 1994:373–411.

2. Frank GC. Assessing diets of children: Environmental influences on dietary data collection methods with children. *Am J Clin Nutr*. Special Issue: First International Conference on Dietary Assessment Methods. 1994;59(Suppl.): 207s–211s.

3. US Department of Agriculture, Human Nutrition Information Service. Food and nutrient intakes by individuals in the United States, one day, 1987–88. Nationwide Food Consumption Survey 1987–88, Report No. 87-I-1. Unpublished manuscript.

4. Berenson GS, McMahan CA, Voors AW, et al. *Cardiovascular Risk Factors in Children—The Early Natural History of Atherosclerosis and Essential Hypertension*. New York, NY: Oxford University Press; 1980.

5. Food Research and Action Center. *Community Childhood Hunger Identification Project*. Washington, DC: Food Research and Action Center; 1991.

6. Food and Nutrition Board, National Academy of Sciences, National Research Council. *Recommended Dietary Allowances*. 10th ed. Washington, DC: National Academy Press; 1989.

7. US Department of Agriculture. *Menu Planning Guide for School Food Service*. Washington, DC: US Department of Agriculture; 1983. Program aid 1260.

8. Frank GC, Berenson GS, Schilling PE, et al. Adapting the 24-hour dietary recall for epidemiologic studies of school children. *J Am Diet Assoc*. 1977;71:26–31.

9. Frank GC. Dietary studies of infants and children. In: *Cardiovascular Risk Factors in Children—The Early Natural History of Atherosclerosis and Essential Hypertension*. New York, NY: Oxford University Press; 1980:289–307.

10. Wotecki CE. Nutrition in childhood and adolescence—Parts 1 and 2. *Contemporary Nutr*. 1992;17(2):1–2.

11. Chan GM. Dietary calcium and bone mineral status of children and adolescents. *Am J Dis Children*. 1991;145: 631–634.

12. Johnson AA. Iron deficiency: Pediatric epidemiology. In: Enwonuw C, ed. *Functional Significance of Iron Deficiency. Annual Nutrition Workshop Series, Volume III*. Nashville, Tenn: Meharry Medical College; 1990; 57–65.

13. Public Law 79-396, 60 Stat 231. 1946.

14. Public Law 89-642, 80 Stat. 1966.

15. Public Law 95-166, 91 Stat 1325, 95th Congress. 1977.

16. Frank GC, Farris RP, Cresanta JL, et al. Dietary intake as a determinant of cardiovascular risk factor variables: Observations in a pediatric population. In: Berenson GS, ed. *Causation of Cardiovascular Risk Factors in Children: Perspectives on Causation of Cardiovascular Risk in Early Life*. New York, NY: Raven Press; 1986:254–291.

17. Parcel GS, Simmons-Morton BG, O'Hara NM, et al. School promotion of healthful diet and exercise behavior: An integration of organizational change and social learning theory interventions. *J School Health*. 1987;57:150–156.

18. Burghardt J, Devaney B. *The School Nutrition Dietary Assessment Study—Summary of Findings*. Princeton, NJ: Mathematica Policy Research, Inc; 1993:3–24.

19. Kirk MC, Gillespie AH. Factors affecting food choices of working mothers with young families. *J Nutr Ed*. 1990; 22:161–168.

20. National Center for Nutrition and Dietetics and International Food Information Council. *Where Do Kids Get Nutrition Information?* Chicago, Ill: American Dietetic Association; 1991.

21. National Center for Nutrition and Dietetics and International Food Information Council. *Kids at the Table: Who's Placing the Orders?* Chicago, Ill: American Dietetic Association; 1991.

22. Bidgood BA, Cameron G. Meal/snack missing and dietary adequacy of primary school children. *J Canad Diet Assoc*. 1992;53:164–168.

23. Lindeman AK, Clancy KL. Assessment of breakfast habits and social/emotional behavior of elementary schoolchildren. *J Nutr Ed*. 1990;22:226–231.

24. Resnicow K. The relationship between breakfast habits and plasma cholesterol levels in schoolchildren. *J School Health*. 1991;61:81–85.

25. Frank GC, Zive M, Nelson J, et al. Fat and cholesterol avoidance among Mexican American and Anglo preschool children and parents. *J Am Diet Assoc*. 1991;91:954–961.

26. Murphy SP, Castillo RO, Martorell R, et al. An evaluation of food group intakes by Mexican-American children. *J Am Diet Assoc*. 1990;90:388–393.

27. Palmer R, Johnson A. Los Angeles County Unified School District Data. University of Southern California. 1991.

28. Sampson H, Buckley R, Matcalf D. Food allergy. *JAMA* 1987;258:2886–2903.

29. May CD. Food allergy: Perspective, principles, practical management. *Nutr Today*. 1980;Nov-Dec:28–31.

30. American Psychiatric Association. *Diagnostic and Statistical Manual (DSM III)*. 3rd ed. Washington, DC: American Psychiatric Association; 1980.

31. American Psychiatric Association. *Diagnostic and Statistical Manual (DSM IV)*. 4th ed. Washington, DC: American Psychiatric Association; 1994.

32. American School Health Association. *The National Adolescent Student Health Survey: A Report on the Health of American's Youth.* Kent, Ohio: American School Health Association; 1989.

33. Frank GC, Deeds S, Cox S, et al. Clusters count—Multirisk taking behaviors of adolescents. Presented at the annual meeting of the American Alliance for Health, Physical Education, Recreation and Dance; April 3-7, 1991; San Francisco, Calif.

34. US Department of Health and Human Services. Office of Disease Prevention and Health Promotion. *Healthy People 2000.* Washington, DC: US Department of Health and Human Services; 1991.

35. Bachman JG, Wallace JM, O'Malley PM, et al. Racial/ethnic differences in smoking, drinking, and illicit drug use among American High school seniors, 1976-89. *Am J Public Health* 1991;81:372-377.

36. Centers for Disease Control and Prevention. Alcohol and other drug use among high school students—United States. *JAMA.* 1991;266:3266-3267.

37. Sarvela PD, Pape DJ, Odulana J, et al. Drinking, drug use, and driving among rural midwestern youth. *J School Health.* 1990;60:215-219.

38. Arbeit ML, Nicklas TA, Frank GC, et al. Caffeine intakes of children from a biracial population: The Bogalusa Heart Study. *J Am Diet Assoc.* 1988;88:466-470.

39. Charney E, Goodman HC, McBride M, et al. Childhood antecedents of adult obesity—Do chubby infants become obese adults? *N Engl J Med.* 1976;295:6-9.

40. Garn, SM, LaVelle M. Two decade follow-up of fatness in early childhood. *Am J Dis Children.* 1985;139:181-185.

41. Kolata G. Obese children: A growing problem. *Science.* 1986;232:20-21.

42. Ross JG, Gilbert GG. The national children and youth fitness study: A summary of findings. *J Phys Ed Rec and Dance.* 1985;56:45-50.

43. US Centers for Disease Control and Prevention. *MMWR.* 1992;41:33-35.

44. Pate RR, Dowda M, Ross G. Associations between physical activity and physical fitness in American children. *Am J Dis Children.* 1990;144:1123-1129.

45. US Department of Health and Human Services. *President's Council on Physical Fitness and Sports Youth Fitness Survey.* Washington, DC: US Government Printing Office; 1986.

46. Suter E, Hawes MR. Relationship of physical activity, body fat, diet, and blood lipid profile in youths 10-15 years old. *Med Sci Sports Exercise.* 1993;25:748-754.

47. Pate RR. Physical activity in children and youth: Relationship to obesity. *Contemporary Nutr.* 1993;18(2):1-2.

48. Sasaki J, Shindo M, Tanaka H, et al. A longterm aerobic exercise program decreases the obesity index and increases the high density lipoprotein cholesterol concentration in obese children. *Int J Obes.* 1987;11:339-345.

49. Epstein LH, Valoski A, Wing RR, et al. Ten year followup of behavioral, family-based treatment for obese children. *JAMA.* 1990;264:2519-2523.

50. Muecke L, Morton-Simons B, Huang IW, et al. Is childhood obesity associated with high-fat foods and low physical activity? *J School Health.* 1992;62:19-23.

51. Stephen A, Wald N. Trends in individual consumption of dietary fat in the United States, 1920-1984. *Am J Clin Nutr.* 1990;52:457-469.

52. Schlicker SA, Borra ST, Regan C. The weight and fitness status of US children. *Nutr Rev.* 1994;52(1):11-17.

53. Tucker LA, Bagwell M. Television viewing and obesity in adult females. *Am J Public Health.* 1991;81:908-911.

54. Gortmaker SL. Increasing pediatric obesity in the US. *Am J Dis Children.* 1987;141:535-541.

55. Story M, Faulkner P. The prime time diet: A content analysis of eating behavior and food messages in television program content and commercials. *Am J Public Health.* 1990;80:738-740.

56. Dietz WH Jr, Gortmaker SL. Do we fatten our children at the television set? Obesity and television viewing in children and adolescents. *Pediatrics.* 1985;75:807-812.

57. Tiwary CM, Holgiun A. Prevalence of obesity among children of military dependents at two major medical centers. *Am J Public Health.* 1992;82:354-357.

58. Hsu LK. Clinical features. In: *Eating Disorders.* New York, NY: Guilford Press; 1990:22-24.

59. Sloan R. Developing an awareness of eating disorders: Identifying the high-risk client. *On the Cutting Edge.* 1994;15(6):21-22.

60. Halmi HK, ed. *The Psychology and Treatment of Anorexia Nervosa and Bulimia Nervosa.* Washington, DC: American Psychiatric Press; 1992.

61. Hsu LK. Epidemiology. In: *Eating Disorders.* New York, NY: Guilford Press; 1990:71.

62. Druss RG, Silverman JA. Body image and perfectionism of ballerinas. *Gen Hosp Psychiatry.* 1979;2:115-121.

63. Centers for Disease Control and Prevention. Body weight perceptions and selected weight-management goals and practices of high school students—United States. *JAMA.* 1991;266:2811-2812.

64. Shisslak CM, Crago M, Neal ME. Prevention of eating disorders among adolescents. *Am J Health Promotion.* 1990;5:100-106.

65. Larson B. Relationship of family communication patterns to eating disorders inventory scores in adolescent girls. *J Am Diet Assoc.* 1991;91:1065-1067.

66. Balentine M, Stitt K, Bonner J, et al. Self-reported eating disorders of black, low-income adolescents: Behavior, body weight perceptions, and methods of dieting. *J School Health* 1991;61:392-396.

67. Desmond SM, Price JH, Hallinan C, et al. Black and white adolescents' perceptions of their weight. *J School Health* 1989;59:353-358.

68. Dodd JM, Bessinger C. Societal issues and nutrition. ADA Research Conference Proceedings. *J Am Diet Assoc.* 1993;77-85.

69. Mitchell JE, Eckert ED. Scope and significance of eating disorders. *J Consult Clin Psychol.* 1987;55:628-634.

70. American Dietetic Association. Position of the ADA: Nutrition intervention in the treatment of anorexia nervosa, bulimia nervosa, and binge eating. *J Am Diet Assoc.* 1994;94:902-907.

71. Rorty M, Yager J, Rossotto E. Why and how do women recover from bulimia nervosa? The subjective appraisals of 40 women recovered for a year or more. *Int J Eating Disorders.* 1993;14:249-260.

72. Vandereycken W, Depreitere L, Probst M. Body-oriented therapy for anorexia nervosa patients. *Am J Psychotherapy.* 1987;41:252-259.

73. Herzog DB, Sacks NR, Keller MB, et al. Patterns and predictors of recovery in anorexia nervosa and bulimia nervosa. *J Am Academy of Child Adolescent Psychiatry.* 1993;32:835 841.

74. Reiff DW, Reiff KKL. *Eating Disorders—Nutrition Therapy in the Recovery Process.* Gaithersburg, Md: Aspen Publishers, Inc; 1992.

75. Story M, Heald F, Dwyer J. Adolescent nutrition: Trends and critical issues for the 1990s. In: Sharbaugh CO, ed. *Call to Action: Better Nutrition for Mothers, Children, and Families.* Washington, DC: National Center for Education in Maternal and Child Health; 1991:169-189.

76. Ventura SJ, Taffel SM, Mosher WD. *Monthly Vital Statistics Report. Trends in Pregnancies and Pregnancy Rates: Estimates for the United States, 1980-1992.* US Department of Health and Human Services. 1995;43:11(S).

77. Story M. Nutrient needs during adolescence and pregnancy. In: Story M, ed. *Nutrition Management of the Pregnant Adolescent: A Practical Reference Guide.* Washington, DC: National Clearinghouse; 1990:21-28.

78. Story M. Eating behaviors and nutritional implications. In: Story M, ed. *Nutrition Management of the Pregnant Adolescent: A Practical Reference Guide.* Washington, DC: National Clearinghouse; 1990:29-35.

79. Newman WP III, Freedman DS, Voors AW, et al. Relation of serum lipoprotein levels and systolic blood pressure to early atherosclerosis: The Bogalusa Heart Study. *N Engl J Med.* 1986;314:138-144.

80. Freedman DS, Newman WP III, Tracy RE, et al. Black-white differences in aortic fatty streaks in adolescence and early adulthood: The Bogalusa Heart Study. *Circulation.* 1988;77:856-864.

81. Wissler RW, Robertson AL, Cornhill JF, et al. Relationship of atherosclerosis in young men to serum lipoprotein cholesterol concentrations and smoking. *JAMA.* 1990;264:3018-3024.

82. Frerichs RR, Webber LS, Voors AW, et al. Cardiovascular disease risk factor variables in children at two successive years—The Bogalusa Heart Study. *J Chronic Dis.* 1979;32:251-262.

83. Voors AW, Webber LS, Berenson GS. Time course study of blood pressure in children over a three-year period—The Bogalusa Heart Study. *Hypertension.* 1980;2(Suppl. 1): 102-108.

84. Webber LS, Cresanta JL, Voors AW, et al. Tracking of cardiovascular disease risk factor variables in school-age children. *J Chronic Dis.* 1983;36:647-660.

85. Clarke WR, Schrott HG, Leaverton PE, et al. Tracking of blood lipids and blood pressure in school age children: The Muscatine Study. *Circulation.* 1978;58:626-634.

86. Oberman A, Lane NE, Harlan WR, et al. Trends in systolic blood pressure in the Thousand Aviator Cohort over a 24-year period. *Circulation.* 1967;36:812-822.

87. Heiss G, Tyroler HA, Hames C. Cholesterol tracking: Prediction over time of serum cholesterol in Evans County, GA. *Advances in Exper and Med Biol.* 1977;82:112-114.

88. Higgins MW, Keller JB, Metzner HL, et al. Studies of blood pressure in Tecumseh, Michigan—II. Antecedents in childhood of high blood pressure in young adults. *Hypertension.* 1980;2(Suppl. 1):117-123.

89. National Cholesterol Education Program. National Heart, Lung, and Blood Institute. *Population Panel Report. Pediatric Panel Report.* Bethesda, Md: National Institutes of Health; April 1991.

90. Carroll MD, Abraham S, Dresser CM. *Dietary Intake Source Data: United States 1976-1980.* Washington, DC: National Center for Health Statistics; March 1983. Vital and Health Statistics Series II, 231 USDHHS, PHS, NCHS, DHHS pub. 83-1681.

91. Wynder EL, Weisburger JH, Ng SK. Nutrition: The need to define "optimal" intake as a basis for public policy decisions. *Am J Public Health.* 1992;82:346-350.

92. Fulgoni VL, Mackey MA. Total dietary fiber in children's diets. In: Williams CL, Wynder EL, eds. Hyperlipidemia and the development of atherosclerosis. *Ann NY Acad Sci.* 1991;623:369-379.

93. *The Food Guide Pyramid.* Washington, DC: US Department of Agriculture; April 1992.

94. *Nutrition and Your Health: Dietary Guidelines for Americans.* 2nd ed. Washington, DC: US Department of Ag-

riculture/US Department of Health and Human Services; 1989. H&G 232 and 322-1.

95. State of California. 1989. Assembly Bill 2109, Speier.

96. California Department of Health Services. *California Daily Food Guide*. Sacramento, Calif: California Department of Health Services; 1990. F-89-559.

97. Gold R, Parcel G, Walberg H, et al. Summary and conclusions of the THTM evaluation: The expert work group perspective. *J School Health.* 1991;61(1):39–42.

98. Harris L. *An Evaluation of Comprehensive Health Education in American Public Schools.* New York, NY: Metropolitan Life Foundation; 1988.

99. Roper WJ. Preface to the Teenage Health Teaching Modules Evaluation. *J School Health.* 1991;61(1):19.

100. Allensworth DD, Kolbe LJ. The comprehensive school health program: Exploring an expanded concept. *J School Health.* 1987;57(10):31.

101. Elder JP. From experimentation to dissemination: Strategies for maximizing the impact and spread of school health education. In: Nutbeam D, Haglund B, Farley P, et al, eds. *Youth Health Promotion: From Theory to Practice in School and Community.* London, England: Forbes Publications Ltd; 1991:22–32.

102. Glanz K, Lewis FM, Rimer BK. *Health Behavior and Health Education.* San Francisco, Calif: Jossey-Bass Publishers; 1991.

103. Cummings K, Becker M, Maile M. Bringing the models together in an empirical approach to combining variables used to explain health actions. *J Behav Med.* 1980;3:123–145.

104. Pentz M, Dwyer J, MacKinnon D, et al. A multicommunity trial for primary prevention of adolescent drug abuse: Effects on drug use prevalence. *JAMA.* 1989; 261:3259–3266.

105. Dhillon HS, Tolsma D. *Meeting Global Health Challenges: A Position Paper on Health Education.* Geneva, Switzerland: World Health Organization; 1991.

106. Dryfoos J. *Adolescents at Risk: Prevalence and Prevention.* New York, NY: Oxford University Press; 1990.

107. Green LW, Krueter MW. *Health Promotion Planning: An Educational and Environmental Approach.* Toronto, Ontario, Canada: Mayfield Publishing; 1991.

108. Perry C. Conceptualizing community-wide youth health promotion programs. In: Nutbeam D, Haglund B, Farley P, et al, eds. *Youth Health Promotion: From Theory to Practice in School and Community.* London, England: Forbes Publications Ltd; 1991; 1–22.

109. Benard B. *An Overview of Community Based Prevention. OSAP Prevention Monograph 3: Prevention Research Findings, 1988.* Washington, DC: US Department of Health and Human Services; 1990. Publication (ADM) 89-1615.

110. National Health Education Organizations. The limitations to excellence in education. *J School Health.* 1984;54:256–257.

111. Lovato CY, Allensworth DD, Chan FA. *School Health in America: An Assessment of State Policies to Protect and Improve the Health of Students.* 5th ed. Kent, Ohio: American School Health Association; 1989.

112. Kolbe LJ. An epidemiological surveillance system to monitor the prevalence of youth behaviors that most affect health. *Health Ed.* 1990;21(6):40–43.

113. Novello AC, DeGraw C, Kleinman DV. Healthy children ready to learn: An essential collaboration between health and education. *Public Health Rep.* 1992;107W:3–14.

114. Frank GC, Vaden A, Martin J. School health promotion: Child nutrition programs. *J School Health.* 1987;57:451–460.

115. Frank GC, Nicklas T, Forcier J, et al. Cardiovascular health promotion of children: The Heart Smart School Lunch Program, Part I. *School Food Serv Res Rev.* 1989;13:130–136.

116. Frank GC, Nicklas T, Forcier J, et al. Cardiovascular health promotion of children: Student behavior and institutional foodservice change, Part II. *School Food Serv Res Rev.* 1989;13:137–145.

117. National Center for Nutrition, and Dietetics and International Food Information Council. *Kids Earn Good Marks for Nutrition Knowledge.* Chicago, Ill: American Dietetic Association; 1991.

118. Levy SR, Iverson BK, Walberg HJ. Nutrition education research: An interdisciplinary evaluation and review. *Health Ed Q.* 1980;7:107–126.

119. *Children's Eating Habits.* Roper Survey Incorporated; 1985.

120. Dubinsky LD, Bodner JH. Food for thought: Starting a K-3 nutrition education program. *J School Health.* 1991;61:181–183.

121. Portland Public Schools. *Fundamental Understanding of Nutrition (FUN) Program. A Comprehensive Nutrition Education Program for Grades K–3.* Portland, Ore: Nutrition Services; 1989.

122. Liang T, Frank GC. Songs to teach nutrition. *J Nutr Ed.* 1994;26:87–92.

123. Green LW, Kreuter MW, Deeds SG, et al. *Health Education Planning—A Diagnostic Approach.* Palo Alto, Calif: Mayfield Publishing Co; 1980:142–158.

124. American School Food Service Association. The Healthy E.D.G.E. in Schools. (supplement). *J Am School Food Service Assoc.* March 1991;45:8.

125. American School Food Service Association. New CN program regs proposed. *J Am School Food Service Assoc.* August 1994;48:12–13.

126. American School Food Service Association. *Youth Advisory Council—At the Starting Line.* Alexandria, Va: American School Food Service Association; 1990.

127. Hong Li-Tsu, Frank GC, Toma R, et al. The nutrient analysis and sensory evaluation of a new recipe for school lunch—modified chinese meat bun. Abstract presented at the California Dietetic Association, April 1992.

128. Simons-Morton BG, Parcel GS, Baranowski T, et al. Promoting physical activity and a healthful diet among children: Results of a school-based intervention study. *Am J Public Health.* 1991;81:986–991.

129. Frank GC, Adsen MA. *Technical Report: California Statewide Census of Child Nutrition Program Employees.* Long Beach, Calif: California State University Long Beach, Child Nutrition Program Management Center; 1992:1–132.

130. Frank GC, Desai S. Shaping healthy meals for school children: Food service employee training curriculum. Long Beach, Calif: California State University Long Beach; 1992:32.

131. Cinciripini PM. Changing food selections in a public cafeteria. *Behavior Mod.* 1984;8:522–539.

132. Schmitz MF, Fielding JE. Point-of-choice nutritional labeling: Evaluation in a worksite cafeteria. *J Nutr Ed.* 1986;18:S65–S68.

133. Davis-Chervin D, Rogers T, Clark M. Influencing food selection with point-of-choice nutrition information. *J Nutr Ed.* 1985;17:18–22.

134. Anderson J, Haas MH. Impact of a nutrition education program on food sales in restaurants. *J Nutr Ed.* 1990; 22:232–238.

135. Computrition, Inc. 1992. Chatsworth, Calif.

136. Dennison D, Dennison KF, Frank GC. The DINE Evaluation Process: Improving food choices of the public. *J Nutr Ed.* 1994;26(2):87–93.

137. LunchByte Systems. NutriKids. Rochester, NY: 1992.

138. Frank GC. Nutrient profile on personal computers—A comparison of DINE with mainframe computers. *Health Ed.* 1985;16:16–19.

139. Mellin LM, Slinkard LA, Irwin CE. Adolescent obesity intervention: Validation of the SHAPEDOWN program. *J Am Diet Assoc.* 1987;87:333–338.

140. American Medical Association. *Guidelines for Adolescent Preventive Services.* Chicago, Ill: American Medical Association; 1992:3.

141. American Medical Association. *Target 2000.* Chicago, Ill: American Medical Association; Fall 1994.

142. California Adolescent Nutrition and Fitness. Berkeley, Calif. 1995.

143. National Institutes of Health. *Heart Memo.* Bethesda, Md: National Institutes of Health; Fall, 1994.

144. Van Horn LV, Stumbo P, Moag-Stahlberg A, et al. The Dietary Intervention Study in Children (DISC): Dietary assessment methods for 8- to 10-year olds. *J Am Diet Assoc.* 93:1396–1403.

145. US Department of Health and Human Services. The President's Council on Physical Fitness and Sports. *The President's Council on Physical Fitness and Sports Newsletter.* 94(1):1–8.

146. Jackson SA. Comprehensive school health education programs: Innovative practices and issues in standard setting. *J School Health.* 1994;64:177–179.

147. Allenworth DD. The research base for innovative practices in school health education at the secondary level. *J School Health.* 1994;64:180–187.

148. Cortese P, Middleton K, eds. *The Comprehensive School Health Challenge: Promoting Health through Education.* Santa Cruz, Calif: ETR Associates; 1993. 95061-1830.

149. National Commission on the Role of the School and the Community in Improving Adolescents' Health. *CODE BLUE: Uniting for Healthier Youth.* Alexandria, Va: National Association of State Boards of Education; 1990.

Appendix 8–A

Anthropometric Measures for School-Age Children

Table 8–A1   Height in Centimeters for Girls 6–19 Years of Age—Number Examined, Mean, Standard Deviation, and Selected Percentiles, by Specified Hispanic Origin and Age: Hispanic Health and Nutrition Examination Survey, 1982–84

				Percentile					
Hispanic Origin/Age	N	Mean	±SD	10th	25th	50th	75th	85th	95th
Mexican-American Girls									
6 years	118	117.6	5.0	111.8	114.8	117.2	120.5	122.5	126.1
7 years	96	123.1	5.9	116.1	119.1	123.0	126.1	128.3	*
8 years	107	127.8	6.6	120.0	123.4	127.9	132.1	134.5	139.6
9 years	124	136.0	6.3	127.2	131.5	136.5	140.6	143.2	146.0
10 years	94	142.0	6.7	133.0	137.6	140.7	146.8	148.2	*
11 years	115	147.3	8.2	135.6	142.2	147.1	152.7	155.8	159.1
12 years	103	152.9	5.5	144.7	150.0	153.2	156.2	158.2	163.0
13 years	89	156.7	5.5	149.6	152.6	157.5	160.4	162.6	*
14 years	75	156.5	5.4	150.5	152.8	157.4	160.3	161.6	*
15 years	85	160.4	5.5	153.1	156.8	160.1	164.3	167.6	*
16 years	99	158.0	7.4	149.4	153.2	158.3	162.7	164.3	*
17 years	75	158.7	5.7	151.7	155.4	158.8	161.5	163.7	*
18 years	77	157.8	5.5	149.6	154.6	158.4	161.7	163.7	*
19 years	75	159.4	5.9	151.9	155.6	159.9	162.9	165.3	*
Puerto Rican Girls+									
6 years	35	120.6	5.1	*	117.0	120.3	124.1	125.0	*
7 years	39	124.7	7.6	*	118.9	123.7	128.2	134.8	*
8 years	30	131.6	6.2	*	126.9	131.7	135.7	*	*
9 years	34	138.2	8.5	*	133.2	136.4	140.7	*	*
10 years	36	142.8	7.9	*	135.6	143.0	151.1	152.1	*
11 years	34	148.9	7.9	*	146.3	151.3	154.4	*	*
12 years	34	154.9	6.1	*	150.0	155.3	158.8	*	*
13 years	46	158.1	6.0	*	154.1	158.1	161.7	163.6	*
14 years	35	158.0	3.7	*	155.5	158.2	160.9	162.0	*
15 years	46	159.2	5.5	*	154.6	158.3	163.4	166.5	*
16 years	43	159.6	6.4	*	154.4	159.7	164.9	167.6	*
17 years	38	160.3	5.6	*	157.5	160.6	163.4	164.0	*
18 years	37	158.3	5.6	*	156.0	157.8	163.1	163.7	*
19 years	35	161.0	6.2	*	156.5	261.7	165.0	167.0	*

+Cuban data not presented because of insufficient sample size.
*No data available.

Source: Reprinted with permission of National Center for Health Statistics. *Vital and Health Statistics: Anthropometric Data and Prevalence of Overweight for Hispanics 1982–1984.* Series 11: data from the National Health Survey. No. 239. March, 1989. Hyattsville, Md. DHHS Publication No. (PHS) 89-1689.

Table 8–A2   Height in Centimeters for Boys 6–19 Years of Age—Number Examined, Mean, Standard Deviation, and Selected Percentiles, by Specified Hispanic Origin and Age: Hispanic Health and Nutrition Examination Survey, 1982–84

Hispanic Origin/Age	N	Mean	±SD	Percentile 10th	25th	50th	75th	85th	95th
Mexican-American Boys									
6 years	109	117.9	5.2	110.1	114.8	118.2	121.2	123.1	126.1
7 years	110	123.5	5.8	115.4	119.5	123.9	127.8	129.4	132.7
8 years	102	129.3	4.6	124.3	125.9	128.5	132.8	134.0	137.5
9 years	106	134.3	6.7	126.7	129.2	133.2	137.4	141.3	147.8
10 years	88	140.0	6.9	130.7	135.2	139.9	145.6	146.7	*
11 years	115	146.4	6.8	138.0	141.6	146.1	151.4	154.4	156.9
12 years	115	152.4	7.5	142.3	146.8	151.5	157.6	161.6	164.7
13 years	97	160.4	8.1	150.4	155.2	161.1	165.7	169.5	*
14 years	97	165.6	7.1	156.5	160.6	166.6	170.4	172.9	*
15 years	69	168.3	7.3	158.7	163.5	168.8	173.7	175.3	*
16 years	76	170.1	6.6	162.2	165.1	171.2	174.6	176.4	*
17 Years	71	171.0	6.8	163.0	166.3	171.1	175.6	177.2	*
18 years	63	169.8	5.8	163.6	165.2	168.1	173.5	175.1	*
19 years	64	169.8	5.6	164.9	166.8	168.5	172.7	176.6	*
Puerto Rican Boys[+]									
6 years	37	119.9	5.0	*	116.0	119.1	123.5	126.3	*
7 years	39	125.8	7.4	*	122.0	124.6	130.7	135.3	*
8 years	41	130.2	6.3	*	125.6	129.1	133.5	138.1	*
9 years	26	136.0	6.4	*	129.6	136.5	141.3	*	*
10 years	38	144.5	7.1	*	138.5	143.7	149.9	152.5	*
11 years	27	145.6	7.4	*	140.5	146.6	151.8	*	*
12 years	37	155.4	7.6	*	151.3	155.8	160.2	163.3	*
13 years	39	160.3	8.6	*	153.2	160.2	166.6	170.6	*
14 years	40	166.4	7.4	*	161.9	165.1	170.8	171.9	*
15 years	37	171.3	7.6	*	167.2	169.6	178.3	180.7	*
16 years	43	172.0	6.3	*	167.5	172.6	177.9	179.1	*
17 years	41	171.4	7.4	*	167.6	172.1	176.2	178.2	*
18 years	35	172.2	7.2	*	169.2	172.6	177.9	179.0	*
19 years	25	173.3	7.0	*	166.1	174.0	178.1	*	*

+Cuban data not presented because of insufficient sample size.
*No data available.

Table 8–A3   Height in Centimeters for Boys and Girls 6–19 Years of Age—Number Examined, Mean, Standard Deviation, and Selection Percentiles, by Sex and Age: United States, 1976–80

Sex and Age	N	Mean	±SD	Percentile					
				10th	25th	50th	75th	85th	95th
Boys									
6 years	133	119.5	5.1	112.6	115.9	120.1	122.6	124.7	126.8
7 years	148	125.1	5.9	117.6	121.8	125.9	128.1	130.2	133.6
8 years	147	129.9	7.0	122.0	125.3	130.6	134.1	136.5	142.0
9 years	145	135.5	5.8	128.4	131.2	136.1	139.6	141.2	144.7
10 years	157	141.6	7.3	132.8	137.0	141.5	146.4	149.6	153.0
11 years	155	146.0	7.8	135.9	141.1	145.6	151.2	153.9	160.2
12 years	145	152.6	7.9	142.6	147.5	152.0	158.0	160.5	164.4
13 years	173	158.9	8.3	147.6	152.6	159.7	165.0	168.7	171.6
14 years	186	167.5	8.3	156.5	162.5	167.5	173.1	176.5	180.6
15 years	184	170.8	6.7	162.0	165.7	171.1	175.5	177.5	181.9
16 years	178	173.8	6.4	164.7	169.8	173.7	178.1	180.3	186.1
17 years	173	175.1	7.1	167.3	170.6	174.9	179.7	182.8	187.5
18 years	164	176.9	6.7	168.8	172.3	176.9	180.9	183.9	189.6
19 years	148	176.5	6.7	168.2	171.8	176.9	181.1	183.5	187.2
Girls									
6 years	135	118.4	6.1	111.1	113.3	118.5	122.2	124.5	128.7
7 years	157	123.7	6.7	116.6	119.6	124.1	128.1	130.1	134.7
8 years	123	130.2	5.7	123.4	125.8	130.6	133.2	135.4	140.5
9 years	149	134.4	7.6	126.4	129.0	134.8	139.0	140.7	147.1
10 years	136	141.9	6.5	133.6	137.6	141.6	146.3	148.1	153.8
11 years	140	147.9	7.8	139.3	142.2	147.9	152.2	154.7	162.7
12 years	147	154.4	7.2	145.7	149.2	154.8	158.6	161.9	165.9
13 years	162	158.9	6.6	150.3	155.3	159.0	163.0	164.5	170.3
14 years	178	160.8	6.4	152.7	156.7	160.9	165.1	166.9	172.3
15 years	145	163.2	6.2	155.2	159.1	163.1	167.1	170.2	173.5
16 years	170	162.9	6.1	154.5	159.1	163.2	166.4	169.4	173.3
17 years	134	163.5	5.7	156.8	160.4	163.1	166.7	169.7	172.2
18 years	170	162.4	6.8	154.2	158.0	162.7	166.2	169.1	174.0
19 years	158	163.5	5.6	156.8	159.7	163.7	167.2	169.5	172.1

Table 8–A4   Triceps Skinfold in Millimeters for Girls 6–19 Years of Age—Number Examined, Mean, Standard Deviation, and Selected Percentiles, by Specified Hispanic Origin and Age: Hispanic Health and Nutrition Examination Survey, 1982–84

Hispanic Origina/Age	N	Mean	± SD	Percentile 10th	25th	50th	75th	85th	95th
Mexican-American Girls									
6 years	118	11.3	4.9	6.5	8.0	10.0	13.0	16.0	22.5
7 years	96	12.7	5.3	7.0	9.0	11.0	15.5	17.5	*
8 years	107	13.7	6.1	7.5	9.0	12.5	16.0	19.0	26.0
9 years	125	15.2	5.8	8.5	11.0	14.5	19.0	21.0	26.0
10 years	94	16.4	7.0	8.0	11.0	15.0	22.0	25.0	*
11 years	115	15.0	6.8	8.0	10.0	14.0	18.0	21.5	26.0
12 years	103	16.9	6.7	9.0	11.5	16.0	21.5	24.0	30.0
13 years	89	18.5	6.7	11.0	12.5	17.0	22.5	26.0	*
14 years	75	19.6	7.1	11.5	15.0	19.5	22.5	24.5	*
15 years	85	19.8	7.5	11.5	14.5	18.5	24.5	26.0	*
16 years	99	20.4	8.5	12.0	14.0	18.0	25.5	28.5	*
17 years	75	19.3	6.6	12.0	13.5	18.5	24.5	26.0	*
18 years	77	21.5	7.5	12.0	17.0	20.5	25.5	27.5	*
19 years	75	21.4	8.4	12.0	15.0	21.5	25.0	28.0	*
Puerto Rican Girls[+]									
6 years	35	13.9	6.2	*	8.0	13.0	18.5	24.0	*
7 years	39	12.0	6.4	*	8.0	9.0	15.0	18.5	*
8 years	30	15.2	6.4	*	10.0	12.5	21.0	*	*
9 years	34	13.7	6.5	*	9.0	11.5	18.0	*	*
10 years	36	13.8	5.6	*	9.0	13.5	18.5	20.0	*
11 years	34	13.6	7.5	*	7.5	11.0	19.0	*	*
12 years	34	17.1	8.9	*	11.0	13.0	23.0	*	*
13 years	46	19.4	7.9	*	13.0	19.0	24.0	26.0	*
14 years	35	19.3	7.6	*	14.0	18.0	23.5	28.5	*
15 years	46	20.4	7.2	*	15.0	20.0	25.5	26.5	*
16 years	43	21.5	8.2	*	16.0	22.5	25.5	28.0	*
17 years	38	18.9	7.8	*	12.0	17.0	25.0	28.0	*
18 years	37	20.6	8.5	*	14.0	19.0	25.5	27.0	*
19 years	35	19.2	8.8	*	13.0	17.5	23.0	25.5	*

+Cuban data not presented because of insufficient sample size.
*No data available.

Table 8–A5   Triceps Skinfold in Millimeters for Boys 6–19 Years of Age—Number Examined, Mean, Standard Deviation, and Selected Percentiles, by Specified Hispanic Origin and Age: Hispanic Health and Nutrition Examination Survey, 1982–84

Hispanic Origin/Age	N	Mean	± SD	Percentile					
				10th	25th	50th	75th	85th	95th
Mexican-American Boys									
6 years	110	8.8	3.2	5.0	7.0	8.0	10.0	11.5	15.0
7 years	110	10.6	5.1	6.0	7.0	9.0	12.5	15.0	24.0
8 years	102	11.1	5.6	6.0	7.0	10.0	13.0	17.0	25.0
9 years	106	12.3	6.6	6.0	7.5	10.0	15.5	20.5	27.0
10 years	88	14.2	7.3	5.5	8.5	11.5	19.0	22.5	*
11 years	115	15.7	7.4	7.5	11.0	14.5	19.5	22.5	32.5
12 years	114	13.4	7.2	7.0	8.5	11.0	17.0	21.0	28.5
13 years	97	12.8	7.3	6.0	8.0	10.5	15.0	20.0	*
14 years	97	13.0	7.8	6.0	7.0	9.5	19.0	21.0	*
15 years	69	11.0	6.6	5.0	7.0	9.0	12.5	16.5	*
16 years	76	12.1	7.4	5.5	7.5	10.0	14.0	17.0	*
17 years	71	10.5	5.5	5.5	6.5	9.0	12.0	15.5	*
18 years	63	12.0	6.5	6.0	7.0	10.5	14.5	17.5	*
19 years	64	13.1	7.0	6.0	7.5	12.5	16.0	20.0	*
Puerto Rican Boys[+]									
6 years	37	*11.2	5.7	*	7.0	9.5	13.0	18.0	*
7 years	39	*10.4	4.7	*	8.0	9.0	12.0	16.0	*
8 years	41	*11.4	5.9	*	8.0	10.0	14.0	18.0	*
9 years	26	*15.1	7.3	*	10.0	12.5	19.5	*	*
10 years	38	*16.4	9.1	*	8.0	13.0	21.5	25.0	*
11 years	27	*12.3	5.6	*	8.0	10.0	15.5	*	*
12 years	37	*12.4	7.8	*	6.5	9.5	14.5	21.5	*
13 years	39	*12.6	6.4	*	8.0	11.0	15.0	18.0	*
14 years	40	*12.1	7.1	*	6.5	9.5	15.0	19.0	*
15 years	37	*10.6	7.2	*	6.0	9.0	12.5	13.5	*
16 years	44	*14.0	8.8	*	8.0	10.0	17.0	25.0	*
17 years	42	*11.3	6.7	*	6.0	9.0	16.0	20.0	*
18 years	35	*11.8	7.1	*	7.0	10.0	13.5	18.0	*
19 years	25	*9.4	4.7	*	6.0	8.0	10.5	*	*

[+]Cuban data not presented because of insufficient sample size.
*No data available.

Table 8–A6 Triceps Skinfold in Millimeters for Boys and Girls 6–19 Years of Age—Number Examined, Mean, Standard Deviation, and Selected Percentiles, by Sex and Age: United States, 1976–80

Sex and Age	N	Mean	± SD	Percentile 10th	25th	50th	75th	85th	95th
Boys									
6 years	133	9.3	4.4	5.5	6.5	8.0	10.5	12.0	17.5
7 years	148	9.2	4.0	5.5	6.5	8.5	11.0	12.0	17.5
8 years	147	10.5	4.9	6.0	7.0	9.0	12.0	16.5	22.0
9 years	145	10.6	5.7	5.0	7.0	9.0	12.5	16.0	23.0
10 years	157	12.6	6.6	6.0	7.5	11.0	16.5	20.0	26.0
11 years	155	13.3	7.7	5.5	7.5	10.5	17.0	22.0	30.0
12 years	145	12.4	6.4	6.0	8.0	11.0	15.0	18.0	26.5
13 years	173	11.2	7.0	5.5	7.0	9.0	12.5	16.5	22.5
14 years	186	10.4	5.8	5.0	6.0	9.0	13.0	15.0	23.0
15 years	184	10.1	7.2	5.0	6.0	7.5	11.0	14.5	22.0
16 years	178	10.9	6.6	5.0	6.5	8.0	13.0	18.5	25.5
17 years	173	8.5	4.6	4.5	5.5	7.0	10.5	12.5	18.0
18 years	164	11.1	6.6	5.0	6.0	9.5	14.5	17.5	22.5
19 years	148	10.9	6.1	5.5	6.5	9.0	13.0	16.0	23.0
Girls									
6 years	135	*11.0	3.9	7.0	8.0	10.0	12.0	14.5	18.5
7 years	157	*11.5	4.5	7.0	9.0	10.5	13.0	15.0	20.0
8 years	123	*11.9	5.2	6.5	8.5	11.0	14.0	16.0	21.0
9 years	149	*14.3	6.5	7.5	10.0	13.0	16.0	20.0	27.0
10 years	136	*14.5	5.9	8.0	10.0	13.5	18.0	21.0	24.5
11 years	140	*15.7	6.9	8.5	11.0	14.0	19.5	21.5	29.5
12 years	147	*15.1	6.0	8.0	11.5	13.5	18.5	21.5	27.0
13 years	162	15.9	7.9	7.5	10.5	15.0	19.0	22.0	30.0
14 years	178	17.6	7.5	10.0	12.0	17.0	21.5	25.0	32.0
15 years	145	17.1	7.1	9.5	11.5	16.5	20.5	24.5	32.1
16 years	170	19.5	7.2	11.5	14.0	18.0	23.0	27.0	33.1
17 years	134	19.8	7.8	11.0	14.0	20.0	24.5	26.5	34.5
18 years	170	19.9	7.6	12.0	14.0	18.0	23.5	27.0	35.0
19 years	158	20.4	7.6	11.5	15.0	19.0	25.0	28.0	33.5

*No data available.

Table 8–A7   Weight in Kilograms for Girls 6–19 Years of Age—Number Examined, Mean, Standard Deviation, and Selected Percentiles, by Specified Hispanic Origin and Age: Hispanic Health and Nutrition Examination Survey, 1982–84

Hispanic Origin/Age	N	Mean	± SD	Percentile					
				10th	25th	50th	75th	85th	95th
Mexican-American Girls									
6 years	118	22.1	4.6	18.0	19.2	20.8	23.2	27.3	31.5
7 years	96	25.4	5.9	19.8	21.3	24.0	27.6	31.6	*
8 years	107	28.2	6.7	21.4	23.9	27.0	30.9	35.2	41.1
9 years	125	33.9	7.9	24.3	28.0	32.7	38.9	42.4	48.7
10 years	94	38.3	9.6	27.7	31.7	36.1	43.7	46.5	*
11 years	115	41.5	10.7	30.3	33.8	39.9	48.7	52.1	60.0
12 years	103	48.2	10.0	37.0	40.7	47.6	54.2	57.4	66.3
13 years	89	52.4	10.0	42.5	45.5	50.4	55.8	61.0	*
14 years	75	54.3	9.9	43.5	47.6	51.8	59.1	63.8	*
15 years	85	57.1	10.8	45.5	49.1	55.7	62.4	70.0	*
16 years	99	57.4	14.8	43.3	49.1	53.3	60.4	70.6	*
17 years	75	56.3	9.6	45.9	49.4	54.2	61.9	68.1	*
18 years	77	57.5	9.2	46.3	51.1	56.4	63.0	67.1	*
19 years	75	60.2	13.7	46.8	51.9	57.7	64.0	69.8	*
Puerto Rican Girls+									
6 years	35	25.1	5.1	*	20.5	24.9	29.7	31.6	*
7 years	39	26.3	7.9	*	22.7	23.5	30.5	33.5	*
8 years	30	32.8	8.9	*	24.8	29.9	39.5	*	*
9 years	34	33.2	8.2	*	27.4	32.1	33.9	*	*
10 years	36	38.0	8.4	*	32.3	36.4	43.6	48.0	*
11 years	34	42.1	10.9	*	36.3	41.3	50.6	*	*
12 years	34	50.1	14.3	*	40.4	46.2	56.4	*	*
13 years	46	55.6	12.4	*	48.3	51.2	62.9	67.3	*
14 years	35	54.9	8.5	*	49.0	52.0	59.6	64.0	*
15 years	46	57.0	10.1	*	49.6	54.4	62.1	67.8	*
16 years	43	59.5	12.1	*	49.7	57.7	64.9	71.1	*
17 years	38	57.5	11.8	*	49.1	56.1	67.8	69.3	*
18 years	37	59.0	14.7	*	49.3	55.7	64.5	69.2	*
19 years	35	57.0	12.1	*	49.4	54.5	61.0	62.4	*

Note: Includes clothing weight, estimated as ranging from 0.09 to 0.28 kilogram.
+Cuban data not presented because of insufficient sample size.
*No data available.

Table 8–A8   Weight in Kilograms for Boys 6–19 Years of Age—Number Examined, Mean, Standard Deviation, and Selected Percentiles, by Specified Hispanic Origin and Age: Hispanic Health and Nutrition Examination Survey, 1982–84

Hispanic Origin/Age	N	Mean	± SD	Percentile					
				10th	25th	50th	75th	85th	95th
Mexican-American Boys									
6 years	110	22.3	4.4	17.8	19.3	21.7	24.4	25.2	29.6
7 years	110	25.7	5.3	19.7	22.5	24.4	28.8	30.6	35.6
8 years	102	28.6	5.8	23.2	24.6	27.1	30.2	32.5	40.5
9 years	106	32.4	8.0	24.9	27.1	30.0	36.4	40.3	47.8
10 years	88	36.8	10.1	26.6	28.5	34.6	43.5	49.3	*
11 years	115	43.2	11.3	31.4	35.7	40.5	48.6	53.5	62.3
12 years	115	45.8	11.1	34.0	38.2	44.6	49.8	52.4	76.4
13 years	96	52.4	10.4	40.4	44.8	50.9	58.0	62.8	*
14 years	97	58.7	13.1	43.8	49.4	56.8	65.0	70.8	*
15 years	69	59.4	10.7	47.5	52.3	57.9	64.6	68.3	*
16 years	76	65.1	13.4	48.2	57.0	62.0	70.6	78.8	*
17 years	71	63.7	9.9	52.4	55.8	61.7	69.8	76.1	*
18 years	63	66.9	11.4	53.1	58.9	67.6	72.0	76.6	*
19 years	64	70.0	15.0	54.1	60.9	64.8	76.2	87.9	*
Puerto Rican Boys									
6 years	37	*24.1	6.4	*	20.1	22.4	25.3	27.1	*
7 years	39	*26.3	5.6	*	23.0	24.4	28.3	30.1	*
8 years	41	*29.5	7.2	*	24.6	28.2	31.9	38.8	*
9 years	26	*36.1	9.3	*	28.2	33.4	45.7	*	*
10 years	38	*41.4	11.0	*	31.0	40.8	54.1	56.2	*
11 years	27	*38.8	8.9	*	32.1	36.3	46.0	*	*
12 years	37	*48.7	14.4	*	37.8	47.3	53.9	57.3	*
13 years	39	*52.8	13.1	*	43.9	48.9	59.1	64.3	*
14 years	40	*61.4	17.2	*	50.5	56.8	65.8	70.7	*
15 years	37	*62.9	15.2	*	51.4	59.6	69.8	73.9	*
16 years	44	*70.9	15.8	*	58.9	66.0	77.4	88.8	*
17 years	42	*68.3	15.3	*	57.02	66.1	76.2	78.8	*
18 years	35	*72.3	16.9	*	61.5	68.5	76.0	94.3	*
19 years	25	*67.1	9.6	*	60.4	66.2	74.8	*	*

Note: Includes clothing weight, estimated as ranging from 0.09 to 0.28 kilogram.
*No data available.

Table 8–A9   Weight in Kilograms for Boys and Girls 6–19 Years of Age—Number Examined, Mean, Standard Deviation, and Selected Percentiles, by Sex and Age: United States, 1976–80

Sex and Age	N	Mean	± SD	Percentile					
				10th	25th	50th	75th	85th	95th
Boys									
6 years	133	23.0	4.0	19.2	20.3	22.0	24.1	26.4	30.1
7 years	148	25.1	3.9	20.8	22.2	24.8	26.9	28.2	33.9
8 years	147	28.2	6.2	22.7	24.6	27.5	29.9	33.0	39.1
9 years	145	31.1	6.3	25.6	27.1	30.2	33.0	35.4	43.1
10 years	157	36.4	7.7	28.2	31.4	34.8	39.2	43.5	53.4
11 years	155	40.3	10.1	28.8	33.5	37.3	46.4	52.0	61.0
12 years	145	44.2	10.1	32.5	37.8	42.5	48.8	52.6	67.5
13 years	173	49.9	12.3	37.0	40.1	48.4	56.3	59.8	69.9
14 years	186	57.1	11.0	44.5	49.8	56.4	63.3	66.1	77.0
15 years	184	61.0	11.0	49.1	54.2	60.1	64.9	68.7	81.3
16 years	178	67.1	12.4	54.3	58.7	64.4	73.6	78.1	91.2
17 years	173	66.7	11.5	53.4	58.7	65.8	72.0	76.8	88.9
18 years	164	71.1	12.7	56.6	61.9	70.4	76.6	80.0	95.3
19 years	148	71.7	11.6	57.9	63.8	69.5	77.9	84.3	92.1
Girls									
6 years	135	*22.1	4.0	17.8	19.3	21.3	23.8	26.6	29.6
7 years	157	*24.7	5.0	19.5	21.4	23.8	27.1	28.7	34.0
8 years	123	*27.9	5.7	22.3	24.4	27.5	30.2	31.3	36.5
9 years	149	*31.9	8.4	25.0	27.0	29.7	33.6	39.3	48.4
10 years	136	*36.1	8.0	27.5	31.0	34.5	39.5	44.2	49.6
11 years	140	*41.8	10.9	30.3	33.9	40.3	45.8	51.0	60.0
12 years	147	*46.4	10.1	35.0	39.1	45.4	52.6	58.0	64.3
13 years	162	50.9	11.8	39.0	44.1	49.0	55.2	60.9	76.3
14 years	178	54.8	11.1	42.8	47.4	53.1	60.3	65.7	75.2
15 years	145	55.1	9.8	45.1	48.2	53.3	59.6	62.2	76.6
16 years	170	58.1	10.1	47.3	51.3	55.6	62.5	68.9	76.8
17 years	134	59.6	11.4	48.9	52.2	58.4	63.4	68.4	81.8
18 years	170	59.0	11.1	49.5	52.8	56.4	63.0	66.0	78.0
19 years	158	60.2	11.0	49.7	53.9	57.1	64.4	70.7	78.1

Note: Includes clothing weight, estimated as ranging from 0.09 to 0.28 kilogram. 66 kg = 145.2 lb.
*No data available.

Appendix 8–B

Strategies To Promote 5-A-Day Messages Using Allensworth and Kolbe's Model for a Comprehensive School Health Education Program

Table 8–B1   Healthy Environment, Health Education Curriculum, Health Services, and Physical Education Strategies

	Healthy Environment	Health Education Curriculum	Health Services	Physical Education
Personnel	Board of Education, Superintendent, Principals	Elementary and Secondary Teachers, Librarians, Health Educators	School Nurses, School Dietitians, Physicians	Physical Education Instructors, Coaches, Trainers
Policy	Develop policies to: (1) Implement the USDA recommendations; (2) Limit competing foods in vending machines and as fundraisers.	Infuse 5-A-Day messages throughout curriculum.	Facilitate policy to implement 5-A-Day messages.	Facilitate policy to implement 5-A-Day messages.
Training/Inservice	Provide inservice training to all school personnel on: (1) the importance of consuming five servings of fruit and vegetables a day; (2) instructional strategies which can deliver the 5-A-Day message throughout the school; (3) their part as role models.			
Instruction	Institute a 5-A-Day Awareness Week. Infuse 5-A-Day messages in other health promotion observances and across curricula.	Institute delivery of the 5-A-Day message using lessons based upon Prochaska's Stages of Change intervention. Provide homework activities for child and family.	Coordinate supplemental instruction for delivery of 5-A-Day messages. Conduct inservice programs for staff and community on the importance of eating five a day.	Use teachable moments to reinforce 5-A-Day message in relation to physical fitness. Develop activities to deliver the 5-A-Day message (e.g., a 5-A-Day dance, a 5-A-Day walk).

continues

Source: Reprinted from Neill K, Allensworth DD. A Model to Increase Consumption of Fruit and Vegetables by Implementing the "5-A-Day" Initiative. *Journal of School Health.* 1994;64(4):152–153.

Table 8–B1 continued

	Healthy Environment	Health Education Curriculum	Health Services	Physical Education
Media	Promote 5-A-Day messages through the school's public address system, bulletin boards, display areas, etc.	Deliver 5-A-Day messages via student newsletters, posters, buttons, bulletin board displays, and videos. Have students stage "5-A-Day" fair for parents and community.	Distribute brochures to students, staff, and communities to deliver the 5-A-Day message.	—
Role Modeling/ Peer Modeling/ Social Support	Attend special events that promote the 5-A-Day message. Consume fruit and vegetables.	Develop peer instruction program with opportunities to teach younger students by direct instruction, through the PA system or video tape. Eat five servings of fruit and vegetables a day.	Eat five servings of fruit and vegetables a day. Model support for students at risk.	Eat five servings of fruit and vegetables a day.
Direct Intervention	Support intervention programs for weight management, nutritional counseling, and education.	Refer students to nutrition education and weight management programs.	Deliver messages of 5-A-Day while screening for height and weight. Institute programs for students at risk (undernourished and overnourished).	Refer students at risk (under-nourished and overnourished).
Environmental/ Facility Change	Provide opportunities for consumption of fresh fruit and vegetables in cafeteria and via vending machines.	Display posters in homerooms and the library to promote 5-A-Day messages.	Display posters and food models to promote 5-A-Day.	Display posters in gym.

Table 8–B2   Counseling, Food Service, Worksite Health Promotion, and Integrated School and Community Strategies

	Counseling	*Food Service*	*Worksite Health Promotion*	*Integrated School and Community*
Personnel	Counselors, Social Workers, Psychologists	Food Service Directors, Dietitians, Cooks	Staff, Faculty	Parents, Peers, Community Members
Policy	Facilitate policy.	Form an interdisciplinary work team to plan a 5-A-Day promotion program with the food service personnel.	Implement 5-A-Day messages in the worksite health promotion program.	Form coalition with key community members to launch a community-wide 5-A-Day promotion campaign.
Training/Inservice	—	Provide inservice on innovative ways to increase offerings of fruit and vegetables in school breakfast and lunch programs.	Include training of this team in 5-A-Day message program.	Have special training sessions for community leaders.
Instruction	Develop a parent training program. Provide confidential counseling to students with weight or eating problems.	Have culinary professionals demonstrate innovative uses of fruit and vegetables. Use marketing experts to show how to advertise and promote fruit and vegetables.	Coordinate inservice programming for staff, teachers, and parents.	Develop programs for delivery of 5-A-Day message to PTA groups. Coordinate parent training programs. Incorporate 5-A-Day messages in community meetings and social events.
Media	—	Print special messages on the menus. Display the 5-A-Day messages on the bulletin boards, table tents, and posters in the cafeteria. Wear aprons or T-shirts with the 5-A-Day message.	Organize cooking demonstrations, cookoffs, food fairs, cooking contests, recipe sharing parties.	Have supermarkets run promotions on consuming fruit and vegetables. Offer free fruit and vegetable samples. Provide radio, TV, and print ads for "5-A-Day" Awareness Week.

continues

Table 8–B2 continued

	Counseling	Food Service	Worksite Health Promotion	Integrated School and Community
Role Modeling/ Peer Modeling/ Social Support	Eat five servings of fruit and vegetables a day. Provide social support for students and staff with weight or eating problems.	Eat five servings of fruit and vegetables.	Eat five servings of fruit and vegetables a day.	Encourage everyone to show exemplary behavior by eating five servings of fruit and vegetables.
Direct Intervention	—	—	Offer more choices of fruit and vegetables. Start breakfast programs if not already in place.	—
Environmental/ Facility Change	—	Purchase new equipment if necessary to offer more fruit and vegetables (e.g., refrigerated salad bar, juice machines, steamer for vegetables).	Display posters promoting 5-A-Day message.	Display posters in community to promote 5-A-Day.

Appendix 8-C

California Adolescent Nutrition and Fitness (CANFit) Grants

The California Adolescent Nutrition and Fitness (CANFit) planning and intervention grants funded initially in 1994 are described briefly below.

- *Community Leadership Development Institute*—The HYPE Advocacy Project, 322 Harbor Way, Suite 24, Richmond, CA 94804. Tel. (510) 215-8292, Fax (510) 215-8294. The HYPE Advocacy Project is a planning process that builds youth leadership and advocacy skills through involving youth in the development of strategies to improve the nutrition, fitness, and overall health of the predominantly African-American early adolescents, aged 10–14.

- *Monterey County Health Department*—Project U-Fit, 1270 Natividad Road, Salinas, CA 93906. Tel. (408) 755-4796, Fax (408) 757-9586. Project U-Fit assesses the nutrition and fitness needs of adolescents, ages 10–14, in a section of Monterey County with a high percentage of low-income Hispanic students.

- *Stanislaus County Department of Public Health*—Multi-Ethnic Youth Nutrition/Fitness Needs Assessment-Project, 2030 Coffee Road, Suite C-4, Modesto, CA 95355. Tel. (209) 558-7400, Fax (209) 558-8315. The Stanislaus County Department of Public Health and the Stanislaus Minority Community Health Coalition are collaborating to: (1) create a community-based task force representative of the ethnic and cultural diver-

sity of Modesto; (2) develop a needs assessment for low-income, multiethnic adolescents (10–14) to assess both their nutrition and fitness status; (3) collect and analyze the assessment data; and (4) create a plan of action with community input to address solutions to identified problems.

- *El Concilio del Condado de Ventura*—Latino Adolescent Nutrition and Physical Activity Planning Group Project, 625 North A Street, 2nd Floor, Oxnard, CA 93030. Tel. (805) 983-2336, Fax (805) 485-1406. This project forms the Latino Adolescent Nutrition and Physical Activity Planning Group, consisting of adolescents from public housing, representatives from Tenant Associations, a Coalition on Alcohol and Drug Issues, City of Oxnard Parks and Recreation, Friday Night Live, El Centrito, the Diagnostic Pediatric Center, and the Ventura County Latino Health Coalition. The planning group will conduct nutrition and physical activity needs assessment activities, set priorities, plan activities, and develop a plan of action.

- *Kalusugan Community Services*—Kabataang Filipino NUTRIFIT Program, c/o MCH Division, Graduate School of Public Health, SDSU, 6505 Alvarado Road, Suite 205, San Diego, CA 92120. Tel. (619) 594-2795, Fax (619) 594-4570. Kabataang Filipino NUTRIFIT Project will conduct a community needs assessment of the nutrition/ fitness needs of Filipino-American youth aged 10–14 years in National City. The methods used will include youth forums, focus groups, surveys, and a resources inventory. Data from the needs assessment will be used as the basis for developing a plan of intervention.

- *Korean Health Education, Information and Referral (KHEIR) Center*–Healthy Youths Project, 981 S. Western Avenue, #404, Los Angeles, CA 90006. Tel. (213) 732-5648, Fax (213) 732-3857. KHEIR's Healthy Youths Project is the first nutrition and fitness program targeting 10-to-14-year-old Korean youths in Los Angeles County. The goal of this project is to shift the attitudes and behaviors of Korean youths regarding nutrition and fitness to reflect a healthier lifestyle. A needs assessment of the target population will develop a program that is responsive to the needs of Korean youths in culturally and linguistically appropriate manners.

- *St. Mary Medical Foundation/Southeast Asian Health Project*–Teens in Good Health Planning Project, 411 E. 10th Street, Suite 207, Long Beach, CA 90813. Tel. (310) 491-9100, Fax (310) 491-9824. This project will extend the Families in Good Health Program, which promotes physical activity and healthy living among Cambodian, Laotian families in Long Beach. The current program targets the family as a whole, but local youth from the target population will be employed to participate directly and extensively in planning a needs assessment for nutrition and fitness.

- *Viejas Indian School, Inc.*–Viejas Indian School CANFit Program, P.O. Box 1389, Viejas Reservation, Viejas Grade and Browns Road, Alpine, CA 91903. Tel. (619) 445-4938, Fax (619) 445-8912. Health-Literate Teens is creating a planning group consisting of parents, students, and staff to educate adolescent Viejas Indian School children and their families on nutrition and fitness values. A total child approach will create a program to incorporate family, peers, traditional foods, and dance. Student planning activities will involve menu planning and hands-

on cooking demonstrations using traditional foods.

A brief description of the California Adolescent Nutrition and Fitness (CANFit) intervention grants follows:

- *Escondido Community Health Center*–Healthy Lives CANFit for Kids Project, 460 North Elm Street, Escondido, CA 92025. Tel. (619) 737-2030, Fax (619) 737-2039. Healthy Lives CANFit for Kids targets Hispanic and American Indian adolescents ages 10–14 in north and east San Diego County. This is a coalition project representing the La Vida Buena, Project LEAN, and Southern Indian Health Council's CAMP existing coalitions.

- *San Bernardino County Department of Public Health*–"Goal for Health" Nutrition and Fitness Project, 351 North Mountain View Avenue, Room 104, San Bernardino, CA 92415. Tel. (909) 387-6320, Fax (909) 387-6228. The "Goal for Health" Nutrition and Fitness Project will promote optimal nutrition, low fat, and physical fitness of low-income Latino youth 10–14 years of age in the Colton Youth Soccer Association (CYSA) and in the community. Peer youth advisors who are representatives of the target youth population will provide direction to the project. Peer youth advisors will develop and distribute "Goal for Health" newsletters, publicize and motivate youth to participate in the Presidential Sports Award Program, assist the project in promoting consumption of fruits and vegetables (5-A-Day), as well as low fat (1% or nonfat) milk, and suggest changes to foods offered at the snack bar.

- *Ventura County Public Health Services/ SPHAC*–Santa Paula "Baile de Vida" Dance of Life Project, 3147 Loma Vista Road, Ventura, CA 93003. Tel. (805) 652-5914, Fax (805) 652-6617. This Dance of Life Project is a collaborative community-based project to improve fitness and nutrition status of low-income Latino youth with quebradita dance classes, a youth snack committee, nutrition/fitness education, cooking and dancing demonstrations, contests and incentives, media support, and development of a video by youth.

- *Girls Incorporated of San Leandro–* Mawiyah Project, 13666 East 14th Street, San Leandro, CA 94577. Tel. (510) 357-5515, Fax (510) 357-5112. This project empowers African-American adolescent girls to recognize their own potential and to adopt healthy nutrition and fitness habits that can help them develop with confidence and skills. Linking nutrition, fitness, and leadership, young women advocates will create positive changes in their own lives and for their future.

9

Adults and Their Nutritional Needs

Learning Objectives

- Describe the major chronic diseases of adult men and women.
- Identify major research initiatives undertaken to evaluate primary and secondary prevention approaches for breast and colon cancer, heart disease, and osteoporosis among women.
- List the major primary and secondary prevention strategies to educate and to interest men in nutrition and eating behavior programs for improved health and wellness.
- Detail community-based nutrition programs that target adults and their health needs.

High Definition Nutrition

Aerobic training—training that increases the body's ability to use oxygen and improves endurance.

Body work—any type of regularly practiced physical activity (e.g., a sport, a special exercise program, or a hobby involving body movement).

Certified lactation educator (CLE)—the individual who completes basic lactation courses successfully and qualifies for a Lactation Educator Certificate. This designation enables the individual to teach breastfeeding education classes to parents and provides health care professionals with a basic understanding to help mothers breastfeed. This provides the foundation for the lactation consultant courses.

Certified lactation specialist (CLS)—an individual who has completed the degree program or the lactation certificate program for those who hold previous master's or doctoral degrees. A lactation specialist is qualified clinically and academically to assist mothers with breastfeeding problems and to teach professionals about breastfeeding (*Source:* The Lactation Institute and Breastfeeding Clinic, 16430 Ventura Blvd., Suite 303, Encino, CA 91436).

Fitness—having adequate muscular strength and endurance to accomplish individual goals, reasonable joint flexibility, an efficient cardiovascular system, and a body composition that falls within the normal range of body weight and percent body fat.

Strength training—training that enhances size and strength of particular muscles and body regions.

The living arrangements of adult men and women in the 1990s vary from single adults living alone or together to adults who are the head of the household or a member of nuclear or extended families. The adult years encompass four decades (from 20 to 60 years of age) and, for some individuals, these years are marked by maturity, financial acumen, and community service. On the other hand, the adult years may reflect single parenting, the onset of chronic disease symptoms, unemployment, or reduced economic independence.

Women during the childbearing years from 20 to 50 often demonstrate a need to remain youthful in appearance, attractive, and vital in the family day-to-day functioning. Health and nutrition may not be priorities. Young adult men generally continue with established sports and athletic interests either from the vantage point of the sports field or from in front of the television. For individuals entering the adult years in the 1990s, a wellness approach to living as part of primary prevention of disease generates more interest than in prior decades. However, disease prevention remains a future and somewhat distance frontier for many of today's adults.

THE ADULT FEMALE AND HER NUTRITION NEEDS

Pregnancy

The United States is 11th in the world in infant mortality. This relatively low ranking is likely due to a lack of nutrition education and prenatal care of women during pregnancy. In fact, inadequate nutrition during pregnancy is linked to the following conditions[1]:

- iron deficiency anemia, which creates low levels of hemoglobin and endangers the health of mother and baby
- gestational diabetes, seen in increased blood sugar levels during pregnancy that may predispose the woman to abnormal blood sugar levels later in life
- toxemia or preeclampsia symptoms of increased blood pressure; swelling in face, hands, and feet; and convulsions
- stillbirths
- birth defects

Current recommendations are that each pregnant woman's eating pattern should be reviewed,

designed, and monitored by a registered dietitian (RD) to ensure that individual needs are being met.[1]

Preconception Nutrition

Future mothers need a watchful approach not only to their eating patterns during pregnancy, but also to their food choices at least three months before conception. Studies of the eating patterns of nonpregnant women of childbearing age reveal possible inadequacies in vitamins and minerals important to a healthy pregnancy.

Women's nutritional status before pregnancy can greatly affect the fetus. Inadequate maternal nutrient stores can prevent the placenta from growing to an adequate size, resulting in a small or a malnourished infant. Pregnant adolescents are at high risk, simply because they are still growing and need extra stores of iron, calcium, and zinc.

Supplements during Pregnancy

The National Academy of Science's Institute of Medicine recommends individual assessment of dietary practices for all pregnant women. A well-balanced eating pattern is generally sufficient for optimal nutrition. Dietary supplements should not replace food. In fact, iron is the only supplement often required during normal pregnancy. Larger amounts are needed in the second and third trimesters, especially for the oldest and the youngest women. The fetus may exhaust the mother's body stores of iron and cause her to become anemic. A low-dose supplement of 30 mg is generally sufficient to provide the extra iron needed.[2]

Calcium Needs

The current Recommended Dietary Allowance (RDA) for calcium during pregnancy and lactation is 1,200 mg/day, regardless of age. Pregnancy creates a significant physiologic stress on maternal skeletal homeostasis. Full-term infants accumulate approximately 30 g of calcium during gestation, mainly during the third trimester. Data suggest that no permanent decline in body calcium occurs with pregnancy if recommended dietary calcium intake is achieved. No association is observed between parity and bone mass, and no evidence has surfaced to support changing the current recommendation of calcium intake for well-nourished, pregnant women.[2,3]

About 160 to 300 mg/day of maternal calcium is lost in breast milk. Longitudinal studies show that healthy women have an acute bone loss during lactation, but this is followed by rapid restoration of bone mass after weaning and return of menses.

The current opinion is that calcium intake does not affect the transient loss of bone mass during lactation. The National Institutes of Health (NIH) Consensus Development Conference stated that calcium intakes exceeding the current RDA of 1,200 mg are not justified for lactating women. Data are not available to show whether calcium requirements differ for pregnant women with closely spaced pregnancies or at the extremes of reproductive years.

Prenatal Weight Gain

The prepregnancy weight dictates the recommended weight gain during pregnancy. The prepregnancy weight, concomitant body mass index (BMI), and recommended weight gain are as follows:

- If underweight (e.g., BMI <19.8), then 28 to 40 pounds is recommended.
- If normal weight (e.g., BMI >19.8 and <26), then 25 to 35 pounds is recommended.
- If overweight (e.g., BMI is 26 to 29), then 15 to 25 pounds is recommended.
- If obese (e.g., BMI >29), then at least 15 pounds is recommended.

Weight gain during pregnancy should be gradual, with 25% of the total weight gain during the first trimester (four to six pounds) and 75% during the second and third trimesters (approximately one-half to one pound a week).[1] Overall rate of gain should remain relatively constant during the last two-thirds of gestation. During the second trimester, weight gain reflects expansion of maternal fluids and tissues. Weight gain during the third trimester represents growth of the fetal compartment (see Figure 9–1).[4]

Young adolescents and African-American women generally are at high risk for low-birth-weight babies. They should gain at the upper end of the recommended weight gain ranges. Nutrition supplementation during a high-risk pregnancy is advised for iron at 30 mg ferrous iron daily during the second and third trimesters. Folate at 300 mg daily may be needed if dietary folate intake is inadequate. Women who do not have an adequate eating pattern, are expecting multiple births (twins, triplets, etc.), smoke, or abuse alcohol or other drugs may need a multivitamin supplement. The supplement should contain 300 mg folate, 30 mg ferrous iron, 15 mg zinc, 2 mg copper, 250 mg calcium, 2 mg vitamin B_6, 50 mg vitamin C, and 5 mg vitamin D. A 600-mg calcium supplement seems to be appropriate for women under 25 years whose dietary intake is less than 600 mg daily. Zinc at 15 mg and 2 mg of copper should be provided when therapeutic levels of iron are given to treat anemia. Preconceptional administration of folate may be effective in reducing the risk of neural tube defect in the fetus.[4]

A healthy eating plan for pregnant women includes the following[1]:

- five servings of fruits and vegetables (one high in Vitamin A [such as apricots, carrots, broccoli] and one high in Vitamin C [oranges, grapefruit, tomatoes])
- seven servings of breads and cereals (four whole grain) (one serving equals one slice bread, ½ bun, ½ cup cooked cereal, ¾ cup dry cereal)
- three servings of milk and milk products (one serving equals 8 ounces milk or yogurt, ½ cup grated cheese, 2 cups cottage cheese)
- seven one-ounce servings of cooked meat, fish, poultry, or other protein foods such as beans, eggs, tofu, and peanut butter
- three teaspoons unsaturated fats, margarine, salad dressing
- one serving of foods rich in folate, such as dark green leafy vegetables, orange juice, liver, dried beans, or peas

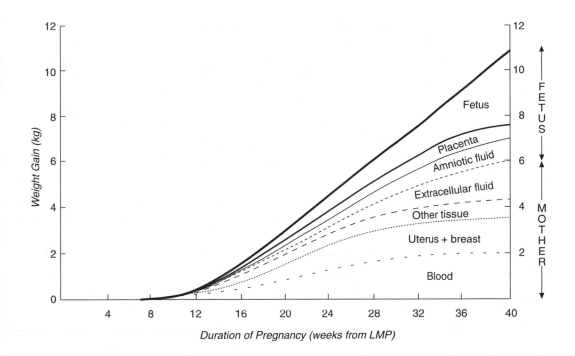

Figure 9-1 Pattern and distribution of weight gain: constant gain during second and third trimester, but different distribution (second trimester to mother and third trimester to fetus). *Source:* Reprinted from Pitkin R. *Nutrition during Pregnancy.* Nutritional Medicine in Medical Practice Symposium. 1993.

Women often experience nausea and vomiting in the first trimester. The following practices may reduce the discomfort[1]:

- Eat small, frequent meals at two-to-three-hour intervals; supplement meals with nutritious between-meal snacks like whole-grain breads or cottage cheese.
- Drink at least 10 glasses of fluid each day but not during meals.
- Eat dry crackers immediately upon feeling nauseous.
- Do not skip meals, as this may cause illness due to a lack of adequate blood sugar.
- Avoid or limit greasy, fried, or spicy foods and caffeinated drinks.
- Eat foods slowly.
- Avoid very hot or very cold foods.
- Do not resort to home remedies or over-the-counter medications without consulting the obstetrician.

Caffeine

Caffeine-containing foods or beverages consumed in moderation do not appear to affect fertility or create adverse health effects for the mother or fetus.[5]

Although studies differ in design and variables examined, the general consensus is that caffeine consumption does not affect the reported time to conceive. One study compared 2,800 women who delivered babies with 1,800 women diagnosed as infertile. A 1992 Canadian study of 40,000 women reported adverse effects of cigarettes and alcohol intake on pregnancy. Nonsmokers did not experience delayed conception, regardless of whether they were high or low caffeine consumers.[6]

The data regarding caffeine and miscarriages vary. Research at McGill University reported an association between the two. However, a study in the United States controlled for nausea, smoking, alcohol intake, and age of the mother reported no association. Moderate caffeine consumption (i.e., about three 8-ounce cups of coffee, tea, or carbonated beverage) has not been shown to cause either early birth or low-birth-weight babies, nor to influence motor development of the infant later in life.[7]

Caffeine transfers into breast milk, but an intake limited to two or three cups of coffee a day does not appear to give a significant amount in breast milk. The American Academy of Pediatrics Committee on Drugs supports this recommendation as an acceptable and safe level.[5,8-10]

Aspartame in Pregnancy

Aspartame, which is sold as NutraSweet brand sweetener, provides the sweet taste of sugar at four calories per individual pack. Aspartame is comprised of the amino acids aspartic acid and phenylalanine.

Since its discovery in 1965, aspartame has been thoroughly reviewed by numerous regulatory agencies and scientific organizations and found safe for consumption by pregnant women and teens. An 8-ounce glass of milk has six times more phenylalanine and 13 times more aspartic acid than an equivalent amount of carbonated beverage sweetened with NutraSweet. An 8-ounce glass of fruit juice contains three to five times more methanol than an equivalent amount of soda sweetened with NutraSweet.[11]

Individuals with phenylketonuria (PKU) cannot properly metabolize phenylalanine and must monitor their intake of this amino acid from all foods. Infants are routinely screened for PKU within 28 days of birth. Foods should contribute nutrients via a variety of foods and beverages. Foods sweetened with aspartame satisfy one's taste for sweets but may not provide a full array of nutrients to support growth of both the fetus and the mother.

Quality Assurance in Prenatal and Postpartum Nutrition

Quality assurance/quality improvement criteria for nutritional well-being of prenatal women and adolescents were developed by the Public Health Nutrition Practice Group of the American Dietetic Association[12] (see Appendix 9-A). The criteria are synonymous with clinical indicators and include women and adolescents at their first postpartum visit and breastfeeding women and adolescents with no chronic medical conditions. Preconception nutrition care does not fall within the scope of the criteria list.

The criteria are based on several sources.[13-15] They were field tested at six sites that served various cultural and geographic populations. A 75% achievement level at a minimum of one test site was required for retention as a final criteria. Implementation of the criteria requires a careful and thorough training of the monitoring staff.

Women's Health Issues

Cardiovascular disease is the major cause of death for US women (see Figure 9-2). It kills approximately 500,000 more women than men each year, with most deaths occurring in the fifth decade.[16] The major risk factors for cardiovascular disease in women are prevalent and modifiable among all ethnic groups (see Figure 9-3).[17] Lung cancer followed by breast cancer are the major causes of cancer death among women.[18] Osteoporosis is more common among women than men, causing over 1.5 million bone fractures annually.[19] Mortality rates differ among women in various ethnic groups.

Women's perceptions of their health risks may differ from reality[20] (see Table 9-1). For example, women of all ethnic groups may carry excess body weight and feel "fat" but not think their weight carries a health risk. African-American women may not participate in cancer screenings and may not practice breast self-exams or think of themselves at high risk for breast cancer. Many women do not make the connection between illness or morbidity and mortality. They do not view themselves as a potential statistic. Nor do they think their eating behavior is poor, since they see no immediate adverse effect. However, women of all ethnic groups face major health issues (see Figure 9-4).

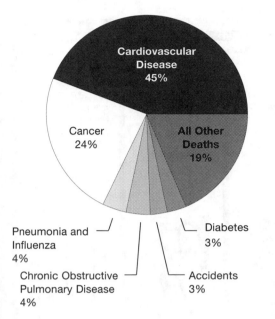

Figure 9-2 Leading causes of death as proportion of all deaths among women, 1991. *Source:* Reprinted from National Heart, Lung, and Blood Institute. *Heart Memo.* 1994, p.23.

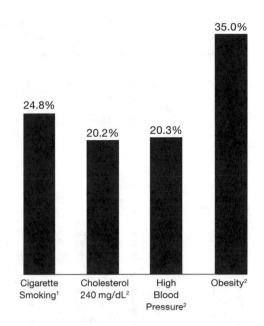

[1]Data from National Health Interview Survey, 1991.
[2]Data from National Health and Nutrition Examination Survey III, 1988–91.

Figure 9-3 Risk factor prevalence among women of all ethnic groups. *Source:* Reprinted from National Heart, Lung, and Blood Institute. *Heart Memo.* 1994, p.24.

Table 9–1 Women's Health—Perceptions versus Reality

Perception*	Reality
Majority of women surveyed cite breast cancer as the main health issue facing women.	Heart disease is the leading cause of death and disability in women today, affecting more women than men.
90% of women surveyed say their diet is healthy.	Only 20% of women today meet contemporary dietary recommendations.
77% of women describe their eating habits today as better than a few years ago.	Incidence of being overweight in women has increased by 32% from 1980 to 1991.
Women surveyed cite smoking as the prime risk factor for breast cancer.	Body weight and dietary habits are also factors that can influence the risk of breast cancer.

*Data from Women's Knowledge and Behavior Regarding Health and Fitness, 1993 Gallup poll conducted for Weight Watchers International, Inc., and The American Dietetic Association.

Source: Adapted from Finn S. ADA's Nutrition and Health Campaign for Women Promotes Research and Behavioral Change. *Perspectives in Applied Nutrition.* Winter 1993;1(3):3–7.

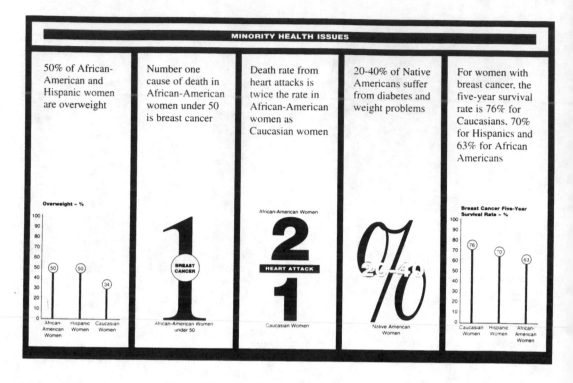

Figure 9-4 Minority health issues facing US women. *Source:* Adapted from Women's Knowledge and Behavior Regarding Health and Fitness, 1993 Gallup poll conducted for Weight Watchers International, Inc., and The American Dietetic Association.

Women's Health Initiative

Cardiovascular diseases, cancer, and osteoporosis have become the most common causes of mortality, disability, and impaired quality of life among postmenopausal women. They respond to primary prevention efforts with dietary, behavioral, and drug interventions. In 1992, under the leadership of NIH Director, Bernadine Healy, NIH initiated the Women's Health Initiative (WHI).[21] The WHI has three major components: a randomized controlled trial of promising but unproven approaches to prevention, an observational study to identify predictors of disease, and a trial of community approaches to develop healthful behaviors. A symbol has been adopted to identify the trial approach for a multicultural representation (see Figure 9-5).

The randomized, controlled clinical trial of the Women's Health Initiative will enroll 60,000 postmenopausal women 50 to 79 years of age between 1993 and 1996. This trial has three interventions, and women can enroll in one or more of the components. One intervention evaluates the effect of a low-fat dietary pattern on prevention of breast and colon cancer and coronary heart disease. A second intervention examines the effect of hormonal-replacement therapy on prevention of coronary heart disease, osteoporosis, and/or increased risk of breast cancer. The third intervention evaluates the effect of calcium and vitamin D supplementation on prevention of osteoporosis and colon cancer. Primary, secondary, and tertiary outcomes for the various arms of the trial are listed in Table 9-2.

The trial will require four years for protocol development and recruitment and nine years of follow up to achieve the goals. The first participants were enrolled in September 1993. Women who are ineligible or unwilling to participate in the trial can enroll in a long-term, 9-to-11-year observational study that will identify new risk

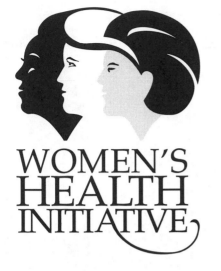

Figure 9-5 Women's Health Initiative emblem used on all communications. *Source:* National Institutes of Health. Bethesda, Maryland, 1995.

factors and biological markers for diseases in women. About 100,000 women will participate in this part of the study for a total of 160,000 women.

WHI studies are performed at 40 clinical centers located throughout the United States (see Table 9-3). One coordinating center, the Fred Hutchinson Cancer Research Center in Seattle, Washington, will manage data collection and analysis.

Each of the 40 clinical centers will recruit 3,490 postmenopausal women over a three-year period for the clinical trial and observational study. The broad geographic distribution of the clinical centers allows recruitment of medically underserved areas or target minority populations, as well as a representative cross-section of the US population (see Figure 9-6). Ten of the clinical centers will recruit primarily minority populations—African Americans, Hispanics, and Native Americans.

Table 9-2 Primary, Secondary, and Tertiary Outcomes for the Women's Health Trial, NIH, 1994

Outcome	Hormone Replacement	Dietary Modification	Vitamin D/Calcium Supplementation	Observational Study
Cardiovascular				
Coronary heart disease	a	b	c	c
Stroke	b	b	c	c
Congestive heart disease	b	b	c	c
Angina	b	b	c	c
Peripheral vascular disease	b	b	c	c
Coronary revascularization	b	b	c	c
Total cardiovascular	b	b	c	c
Cancer				
Breast cancer	b	a	b	c
Endometrial cancer	b	b	c	c
Colorectal cancer	c	a	b	c
Ovarian cancer	b	b	c	c
Total cancers	b	b	b	c
Fractures				
Hip	b	c	a	a
Other fractures	b	c	b	a
Total fractures	b	c	b	a
Venous thromboembolic disease				
Pulmonary embolism	b	c	c	a
Deep vein thrombosis	b	c	c	a
Diabetes mellitus requiring therapy	b	b	c	a
Death from any cause	b	b	b	a

Note: a = primary, b = secondary, c = tertiary end point.

Source: Adapted from National Institutes of Health, Women's Health Initiative. Protocol Vol 1, Section 2, pp. 2–22, 1993.

Table 9–3 Clinical Centers for the Women's Health Initiative

Location (N = 40)	Minority Population*
Albert Einstein College of Medicine	
Baylor College of Medicine	
Bowman Gray School of Medicine	
Brigham and Women's Hospital	
Emory University	a
Fred Hutchinson Cancer Research Center	
George Washington University	
Harbor-UCLA Research and Education Institute	
Kaiser Foundation Research Institute, Portland	
Kaiser Permanente Medical Care Program	
Medical College of Wisconsin	
Medlantic Research Institute	a
Memorial Hospital of Rhode Island	
Northwestern University	
Ohio State University	
Rush Presbyterian-St. Luke's Medical Center	a
Stanford University	
State University of New York at Buffalo	
State University of New York at Stony Brook	
University of Alabama at Birmingham	a
University of Arizona	d
University of California, Davis	
University of California, Irvine	
University of California, Los Angeles	
University of California, San Diego	b
University of Cincinnati Medical Center	
University of Florida	
University of Hawaii	c
University of Iowa	
University of Massachusetts Medical Center	
University of Medicine and Dentistry of New Jersey	
University of Miami	b
University of Minnesota	
University of Nevada, Reno	
University of North Carolina, Chapel Hill	
University of Pittsburgh	
University of Tennessee, Memphis	
University of Texas Health Science Center, San Antonio	b
University of Wisconsin, Madison	
Wayne State University	a

*60% minority population recruited: a = African American, b = Hispanic, c = Asian-Pacific Islander, d = American Indian.

Source: Adapted from National Institutes of Health. Women's Health Initiative. Protocol Vol 1, Section 2, pp. 2–25, 1993.

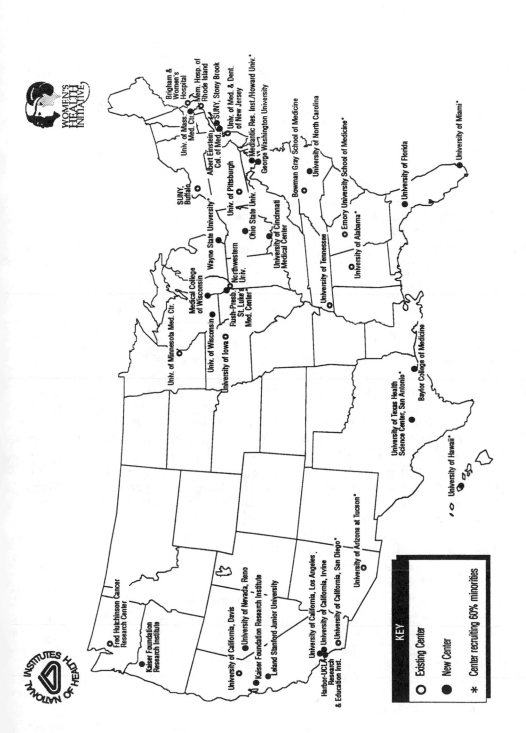

Figure 9–6 Location of Women's Health Initiative clinical centers, National Institutes of Health. *Source:* Reprinted from National Institutes of Health, Women's Health Initiative, 1994.

Implementation includes strategies to enhance adoption of healthful behaviors. Studies will mobilize community resources to enhance adoption of these behaviors by providing education, removing barriers, and improving social support. The behaviors target national goals described in *Healthy People 2000*.[22] As noted above, 10 clinical centers focus on minorities and the medically underserved because these groups have not received sufficient attention and have lagged in adoption of preventive behaviors.

The Women's Health Initiative will provide important, scientific, valid information for women, their health care providers, and their communities. This information will indicate the benefits and risks of preventive approaches and the means of achieving successful adoption of these behaviors. WHI will require 14 years and the investment of over $680 million.[21]

Part of the rationale for the study is to expand the database regarding the effect of women's lifestyles, habits, and response to therapies on health, morbidity, and mortality. Many national studies and clinical trials have not included women. Studies involving men have based their design on the premise that the results could be extrapolated to women.[23]

According to a June 1993 Gallup survey sponsored by the American Dietetic Association and Weight Watchers International, 87% of women believe they can reduce their risk for heart disease, 70% believe they can help alter their chances of developing osteoporosis, and 59% think they can slow their chances of developing breast cancer. The current problem is that few women take action to reduce their risk for these diseases. Only 55% of the women who were surveyed reported taking action to prevent heart disease risk, 44% reported action to prevent breast cancer, and 42% reported action against osteoporosis.[20]

As a result, the American Dietetic Association initiated the Nutrition and Health Campaign for Women, which includes research, public policy, industry, media, and grassroots efforts. The campaign recognizes that for each of these efforts, attention must be given to ethnic diversity, special needs of women, low-income women, young girls and teens, older women, and women with disabilities.[23]

Three key messages form the basis of the campaign:

1. Nutrition has a critical role in fitness and prevention of disease.
2. A low-fat diet is a preventive approach to high cholesterol and breast cancer. Regular exercise can enhance the effects.
3. Calcium can help prevent osteoporosis if girls between the ages of 8 and 18 years and older women consume adequate calcium.

Osteoporosis

Osteoporosis affects more than 25 million people in the United States, resulting primarily in bone fractures among postmenopausal and elderly women. In the absence of primary prevention during the next decades, women over 45 years old will experience 5.2 million fractures and incur $45.2 billion in health care costs.

There are about 195,000 vertebral fractures in the United States annually. At 50 years of age, a US Caucasian woman has a 32% chance of a vertebral fracture, 16% chance of a hip fracture, and 15% chance of a wrist fracture.[24] Peak bone mass achieved in the first 30 years of life and the rate at which bone is lost later in life are the major predisposing factors for osteoporosis. Adequate calcium intake, hormones, and lifestyle (mainly exercise) are critical to the process (see Chapter 16).

Obesity

More than one-third of US adults are considered obese. Approximately 35% of white females, 49% of African-American females, and 47% of Hispanic females are overweight or obese.[23] Excess weight is linked to five of ten leading causes of death in the United States: coronary heart disease, some cancers, diabetes, stroke, and atherosclerosis.

Studies have examined women's body weights and their personal values about their body size. One study reported the results of an open-ended interview completed by 36 Caucasian and 31 African-American women of varying socioeconomic status (SES).[25] The women's body size values and body mass index were assessed. Black women of lower SES were heavier, perceived themselves as heavier, and perceived attractive body size as heavier than black women of higher SES and white women of all SES levels. The body weight they considered overweight was considerably higher for black women of lower SES than for other cohorts.

Over one-third of black women perceived themselves as thinner than their actual size. White and black women at a higher SES reported more pressure to be thin because of lifestyle and their environment, especially the media. Black women tend to view obesity as the result of their capacity and opportunity for physical activity, and not a function of their eating behavior. Black women do believe obesity places them at risk for health problems. White women see obesity as a major threat to their self-esteem and social acceptance.[25]

It appears that black women of lower SES have a wider range of perceptions about "normal" and "attractive" body size. Their ideas of normal weight versus excess weight are more affected by social status, family, and peers when compared to white women and black women at higher SES, who are affected by images in the media. This type of study needs to be extended to larger samples of women in various ethnic groups. Diverse approaches to weight management require an understanding of the meaning of weight for individuals and their social context[25] (see Chapter 15).

Hypertension

Hypertension, a major risk factor in cardiovascular disease, is two to three times more common in women than in men, and is highest among African-American women.[23] Hypertension occurs nearly three times more frequently among overweight adults than normal-weight adults, and data suggest that one-third of all cases are caused by excess weight. Likewise, elevated blood pressure in overweight adults leads to an increased rate of stroke.

The National Health and Nutrition Examination Survey (NHANES) III data show a decline in the age-adjusted prevalence of hypertension for women, 20 to 74 years of age, from 34% (NHANES II) to 20% (NHANES III). The age-adjusted prevalence rate of hypertension is 31% among African-American women and 19% among white women[26] (see Chapter 14).

Diabetes

Diabetes mellitus, or high blood sugar, is a serious disorder that increases the risk of coronary heart disease. Diabetes is often called a "woman's disease" because, after age 45, about twice as many women as men develop diabetes. Over 80% of individuals with diabetes die of some type of cardiovascular disease (e.g., myocardial infarction). The risk of death from coronary heart disease is twice as common among women than men with diabetes. Compared with nondiabetic women, diabetic women tend to experience more hypertension and dyslipidemia. Untreated diabetes can also contribute to the development of kidney disease, blindness, problems in pregnancy and childbirth, neuropathy, and gangrene. For unknown reasons, the risks of heart disease and heart-related death are higher for diabetic women than for diabetic men.

Non-insulin-dependent diabetes mellitus or Type II diabetes develops in adulthood and is the most common form of the disease. Of all individuals with non-insulin-dependent diabetes mellitus, 85% are at least 20% overweight[27] (see Chapter 13).

Coronary Heart Disease and Cancer

Women with high total cholesterol and high LDL (low-density lipoprotein) cholesterol levels have significantly higher heart disease rates. Low HDL (high-density lipoprotein) cholesterol is associated with a high risk for heart disease; each milligram percent decline in HDL cholesterol produces a 2 to 3% increase in coronary disease risk. The National Cholesterol Education Panel recommendation is greater than

50 mg% HDL; less than 35 mg% HDL is a strong risk factor for coronary heart disease (CHD). With this backdrop, women seek to raise or to sustain their HDL levels beyond the impact of genetics. Weight loss, exercise, alcohol, and estrogen replacement enhance HDL cholesterol. Every pound of weight loss increases HDL cholesterol by one-half of a percent. Moderate, consistent exercise increases HDL cholesterol by 10%.[28]

The placement of body fat influences disease risk. A waist-to-hip ratio greater than 1.0 increases a women's risk for CHD, cancer, and other chronic diseases. It appears that stability of weight, especially in peri- and postmenopausal years, is associated with increased breast cancer risk. Several large cohort studies in the United States (N = 89,494 nurses 34 to 59 years old) and in the Netherlands (N = 62,573 women 55 to 69 years old) did not report significant associations between risk of breast cancer and fat intake.[28] It is thought that the vast majority of these women had a consistently high fat intake. A true test of the effect of low-fat eating behaviors on cancer risk with a sufficiently large sample has not been conducted, but will be addressed in the WHI.

Alcohol, vitamins and minerals, and aspirin are being investigated for their role in cancer and CHD risk. Alcohol intake increases risk of breast cancer; but moderate alcohol intake of two servings a day increases HDL cholesterol levels, which may lower overall CHD risk. The alcohol and breast cancer association appears to be dose-related, beginning with as few as two drinks a day. Vitamins A, C, and E and selenium are being examined for their role in breast cancer risk, whereas the role of vitamins in CHD has resulted in recommendations for behavioral changes. For example, Vitamin E supplementation for more than two years gave healthy women a relative risk for major coronary disease of 0.59 (95% CI; 0.38 to 0.91) after adjusting for age, smoking status, and use of other antioxidants.[29] A recent study reported that women who took low-dose aspirin regularly were less likely to have a first heart attack than women who did not take aspirin.[30]

Physical Activity

The 1990 National Health Interview Survey data estimate that 37.7% of women at least 18 years of age exercise regularly. Caucasian women exercise more often than African-American women (39% versus 28%). As age increases, irrespective of race, fewer women report exercising regularly.[26]

A major concern about physical activity programs for women is that the programs generally offer approaches for women already physically active. Marcus and Stanton[31] recommend a theoretical model to develop appropriate exercise programs. Their model links stages of change with stages of readiness to adapt a new behavior such as a physical activity program. In the "Imagine Action" model, individuals can be classified in one of several stages, as follows[31]:

- *Precontemplator:* Individual is not thinking about change. Common comment is "Do I need this?"
- *Contemplator:* Individual is thinking but not doing. Common incentive is "Try it, you'll like it!"
- *Preparer:* Individual is participating but not regularly. Common comment is "I'll try it once."
- *Person in action:* Individual is regular participant. Common incentive is "Keep it going."
- *Maintainer:* Physical activity has become a regular part of lifestyle. Common response is "I won't stop now."

This model has been used to define and to tailor exercise programs to meet people at their level of need. For example, low-impact aerobics are suitable for individuals who have never exercised and don't wish to show their lack of activity.[31] Women with hypertension, Type II diabetes mellitus, or any joint disease may also benefit from low-impact aerobics.

Average energy expenditure during various types of physical activities is shown in Table 9–4.[32] Women are encouraged to select physical activities they enjoy and can place into their lifestyle. Consistent, frequent participation in activities women enjoy has a positive influence on their long-term adherence.

A sample walking program from the National Heart, Lung, and Blood Institute is outlined in Table 9–5. Individuals should strive for a minimum of three exercise sessions each week of the program. If they find a particular week's pattern tiring, they should repeat it before moving to the next pattern. The walking program does not have to be completed in 12 weeks.

Individuals should check their pulse periodically to see if they are exercising within a target zone (see Table 9–6). As individuals become more physically fit, they should try exercising within the upper range of the target zone. Encourage individuals to increase their brisk walking time gradually from 30 to 60 minutes, three or four times a week. Remind them that their goal is to acquire both cardiovascular benefits and enjoyment.

Use the following method to check if individual is within target heart rate zone:

1. Immediately after exercising stops, have individual take her pulse. Place the tips of her first two fingers lightly over one of the blood vessels on the neck, just to the left or right of the Adam's apple. Or try the pulse spot inside the wrist just below the base of the thumb.
2. Count the pulse for 10 seconds, and multiply the number by 6.
3. Compare the number to the target heart rate in Table 9–6. Look for the age grouping that is closest to the individual's age, and read the line across. For example, if she is 43, the closest age on the chart is 45; the target zone is 88–131 beats per minute.

Table 9–4 Relative Energy Expenditure of 14 Common Physical Activities

Physical Activity	Energy Expenditure*
Bicycling 6 mph	240 cals/hr
Bicycling 12 mph	410 cals/hr
Cross-country skiing	700 cals/hr
Jogging 5½ mph	740 cals/hr
Jogging 7 mph	920 cals/hr
Jumping rope	750 cals/hr
Running in place	650 cals/hr
Running 10 mph	1280 cals/hr
Swimming 25 yds/min	275 cals/hr
Swimming 50 yds/min	500 cals/hr
Tennis-singles	400 cals/hr
Walking 2 mph	240 cals/hr
Walking 3 mph	320 cals/hr
Walking 4½ mph	440 cals/hr

*Energy expended varies in proportion to body weight; a 100-pound person burns one-third fewer calories (i.e., multiply the number of calories by 0.7); for a 200-pound person, multiply by 1.3. A preferred way to increase calories per activity is to increase the time spent per activity.

Source: Adapted from *Exercise and Your Heart*, National Heart, Lung, and Blood Institute/American Heart Association, NIH Publication No. 93-1677. August 1993.

Info Line

Three reproducible fact sheets, developed by the National Heart, Lung, and Blood Institute and the Indian Health Service, are designed for American Indian and Alaska Native women.

- "Keep the Harmony Within You—Check Your Blood Pressure" offers useful tips for people who have high blood pressure.
- "Treat Your Heart to a Healthy Celebration" emphasizes that native foods and traditional ways of preparing foods can help people stay healthy. Tips for making healthy food choices are offered.
- "Give Your Heart a Workout" stresses the importance of being a gift of the earth; it should be used to show respect and honor and should not be abused. The harmful effects of tobacco are described.

To order a free copy of the fact sheets, write to NHLBI Information Center, PO Box 30105, Bethesda, MD 20824-0105.

Table 9–5 A Sample Walking Program

	Warm Up	Target Zone Exercising	Cool Down Time	Total Time
Week 1				
Session A	Walk normally 5 minutes	Then walk briskly 5 minutes	Then walk normally 5 minutes	15 minutes
Session B	Repeat above			
Session C	Repeat above			
Week 2	Walk 5 minutes	Walk briskly 7 minutes	Walk 5 minutes	17 minutes
Week 3	Walk 5 minutes	Walk briskly 9 minutes	Walk 5 minutes	19 minutes
Week 4	Walk 5 minutes	Walk briskly 11 minutes	Walk 5 minutes	21 minutes
Week 5	Walk 5 minutes	Walk briskly 13 minutes	Walk 5 minutes	23 minutes
Week 6	Walk 5 minutes	Walk briskly 15 minutes	Walk 5 minutes	25 minutes
Week 7	Walk 5 minutes	Walk briskly 18 minutes	Walk 5 minutes	28 minutes
Week 8	Walk 5 minutes	Walk briskly 20 minutes	Walk 5 minutes	30 minutes
Week 9	Walk 5 minutes	Walk briskly 23 minutes	Walk 5 minutes	33 minutes
Week 10	Walk 5 minutes	Walk briskly 26 minutes	Walk 5 minutes	36 minutes
Week 11	Walk 5 minutes	Walk briskly 28 minutes	Walk 5 minutes	38 minutes
Week 12	Walk 5 minutes	Walk briskly 30 minutes	Walk 5 minutes	40 minutes
Week 13	Gradually increase brisk walking time from 30 to 60 minutes.			

Source: Adapted from *Exercise and Your Heart*, National Heart, Lung, and Blood Institute/American Heart Association, NIH Publication No. 93-1677. August 1993.

In Part III of this book, separate chapters address different chronic diseases. Issues relevant to both women and men are included.

THE ADULT MALE AND HIS NUTRITION NEEDS

Significant changes in the roles of men and women in the 1980s led to new challenges in the 1990s regarding health and nutrition of men. More than 75% of men stated in a Gallup Poll that they are concerned about the effect of eating on their health. The strange twist was that only 23% of the men could name the major food groups. Men appear to have ideas or assumptions about the components of healthy eating, but limited knowledge to help them make informed food choices.[33]

Men have many of the same risk factors as women for chronic disease, but some differences exist. Due to a greater muscle mass, men have higher metabolic rates, which result in a higher calorie expenditure than women for the same activity. Men accumulate fat in their midsection rather than in the upper or lower body as ob-

served for women. The midsection location for fat deposition increases a man's waist-to-hip ratio and his risk for cardiovascular disease, hypertension, and diabetes. Conversely, men appear to be more successful than women at losing weight; however, their lifestyle and work habits may invite excess weight gain.[33]

Eating on the run and choosing high-fat and high-sugar baked products adds excessive fat calories. Approximately 30% of a man's energy and fat intake is ingested outside his home. This includes snacks that come from vending machines, snack bars, and airport terminals. Business meals, entertaining, and relaxing after work often include alcoholic beverages, which increase the total number of calories ingested, stimulate insulin, and promote weight gain. High-fat food selections at meals and snacks instead of abundant carbohydrate foods promote a higher weight gain.

Men who consistently participate in a physical activity, fitness program, or team sports may demonstrate a keener sense about food selections to enhance performance. The desire to remain physically fit opens the door for focused nutrition education and primary prevention efforts.[33]

Table 9–6 Target Heart Rate Zone by Age for Men and Women

Age	Target Heart Rate Zone (Beats/Minute)
20 years	100–150
25 years	98–140
30 years	95–142
35 years	93–138
40 years	90–135
45 years	88–131
50 years	85–127
55 years	83–123
60 years	80–120
65 years	78–116
70 years	75–113

Source: Reprinted from *Exercise and Your Heart*, National Heart, Lung, and Blood Institute/American Heart Association, NIH Publication No. 93-1677. August 1993.

Once men have been diagnosed with a chronic disease (e.g., hypertension or diabetes) or identified as having a risk factor for coronary heart disease (CHD) (e.g., hyperlipidemia), they may be more receptive to dietary instruction and behavioral change. Data from numerous randomized clinical trials have shown that lowering cholesterol levels among men at high risk for CHD reduces the incidence of CHD.[34-54] These studies have been summarized by Kris-Etherton[34] and include the following:

- The Lipid Research Clinics Coronary Primary Prevention Trial showed a 19% lower incidence of CHD among men in the cholestyramine and diet arm of the trial versus those in the placebo and diet group. Total plasma cholesterol and LDL cholesterol were 8% and 12% lower, respectively, in the cholestyramine and diet group compared with the placebo and diet group.[53,54]

- In the Multiple Risk Factor Intervention Trial, the effect of a multifactor intervention over seven years on mortality from CHD was observed in 12,866 high-risk men, aged 35 to 57. The men were randomized into either (1) special intervention, including stepped-care hypertension reduction, nutrition modi-

fication to reduce serum total cholesterol, and smoking cessation; or (2) the usual care from their own physicians. A 7.1% decrease in mortality (which was not significant) was observed in the special-intervention group compared to the usual-care group. CHD mortality was 17.9 per 1,000 in the special-intervention group and 19.3 per 1,000 in the usual-care group.[51]

- The Cholesterol-Lowering Atherosclerosis Study assessed the effects of decreasing LDL cholesterol and increasing HDL cholesterol on the growth of atherosclerotic lesions. Participants included 162 eligible men who had coronary bypass surgery; they were randomized into a treatment or control group. Treatment group participants ($N = 80$) received colestipol-niacin and instruction for a low-fat diet (i.e., 22% calories from fat; 10% as polyunsaturated, 4% as saturated, and 125 mg of cholesterol a day). The control group ($N = 82$) received placebo pills and instruction on a low-fat diet comprised of 250 mg of cholesterol per day, 26% calories from fat, 10% as polyunsaturated and 5% as saturated. For the colestipol group, plasma total cholesterol and LDL cholesterol were lowered by 26% and 43%, respectively, and HDL cholesterol was increased by 37% within two years. This is in contrast to the placebo group, whose total cholesterol and LDL cholesterol were lowered by 4% and 5%, respectively. The colestipol group had significantly less lesion progression and new atheroma development in the native coronary arteries. Atherosclerotic regression was noted in 16.2% of the colestipol men versus 2.4% in the placebo group.[55]

Data show that the incidence of CHD morbidity and mortality can be reduced in men at high risk for CHD, and also that primary and secondary prevention efforts are effective in reducing CHD mortality. The incidence of recurrent myocardial infarction and death due to CHD can be reduced. Lowering plasma total cholesterol levels and LDL cholesterol levels (e.g., by a fat-modified eating pattern) can lower the incidence of CHD among men either with or prior to a diagnosis of CHD.[34]

The extent of the reduction in CHD has been defined by baseline serum cholesterol level. That is, individuals in the 250 to 300 mg/dL range can expect for each 1% reduction in the serum cholesterol level, a 2% reduction in the incidence of CHD.[53,54] This means that a 10% to 15% reduction in the serum cholesterol level can reduce CHD risk by 20% to 30%. Men who smoke or have hypertension can greatly benefit from cholesterol lowering.

Intervention and longitudinal studies demonstrate a benefit of both minimal and average increases in HDL cholesterol levels. Every 1 mg/dL increment in baseline HDL cholesterol produced a 3.5% to 5.5% decrease in CHD as noted in the Lipid Research Clinic's Coronary Primary Prevention Trial,[53,54] the Lipid Research Clinic's Prevalence Study, and the Framingham Study.[56] Specifically, each 1 mg/dL increase in HDL cholesterol from baseline equaled a 4.4% reduction in CHD risk.[56]

- For men in the Veterans Administration Cooperative Study Group on Antihypertensive Agents,[57-59] a positive benefit was noted when blood pressure was controlled. For middle-aged men having average diastolic levels of 115 to 129 mm Hg, a 93% reduction in the rate of nonfatal plus fatal complications of CHD was noted. If men had a diastolic blood pressure of 105 to 114 mm Hg, the reduction was 69%. For most of the clinical trials with antihypertensive drugs, the men who received the drug had a significant reduction in the incidence of stroke.[60]

For men who stop smoking, CHD risk status improves.[61] Stopping after one or more myocardial infarctions also improves the prognosis of fatal and nonfatal CHD.[62] Further, the Physician's Health Study with 22,071 men observed that taking one aspirin every other day can lower heart disease risk. In addition, the Baltimore Longitudinal Study of Aging has yielded important data regarding the natural aging process (see Chapter 10).

Adult men do experience osteoporosis and fractures of the hip and vertebrae but at a lower frequency than women. Calcium intake, exercise, and overall eating pattern is as important for men as for women. The calcium RDA for adult men is 800 mg per day.[3]

Obesity and Healthy Body Weight

The risk of diabetes increases about twofold in people who are mildly overweight, fivefold in those who are moderately overweight, and tenfold in those who are obese. Medical professionals strongly recommend achieving a healthy weight, which is considered the single most important strategy for adults to improve their health status. A 10% weight loss promotes positive health benefits. Overweight people who lose only two pounds can lower blood cholesterol, and a seven-pound weight loss can lower high blood pressure to normal.

The *Dietary Guidelines for Americans* contain a suggested healthy body weight range based on an individual's height[63] (see Chapter 15). It is recommended that women attain the lower weight in a range unless they are physically active, in which case they are recommended to attain the higher weight in a range.

Info Line

A quick way to estimate healthy body weight for women, 18 to 25 years old, is to use the formula of 100 pounds plus 5 pounds for every inch over 5 feet. For example, a woman who is 5 feet 7 inches would have a healthy body weight of 135 pounds. The weight range is ± 10%, and for each year under 25, subtract 1 pound. For men, the formula is 110 pounds at 5 feet plus 5 pounds for every inch over 5 feet.

Source: Hamilton EMN, Whitney EN, and Sizer FS. *Nutrition: Concepts and Controversies.* 4th ed. Los Angeles, CA. West Publishing Company. 1988.

Millions of men and women in the United States strive to control their body weight. One of the most controversial weight-loss methods is the very-low-calorie diet (VLCD), a diet containing no more than 800 kcal per day or no more than 12 kcal per kg of ideal body weight per day. The VLCD is designed to promote significant short-term weight loss rapidly, while avoiding the risks of total fasting.[64]

Very-low-calorie diets are provided in the context of comprehensive treatment programs, in the course of which the patient's usual intake is totally replaced by specific foods or liquid formulas. Weight loss on a VLCD averages 1.5 to 2.5 kg/week, with total losses averaging 20 kg after 12 to 16 weeks of treatment. In contrast, standard low-calorie diets that provide 1,200 kcal/day produce losses of 0.4 to 0.5 kg/week and an average total loss of 6 to 8 kg. There is little evidence that an intake of less than 800 kcal/day leads to even greater weight loss. To preserve lean body mass, it appears necessary to provide protein of high biological value in an amount of at least 1 g/per kg of ideal body weight per day. Serious complications are infrequent with modern VLCDs; the most common complication is cholelithiasis.[34]

It appears that modern VLCDs are generally safe under proper medical supervision. They may be used with adults who are moderately or severely obese, and they may be expected to promote significant short-term weight loss and to improve obesity-related disorders. Long-term weight loss, however, is not very impressive. It appears helpful to accompany a VLCD with behavioral measures and physical activity.

THE CONSUMER IN THE HEALTH AND FITNESS MARKET

When individuals accept a personal responsibility for their health, they often find their participation in aerobic exercise and physical conditioning more likely if they can work amid family and friends. Many of today's health-conscious consumers consider joining a health club as important as paying for medical services. There are a variety of facilities from private club memberships with fitness rooms, to fitness centers for families, to facilities located in large business centers. The location and hours of operation often influence attendance. The extent of programs offered (e.g., aerobics and child care) may determine whether women participate.

Facilities may have highly automated equipment in addition to free weights, stationary exercise bikes, treadmills, stair climbers, and rowing machines. Qualifications of personnel determine the level of counseling, instruction, and follow up to defined programs. Personal trainers are generally available to assist clients with programs.

Most fitness centers require monthly or annual contracts; special reduced entrance fees are often available two or three times a year. Membership may include a trial period or the opportunity to add additional services to a basic membership packet. This may include racquetball or aerobic exercise fees.

Passive exercise devices and techniques are still available in most facilities for strength training (e.g., barbells, dumbbells, and exercise machines). Isometric training requires a person to push against an immovable object. Vibrating equipment and rubberized inflatable suits do not cause the body to expend appreciable energy. Strength training has a small impact on cardiovascular fitness and only expends about 4 calories per minute.[65] Other equipment available includes motion machines, motor-driven exercise bikes, vibrating belts, rolling machines, massage, rubberized inflatable suits, and electrical stimulation devices. Cosmetic additions to health clubs may include spas, steam baths, and saunas. Tanning beds may be available, but their use is a concern due to the exposure to two types of ultraviolet radiation, ultraviolet B (UVB) and ultraviolet A (UVA). The light is similar to sunlight but is more intense and can produce an effect in a relatively short period of time. Because tanning booths are not inspected, users should take caution.

The overall purpose of regular physical activity is to condition the heart and blood vessels. Other benefits include the following[65]:

- maintaining normal blood pressure or reducing blood pressure in people with hypertension
- maintaining a healthy body weight
- preventing or reducing chronic low-back pain
- improving sleep habits
- reserving energy for work and leisure
- increasing ability to cope with illness or accidents
- reducing fatigue

Both women and men have a greater chance of dying from heart disease, cancer, and several other causes when they have sedentary lifestyles than when they have a modest amount of activity. Greater longevity is associated with a daily brisk walk lasting 30 to 60 minutes. Strength training generally is not aerobic, but isometric. What is important to note is that strenuous exercise, such as long-distance running, is not required for good health.[65] Persistent and consistent aerobic exercise can create a training effect or real physiologic changes, but a sufficient amount and duration of exercise is required for a training effect (see Table 9–7).[66]

Selecting appropriate clothing and shoes for exercise are important. Cotton clothing for comfort is needed for exercise in hot, humid weather. Sufficient clothing is needed for exercise in cold weather to retain the body heat without creating excess sweat. Shoes should be selected to provide ample support and a comfortable fit during activities such as running, jogging, biking, etc.

During pregnancy, the major concern regarding exercise is whether there is a possibility of injury to the fetus or to the mother. During the first trimester, a possible teratogenic effect of high maternal body temperature can occur. Keeping a core body temperature is important. It is not known if certain exercises are potentially more harmful or if a threshold of intensity of an exercise is an issue.[67]

Info Line

DINE Healthy—a dietitian's personal trainer for nutrition and fitness—is a comprehensive nutrition software designed to help dietitians and health care professionals teach clients how to modify their eating behaviors and improve their exercise levels. With the software, clients can do the following:

- set their own nutrition and exercise goals
- learn to change their current eating habits by changing the type and amount of food they eat
- use the DINE Score to choose healthy foods to improve their eating pattern (see Figure 9–7)
- print reports

DINE Healthy sorts foods by nutrient content from either highest to lowest amount or lowest to highest amount. The database contains more than 7,200 foods. Fast foods, fat-free and low-sodium foods, and an exercise database are included. Clients' weight changes can be tracked on a daily or weekly basis. The software provides a sample seven-day perfect meal plan and recipes for clients trying to improve their food and beverage choices.

Source: DINE Systems, 586 North French Road, Amherst, New York 14228, 1-800-688-1848.

HEALTH BELIEFS, HEALTH STATUS, AND VITAMIN/MINERAL SUPPLEMENTATION

Health beliefs, self-reported health status, and vitamin/mineral supplementation were assessed with a random sample of 1,730 adults in seven western US states.[68] Chi-square analysis was used

Table 9–7 Popular Aerobic Activities and Fitness Points Achieved

Points	Exercise	Amount	Duration
11	Walking/running	3.0 miles	30–36 minutes
10.5	Swimming	1,000 yards	17–25 minutes
10	Walking/running	1.5 miles	Under 9 minutes
9	Running in place	100–110 steps/minute	15–17 minutes
9	Cycling	6 miles	Less than 18 minutes
9	Rope skipping	—	30 minutes
8	Rowing	20 strokes/minute	36 minutes

Source: Data from K. Cooper, *The New Aerobics*. New York: Bantam Books, 1970.

on pooled data to evaluate significant differences in demographic and personal characteristics across frequency of vitamin/mineral supplement use. Three frequency categories were nonuser, regular user, and occasional user. Health status was a self-reported measure, described as excellent, very good, good, fair, or poor.

Of the respondents, 35% reported their health as very good, 21% responded excellent, 8% said fair, and 3% said poor. A significant difference was noted in eating patterns for different ethnic groups and different educational levels. More Caucasians considered themselves in better health (p <0.001). Adults with a higher education reported having better health (p <0.01). A significant difference was noted in reported health status by income and marital status. Married adults and individuals at higher income categories reported a higher health rating ($p \leq 0.01$ and $p \leq 0.001$, respectively). A positive association was found between vitamin/mineral supplement users and perception of reduced susceptibility and/or severity of health problems (p <0.01). Specific illnesses cited were stress, colds, skin problems, heart attacks and cancer.

Findings from this study are consistent with earlier findings. Supplement use was common among individuals who followed an exercise regimen or believed that supplement use provided a health benefit.[69-71] In fact, taking a vitamin supplement may fulfill the general public's need to be proactive about their health. Recently, the American Dietetic Association's Survey of American Dietary Habits explored US eating patterns and attitudes about eating to influence health.[72] Three population subgroups were identified: Group A—"I'm doing it" (26%); Group B—"I know, but" (38%); and Group C—"Leave me alone" (36%).

Individuals in Group A believe nutrition and foods are important but tend to have misconceptions about the interactions; 93% of this group feel they are doing all they can. In Group B, only 32% of members are willing to give up favorite foods. For Group C, 83% are adamant about not giving up their favorite foods.

A consumer profile study on produce use revealed that people tried a new type of produce for the following reasons: a friend recommended (29%), a household member requested (21%), it was needed for a recipe (18%), and they heard or read about it in a magazine (16%).[73]

Cholesterol and fat content of foods continue to be major concerns of the US consumer. Vitamins and minerals rank high. Although balance, variety, and moderation are key concepts that Americans believe influence the health quality of their eating pattern, two-thirds of Americans choose food based on a "good" or "bad" perception (see Figure 9–8). Overall, 80% of US adults are concerned about the effect of what they eat on their future health.[72]

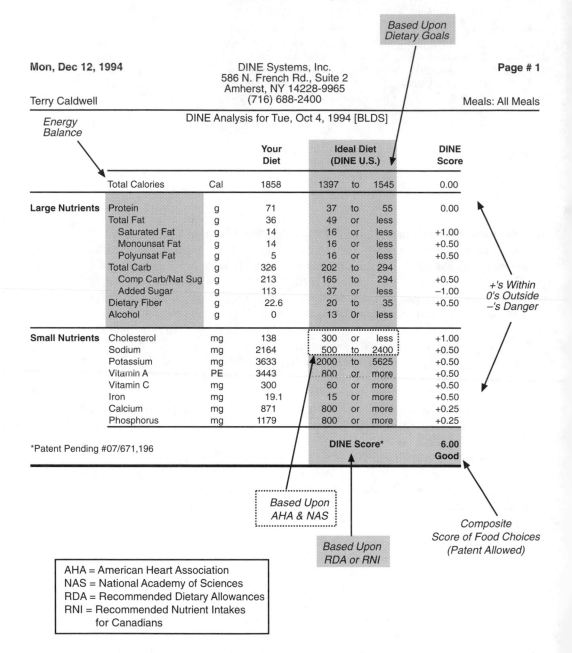

DINE Score Analysis

Based Upon Dietary Goals

Mon, Dec 12, 1994

DINE Systems, Inc.
586 N. French Rd., Suite 2
Amherst, NY 14228-9965
(716) 688-2400

Page # 1

Terry Caldwell

Meals: All Meals

Energy Balance

DINE Analysis for Tue, Oct 4, 1994 [BLDS]

			Your Diet	Ideal Diet (DINE U.S.)			DINE Score
	Total Calories	Cal	1858	1397	to	1545	0.00
Large Nutrients	Protein	g	71	37	to	55	0.00
	Total Fat	g	36	49	or	less	
	Saturated Fat	g	14	16	or	less	+1.00
	Monounsat Fat	g	14	16	or	less	+0.50
	Polyunsat Fat	g	5	16	or	less	+0.50
	Total Carb	g	326	202	to	294	
	Comp Carb/Nat Sug	g	213	165	to	294	+0.50
	Added Sugar	g	113	37	or	less	−1.00
	Dietary Fiber	g	22.6	20	to	35	+0.50
	Alcohol	g	0	13	Or	less	
Small Nutrients	Cholesterol	mg	138	300	or	less	+1.00
	Sodium	mg	2164	500	to	2400	+0.50
	Potassium	mg	3633	2000	to	5625	+0.50
	Vitamin A	PE	3443	800	or	more	+0.50
	Vitamin C	mg	300	60	or	more	+0.50
	Iron	mg	19.1	15	or	more	+0.50
	Calcium	mg	871	800	or	more	+0.25
	Phosphorus	mg	1179	800	or	more	+0.25

*Patent Pending #07/671,196

DINE Score* — **6.00 Good**

+'s Within 0's Outside −'s Danger

Based Upon AHA & NAS

Based Upon RDA or RNI

Composite Score of Food Choices (Patent Allowed)

AHA = American Heart Association
NAS = National Academy of Sciences
RDA = Recommended Dietary Allowances
RNI = Recommended Nutrient Intakes
      for Canadians

Figure 9–7 DINE score analysis. A sample printout that profiles a food intake by large and small nutrients and a composite score. *Source:* Reprinted from DINE Systems, Inc. Amherst, NY. Copyright © 1994.

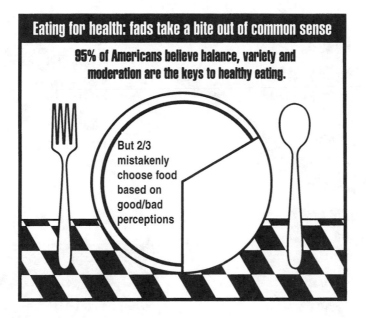

Eating for health: fads take a bite out of common sense

95% of Americans believe balance, variety and moderation are the keys to healthy eating.

But 2/3 mistakenly choose food based on good/bad perceptions

Figure 9-8 Eating for health: fads take a bite out of common sense. *Source:* Gallup Survey for International Food Information Council and The American Dietetic Association. 1992.

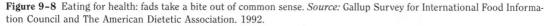

Men eat out slightly more often than women. The average number of meals eaten away from home in a week increases for men after 24 years of age and as the family income increases. Lunch is the most common commercially prepared meal; breakfast is the most frequently skipped meal. About 54% eat one or more dinner meals away from home each week.[74] The International Food Information Council and the American Dietetic Association have developed "10 Healthy Eating Tips" for Adults (see Figure 9-9).

COMMUNITY-ORIENTED PROGRAMS

Several community-based organizations provide direct service to adults on a national basis. Only two of the programs are described here—the Cooperative Extension System and the Women, Infants and Children Program.

The Cooperative Extension System

The Cooperative Extension (CE) System is a nationwide, tax-supported, educational program that enables people to make practical decisions in life. The CE mission is to help people improve their lives through an educational process using scientific knowledge focused on issues and needs. The CE System is based on a funding partnership of federal, state, and county governments. The Smith Lever Act of 1914 established a partnership between the US Department of Agriculture (USDA) and land grant universities. Legislation in various states allowed governments or organized groups at the county level to become a third legal partner.[75]

This educational system includes professionals in each US land grant university, at Tuskegee University, and in American Samoa, the District of Columbia, Guam, Micronesia, Northern Marianas, Puerto Rico, and the US Virgin Islands.

HOW ARE AMERICANS MAKING FOOD CHOICES?

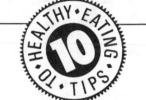

HOW ARE AMERICANS MAKING FOOD CHOICES?

1. Eat a variety of nutrient-rich foods.

2. Enjoy plenty of whole grains, fruits and vegetables.

3. Maintain a healthy weight.

4. Eat moderate portions.

5. Eat regular meals.

6. Reduce, don't eliminate, certain foods.

7. Balance your food choices over time.

8. Know *your* diet pitfalls.

9. Make changes gradually.

10. Remember, foods are not good or bad.

Source International Food Information Council and The American Dietetic Association.

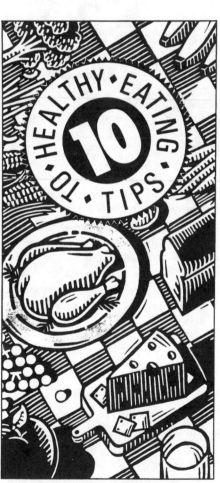

For a free copy send a self-addressed, business-size envelope to: 10 Tips, P.O. Box 1144, Rockville, MD 20850

Figure 9–9 10 Healthy Eating Tips. *Source:* International Food Information Council and The American Dietetic Association. 1992.

The land grant universities are listed in Appendix 9–B.

Basic programs of the CE System include the following:

- agriculture competitiveness and profitability
- community resources and economic development
- family development and resource management
- 4-H and youth development
- leadership and volunteer development
- natural resources and environmental management
- nutrition, diet, and health

From these basic programs and with strategic planning, national initiatives are developed every five years. The current national initiatives are:

- food safety and quality
- international marketing
- plight of young children
- revitalizing rural America
- sustainable agriculture
- waste management
- water quality
- youth at risk

In most states, the CE System is the university's service window to each county. Research information flows from the university to help a diversified audience to (1) improve the quality of their lives, (2) develop problem-solving skills, (3) become more competent consumers, (4) conserve and wisely use the natural resources, and (5) build better communities.

Resident professional researchers and educators are located in county offices. These professionals include farm advisors, home economists, and 4-H youth development advisors. The county-based advisors link with land grant university research programs through CE specialists who are faculty.[75]

Cooperative Extension programs differ from most programs offered by universities and community-based organizations in three important ways[75]:

1. All of CE training activities and programs are offered free or for a small fee to cover the cost of materials used in the program.
2. Most of CE's educational programs do not offer college credit.
3. CE programs are held at off-campus locations throughout the county, at times and places convenient to the clientele.

Besides offering workshops, seminars, and field days, CE publishes information on various topics of interest to consumers, homemakers, business people, farmers, educators, and researchers. Businesses and industries receive CE information and training principally in the areas of agronomy and range management, environmental horticulture, and consumer marketing.

Major programs in CE include the Adult and Youth Expanded Food and Nutrition Education Program, the Home Economics Program, the Environment Horticulture Program, the 4-H Youth Development Program, and the Urban Horticulture Program.

Consumer Program

This program responds to consumer needs for sound, objective information on food safety, food fads, prenatal and infant information, food quality, and childhood obesity. Consumers receive information on financial planning and management skills through MONEY SENSE programs. New parents and parents of school-age children benefit from age-appropriate home-learning programs such as "Parent Express" and the "Caring" series.

Expanded Food and Nutrition Education Program (EFNEP)

This program was established in 1969 when the federal government officially realized that hunger existed in the United States. The program's mission is to improve the dietary well-being of low-income families. The goal of EFNEP is to help low-income families, especially those with young children, to acquire the knowledge, skills, attitudes, and behavior changes necessary to improve their food intake. The target audience includes low-income families living in rural or urban areas and, specifically, family members who are responsible for planning and/or preparing their family's meals. Nutrition education assistants are recruited from the community and receive a six-week training session before placement in an assigned work area. They receive training in basic nutrition, food purchasing, budgeting, menu planning, and community resources, and monthly inservice training as needed.

Working with small groups of six to eight people, EFNEP makes serial presentations to introduce basic nutrition, meal planning, food preparation, sanitation, food storage, food preservation, and food buying to participants. Food demonstrations and food sampling help partici-

pants learn additional key nutritional concepts and practices. Six to eight class sessions are held, with the last session consisting of a visit to a local supermarket to practice wise shopping (see Figure 9–10). Upon completion of six to eight group sessions, a certificate of participation is presented to each participant.

Since 1986, EFNEP has expanded to include training in local emergency food distribution systems. Training is also available for staff and volunteers in related agencies that work with low-income groups. EFNEP has developed a creative media approach that includes a food stamp hotline, a Spanish language radio program, and videotapes to disseminate nutrition information.

In 1970, a youth component of EFNEP was implemented to instill positive behaviors in children at an earlier age. The youth component of

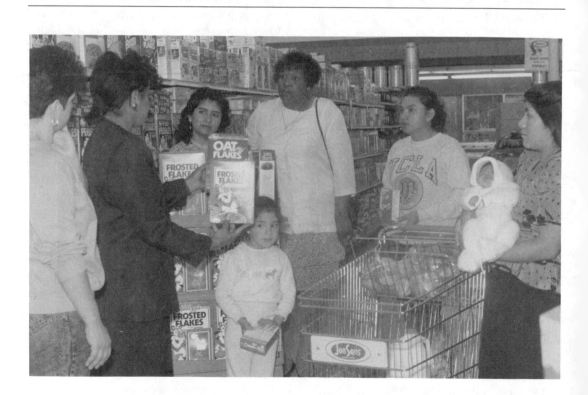

Figure 9–10 EFNEP nutrition education assistant conducts supermarket tour to teach women about unit prices and food selection, Los Angeles, California, 1991. *Source:* Reprinted with permission from Los Angeles County Cooperative Extension System. 1995.

EFNEP operates under the 4-H Youth Development Program. The target audience includes youths, 5 to 18 years old, who live in low-income geographic areas; youths from families participating in Adult EFNEP; youths who receive free or reduced-price school lunch and free breakfast; youths from families receiving Aid to Families with Dependent Children (AFDC); and youths from families enrolled in other low-income programs.

The CE staff provide an educational curriculum that reflects the nutritional needs and cultural heritage of the audience. The curriculum also includes information on food safety, shopping, and developing job skills. The programs can be tailored to meet special educational needs, such as the needs of developmentally disabled children; soon-to-be emancipated foster children; low-literacy youths; pregnant adolescents; and immigrant children. Programs are also delivered via summer day camps and after-school programs. Volunteer and extenders for the programs include parents, teachers, agency staff, college and university students, and recreation leaders.[75]

Women, Infants and Children

The Special Supplemental Food Program for Women, Infants and Children (WIC) is a federal nutrition program that provides nutritious food, individual counseling, and health care referrals to high-risk, low-income women and children up to the age of five. The purpose of the WIC program is to prevent poor birth outcomes, such as infant mortality and low birth weight, and to improve the nutrition and health of participants. Many studies report WIC to be a cost-effective and positive primary prevention strategy.

Nationwide, WIC currently serves about 6.4 million low-income, nutritionally at-risk participants (49% are children) with a $3.1 billion budget. Participation varies across states. In California, for example, 80 local agencies served 850,000 participants in May 1994, with a 1994 food budget of $296 million. Approximately 32% of the participants were pregnant and postpartum

women, 34% were infants, and 34% were children ages 1 to 5.[76]

Millions of low-income, nutritionally at-risk women, infants, and children do not receive program benefits. Nationally, WIC serves only about 60% of the eligible women, infants, and children. Several US states provide supplemental funding to WIC programs to increase the number of eligible participants. In 14 states, the state legislatures have appropriated funds for food and nutrition services and program administration. In seven states, funds have been appropriated for either food or for nutrition services and program administration. In five states (New York, Pennsylvania, Illinois, Massachusetts, and Texas), the legislatures have provided from $6 million to $42 million to enable WIC to reach substantially more low-income, nutritionally at-risk pregnant women, infants, and young children.

When a state reaches the maximum number of participants that it can serve with its annual budget, individuals applying for program benefits are served on a highest-need basis, in compliance with a seven-tiered priority system. The priority system ranks most pregnant women and infants before children, including children with documented health problems. When the priority system is implemented, WIC agencies must turn away eligible applicants who are in lower-priority categories.

FEDERALLY FUNDED RESEARCH ON US ADULTS

In the United States, the National Heart, Lung, and Blood Institute funds various programs in adult research. Projects address major health concerns. The currently funded investigations are described briefly below.[26]

Atherosclerosis Risk in Communities

Initiated in July 1985, the Atherosclerosis Risk in Communities study measures the association of CHD risk factors with both atherosclerosis and new CHD. The target population is a representative cohort from four diverse communities. The study population comprises men and women, ages 35 to 74, residing in four communities, each with a cohort of 4,000 participants; one community cohort is only African-American participants. Hospital records, death certificates, and out-of-hospital deaths are compiled.

Epidemiology of Cardiovascular Risk Factors in Women—Healthy Women Study

The Healthy Women Study began in April 1993 and continued until 1995 to determine cardiovascular risk factors and the change in risk factors during and following menopause. The study population was 541 healthy, premenopausal women, age 42 and above. Premenopausal women served as controls.

Observations to date are that menopause, especially without subsequent hormonal-replacement therapy, produces a more atherogenic lipid profile. High-density lipoprotein (HDL) cholesterol levels decreased and low-density lipoprotein (LDL) cholesterol levels increased in women with natural menopause who did not receive hormonal-replacement therapy for a period of at least 12 months. Natural menopause did not affect blood pressure, plasma glucose or insulin levels, body weight, or the total number of calories consumed in food or expended in physical activity. HDL and LDL cholesterol levels did not change in menopausal women who received hormonal-replacement therapy. Levels of triglycerides, apolipoprotein A-I, and apolipoprotein A-II increased compared with premenopausal controls.

Risk Factors for Cardiovascular Disease in Women (Nurses' Health Study)

The Nurses' Health Study began in August 1980 to determine the relationships of hormonal factors, a variety of nutrients, diabetes, exercise, and brand of cigarettes smoked with the subsequent risk of heart disease, pulmonary embolism, and stroke. Female registered nurses, 42 to 67 years old, comprise the study sample of 121,700 women. Observations to date are that current estrogen use is associated with reduction in the incidence of CHD as well as mortality from cardiovascular disease. However, estrogen use is not associated with any change in the risk of stroke. Reproductive experience (number of births, age at menarche, and age at first birth) had no important association with heart disease risk. For middle-aged women, moderate alcohol consumption appeared to decrease the risk of heart disease and ischemic stroke and increase the risk of subarachnoid hemorrhage. Mild to moderate overweight status increased the risk of heart disease in middle-aged women.

Tamoxifen Study (Breast Cancer Prevention Trial)

The Tamoxifen Study was initiated in April 1992 to assess the impact of tamoxifen on the development of breast cancer, heart disease, and bone fractures. The study population comprises 16,000 women aged 35 and above, approximately 10,000 of whom will be over the age of 50.

The trial was initiated by the National Cancer Institute; the National Heart, Lung, and Blood Institute provides support to obtain blood pressure and lipid measurements as well as lipoprotein level. Tamoxifen is referred to as an "antiestrogen" and "estrogen-like" and has been shown to decrease plasma total cholesterol and LDL cholesterol levels in women with breast cancer.

HEALTHY PEOPLE 2000 ACTIONS

The major objectives to promote health among adults include several diet-related behaviors (see Exhibit 9–1). These include reducing weight; lowering sodium intakes; increasing complex carbohydrates; and reducing total fat, alcohol, and saturated fat. To achieve these objectives, worksite wellness programs, as well as drug and alcohol policies, are necessary. Education and access to programs ranging from breastfeeding promotion to dental health must be available to individuals from all ethnic groups. Community nutrition pro-fessionals have an important role in the transfer of nutrition knowledge and the integration of positive nutrition behaviors into the daily lives of adults, especially pregnant and lactating women[77] (see Exhibit 9-2).

Exhibit 9-1 *Healthy People 2000* Objectives for Adults

2.3	Reduce overweight to a prevalence of no more than 20% among people aged 20 and older and no more than 15% among adolescents aged 12 through 19.
2.5	Reduce dietary fat intake to an average of 30% of calories or less and average saturated fat intake to less than 10% of calories among people aged 2 and older. (Baseline: 36% of calories from total fat and 13% from saturated fat for people aged 20 through 74 in 1976-80; 36% and 13% for women aged 19 through 50 in 1985.)
2.6	Increase complex carbohydrate and fiber-containing foods in the diets of adults to 5 or more daily servings for vegetables (including legumes) and fruits, and to 6 or more daily servings for grain products. (Baseline: 2½ servings of vegetables and fruits and 3 servings of grain products for women aged 19 through 50 in 1985.)
2.7	Increase to at least 50% the proportion of overweight people aged 12 and older who have adopted sound dietary practices combined with regular physical activity to attain an appropriate body weight.
2.8	Increase calcium intake so at least 50% of youth aged 12 through 24 and 50% of pregnant and lactating women consume 3 or more servings daily of foods rich in calcium, and at least 50% of people aged 25 and older consume 2 or more servings daily.
2.9	Decrease salt and sodium intake so at least 65% of home meal preparers prepare foods without adding salt, at least 80% of people avoid using salt at the table, and at least 40% of adults regularly purchase foods modified or lower in sodium.
2.13	Increase to at least 85% the proportion of people aged 18 and older who use food labels to make nutritious food selections.
2.20	Increase to at least 50% the proportion of worksites with 50 or more employees that offer nutrition education and/or weight management programs for employees.
4.8	Reduce alcohol consumption by people age 14 and older to an annual average of no more than 2 gallons of ethanol per person. (Baseline: 2.54 gallons of ethanol in 1987.)
4.14	Extend adoption of alcohol and drug policies for the work environment to at least 60% of worksites with 50 or more employees. (Baseline data available in 1991.)
8.5	Increase to at least 50% the proportion of postsecondary institutions with institutionwide health promotion programs for students, faculty, and staff. (Baseline: At least 20% of higher education institutions offered health promotion activities for students in 1989-90.)
8.6	Increase to at least 85% the proportion of workplaces with 50 or more employees that offer health promotion activities for their employees, preferably as part of a comprehensive employee health promotion program. (Baseline: 65% of worksites with 50 or more employees offered at least one health promotion activity in 1985; 63% of medium and large companies had a wellness program in 1987.)
13.5	Reduce the prevalence of gingivitis among people aged 35 through 44 to no more than 30%. (Baseline: 42% in 1985-86.)

continues

Exhibit 9-1 continued

Special Population Targets

Gingivitis Prevalence	1985 Baseline	2000 Target
13.5a Low-income people (annual family income <$12,500)	50%	35%
13.5b American Indians/Alaska Natives	95%[+]	50%
13.5c Hispanics		
Mexican Americans	74%[++]	50%
Cubans	79%[++]	
Puerto Ricans	82%[++]	

[+]1983–84 baseline.
[++]1982–84 baseline.

13.6   Reduce destructive periodontal diseases to a prevalence of no more than 15% among people aged 35 through 44. (Baseline: 24% in 1985–86.)

Note: Destructive periodontal disease is one or more sites with 4 millimeters or greater loss of tooth attachment.

14.9   Increase to at least 75% the proportion of mothers who breastfeed their babies in the early postpartum period and to at least 50% the proportion who continue breastfeeding until their babies are 5 to 6 months old. (Baseline: 54% at discharge from birth site and 21% at 5 to 6 months in 1988.)

Special Population Targets

Mothers Breastfeeding Their Babies: during Early Postpartum Period	1988 Baseline	2000 Target
14.9a Low-income mothers	32%	75%
14.9b Black mothers	25%	75%
14.9c Hispanic mothers	51%	75%
14.9d American Indian/Alaska Native mothers	47%	75%
At Age 5–6 Months		
14.9a Low-income mothers	9%	50%
14.9b Black mothers	8%	50%
14.9c Hispanic mothers	16%	50%
14.9d American Indian/Alaska Native mothers	28%	50%

14.11   Increase to at least 90% the proportion of all pregnant women who receive prenatal care in the first trimester of pregnancy. (Baseline: 76% of live births in 1987.)

Special Population Targets

Proportion of Pregnant Women Receiving Early Prenatal Care	1987 Baseline	2000 Target
14.11a Black women	61.1[+]	90[+]
14.11b American Indian/Alaska Native women	60.2[+]	90[+]
14.11c Hispanic women	61.0[+]	90[+]

[+]Percent of live births.

---

continues

Exhibit 9-1 continued

15.6   Reduce the mean serum cholesterol level among adults to no more than 200 mg/dL. (Baseline: 213 mg/dL among people aged 20 through 74 in 1976-80, 211 mg/dL for men and 215 mg/dL for women.)

17.10   Reduce the most severe complications of diabetes as follows:

Complications among People with Diabetes	1988 Baseline	2000 Target
End-stage renal disease (ESRD)	1.5/1,000[+]	1.4/1,000
Blindness	2.2/1,000	1.4/1,000
Lower extremity amputation	8.2/1,000[+]	4.9/1,000
Perinatal mortality[++]	5%	2%
Major congenital malformations[++]	8%	4%

[+]1987 baseline.
[++]Among infants of women with established diabetes.

Special Population Target for ESRD

	ESRD Due to Diabetes (per 1,000)	1983-86 Baseline	2000 Target
17.10a	Blacks with diabetes	2.2	2
17.10b	American Indians/Alaska Natives with diabetes	2.1	1.9

Special Population Target for Amputations

	Lower Extremity Amputations Due to Diabetes (per 1,000)	1984-87 Baseline	2000 Target
17.10c	Blacks with diabetes	10.2	6.1

Note: End-stage renal disease (ESRD) is defined as requiring maintenance dialysis or transplantation and is limited to ESRD due to diabetes. Blindness refers to blindness due to diabetic eye disease.

17.11   Reduce diabetes to an incidence of no more than 2.5 per 1,000 people and a prevalence of no more than 25 per 1,000 people. (Baseline: 2.9 per 1,000 in 1987; 28 per 1,000 in 1987 respectively.)

Special Population Targets

	Prevalence of Diabetes (per 1,000)	1982-84 Baseline[+]	2000 Target
17.11a	American Indians/Alaska Natives	69[++]	62
17.11b	Puerto Ricans	55	49
17.11c	Mexican Americans	54	49
17.11d	Cuban Americans	36	32
17.11e	Blacks	36[+++]	32

[+]1982-84 baseline for people aged 20-74.
[++]1987 baseline for American Indians/Alaska Natives aged 15 and older.
[+++]1987 baseline for blacks of all ages.

Source: Reprinted with permission from *Healthy People 2000: National Health Promotion and Disease Prevention Objectives.* Washington, DC: US Department of Health and Human Services; 1991. DHHS (PHS) publication 91-50212.

Exhibit 9-2 Model Nutrition Objectives for Reduced Risk Factors

By 19__, ____% of pregnant women will avoid the harmful substance (tobacco, alcohol, drugs, caffeine) during pregnancy.

By 19__, ____% of women will breastfeed upon hospital discharge and ____% will continue breastfeeding for ____ months.

By 19__, ____% of (pregnant women, lactating women, infants, women of childbearing age, adults) will consume a nutritionally adequate and prudent diet consistent with established state or federal recommendations.

Source: Model State Nutrition Objectives. Association of State and Territorial Public Health Nutrition Directors, June 1988. Adapted from Kaufman M. *Nutrition in Public Health—A Handbook for Developing Programs and Services.* Gaithersburg, Md: Aspen Publishers, Inc; 1990:570.

REFERENCES

1. *Eating for Two: Pregnancy and Nutrition Guidelines from the California Dietetic Association.* San Diego, Calif: California Dietetic Association; 1993.

2. National Academy of Science. Institute of Medicine. *Consensus Development Conference Statement: Optimal Calcium Intake.* Bethesda, Md: National Academy of Science; 1994.

3. National Research Council, Committee on Dietary Allowances, Food and Nutrition Board. *Recommended Dietary Allowances.* 9th ed. Washington, DC: National Academy Press; 1980.

4. Pitkin R. Nutrition during pregnancy. Presented at Nutritional Medicine in Medical Practice Symposium; 1993; University of California Los Angeles.

5. Infante-Rivard C, Fernandex A, Gauthier R, et al. Fetal loss associated with caffeine intake before and during pregnancy. *JAMA.* 1993;270:2940–2943.

6. Olsen J. Cigarette, tea and coffee drinking and subfecundity. *Am J Epidemiol.* 1991;133:734–739.

7. Barr HM, Streissguth AD. Caffeine use during pregnancy and child outcome: A 7-year prospective study. *Neurotoxicology and Teratology.* 1991;13:441–448.

8. American Academy of Pediatrics' Committee on Drugs. The transfer of drugs and other chemicals into human milk. *Pediatrics.* 1994;93:137–150.

9. Armstrong BG, McDonald AD, Sloan M. Cigarette, alcohol, and coffee consumption and spontaneous abortion. *Am J Public Health.* 1992;82:85–90.

10. Mills JL, Holmes LB, Aarons JH, et al. Moderate caffeine use and the risk of spontaneous abortion and intrauterine growth retardation. *JAMA.* 1993;269:595–597.

11. American Dietetic Association. National Center for Nutrition and Dietetics. *Nutrition Fact Sheet—Aspartame in Pregnancy.* Chicago, Ill: American Dietetic Association; 1994.

12. Caldwell M, ed. Quality assurance/quality improvement criteria for nutritional care of pregnant and postpartum women and adolescents. Public Health Nutrition Practice Group of the American Dietetic Association, and USDHHS, DHS, CDC, NCCDPHP, Division of Nutrition. ADA: Chicago, Ill, 1993.

13. Mitchell MC, Lerner E. Weight gain and pregnancy outcome in underweight and normal weight women. *J Am Diet Assoc.* 1989;89:634–638.

14. Institute of Medicine. *Nutrition During Pregnancy. Part I: Weight Gain. Part II: Nutrient Supplement.* Washington, DC: National Academy Press; 1990.

15. *Primer on Indicator Development and Application. Measuring Quality in Health Care.* Oakbrook Terrace, Ill: Joint Commission on Accreditation of Healthcare Organizations; 1990.

16. American Heart Association. *1993 Heart and Stroke Statistics.* Dallas, Tex: American Heart Association; 1992.

17. National Center for Health Statistics. *Vital Statistics of the US.* Washington, DC: US Government Printing Office; 1991.

18. *Cancer Facts and Figures.* Atlanta, Ga: American Cancer Society; 1994.

19. Avioli LV. Significance of osteoporosis: A growing international health care problem. *Calcif Tissue Int.* 1991;49(suppl. 5-7):25–45.

20. The Gallup Organization. Women's knowledge and behavior regarding health and fitness. Survey conducted for the American Dietetic Association and Weight Watchers International; June 1993.

21. National Institutes of Health. *Women's Health Initiative Protocol.* Bethesda, Md: National Institutes of Health; 1993: volume 1, section 1: 1–58.

22. *Healthy People 2000: National Health Promotion and Disease Prevention Objectives.* Washington, DC: US Department of Health and Human Services; 1991. Public Health Service publication 91-50212.

23. Finn S. ADA's nutrition and health campaign for women promotes research and behavioral change. *Perspec in Applied Nutr.* 1993;1(3):3-7.

24. Black DM, Cummings SR, Genant HK, et al. Axial and appendicular bone mineral and a woman's lifetime risk of hip fracture. *J Bone Min Res.* 1992;7:633-638.

25. Allan JD, Mayo K, Michel Y. Body size values of white and black women. *Res Nurs Health.* 1993;16:323-333.

26. National Health, Lung, and Blood Institute. *Heart Memo. Special Edition.* Bethesda, Md: National Heart, Lung, and Blood Institute; 1994.

27. National Institutes of Health. *The Healthy Heart Handbook.* Washington, DC: US Department of Health and Human Services; 1992. NIH publication 92-2720.

28. National Cholesterol Education Program. *Report of the Expert Panel on Detection, Evaluation, and Treatment of High Blood Cholesterol in Adults.* Bethesda, Md: US Department of Health and Human Services, Public Health Service, National Institutes of Health, National Health, Lung, and Blood Institute; January 1988. NIH publication 88-2925.

29. Stampfer MJ, Hennekens CH, Manson JE, et al. Vitamin E consumption and the risk of coronary disease in women. *N Engl J Med.* 1993;328:1444-1449.

30. Barnett HJM, Eliasziw M, Meldrum HE. Drugs and surgery in the prevention of ischemic stroke. *N Engl J Med.* 1995;332:238-248.

31. Marcus BH, Stanton AL. Evaluation of relapse prevention and reinforcement to promote exercise. *Res Q Ex Sp.* 1993;64:447-452.

32. *Exercise and Your Heart.* Washington, DC: US Department of Health and Human Services and the American Heart Association; August 1993. NIH publication 93-1677.

33. American Dietetic Association. *Men's Health Campaign.* Chicago, Ill: American Dietetic Association; 1991.

34. Kris-Etherton P, ed. *Cardiovascular Disease: Nutrition for Prevention and Treatment.* Chicago, Ill: American Dietetic Association; 1990;98-107.

35. Morrison JA, Nambodiri K, Green P, et al. Familial aggregation of lipids and lipoproteins and early identification of dyslipoproteinemia: The Collaborative Lipid Research Clinics Family study. *JAMA.* 1993;250:1860.

36. Moll PP, Sing CF, Weidman WH, et al. Total cholesterol and lipoproteins in school children: Prediction of coronary heart disease in adult relatives. *Circulation.* 1993;67:127.

37. Kannel WB, Doyle JT, Ostfeld AM, et al. *Optimal Resources for Primary Prevention of Atherosclerotic Disease.* Dallas, Tex: American Heart Association; 1984.

38. National Institute of Health Consensus Development Conference Statement, 1985: Lowering blood cholesterol to prevent heart disease. *JAMA.* 1985;253:2080.

39. Dawber TR, Kannel WB. Susceptibility to coronary disease. *Mod Concepts Cardio Dis.* 1961;30:671.

40. Grundy SM, Bilheimer D, Blackburn H, et al. Rationale of the diet-heart statement of the American Heart Association. *Circulation.* 1982;65:839A.

41. Pooling Project Research Group. Relationship of blood pressure, serum cholesterol, smoking habits, relative weight, and ECG abnormalities to incidence of major coronary events: Final report. *J Chronic Dis.* 1978;31:201.

42. Rifkin BM, Segal P. Lipid Research Clinics Program reference values for hyperlipidemia and hypolipidemia. *JAMA.* 1983;250:1869.

43. Newman WP, Freedman DS, Voors AW. Relation of serum lipoprotein levels and systolic blood pressure to early atherosclerosis: The Bogalusa Heart Study. *N Engl J Med.* 1986;314:138.

44. Kannel WB. Lipids, diabetes, and coronary heart disease: Insights from the Framingham Study. *Am Heart J.* 1985;110:1100.

45. Reaven GM. Looking at the world through LDL-cholesterol glasses. *J Nutr.* 1986;116:1143.

46. Kannel WB, Gordon T, Castelli WP. Obesity, lipids, and glucose tolerance: The Framingham Study. *Am J Clin Nutr.* 1979;32:1238.

47. Stamler J. Research related to risk factors. *Circulation.* 1979;60:1575.

48. West RJ, Shaw A. Dietary management of familial hyperlipidemia. *Proc Nutr Soc.* 1979;38:325.

49. Knuiman JT, West CE, Burema J. Serum total and high density lipoprotein cholesterol concentrations and body mass index in adult men from thirteen countries. *Am J Epidemiol.* 1982;116:631.

50. Miettinen TA, Huttunen JK, Naukkarinen V, et al. Multifactorial primary prevention of cardiovascular disease in middle-aged men: Risk factors, changes, incidence and mortality. *JAMA.* 1985;254:2097.

51. Multiple Risk Factor Intervention Trial Research Group. Multiple Risk Factor Trial: Risk factor changes and mortality results. *JAMA.* 1982;248:1465.

52. Watkins LO, Neaton JD, Kuller LH. Racial differences in high-density lipoprotein cholesterol and coronary heart disease incidence in usual care group of multiple risk factor intervention trial. *Am J Cardiol.* 1986;57:538.

53. Lipid Research Clinics Program. The Lipid Research Clinic's Coronary Primary Prevention Trial Results, II: The relationship of reduction in incidence of coronary heart disease to cholesterol lowering. *JAMA.* 1984;251:365.

54. Lipid Research Clinics Program. The Lipid Research Clinic's Coronary Primary Prevention Trial Results, I: Reduction in incidence of coronary heart disease. *JAMA.* 1984;251:351.

55. Illingworth DR. Meninolin plus colestipol in therapy for severe heterozygous familial hypercholesterolemia. *Ann Intern Med.* 1984;101:598-604.

56. Gordon DJ, Ekelund LG, Karon JM, et al. Predictive value of the exercise tolerance test for mortality in North American men: The Lipid Research Clinic's Mortality Follow-Up Study. *Circulation.* 1986;74:252.

57. Veterans Administration Cooperative Study Group on Antihypertensive Agents. Effects of treatment on morbidity in hypertension: Results in patients with diastolic blood pressure averaging 115 through 129 mm Hg. *JAMA.* 1967;202:1028.

58. Veterans Administration Cooperative Study Group on Antihypertensive Agents. Effects of treatment on morbidity in hypertension, II: Results in patients with diastolic blood pressure averaging 90 through 114 mm Hg. *JAMA.* 1970;213:1143.

59. Veterans Administration Cooperative Study Group on Antihypertensive Agents. Effects of treatment on morbidity in hypertension, III: Influence of age, diastolic blood pressure and prior cardiovascular disease; further analysis of side effects. *Circulation.* 1972;45:991.

60. Castelli WP. Epidemiology of coronary heart disease: The Framingham Study. *Am J Med.* 1984;76:4.

61. Stamler J. Lifestyles, major risk factors, proof and public policy. *Circulation.* 1978;58:3.

62. Stamler J. Introduction to risk factors in coronary artery disease. In: McIntosh HO, ed. *Cardiology Series.* Northfield, Ill: Medical Communications Inc; 1978;1 (part 3).

63. US Department of Agriculture/US Department of Health and Human Services. *Nutrition and Your Health: Dietary Guidelines for Americans.* 2nd ed. Washington, DC: US Government Printing Office; 1985. HG-232.

64. Schapell DS. A critical evaluation of popular low calorie diets in America: Part I. *Top Clin Nutr.* 1988;3:36–40.

65. Edlin G, Golanty E. *Health and Wellness—A Holistic Approach.* 4th ed. Boston, Mass: Jones and Bartlett Publishers; 1992:111–112.

66. Cooper K. *The New Aerobics.* New York, NY: Bantam Books; 1970.

67. National Center for Health Statistics. *Assessing Physical Fitness and Physical Activity in Population-Based Surveys.* Drury TF, ed. Washington, DC: US Department of Health and Human Services; 1989. Public Health Service publication 89-1253.

68. Read MH, Bock MA, Carpenter K, et al. Health beliefs and supplement use: Adults in seven western states. *J Am Diet Assoc.* 1989;89:1812–1813.

69. Gray GE, Pagnini-Hill A, Ross RK, et al. Vitamin supplement use in a southern California retirement community. *J Am Diet Assoc.* 1986;86:800.

70. Levy AS, Schuchez RE. Patterns of nutrient intake among dietary supplement users: Attitudinal and behavioral correlates. *J Am Diet Assoc.* 1987;87:754.

71. Ranno BS, Wardlaw GM, Geiger CJ. What characterizes elderly women who overuse vitamin and mineral supplements? *J Am Diet Assoc.* 1988;88:347.

72. American Dietetic Association. *Survey of American Dietary Habits.* Chicago, Ill: American Dietetic Association; October 1991.

73. Fresh trends '92: A profile of fresh produce consumers. *The Packers Focus.* 1992.

74. National Restaurant Association. *Meal Consumption Behavior.* Washington, DC: National Restaurant Association; 1991.

75. US Department of Agriculture. *Cooperative Extension System.* Washington, DC: US Department of Agriculture; 1994.

76. US Department of Agriculture. *Women, Infants, and Children. Fiscal Year Closeout Summary, 1983–1991.* Washington, DC: US Department of Agriculture; 1983–1991.

77. Kaufman M. *Nutrition in Public Health—A Handbook for Developing Programs and Services.* Gaithersburg, Md: Aspen Publishers, Inc; 1990:570.

Appendix 9-A

Quality Assurance/Quality Improvement Criteria for Nutritional Care of Pregnant Women and Adolescents

Criteria	Critical Time (CT) and Exception (Ex)	Required Data Elements
1. Nutrition assessment completed, including:	CT: First trimester or by the second prenatal visit	
• Gynecological age (adolescent)	Ex: None	a. Calculation of chronological age minus age of menarche (adolescent)
• Height		b. Height
• Estimate of prepregnancy weight status as percent of standard weight for height or body mass index (BMI)		c. Prepregnancy weight expressed as percent of standard or BMI, or classified as underweight, standard weight, overweight, or obese
• Current weight for gestational age		d. Current weight and estimated weeks of gestation
• Hemoglobin or hematocrit		e. Hemoglobin or hematocrit
• Estimate of dietary pattern/food intake		f. Diet recall, diet record, or food frequency or nutrient analysis
• Use of nutrient supplements		g. Documentation of nutrient supplements used
• Access to adequate food		h. Documentation of food access
• Substance use: tobacco, alcohol, other drugs (OTC, prescription, and illicit)		i. Documentation of other substance use/abuse
• History of pregnancy involving an infant or fetus with a neural tube defect		j. Obstetrical history documenting prior pregnancy outcomes
		k. Date of nutrition assessment
		l. Number of weeks gestation or date of second prenatal visit
2. If women has a history of pregnancy involving an infant or fetus with a neural tube defect, she receives 4 mg folic acid/day for the first 12 weeks of pregnancy.	CT: First 12 weeks of pregnancy Ex: None	a. Entry in medications section of chart b. Week of gestation c. Chart note of history of infant with neural tube defect

Source: Caldwell, M. (ed.). "Quality Assurance/Quality Improvement Criteria for Nutritional Care of Pregnant and Postpartum Women and Adolescents," Public Health Nutrition Practice Group of the American Dietetic Association, and USDHHS, DHS, CDC, NCCDPHP, Division of Nutrition. September, 1993.

Criteria	Critical Time (CT) and Exception (Ex)	Required Data Elements
3. If woman is identified by assessment to need food assistance, she is referred to food assistance program.	CT: When need is identified or by second prenatal visit Ex: None	a. Documentation of need for food assistance b. Referral to food assistance program c. Date of referral to food assistance program d. Date of second prenatal visit
4. If woman is identified by assessment to need smoking cessation or substance use/abuse counseling/treatment, she receives counseling/treatment or is referred to resource.	CT: When need is identified or by second prenatal visit Ex: None	a. Documentation that woman smokes more than 1 pack (20 cigarettes/day) or documentation that woman abuses alcohol/drugs (OTC or illicit) b. Referral to counseling/treatment resource c. Date of referral d. Date of second prenatal visit
5. Woman receives instruction on recommended dietary intake for pregnancy.	CT: First trimester or by second prenatal visit Ex: None	a. Documentation of education using written, verbal, or audiovisual methods; classes; or individual counseling b. Date of education c. Number of weeks gestation or date of second prenatal visit
6. Nutrition education and counseling is provided in a manner consistent with the cultural, linguistic, and literacy needs of the pregnant woman.	CT: Throughout pregnancy Ex: None	a. Publication provided in client's language or interpreter used b. Publication provided at client's reading level
7. Weight gain is plotted on prenatal grid.	CT: At regular visits Ex: None	a. Weight plotted on prenatal weight gain grid b. Dates of regularly scheduled visits
8. Woman receives counseling/education on individualized weight gain goals and rate of weight gain for pregnancy.	CT: First trimester or by second prenatal visit Ex: None	a. Documentation of total weight gain goal b. Documentation of education on weight gain goal and rate of weight gain c. Date of education d. Number of weeks gestation or date of second prenatal visit
9. Woman receives counseling if pattern of weight gain is inadequate or excessive. • Excessive weight gain of greater than 6.5 lbs (3 kg)/month especially after 20 weeks gestation • Inadequate weight gain of less than 2 lbs (1 kg)/month for women of normal weight after the first trimester	CT: When need identified Ex: None	a. Documentation of excessive or inadequate weight gain b. Date identified c. Documentation of counseling on weight gain d. Date of counseling

Criteria	Critical Time (CT) and Exception (Ex)	Required Data Elements
10. Vitamin/mineral supplementation is provided to pregnant women with multiple fetuses; pregnant women who smoke 20 cigarettes/day; alcohol and drug abusers; and pregnant women at nutritional risk because of poor nutrition history/dietary intake.	CT: Second trimester or when identified after first trimester Ex: None	a. Chart note indicating multiple fetuses, if woman smokes 20 cigarettes/day, alcohol or substance abuse, or poor nutrition history/dietary intake b. Documentation of recommendation or supplement given c. Date of recommendation or supplementation d. Week of gestation
11. Woman receives education on harmful effects of substance use: tobacco, alcohol, other drugs (OTC, prescription, illicit).	CT: First trimester or by second prenatal visit Ex: None	a. Documentation of education on tobacco/alcohol/drugs using written, verbal, or audiovisual methods; classes; or individual counseling b. Date of education by first trimester or by second prenatal visit
12. Woman receives education on benefits of breastfeeding.	CT: First trimester or by second prenatal visit Ex: Adoption plan made; woman is HIV positive; woman has history of mastectomy or is taking antimetabolites or radiotherapy; or woman is substance abuser	a. Documentation of education using written, verbal, or audiovisual methods; classes; or individual counseling b. Date of education c. Number of weeks gestation or date of second prenatal visit or exception is documented
13. Diet is adequate/improved based on dietary assessment.	CT: By the third nutrition visit Ex: None	a. Initial nutrition assessment b. Documentation of dietary improvement/adequacy c. Number of nutrition visits
14. Woman maintains acceptable hemoglobin or hematocrit: • $\geq$11.0 gm/dL Hgb or >33% Hct • $\geq$10.5 gm/dL Hgb or $\geq$32% Hct • $\geq$11.0 gm/dL Hgb or $\geq$33% Hct	CT: First trimester CT: Second trimester CT: Third trimester Ex: Smokers, women living at high altitude (see CDC reference)	a. Hgb $\geq$11.0 gm/dL or Hct $\geq$33% at first trimester b. Hgb $\geq$10.5 gm/dL or Hct $\geq$32% at second trimester c. Hgb $\geq$11.0 gm/dL or HCT $\geq$33% at third trimester or d. Documentation of exception
15. All pregnant women receive 30 mg elemental iron after the first trimester.	CT: By second trimester or first prenatal visit Ex: Anemia	a. Documentation of recommendation or supplement given b. Week of gestation or c. Documentation of anemia
16. If woman is anemic, she receives 60–120 mg elemental iron and a multivitamin/mineral supplement containing 15 mg Zn and 2 mg Cu.	CT: When identified Ex: None	a. Chart note indicating anemia b. Entry in medications section of chart c. Date supplement given

Criteria	Critical Time (CT) and Exception (Ex)	Required Data Elements
17. All women receive serum glucose screen.	CT: By 24–28 weeks Ex: Known diabetic or gestational diabetes	a. Diagnosis of diabetes or gestational diabetes b. Weeks gestation at entry into care c. Date of glucose screen
18. Woman with serum glucose screen $\geq$140 mg/dL ($\geq$7.8 mm) is scheduled for three-hour oral glucose tolerance test.	CT: Within two weeks of abnormal glucose screen Ex: None	a. Date of abnormal glucose screen b. Date oral glucose tolerance test scheduled
19. Woman receives education regarding selected method of infant feeding.	CT: By the end of the third trimester Ex: Adoption plan made	a. Documentation of education using written, verbal, or audiovisual methods; classes; or individual counseling b. Date of education c. Weeks of gestation or d. Exception is documented
20. Woman who has chosen to breastfeed receives information on lactation management.	CT: By end of the third trimester Ex: None	a. Documentation of education using written, verbal, or audiovisual methods; classes; or individual counseling b. Date of education c. Weeks of gestation
21. Woman achieves appropriate weight gain based on prepregnant body mass index (BMI) or percent of standard (std) height: • Normal: (BMI 19.8 to 26.0 or 90–120% std wt/ht): 25–35 lbs • Low: (BMI <19.8 or <90% std wt/ht): 28–40 lbs • High: (BMI >26.0–29.0 or >120–135% std wt/ht): 15–25 lbs • Very high: (BMI >29.0 or >135% std wt/ht): minimum 15 lbs *Note 1:* Adolescents (gynecological age <2) and black women should gain at upper end of range. *Note 2:* Short women (<62 inches) should gain at lower end of range.	CT: By delivery Ex: Gestation <37 weeks or entry into care after 24 weeks	a. Total weight gain b. Height c. Prepregnant weight d. Body mass index or percent of standard weight/height e. Chronological age f. Age at menarche g. Date of entry into care h. Week of gestation
22. Women delivers infant weighing 3,000–4,000 grams.	CT: At delivery Ex: Gestation less than 37 weeks	a. Birth weight of infant b. Length of gestation, or c. Documentation of gestational age of infant less than 37 weeks

Criteria	Critical Time (CT) and Exception (Ex)	Required Data Elements
23. Nutrition assessment was completed, including • Height • Current weight • Estimate of weight/height as percent of standard or BMI • Hematocrit/hemoglobin • Estimate of dietary pattern/ food intake • Use of nutrient supplements • Infant feeding method • Method of birth control • Estimate of access to adequate food • Substance use/abuse: tobacco, alcohol, other drugs (OTC, prescription, and illicit) • History of pregnancy involving an infant or fetus with neural tube defect *Note:* Height must be measured for adolescents (gynecological age <2) and for adults if height is not available from prenatal record.	CT: Postpartum visit Ex: None	a. Height b. Weight and date of measurement c. Weight expressed as percent of standard or BMI d. Hematocrit or hemoglobin e. Diet recall or diet record or food frequency or nutrient analysis f. Documentation of nutrient supplements used g. Documentation of infant feeding method h. Documentation of method of birth control i. Documentation of food access j. Documentation of substance use/ abuse k. Obstetrical history documenting prior pregnancy outcomes l. Date of assessment m. Date of postpartum visit
24. Woman identified by assessment to need food assistance is referred to food assistance program.	CT: When need is identified prior to or at first postpartum visit Ex: None	a. Documentation of need for food assistance b. Date of documentation of need c. Referral to food assistance program d. Date of referral
25. Woman identified by assessment to need smoking cessation or substance counseling/treatment receives counseling/treatment or is referred to resource.	CT: When need is identified prior to or at first postpartum visit Ex: None	a. Documentation that woman smokes more than 1 pack (20 cigarettes)/day or documentation that woman abuses alcohol/drugs (OTC, prescription, or illicit) b. Referral to counseling/treatment resources c. Date of referral
26. Woman receives counseling on individualized weight goals.	CT: Postpartum visit Ex: None	a. Documentation of weight counseling b. Documentation of weight goal c. Date of counseling d. Date of postpartum visit
27. Woman receives counseling/ education on dietary intake to achieve stated weight goals and adequate nutrient intake.	CT: Postpartum visit Ex: None	a. Documentation of education on dietary intake using written, verbal, or audiovisual methods; classes; or individual counseling b. Date of counseling/education c. Date of postpartum visit

Criteria	Critical Time (CT) and Exception (Ex)	Required Data Elements
28. Woman receives education on harmful effects of substance use (tobacco, alcohol, and other drugs—OTC, prescription, and illicit) on health/nutritional status of woman.	CT: Postpartum visit Ex: None	a. Documentation of education on tobacco/alcohol/drugs using written, verbal, or audiovisual methods; classes; or individual counseling b. Date of education c. Date of postpartum visit
29. Woman receives counseling on physical activity goals.	CT: Postpartum visit Ex: None	a. Documentation of education on physical activity using written, verbal, or audiovisual methods; classes; or individual counseling b. Date of counseling
30. Woman receives counseling or education on infant feeding practices/problems.	CT: Postpartum visit Ex: Adoption or perinatal death	a. Documentation of education on infant feeding using written, verbal, or audiovisual methods; classes; or individual counseling b. Date of counseling or education c. Date of postpartum visit or d. Adoption or e. Perinatal death
31. Woman receives education or counseling on recommended vitamin/mineral supplements.	CT: Postpartum visit Ex: No supplements recommended	a. Documentation of education on use of supplements using written, verbal, or audiovisual methods; classes; or individual counseling b. Date of education/counseling c. Documentation of recommended supplements d. Date of postpartum visit
32. Nutrition education and counseling is provided in a manner consistent with the cultural, linguistic, and literacy needs of the postpartum woman.	CT: Postpartum visit Ex: None	a. Publication provided in client's language or interpreter used b. Publication provided at client's reading level c. Dates of education/counseling d. Date of postpartum visit
33. Woman identified with anemia receives individualized nutrition counseling or education.	CT: Postpartum visit Ex: None	a. Documentation of Hgb <12 gm/dL; Hct <36% b. Documentation of education using written, verbal, or audiovisual methods; classes; or individual counseling c. Date of counseling/education d. Date of postpartum visit
34. Woman who is anemic is given or prescribed 60–120 mg iron, 15 mg Zn, and 2 mg Cu.	CT: When anemia is diagnosed Ex: None	a. Lab data or chart note indicating anemia b. Chart note indicating supplement or prescription given c. Date of chart note
35. Woman who had gestational diabetes is scheduled for a two-hour oral glucose tolerance test.	CT: 6–12 weeks postpartum Ex: None	a. Date of delivery b. Date two-hour oral glucose tolerance test scheduled c. Diagnosis of gestational diabetes at last pregnancy

Criteria	Critical Time (CT) and Exception (Ex)	Required Data Elements
36. Woman identified with breastfeeding problems receives counseling on resolution of problem.	CT: Postpartum visit Ex: None	a. Documentation of breastfeeding problems. b. Documentation of counseling to resolve identified problems c. Date of education/counseling d. Date of postpartum visit
37. Woman receives education or counseling on breastfeeding maintenance, support/ resources.	CT: Postpartum visit Ex: None	a. Documentation of education using written, verbal, or audiovisual methods; classes; or individual counseling b. Date of counseling/education c. Date of postpartum visit
38. Woman receives counseling or education on dietary needs of breastfeeding.	CT: Postpartum visit Ex: None	a. Documentation of education using written, verbal, or audiovisual methods; classes; or individual counseling b. Date of counseling/education c. Date of postpartum visit
39. Woman receives education on harmful effects of substance use (tobacco, alcohol, and drugs) on quality and quantity of breast milk and effects on infant.	CT: Postpartum visit Ex: None	a. Documentation of education on use of tobacco, alcohol, and drugs using written, verbal, or audiovisual methods; classes; or individual counseling b. Date of education c. Date of postpartum visit
40. Woman receives education/ counseling on weight goals in relation to breastfeeding.	CT: Postpartum visit Ex: None	a. Documentation of weight goals b. Documentation of education using written, verbal, or audiovisual methods; classes; or individual counseling c. Date of education d. Date of postpartum visit
41. Multivitamin/mineral supplements are provided to breastfeeding woman who smokes more than 20 cigarettes/day or is a vegan or has inadequate or severely restricted diet.	CT: When identified Ex: None	a. Documentation that woman smokes more than 20 cigarettes/day, is a vegan, or has severely restricted diet b. Date of identification of problem c. Chart note that supplement is provided or prescribed d. Date of provision or prescription of supplements

Appendix 9-B

State Cooperative Extension System
Land Grant Universities

State	University
Alabama	Auburn University, Auburn 36849
	Alabama A & M University, Normal 35762
	Tuskegee University, Tuskegee 36088
Alaska	University of Alaska, Fairbanks 99775-5200
American Samoa	American Samoa Community College, Pago Pago 96799
Arizona	University of Arizona, Tucson 85721
Arkansas	University of Arkansas, Little Rock 72203
	University of Arkansas, Pine Bluff 71601
California	University of California, Oakland 94612-3560
Colorado	Colorado State University, Fort Collins 80523
Connecticut	University of Connecticut, Storrs 06269-4066
Delaware	University of Delaware, Newark 19717-1303
	Delaware State College, Dover 19901
District of Columbia	University of the District of Columbia, Washington, DC 20008
Florida	University of Florida, Gainesville 32611
	Florida A & M University, Tallahassee 32307
Georgia	University of Georgia, Athens 30602
	Fort Valley State College, Fort Valley 31030
Guam	University of Guam, Mangilao 96913
Hawaii	University of Hawaii, Honolulu 96822
Idaho	University of Idaho, Moscow 83843
Illinois	University of Illinois, Urbana 61801
Indiana	Purdue University, West Lafayette 47907
Iowa	Iowa State University, Ames 50011
Kansas	Kansas State University, Manhattan 66506
Kentucky	University of Kentucky, Lexington 40546
	Kentucky State University, Frankfort 40601
Louisiana	Louisiana State University, Baton Rouge 70803-1900
	Southern University, Baton Rouge 70813
Maine	University of Maine, Orono 04469
Maryland	University of Maryland, College Park 20742
	University of Maryland, Eastern Shore 21853
Massachusetts	University of Massachusetts, Amherst 01003
Michigan	Michigan State University, East Lansing 44824

Source: Adapted from *Cooperative Extension System*, U.S. Department of Agriculture, Washington, DC 20250-0900, p. 3.

State	University
Micronesia	College of Micronesia, Kolonia, 96941
Minnesota	University of Minnesota, St. Paul 55108
Mississippi	Mississippi State University, 39762
	Alcorn State University, Lorman 39096
Missouri	University of Missouri, Columbia 65211
	Lincoln University, Jefferson City 65101
Montana	Montana State University, Bozeman 59717
Nebraska	University of Nebraska, Lincoln 68583-0703
Nevada	University of Nevada, Reno 89557
New Hampshire	University of New Hampshire, Durham 03824
New Jersey	Rutgers State University, New Brunswick 08903
New Mexico	New Mexico State University, Las Cruces 88003
New York	Cornell University, Ithaca 14853
North Carolina	North Carolina State University, Raleigh 27695-7602
	North Carolina State University, Greensboro 27420
North Dakota	North Dakota State University, Fargo 58105
Northern Marianas	Northern Marianas College, Saipan 96950
Ohio	Ohio State University, Columbus 43210
Oklahoma	Oklahoma State University, Stillwater 74078
	Langston University, Langston 73050
Oregon	Oregon State University, Corvallis 97331
Pennsylvania	Penn State University, University Park 16802
Puerto Rico	University of Puerto Rico, Mayaguez 00708
Rhode Island	University of Rhode Island, Kingston 02881
South Carolina	Clemson University, Clemson 29634
	South Carolina State College, Orangeburg 29117
South Dakota	South Dakota State University, Brookings 57007
Tennessee	University of Tennessee, Knoxville 37901
	Tennessee State University, Nashville 37209-1561
Texas	Texas A & M, College Station 77843
	Prairie View A & M, Prairie View 77446-2867
Utah	Utah State University, Logan 84322-4900
Vermont	University of Vermont, Burlington 05405
Virginia	Virginia Polytechnic Institute, Blacksburg 24061-0220
	Virginia State University, Petersburg 23803
Virgin Islands	University of the Virgin Islands, St. Croix 00850
Washington	Washington State University, Pullman 99164-6230
West Virginia	West Virginia University, Morgantown 26506
Wisconsin	University of Wisconsin, Madison 53706
Wyoming	University of Wyoming, Laramie 82071

10

Older Adults

Learning Objectives

- Characterize the nutritional needs of older adults in the United States.
- Describe the nutrition program components of Title IIIC of the Older Americans Act.
- Outline the qualifications of a community nutrition professional who functions in a congregate food service setting.
- Specify primary, secondary, and tertiary intervention for older adults at different stages of health.
- List the reasons for expanding the Recommended Dietary Allowances for the decades of life after 50 years of age.
- Describe the Nutrition Screening Initiative and the different levels of screening.
- Discuss compressed morbidity, syndrome X, and ageism.

High Definition Nutrition

Ageism—the feelings of prejudice that result from misconceptions and myths about older people. This prejudice generally evolves from beliefs that aging makes people senile, unattractive, asexual, weak, and useless.
Compressed morbidity—a few years of major illness among the very old.
Old-old—age 75 to 84.

Oldest-old—age 85 and over.
Social gerontologists—professionals who study how the older population and the aging process is affected by and affects the social structure.
Social gerontology—the area of gerontology concerned not only with the impact of social and sociocultural conditions on the process of aging but also with the social consequences of this process.
Young-old—age 65 to 74.

OLDER ADULTS IN THE UNITED STATES

Members of the newest generation of older adults have broken out of the "rest home" image and generated some unrest of their own by their desire to remain healthy and vital into their 90s and 100s. Over 40,000 older adults (or elders, as many prefer being called) have reached their 100th birthday. This growing and graying portion of our population has far from a "rest home" mentality. With an estimated 22% of the US population at age 65 or older by 2050, the upper limit for being old has increased.[1]

History will be made by the way the United States cares for its older adult population. The stage has been keenly described by Daniel Perry, Executive Director of the Alliance for Aging Research:

The US cannot afford to find itself in the 21st century with vastly larger populations of older persons but without a much higher level of knowledge about the biology of aging and health than we have in the 1990s. The senior citizens of 2020 and beyond—today's "Baby Boomers"—must benefit from as-yet-undiscovered insights in health, medicine, and nutrition. Otherwise the future may be marked by excessive demand for long-term nursing care and severe rationing of medical care.

A more positive alternative future, one marked by improved health, vitality, and personal independence for older Americans, is an achievable goal. Already nursing home admissions are falling relative to the growing numbers of people in their 70s, 80s, and 90s. The newest figures show that the dependency rate among the very old declined in the 1980s, catching even professional demographers by surprise. Among the reasons cited: a higher level of education among those now entering old age, higher economic status, the applications of new technologies such as joint replacements and cataract surgery, and better nutrition than that experienced by the elderly in the past.

If we are to achieve healthy and successful aging on a mass scale in our society, the role of good nutrition will be a key to success.[2]

Gerontologists view aging in terms of four distinct processes:

- *Chronological aging* is aging on the basis of a person's years from birth. Ages of individuals are defined as the "young-old," the "old-old," and the "oldest-old."[1]
- *Biological aging* refers to the physical changes that reduce the efficiency of organ systems such as the lungs, heart, and circulatory system.

- *Psychological aging* includes the changes that occur in sensory and perceptual processes and mental functioning involving memory, learning, and intelligence. Changes in adaptive capacity, personality, drives, and motives also demonstrate psychological aging.
- *Social aging* refers to an individual's changing roles and relationships in the social structure. These roles and relationships involve interactions with family and friends; with the working world; and within religious, professional, and political organizations.

Senescence is the period of life generally beginning after age 30 when changes occur that reflect normal declines in all organ systems. It occurs gradually throughout the body, ultimately reducing the viability of different body systems and increasing their vulnerability to disease. This is the final stage in the development of an organism.

Gerontologists study the ability of older adults to remain independent and to maintain their competence. Competence is considered the theoretical upper limit of an individual's abilities to function in the areas of health, social behavior, and cognition.[3] Some of the abilities needed to adapt to environmental pressure and change include problem solving and learning; performing on the job; and managing the basic activities of daily living such as dressing, grooming, and cooking.[3,4]

A rapid increase occurred in the median age of the US population from 1970 to 1990: it increased from 28 to 33 years of age. This five-year increase in the median age during a 20-year period is a noteworthy demographic event.[5] Key factors creating this rise include a steep decline in the birth rate after the mid-1960s, coupled with high birth rates from 1890 to 1915 and just after World War II, which yielded the "baby boomers." Additional factors include the large number of immigrants entering the United States via Ellis Island, New York, before the 1920s.

A dramatic demonstration of the changing US age distribution is the shift in the proportion of older adults compared to young persons. In 1970, about 4% of the US population was 65 or more years of age. Young persons 0 to 17 years of age comprised 40% of the population. By 1980, the reduced birth rates of the 1970s created a decline of young persons to 28% percent of the population. By 2030, there will be an almost equal proportion of young persons 0 to 17 years compared with elderly (22% and 21% percent, respectively).[6] After 2030, current trends will create a death rate that is greater than the birth rate.

The population aged 85 and older is called the "oldest-old."[7] This group has grown more rapidly than any other age group in the United States. In 1990, of the 31.2 million persons aged 65 and over in the United States, 32% were age 75 to 84, and 10% were age 85 and over.[8] Mortality rates among adults have declined significantly since the mid-1940s. The result is an unprecedented number of individuals reaching advanced old age and requiring health and social services.[7] The population of "oldest-old" Americans has thereby increased 23-fold, compared to a 12-fold growth in the 75 to 84 age group and an 8-fold increase among individuals 65 to 74 years of age. Individuals over 85 years of age have increased by 300 percent from 1960 to 1990.[6] This age group is expected to reach 4.6 million in 2000 and 8 million in 2030 before the baby boomers reach old age. The baby boomers will not begin to turn 85 until after 2030.

Due to the graying of the nation, new studies seek to identify the processes that promote successful aging and keep aging adults independent and functional. Characteristics of normal aging are listed in Exhibit 10-1. Almost 43% of the remaining years of men and women currently between the ages of 65 and 69 will be spent depending on others. Their dependence will involve activities of daily living including rising from bed or a chair, bathing, dressing, and eating (see Table 10-1). A decrease in functional capacity corresponds to the time when the most drastic reductions in muscle mass and strength are observed. Further, there is a strong association between functional dependency and nutritional status in elders with chronic illness.[9]

Framingham Study data indicate that 40% of women from 55 to 64, 45% from 65 to 75, and 65% from 75 to 84 could not lift 4.5 kg, and a

Exhibit 10-1 Characteristics of Normal Aging

Individuals age at very different rates. Even for one person, organs and organ systems have different rates of decline. Data from the Baltimore Longitudinal Study of Aging suggest these general changes:

- *Heart*: The heart grows slightly larger with age. Maximal oxygen consumption during exercise declines in men by about 10% with each decade of adult life, and in women by about 7.5%. Cardiac output remains basically the same, even with increased efficiency of the heart.
- *Lungs*: Maximum vital capacity declines by about 40% between 20 and 70 years of age.
- *Brain*: The brain loses neurons but increases connections between cell synapses and regrows branch-like extensions called dendrites and axons, which transmit brain messages.
- *Kidneys*: The kidneys lose efficiency extracting wastes from the blood, accompanied by a decline in bladder capacity. Urinary incontinence occurs with tissue atrophy.
- *Body fat*: The body redistributes fat from under the skin to deeper parts of the body. Women tend to store fat in the hips and thighs, whereas men store fat in the abdominal area.
- *Muscles*: Muscle mass decreases by about 22% for women and 23% for men between 30 and 70 years of age.
- *Sight*: Vision acuity and difficulty focusing begin in the 40s. Susceptibility to glare, and difficulty seeing at low levels of illumination increase with aging.
- *Hearing*: Hearing declines more quickly in men than in women, with an additional decline in the ability to hear higher frequencies.
- *Personality*: Personality is consistent unless it is altered by a disease process.

Source: Adapted from "What is Normal Aging?" National Institutes of Health, National Institute on Aging. Publication No. 93-2756, *In Search of the Secrets of Aging*, 1993, p. 25.

similar percentage could not perform heavy household work.[10] This decreased capacity places older persons at increased risk of dependence and institutionalization.

Among the very old, muscle strength is highly related to function and significantly and positively correlated to normal walking speed for males and females. Among very frail, institutionalized men

Table 10–1 Range of Functional Status of Older Adults

Activities	Independent	Dependent
Personal Activities		
Bathing	Bathes self completely or requires help with hard to reach part (i.e., back).	Does not bath self; requires assistance with more than one body part; requires help getting into or out of bath or shower.
Dressing	Dresses self including getting clothes from closet or drawers and manages fasteners.	Does not dress self.
Toileting	Manages toileting and hygienic activities by self.	Needs assistance getting to and using toilet or uses commode or bedpan.
Transferring	Gets in and out of bed and chair without assistance.	Needs assistance getting in and out of bed or chair.
Continence	Self-controlled.	Partial or total.
Feeding	Gets food from plate to mouth.	Needs assistance eating or is dependent on tube or parenteral feeding.
Instrumental Activities		
Telephone use	Finds and dials numbers.	Cannot use telephone.
Shopping	Manages shopping for needs.	Unable to shop.
Food preparation	Plans, prepares, and serves meals.	Requires meals prepared and served by someone else.
Housekeeping	Can maintain living quarters alone.	Does not perform housekeeping tasks.
Laundry	Does own laundry.	Needs laundry done by others.
Transportation	Travels independently by public transportation or car.	Does not travel at all.
Medications	Manages dose and time of medications.	Cannot manage medications.
Finances	Manages all financial matters.	Cannot handle money.

Source: Adapted from Chernoff R. Meeting the Nutritional Needs of the Elderly in the Institutional Setting. *Nutrition Reviews.* 1994;52(4):133.

and women, muscle strength is associated with walking speed, chair stand time, and the ability to climb stairs.

Nursing home residents classified as "fallers" are significantly weaker in the knees and ankles. Of a sample of 1,042 home-dwelling men and women over 60 years of age, 365 (35%) reported one or more falls in the prior year. Factors that separated fallers from nonfallers were polypharmacy (the practice of taking multiple medications), leg muscle power, arthritis, and handgrip strength of the dominant hand. Handgrip strength was the most important factor and can be predictive of lower-extremity strength.[11]

Because age-related loss in muscle mass may be an important determinant in the reduced maximal aerobic capacity seen in elderly men and women, researchers have applied muscle strengthening and training programs to frail, institutionalized, elderly men and women. One program involved 10 individuals whose mean age was 90 ± 3 years (range 86 to 96 years).[11] Muscle strength increased by almost 180%, and muscle size increased by 11% after eight weeks of training. Increased muscle strength promoted gait, speed, and balance. Significant muscle hypertrophy was observed. Aging does not decrease the ability to adapt to a progressive resistance training program, if the training has sufficient intensity to elicit significant gains in strength and muscle mass. Sufficient intensity is defined as above 60% of maximal lifting capacity.

Assessing and correcting any nutritional deficiencies is essential because specific nutritional deficiencies can place older adults at risk or decrease their ability to respond to the exercise. Dehydration, due to a decreased sensation of thirst and a decreased ability to concentrate urine, affects muscle response. Vitamin D deficiency due to decreased exposure to the sun and decreased consumption of milk is likewise associated with decreased muscle strength.

Undernutrition of older adults has been shown to have a positive association with dysphagia, slow eating, low protein intake, poor appetite, the presence of a feeding tube, and chronological age. Overnutrition, commonly seen as excess food intake, has been shown to be inversely associated with poor appetite, number of feeding impairments, protein intake, and mental state.[12]

Chronic diseases may predispose older adults to impaired mobility and falls. The reduced physical activity linked with institutionalization may increase their functional impairment. However, increased levels of physical activity through walking and/or strengthening exercises may reverse the effects of a very sedentary life.[11]

THEORIES OF AGING

Theories of aging range from "programmed" theories to "error" theories about the process.[12] Programmed theories propose that aging progresses through a biological timetable, perhaps continuing the one that regulates childhood growth and development. Error theories emphasize environmental damage to body cells, organs, and systems, which gradually causes them to function inadequately. These theories overlap, have unique characteristics, and are discussed below.[13,14]

No single theory explains all the changes accompanying aging. Aging involves many processes, interactive and interdependent, that influence life span and health. Gerontologists are studying the multitude of factors that may be involved, including environmental factors that affect aging cells, tissues, and organs, and the body's genetic response to such factors.[15]

Programmed Theories

The *programmed senescence theory* views aging as the result of the sequential switching on and off of certain genes. Senescence becomes the time when age-associated deficits are manifested. The *endocrine theory* proposes that biological clocks controlled by hormones set the pace of aging. *Immunological theory* suggests sequential decline in immune system functions, leading to an increased vulnerability to infectious disease, aging, and death.

Error Theories

The *wear and tear theory* proposes that cells and tissues have vital parts that wear out, whereas the *rate of living theory* suggests that the greater an organism's rate of oxygen basal metabolism, the shorter its life span. The *cross-linking theory* proposes that an accumulation of cross-linked proteins damages cells and tissues, thereby slowing bodily processes. The *free radicals theory* suggests that accumulated damage caused by oxygen radicals causes cells and then organs to stop functioning. The *error catastrophe theory* links damage to mechanisms that synthesize proteins, resulting in faulty proteins that accumulate and cause catastrophic damage to cells, tissues, and organs. The *somatic mutation theory* proposes that genetic mutations occur and accumulate with increasing age, which causes cells to deteriorate and malfunction.[16]

AGING PROCESSES

Aging processes can be divided into three general categories: genetic, biochemical, and physiological.[15]

Genetic Processes

The proteins produced by genes have many functions in each cell and tissue in the body. Some of their actions relate to aging. Antioxidants appear to prevent damage to cells, and some proteins may repair damaged DNA or help cells respond to stress. Some proteins appear to have direct control of cell senescence.

Cell senescence can be visually observed. Inside a cell, threadlike pairs of chromosomes float in cytoplasm along with other tiny organelles that perform the cell's work. The cell is surrounded by a membrane whose surface sends and receives messages from other cells. The chromosomes are rodlike structures that divide into two chromosomes, which migrate to opposite sides of the cell and form a nucleus. The entire process repeats itself over and over.[17]

This process of mitosis or asexual cell division occurs in nearly all of the 100 trillion or so cells composing the human body. However, after a certain number of divisions, cells experience a state of cell senescence and they do not divide or proliferate. DNA synthesis is blocked.[18] An example is the young human fibroblasts or collagen-producing cells, which divide about 50 times and then stop. This phenomenon has been named the *Hayflick limit*, after Leonard Hayflick.[19]

Gerontologists have found links between senescence and human life spans based on the Hayflick limit. Fibroblasts taken from 75 year olds have fewer divisions remaining than cells from a child, and the longer the life span of a species, the higher its Hayflick limit. (For example, human fibroblasts have a higher Hayflick limit than mice fibroblasts.)

Biochemical Processes

The biochemistry of aging remains fascinating and involves research about the damage of cells by oxygen radicals, glucose cross-linking of proteins, and even the differing role of proteins (e.g., heat shock proteins, hormones, and growth factors).

Oxygen Radicals

Oxygen radicals demolish proteins and damage nucleic acids in cells. The free radical theory of aging suggests that damage caused by oxygen radicals is responsible for many of the bodily changes that come with aging, as well as for degenerative disorders (including cancer), atherosclerosis, cataracts, and neurodegeneration.[20]

Glucose Cross-linking

Blood sugar or glucose is also suspected as a cause of cellular deterioration. During glycosylation, glucose molecules attach themselves to proteins, and initiate a chain of chemical reactions that results in proteins binding together or cross-linking. This alters their biological and structural roles. Cross-links, which have been termed advanced glycosylation end products, appear to toughen tissues and are linked to stiffening connective tissue (collagen), hardened arteries, clouded eyes, reduced nerve function, and inefficient kidneys.

These deficiencies often accompany aging and appear at younger ages in people with diabetes. Thereby, much research has focused on the relationship of cross-linking to diabetes and aging.[15]

DNA Repair

In the normal life of a cell, DNA undergoes continual damage from oxygen radicals, ultraviolet light, and other toxic agents. Damage involves deletions or destroyed sections, mutations, or changes in the sequence of DNA bases comprising the genetic code. Biologists suggest that the DNA damage accumulates and deteriorates tissues and organs. Heat-shock proteins are produced when cells are exposed to various stressors including heat, toxic heavy metals, chemicals, and behavioral and psychological stress.

Hormones

In 1989, at Veterans Administration hospitals in Milwaukee and Chicago, a small group of men 60 years and over received recombinant human growth hormone injections three times a week. These injections dramatically reversed some signs of aging and increased their lean body mass, reduced excess fat, and thickened their skin. Signs of aging returned when the injections stopped.[15]

Hormone replacement using estrogen alleviates the discomforts of menopause. Estrogen lessens the accelerated bone loss and may contribute to a decrease in cardiovascular disease among older adults. Testosterone replacement may benefit aging men by increasing bone mass, muscle mass, and strength. Hormones are affected by growth or trophic factors, such as insulin-like growth factor (IGF-1) and the growth hormone, which modulate cell activities.[15]

Physiological Processes

Many answers to questions about normal aging are coming from the Baltimore Longitudinal Study of Aging. This longitudinal study began in 1958 and is studying the aging process in more than 1,000 people (primarily men) from age 20 to age 90 and beyond.[21]

Researchers have found that variations in human development increase as people age and that organ systems within a single individual can change at different rates. These findings suggest that aging is a multifactorial process that is influenced by genetic factors, lifestyle, and disease processes.

The National Institute of Aging's Biomarkers of Aging project began in 1987. It is a 10-year project to identify key biological signs that characterize the aging process. Researchers believe that biomarkers are a better measure of an organism's aging status than chronological age. Biomarkers improve the ability to study normal aging, diseases, and antiaging interventions. Two organ systems, the endocrine system and the immune system, are the focus of much of the physiological research on aging.[15-22] Other factors include energy consumption and behavioral factors.

The Immune System

Many cells, substances, and organs compose the immune system. The thymus, spleen, tonsils, bone marrow, and lymphatic system produce, store, and transport B lymphocytes and T lymphocytes, antibodies, interleukins, and interferon. White blood cells are lymphocytes that fight invading bacteria and other foreign cells.

Lymphocytes are classified as either B cells or T cells. B cells mature in the bone marrow. One of their functions is to secrete antibodies in response to infectious agents or antigens. T cells develop in the thymus and are classified as cytotoxic T cells and helper T cells. Cytotoxic T cells attack infected or damaged cells. Helper T cells produce chemicals called lymphokines, which mobilize other immune system substances and cells.[22]

The Endocrine System

The thymus shrinks in size as people age. The number of T cells remains fairly constant, while the proportion of proliferation and function decline. In older adults, T cells destroyed by trauma (such as decubitus ulcers) take longer to renew than they do in younger people.

The interleukins are one group of T-cell products that relay signals regulating the immune response. Interleukin-6, which increases with age, may interfere with the immune response. Interleukin-2 stimulates T-cell proliferation but declines as people age.

Energy Restriction

Mice fed diets with all essential nutrients but 30 to 60% fewer calories survive several months longer than mice on a normal feeding schedule. Energy restriction has been shown to increase the life spans of nearly every animal species, including protozoa, fruit flies, mice, rats, and other laboratory animals. Primates are currently being studied.[15]

Behavioral Factors

Other aspects of eating and exercise influence changes commonly seen with aging. High blood lipid levels, alteration of blood glucose and insulin, obesity, and increased body fat at the waist and abdomen are common among older people. This constellation has been given the name *syndrome X* (see Chapter 17). The relationship of syndrome X to heart and other cardiovascular diseases is being studied.[22]

Syndrome X may be prevented with low-fat and low-cholesterol eating patterns and physical activity regimens. Overall nutrient intake, such as calcium and vitamin D, slows the thinning of bones that is common with aging in older women and predisposes them to osteoporosis. Vitamin E may be important to the immune system and beta-carotene, vitamin C, and vitamin E may retard oxidative damage.[22]

What is startling to many experts is the finding that most older people are not getting the Recommended Dietary Allowances (RDAs) for some nutrients. The Baltimore Longitudinal Study on Aging found deficiencies among elderly people in calcium; zinc; iron; magnesium; vitamins B_6, B_{12}, D, and E; and folic acid.[21] The US Department of Agriculture (USDA) Human Nutrition Research Center on Aging confirmed the finding; however, it is compounded by the fact that RDAs are not delineated for older people. RDAs are identified as a composite for adults 51 years of age and above.[23]

ETHNIC MINORITIES AND OLDER ADULTS

Ethnic minorities comprise 14% of the US population over 65 years of age. Ethnic minorities include a smaller proportion of elderly and a larger proportion of younger adults than the white population. In 1990, 13% of whites, 8% of African Americans, and 5% of Hispanics were 65 years of age or older. Higher fertility and mortality rates exist for the nonwhite population under age 65 compared to the white population under 65 years of age. In the year 2000, the proportion of older persons should increase at a higher rate for the nonwhite population than for the white population. This is in part due to the large proportion of children in comparison to their parents and especially their grandparents, who will reach old age. By 2020, 22% of the older population will be nonwhite; by 2050, 32% will be nonwhite.[24,25]

African-American Older Adults

The young outnumber the old among this ethnic group because of the higher fertility rates and higher mortality rates at midlife. The median age of African Americans is 24.9 years, which is almost seven years younger than the median age for whites. Mortality rates in childhood and youth for African Americans are higher than for whites. The fastest-growing segment of the African-American population is individuals over 65 years of age. The life expectancy for black men and women was 65.3 and 73.7 years in 1985, respectively; this is in contrast with the life expectancy of 71.9 years for white men and 78.8 years for white women.[25] The difference between these ethnic groups in life expectancy after age 65 is less dramatic.

Hispanic-American Older Adults

After African Americans, Hispanic Americans are the next largest ethnic minority population. Over 85% live in metropolitan areas. Hispanic Americans are the fastest-growing population group in the United States.[26,27] During the 10-year period from 1970 to 1980, older Hispanics in the United States increased by 74%, while there was only a 25% increase among all older adults. Hispanic Americans represent many different groups, and each group has its own distinct national and cultural heritage. These groups include Mexicans, Puerto Ricans, Cubans, Central or South Americans, and the US-born Mexican-American (Chicano) population. The Chicano population has a history in the United States that predates the entrance of English-speaking groups.

These Hispanic groups are bonded by a common language, but differ substantially in terms of geographic concentration, income, and education. Mexican Americans are the largest yet poorest group. They constitute 64% of the Hispanic population. Cubans represent the wealthiest and most educated Hispanic group. They have the largest proportion of foreign-born older adults among the three major Hispanic groups. The largest populations of Puerto Ricans and Cubans live in New York City, New Jersey, and Florida. The Hispanic populations are concentrated in California, Texas, and Florida.[28]

The median age of the Spanish-speaking population is 23.2 years, which is seven years younger than the US median age.[29] Only 3.5% of the Spanish-speaking population is 65 years of age and over. This percentage has remained stable over the past decade.[30]

Pacific-Asian Older Adults

About 6% of the Pacific-Asian population is 65 years of age and over. This group increased rapidly between 1965 and 1975 because of the 1965 repeal of quotas based on race and nationality and the immigration of Southeast Asians in the 1970s.[28] Asian Americans have a diversity of language, culture, acculturation to the United States, and socioeconomic status. Due to previous immigration patterns, many Japanese-American and Chinese-American elders have lived in this country for 40 to 50 years. This contrasts with older adults from Vietnam, Cambodia, and other Southeast Asian countries who immigrated after the Vietnam war. The Vietnam war immigrants tend to be less acculturated and have lower income levels than earlier immigrants.

In contrast to other ethnic minority groups and to white older adults, Pacific Islanders have a larger percentage of men living alone. This is due to a high male immigration in the early 1900s, coupled with previous restrictions on female immigration. It is not due to a higher life expectancy for Asian-Pacific men.

DEMOGRAPHIC CHARACTERISTICS

Older adults live in every US state, but they are not evenly distributed. In 1988, 31% of the older population lived in cities, 43% in suburbs, and 26% in rural areas. The Northeast is home to the oldest population of adults over 65, represented by 13.6% of its population. This contrasts with 12.6% for the total United States.[31] Florida has the highest median age in the United States (36.4 years) and Utah the lowest (25.7 years).

Change of residence is relatively rare for older people in the United States. Of the older population, 23% moved between 1975 and 1980, compared with 48% of individuals under 65 years of age. When older Americans move, they tend to move to a similar environment, such as rural to rural or large town to large town.[32]

For whites 65 years of age and older in 1988, the median level of education was 12.2 years; for African Americans it was 8.4 years, and for Hispanic Americans it was 7.5 years.[5] A disproportionate ratio of older minorities today have less than a high school education. Educational level is closely associated with economic well-being, and ethnic differences in education have a major impact on poverty levels of older adults.

Due to past mandatory retirement practices and incentives of early retirement, only 16% of men and 7% of women over age 65 are in the labor force. Part-time work is popular, and more than 50% of retired workers are employed in part-time or temporary jobs. Social Security remains the major source of income for older Americans. Increases in Social Security benefits with annual cost-of-living adjustments have improved the economic status of older Americans. Approximately 12% of senior citizens live on incomes below the poverty level, compared to 35% living below poverty level in the late 1950s.[30]

NUTRITIONAL STATUS OF NURSING HOME RESIDENTS

About 1.5 million US residents over 65 years of age (5%) live in one of the 20,000 nursing homes across the country. Nutritional status of older Americans, whether residing in an institution or living independently has been profiled using various study designs. Results of these studies indicate energy intakes below the RDAs for about one-third of elders, and vitamin and mineral intake below the RDAs for as many as 50% with 10 to 30% confirmed by serum analysis.[33-35] A fairly consistent picture of low energy and protein intake among institutionalized older adults, and over 50% at high nutritional risk due to physical and serum measures have been noted.[35-37]

A prospective study of older adults in the North Chicago Veterans Affairs Medical Center included a 67-item clinical database. In univariate analysis, seven items were significant predictors of death among the 55 men who died: age, functional level, triceps skinfold, midarm circumference, albumin, cholesterol, and hematocrit. A threshold level was defined for each variable. That is, a significant increase in mortality occurred when the level fell below the threshold. For albumin, cholesterol, and hematocrit, the threshold was within generally acceptable limits (albumin concentration of less than 4.0 g/dL, total serum cholesterol level below 160 mg/dL, and hematocrit less than 41%). Similar results have been reported by others.[38,39] An additional multivariate analysis identified serum total cholesterol and hematocrit as the strongest primary and secondary predictors of mortality, respectively.

This study recommended reformulating nutritional status indicators of older adults at different decades of life after 50 and considering their major residence. The nursing home environment may not be conducive to the maintenance of nutritional status above nonthreatening levels.[35] Two major categories of factors that predispose institutionalized older adults to a nutritional risk status have been identified as follows[35]:

1. factors causing inadequate intake
   - psychosocial setting
   - sensory perception—taste, smell, cognition, attention, manual dexterity
   - ability to chew and swallow (30 to 80% of nursing home residents are edentulous,[40] and 20 to 40% have dysphagia[41,42])
   - mood (33% of nursing home residents have depression[43,44])
   - appetite
   - inability to feed self and lack of assistance with eating
2. factors causing increased nutritional requirements
   - hyperactivity such as Parkinson's disease
   - infection (15 to 20% experience active urinary, respiratory, skin, or eye infection)
   - fever
   - wounds
   - anorexia

Protein-calorie undernutrition has been frequently observed among institutionalized older adults. Modifiable causes, a means to identify the cause, and corrective actions have been enumerated[35] (see Table 10-2). Aggressive but often simple forms of medical nutrition therapy may tilt the nutritional status of institutionalized elders in a positive direction. Taste-free supplements and calorie-dense foods such as chocolate and candy have been used to improve the overall energy intake and nitrogen balance of institutionalized elders.[45] The community nutrition professional may find these observations and results instructive when designing and implementing nutrition programs for older adults who live independently.

COMMUNITY NUTRITION PROFESSIONALS IN HOME CARE

Home care is an acceptable alternative to care and rehabilitation received within a hospital or medical environment. Services may include personal hygiene, assistance with homemaking and shopping, technical care including dialysis, and medical nutrition therapy (e.g., parenteral nutrition). This type of service has been one of the fasting growing sectors of the health care system.[46-48]

Tailored medical nutrition therapy at home may involve older adults with gastrointestinal disorders (e.g., Crohn's disease, short bowel syndrome, and ischemic bowel disease), HIV, cancer, end-stage renal disease, or amputation from diabetes. Using home visits, screening, and monitoring, community nutrition professionals can identify problems associated with an individual's inability to receive the required daily food pattern. The feedback, status, and care plan to rectify any problems can be directed back to the physician for continuity and efficient delivery of the medical nutrition therapy.

Generally, community nutrition professionals who are registered dietitians (RDs) may receive reimbursement from some insurance companies if the following occurs[49]:

Table 10–2 Fourteen Modifiable Causes of Protein-Calorie Undernutrition in an Institutional Environment

Cause	Method of Identification	Corrective Action
Staff unawareness	Lack of documentation in chart by MD, RN, or RD	Staff education
Inappropriate use of restricted diets	Patient receiving a restricted diet no longer indicated	Replace by ad lib diet
Use of drugs which impair desire or ability to eat	Review of medications	Discontinue or replace offending drug
Unmet need for eating assistance or self-help eating devices	Observation and calorie count	Provide assistance or devices
Suboptimal technique of assistance	Observation	Retrain the nursing aide
Suboptimal dining environment	Observation	Improve the environment
Prescription of maintenance instead of repletion dietary intakes (oral or enteral)	Less than 1.5 x RDA of calories and protein prescribed[a]	Increase prescription to 1.5 x RDA calories and protein
Inadequate nutritional support during intercurrent illness	Weight and/or albumin decline during illness; inadequate nutrition support	Project MD will consult on each patient during intercurrent illness
Unrecognized febrile illness	Daily temperatures reveal elevations	Identify and treat infections
Unmet need for modified diet	Clinical review	Prescribed indicated modified diet
Inadequate management of tube-feeding complications	Prescribed tube-feeding volume not being administered or absorbed	Correct management of complication
Poor dental status	Oral examination	Prompt dental care
Unmet need for dysphagia workup	Clinical signs suggest dysphagia; workup not requested	Consult speech pathology for swallowing evaluation
Suboptimal treatment of dysphagia	Recommendations of speech pathology not being followed	Speech pathologist retrains ward staff

[a]RDAs are the standards used to calculate an adequate eating pattern for an individual; the standards, however, are more accurately used to evaluate intake of groups.

Source: Reprinted from Abbasi AA and Rudman D. Undernutrition in the Nursing Home: Prevalence, Consequences, Causes and Prevention. *Nutrition Reviews*. 1994;52(4):119.

- The RD is employed by the physician.
- The RD services are medically supervised.
- The RD services are medically necessary.

With the blossoming of the home health industry, it is imperative to blend the skill of professionals with programs that target the nutrition needs of older individuals in the community. The extent to which older adults can maintain their independence (for example, through home-delivered meals) may depend on their ability to be linked with the services they need. Commu-

nity nutrition professionals can function as a conduit to connect older adults with the services they need.

SPECIAL DIETARY NEEDS OF OLDER ADULTS

Thirst and Fluid Requirements

Renal mass, renal blood flow, and fluid excretion decrease with age.[50,51] The regulation of body water relies on thirst and an individual's response to that thirst. Thirst is reduced in elders in general, and specifically in those with an elevated serum sodium and osmolality. Illness compounds the problem, as the lack of thirst may lead to severe dehydration and reduced mental acuity.[52]

Dehydration among older adults expresses itself as a swollen tongue, constipation, electrolyte disturbance, nausea and vomiting, hypotension, mental confusion, sunken eyeballs, increased body temperature, and decreased urine output. Older adults who are immobile may decrease water and fluid intake so they do not need to ask for assistance with toileting functions.[52]

For normal hydration, eight 8-ounce glasses of water or fluid is needed each day. Common sources include plain water, milk, juice, carbonated beverages, soups, and hydrous fruits. Caffeine-containing beverages such as coffee and tea are not good water sources.

Appetite and Satiety

Age has an inverse effect on the variety of foods eaten.[53,54] How this may occur is interesting. The change in palatability of a food once an individual begins to eat it is called sensory-specific satiety. This type of satiety is associated with a decreased intake of one food and a switch to another food during that ingestion period. The sensory-specific satiety mechanism promotes more variety and potentially a more well-balanced eating pattern.[55]

The mechanism has been shown to diminish among individuals as they age when comparing groups 12 to 15 years, 22 to 35 years, 45 to 60 years, and 65 to 82 years.[56] It is not known whether this is the result of a rather monotonous selection of foods, a lower calorie content of foods, denture problems, or lack of taste or seasoning of food. This area of research is relatively new but of interest to community nutrition professionals who plan and prepare meals and snacks for older adults.

Taste and Smell

Taste buds turn over constantly every 10.5 days; olfactory receptors in the nasal cavity have an average turnover time of 30 days.[57] Losses in taste and smell begin at about 60 years of age and may peak by age 70. Chemosensory losses include the following[57]:

- ageusia—absence of taste
- hypogeusia—diminished sensitivity of taste
- dysgeusia—distortion of normal taste
- anosmia—absence of smell
- hyposmia—diminished sensitivity of smell
- dysosmia—distortion of normal smell

The detection threshold for taste and smell varies with the molar conductivity values of the anions. The threshold for distinguishing odors among elders may be as much as 11 times higher than that of younger individuals. In addition, the ability to distinguish the odors of certain items varies. For example, the ability to distinguish the odor of breads, vegetables, and coffee declines greatly with age, but elders retain the ability to identify green bell pepper.[57]

Several medical conditions affect the sense of taste and smell (see Table 10–3). Drugs such as local anesthetics, opiates (codeine, morphine), antihypertensive agents (diltiazem and nifedipine), and antimicrobial agents (allicin, streptomycin, tyrothricin) also influence the sense of smell. Certain types of drugs affect the sense of taste, including anesthetics (benzocaine, lidocaine), antihistamines (chlorpheniramine maleate), antirheumatics (allopurinol, colchicine, hydrocortisone, salicylates), drugs for Parkinson's disease (levodopa, baclofen), vasodilators (nitroglycerin patch), and amphetamines. As taste and smell sensitivities decrease, decreases in stimulation of salivary glands, gastric acid, and pancreatic secretions occur and increases in plasma insulin and pancreatic polypeptide occur. When the senses are stimulated by food, plasma-free fatty acids may decline and sympathetic nervous system activity and metabolic rate may increase. With a reduction of taste and smell, metabolic processes can be altered.[57]

Potassium Loss

Many potent diuretics produce significant potassium losses. Potassium is the main ion inside

Table 10–3 Medical Conditions That Affect the Sense of Taste and Smell

	Effect on	
Condition	Taste	Smell
Nervous	Bell's palsy Damage to chorda tympani Familial dysautonomia Head trauma Multiple sclerosis Raeder's paratrigeminal syndrome	Head trauma Korsakoff's syndrome Multiple sclerosis Parkinson's disease Tumors and lesions
Nutritional	Cancer Chronic renal failure Liver disease including cirrhosis Niacin (vitamin B$_3$) deficiency Thermal burn Zinc deficiency	Chronic renal failure Liver disease including cirrhosis Vitamin B$_{12}$ deficiency
Endocrine	Adrenal cortical insufficiency Congenital adrenal hyperplasia Pseudohypoparathyroidism Panhypopituitarism Cushing's syndrome Cretinism Hypothyroidism Diabetes mellitus Gonadal dysgenesis (Turner's syndrome)	Adrenal cortical insufficiency Cushing's syndrome Hypothyroidism Diabetes mellitus Gonadal dysgenesis (Turner's syndrome) Hypogonadism (Kallman's syndrome) Primary amenorrhea Pseudohypoparathyroidism
Local	Facial hypoplasia Glossitis and other oral disorders Leprosy Oral Crohn's disease Radiation therapy Sjögren's syndrome	Adenoid hypertrophy Allergic rhinitis and atopy Bronchial asthma Leprosy Ozena Sinusitis and polyposis Sjögren's syndrome Viral infections Acute viral hepatitis Influenza-like infections
Other	Hypertension Influenza-like infections Laryngectomy	Familial (genetic) laryngectomy Olfactory sarcoidosis

Source: Adapted from Schiffman S. Changes in Taste and Smell: Drug Interactions and Food Preferences. *Nutrition Reviews.* 1994;52(8):(II)S11–S14.

---

body cells; it maintains fluid balance, electrolyte balance, and cell integrity. Potassium is essential to maintaining the heartbeat; a lack of potassium from fasting or severe diarrhea may cause heart failure. Dehydration is dangerous, because the loss of potassium from brain cells makes the victim unaware of the need for water.[58]

Most eating patterns do not provide enough potassium to compensate for the amount lost due to diuretics. Proper choice of foods can effectively replace potassium losses. Food sources that are high in potassium are listed in Exhibit 10-2.

Dyslipidemia

Data based on a sample of older adults between 70 and 104 years (N = 610 women and 387 men)

Exhibit 10-2 Common Foods That Are Good Sources of Potassium

- bran cereals
- cooked dried fruit such as apricots, peaches, prunes
- bananas
- potatoes, baked or boiled
- sweet potatoes, pumpkin, winter squash
- stewed tomatoes
- spinach, asparagus, cantaloupe, and watermelon
- lima beans
- cooked dry beans, peas, lentils
- milk and yogurt (all types)

Source: Adapted from Hamilton EMN, Whitney EN, and Sizer FS. *Nutrition Concepts and Controversies.* 5th Ed. Whitney EN and Sizer FS (eds.). 1991. West Publishing Company, New York. p. 252.

suggest that elders do not incur an increased risk of heart attack, angina, or death from any cause if they have either low high-density lipoprotein (HDL) cholesterol or high total serum cholesterol levels. Baseline measures in 1990 showed 32% of women and 16% of men with cholesterol levels greater than 240 mg/dL versus 9% of women and 26% of men with low HDL levels. Women with total cholesterol levels greater than 240 mg% had the longest survival; women with 200 to 240 mg% had the lowest survival. There was no significant effect of total cholesterol or HDL on heart attacks or mortality rates for men or women.[59]

Constipation

The prevalence of constipation among older adults may be about 34%. Defined medically as defecation less than three 3 times a week or every third day, constipation is a daily problem for many older adults. In a study of 211 frail elders receiving home care, 45% reported constipation as a problem and 11% felt it was a major problem. The major strategies to overcome constipation cited by 70 respondents were as follows: 4% changed bowel habits, 7% increased exercise, 34% changed what they ate, and 88% used medications. Of the 62 respondents who used medica-

tions, the types commonly used were as follows: 50% stool softeners, 24% bulk agents, 19% stimulants, 19% osmotics, 14% unknown, 10% combination laxatives, 8% cathartics, 2% lubricants, 10% enemas, and 2% suppositories.[60] These data suggest that public education about the role of fiber, especially the laxative effect of fresh fruit, is warranted.

Bereavement

Loneliness at mealtime may influence the amount and frequency of meal and snack consumption. For older adults who live alone, a question for those who may not meet their energy or nutrient needs is whether mealtime is viewed as a chore or a reminder of what meals used to be like.

Eating behaviors of 50 individuals over 60 years who were widowed within the past two years were contrasted with eating behaviors of 50 married elders. Responses showed that 72% of the widowed elders felt that eating was a chore, and a favorite substitute for meals was low-nutrient-dense snacks; 84% experienced weight loss with an average of 7.6 pounds of body weight. The widowed group averaged 35% of total energy intake from fat, compared with 32% for the married respondents. Grief resolution showed a positive association with dietary components, which suggests that emotional and nutritional status may be mediated by the eating pattern.[61]

Oral Health

Dental caries, missing teeth, infections, mucosal lesions, and diseased gums make chewing difficult and decrease the variety and amount of food ingested. Inadequate oral health care, which increases weight loss and the onset of malnutrition, can be resolved with regular dental care.[9,52]

Alzheimer's Disease

Alzheimer's disease was identified in 1907 by Alois Alzheimer, who uncovered abnormal structures of amyloid plaques and neurofibrillary tangles in the brain of a woman. The disease affects four million Americans who are over 65 years of age and is among the top five causes of death among the elderly.[62-65] About 60% of the elderly in long-term care facilities have Alzheimer's disease.[62,64]

Alzheimer's disease is slow and progressive. The cause is unknown.[64-67] The process involves degeneration of neurons in the hippocampus and cerebral cortex due to a 40 to 90% decline in choline acetyltransferase activity.[62-69] There is an association between the number of plaques and the degree of cell loss with the severity of dementia expressed as memory loss, decline in cognition, and distant-type behavior.[67,68]

There is no known cure for Alzheimer's disease, but drugs are used to treat symptoms of depression, agitation, or sleep disorders.[66] Symptoms occur for an average of 6 to 10 years, but the span from onset to death can be from 3 to 20 years. Respiratory diseases and bronchopneumonia are the major causes of death.[68,70]

Alzheimer's disease has three stages that are summarized in Table 10-4.[62,63,68,71] The need for nutritional support increases with each stage. During stage 1, individuals may need assistance shopping, storing, or cooking food. In stage 2, individuals often begin to pace, have chewing or swallowing problems, and need assistance feeding themselves. In stage 3, individuals may not recognize foods, forget to eat, or forget what to do with the food. A loss of muscle mass and body fat results from the reduced eating.[70-72] The need for home care increases, until 24-hour care is appropriate.

Limited nutritional data are available for Alzheimer's disease, because few studies exist and there is a lack of standard criteria used to evaluate nutritional status of patients. The Recom-

Table 10-4 Major Stages of Alzheimer's Disease

Stage	Symptoms
1	Is still alert. Purchases and prepares own food; feeds self. Complains of memory loss. Has decreased vocational abilities. Is increasingly unable to think abstractly and make proper judgments. Displays mood and personality changes, irritability, hostility, and agitation.
2	Is completely unable to learn and recall information. Is disoriented with time and place; needs assistance for daily living. Can feed self, but needs direction and assistance at mealtime. Is at risk of falling. Shows signs of depression, agitation, hostility, uncooperativeness, and physical aggressiveness. Begins pacing needlessly.
3	Is severely impaired intellectually. Is completely disoriented. Requires total assistance. Cannot feed self; may refuse to chew and swallow food. May become incontinent and bedridden. Is at risk for malnutrition, infection, pneumonia, and pressure sores. Coma may occur.

Source: Huey E. *Nutritional Assessment of Patients with Alzheimer's Disease in Three Stages of the Disease.* Master's Thesis 1995. California State University Long Beach. p. 2.

mended Dietary Allowances (RDAs) evaluate food intake, but standards exist only for healthy adults up to 50 years of age and above.[23] Community nutrition and health care professionals must recognize this limitation when they are using the RDAs to evaluate eating patterns, because individuals with Alzheimer's often exceed age 65 and may have different nutritional needs. Huey reported below normal hemoglobin and hematocrit levels for stage 2 patients; stage 3 patients had lower energy intakes than patients in stages 1 and 2, even when the stage 3 patients had nutritional supplements.[65]

"The Dwindles" or Failure to Thrive

Failure to thrive is neither a normal part of aging nor the inevitable result of chronic disease. It is a consequence of a number of factors: normal aging; malnutrition; and specific physical, psychological, and/or social determinants (see Figure 10–1). Medical nutrition therapy is the cornerstone of the treatment of elder adults with failure to thrive. Several factors enhance failure to thrive. Each may be relatively mild, but in combination with malnutrition and aging the synergy is lethal. The factors that enhance failure to thrive include the following[73]:

- physical diseases (chronic obstructive lung disease, heart failure, cancer, infections, hyperthyroidism, hypothyroidism, or uncontrolled diabetes)
- dementia
- delirium
- alcohol consumption
- drug use
- dysphagia
- sensory deficits such as deafness and blindness
- depression
- desertion by family and friends
- poverty
- despair

Normal changes of aging plus physical, psychological, and social precipitants

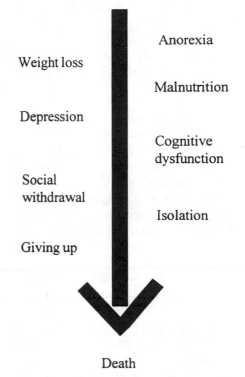

Figure 10–1 The downward spiral of geriatric failure to thrive. *Source:* Egbert AM. "The Dwindles": Failure to Thrive in Older Patients. *Postgrad Med* 1993;94:199–212.

Info Line

The 11 D's of "the dwindles" is a clever mnemonic for remembering the primary causes of geriatric failure to thrive: diseases (medical illnesses), dementia, delirium, drinking alcohol, drugs, dysphagia, deafness (or other sensory deficits), depression, desertion by family and friends (social isolation), destitution (poverty), and despair (giving up).[73]

RDAs FOR HEALTHY OLDER ADULTS

Many nutritional surveys of elders report only a low or moderate prevalence of clear nutrient deficiency but show an increased risk for malnutrition and subclinical deficiencies. This has a cyclic effect: nutritional status influences the age-related rate of functional decline for body organs, influences body composition, and predisposes to chronic diseases.[74-76]

The nutritional needs of older adults vary due to the age range of this population. One notices this when contrasting 50-to-60 year olds with 80-to-90 year olds in terms of habits, activities, and abilities. The need to rethink specific RDAs for each decade after 50 years of age is gaining support,[77] but the criteria for establishing new and extended RDAs remains a critical issue. Relevant questions are as follows[78]:

- Should RDAs for elders be based on observed age-associated changes in body composition and physiologic function?
- Should RDAs be based on optimal body composition and function by chronological age strata?
- Should RDAs be based on level of dietary intake needed to maintain current health?
- Should RDAs be based on intake that creates maximum reduction of chronic disease risk?

Nutrient needs are related to observed body functions and changes that take place after a person passes 50 years of age. The rationale for variations in nutrient requirements for individuals over 50 years of age is based on the following needs and/or changes[78]:

- the need for vitamins B_6 and E to promote immune response
- reduced ability to absorb vitamin B_{12} and folic acid due to less hydrochloric acid produced
- the need for vitamin B_6 for glucose tolerance and normal cognitive function

- the need for vitamin B_6, B_{12}, and folate to protect against homocysteine
- decreased ability to convert vitamin D to an active form
- the need for vitamins C and E and beta-carotene to reduce risk for coronary heart disease, cancer, and cataracts
- marginal zinc deficiency leading to mental lethargy, delayed wound healing, and loss of taste
- vitamin-disease associations (e.g., folate with cervical dysplasia, and vitamin C with atrophic gastritis)

Even though the scientific data are not available to make definitive decisions and choose exact criteria, the United States has recognized the need to address uniqueness of the graying population and various requirements at different stages of elder life.

OLDER AMERICANS ACT OF 1965

The Nutrition Program for Older Americans was mandated by the 1972 Title VII Amendment to the Older Americans Act of 1965. In the United States, nutrition services assist older Americans to live independently by promoting better health through improved nutrition and reduced isolation. In 1977, the US Congress approved funding of home-delivered meals under Title IIIC of the Older Americans Act. Title IIIC is a federal program coordinated with other supportive services.[79]

Nutrition services include the procurement, preparation, transport, and service of meals; nutrition education; and nutrition counseling to older persons at congregate sites or in their homes. Nutrition-related supportive services include outreach, transportation, and escort of older persons to nutrition sites, and food shopping assistance.

In most states, Title IIIC is administered through a department of aging or a nutrition section. Program goals are generally to maintain or improve the physical, psychological, or social well-being of elders by providing or securing appropriate nutrition services. Program objectives may include the following[79]:

- to give preference to elders in greatest economic or social need, with particular attention to low-income minority individuals
- to maintain or increase the number of meals served consistent with funding levels and inflation rates
- to serve meals that are nutritious, safe, of good quality, at the lowest reasonable cost
- to promote increased cost-effectiveness through improved program and food service management
- to promote or maintain high food safety and sanitation standards
- to promote or maintain coordination with other supportive services

To be eligible for congregate meals, a person must be either 60 years old or over, the spouse of any person aged 60 or over, or a disabled person under age 60 who resides in housing facilities occupied primarily by elderly persons who receive congregate nutrition services. To be eligible to receive a home-delivered meal, the above criteria apply, and a telephone interview or a home visit to the applicant is usually required. Verification of need for the service is determined through home assessment and, if eligible, the recipient receives meal service within one week.

In most states, the following criteria must be met for individuals to be eligible to receive a home-delivered meal[79]:

- any person aged 60 or over
- the spouse of any person aged 60 or over
- any person aged 60 or over who is frail, homebound by reason of illness or incapacitating disability, or otherwise isolated
- a spouse of a recipient above may receive a home-delivered meal if the agency concludes that it is in the best interest of the homebound older person

The following individuals are also eligible to receive a congregate or home-delivered meal:

- a nonelderly, disabled person who resides with an elderly person who receives either home-delivered or congregate meals
- a volunteer of any age who provides essential services during program hours (may be offered a meal and the opportunity to contribute to the meal cost)
- a guest less than 60 years of age (may be offered a meal and shall pay a fee)
- nutrition service staff

Each congregate and home-delivered meal is planned to supply one-third of the Recommended Dietary Allowances (RDAs) as established by the Food and Nutrition Board of the National Academy of Sciences-National Research Council.[23] When feasible and appropriate, the cultural and religious preferences and special dietary needs of eligible persons are considered (see Table 10–5).

In most communities, a local agency is set up to develop, implement, and monitor policies, procedures, and standards that comply with all applicable laws and regulations of the state and county, including health and fire safety inspections. The staff at an agency generally includes a nutrition services director. If the agency provides its own meal and delivery service, then it may employ its own project community nutrition professional, food service manager, and diet technician.

The community nutrition professional usually has a bachelor's degree in nutrition, dietetics, institutional food service management, or a closely-related field from an accredited college or university. Postgraduate course work and/or a graduate degree is desirable in nutrition, dietetics, institutional food service management, public health nutrition, home economics with an emphasis in nutrition and food service management, or gerontology. A master's degree is encouraged but not mandatory. The commu-

Table 10–5 Minimum Menu Requirements for Congregate and Home-Delivered Meals, Title IIIC

Meal Component	Food Sources
Protein	A three-ounce cooked edible portion of meat, fish, fowl, eggs, or cheese. Meat alternatives may be used only once per week and include cooked dried beans, peas, lentils, nuts, nut butter (peanut butter and others), or products made from these foods.
Vegetable/Fruit	Two (2) one-half cup servings of vegetables or fruits or their juices.
Bread or Alternate	One serving of whole-grain or enriched bread, biscuits, muffins, rolls, sandwich buns, corn bread, or other hot breads. Bread alternates include enriched or whole-grain cereals, rice, spaghetti, macaroni, noodles, dumplings, pancakes, waffles, and tortillas.
Milk	Eight ounces of fortified skim, low-fat, or buttermilk, or the calcium equivalent.
Margarine	One teaspoon of fortified margarine or butter. Each meal shall contain one (1) one-half cup serving of a dessert such as fruit, pudding, gelatin dessert, ice cream, ice milk, or sherbet. Cake, pie, cookies, and similar foods shall be limited to once per week. Coffee, tea, or decaffeinated beverages may be used, but shall not be counted as fulfilling any part of the meal pattern requirements.

Source: Adapted from Older Americans Act Title IIIC. U.S. Congress, 1965.

---

nity nutrition professional or nutritionist is generally required to be a registered dietitian (RD) with the American Dietetic Association and have three years of professional experience in nutrition and dietetics, food service management, geriatric nutrition, or community nutrition. A minimum of one year of experience in food service management is often required. Completion of a one-year dietetic internship may be substituted for one year of experience.

The job responsibilities of the professional generally include participating in developing policies, procedures, and standards; annually assessing each nutrition service provider on-site; and providing technical assistance to other agency personnel and nutrition service providers. The nutritionist provides nutrition education to participants in congregate and home-delivery meal programs, and approves and certifies menus prior to use. He or she participates in needs assessments for applicants and the development of

public service announcements for local radio, television, and newspaper.

The nutritionist regularly schedules on-site monitoring of nutrition service providers and evaluates how efficiently and effectively services are provided. He or she conducts problem solving, information sharing, and continuing education activities among service provider staff. The nutritionist reviews and approves nutrition-related contracts and monitors contracts for adherence, quality, and effectiveness.

The number of hours needed for nutrition consultation to perform all duties is usually determined by the administrator, but it may vary from one day per week to full-time. Often the nutritionist and all nutrition service contracts are selected through a competitive bid process. Providers who apply often furnish the appropriate congregate or home-delivered meals and a nutrition consultant or a food service manager.

Info Line

**Nutrition Education Services for
Congregate and Home-Delivered Meal Participants**

Nutrition education is generally required no less than once every other month per fiscal year, and preferably monthly at each congregate site. The nutrition education for congregate sites is defined as demonstrations, audiovisual presentations, lectures, or small group discussions, which are planned, approved, and coordinated by a qualified nutritionist. Home-delivered nutrition education occurs no less than quarterly. Home-delivered education is usually an educational brochure, questionnaire, or fact sheet on nutrition. The Gerontological Nutrition Dietetic Practice Group provides camera-ready nutrition education sheets as inserts in its monthly newsletter (see Figures 10–2 and 10–3).[80]

The purpose of nutrition education is to inform individuals about available facts and information that will promote improved food selection and eating habits. One nutrition education session per year addresses the sources and prevention of food-borne illness. The education may guide older persons in making sound food choices and in obtaining the best food to meet nutritional needs for the least money. Or, the education can make older persons aware of community-sponsored health programs that encourage and promote sound nutritional habits and good health. Often the education assists older persons with special diets.

Nutrition education services are based on the particular needs of congregate and homebound older persons. This is usually determined by an annual needs assessment and evaluation of the service. All nutrition education activities are documented with signatures of attendees, a copy of any handout material, and a description of the verbal presentation or talk kept on file in the agency office.

MEAL SERVICE REQUIREMENTS

The *Dietary Guidelines for Americans* are used throughout the United States for Title IIIC menus.[81] California has developed the *California Daily Food Guide* to give additional meal planning direction.[82] These guidelines include increasing the consumption of complex carbohydrates and fiber and lowering intake of fat, sodium, and simple sugars. Low-sodium meats, flavorings, and stocks are strongly encouraged, as well as whole grains, meat alternates, and raw fruits and vegetables to increase the fiber content of menus. Low-fat salad dressings, cheeses, and gravies made without drippings and fats are strongly recommended, as well as baking, broiling, and steaming foods rather than frying them in fat.

Detailed nutritional analyses must accompany the menus. The menus must meet one-third of the RDAs for males age 51 and above for these nutrients: protein, thiamin, riboflavin, niacin, vitamin B_6, folacin, vitamin B_{12}, vitamin A, vitamin C, vitamin D, calcium, iron, phosphorus, magnesium, zinc, and vitamin E (see Appendix 10–A and Appendix 10–B). The menus must provide a protein source, vegetable and/or fruit, bread or bread alternate, and milk, and provide more than 500 kilocalories per meal.

All foods for congregate and home-delivered meals are packaged and transported in a manner that protects them from potential contamination including dust, insects, rodents, unclean equipment and utensils, and unnecessary handling. Hot food is maintained at or above 140°F, and cold

30 Snacks for less than 1 gram of fat

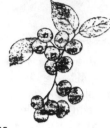
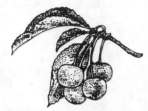
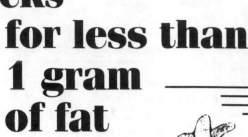
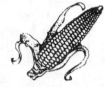

When you cut the fat out of your diet, there is still plenty of room for fun and tasty snacks. Try one of the following when you need a snack or a quick meal. Each contains less than one gram of fat.

○ Two pretzel rods

○ Fresh fruit chunks sprinkled with cinnamon

○ Two rice cakes spread with fruit spread

○ A small whole wheat pita stuffed with sliced tomatoes, cucumbers, sprouts, and a sauce of lemon juice and Dijon mustard

○ A cinnamon-raisin bagel spread with apple butter

○ A flour tortilla wrapped around vegetarian "refried" beans

○ Eight ounces of Bloody Mary mix with a stalk of celery (and without the vodka)

○ Popcorn sprinkled with salt and chili powder

○ One cup of Wheat Chex sprinkled with Cajun seasoning mix and baked in an oven until crisp

○ One-half cup of applesauce sprinkled with nutmeg

○ A juicy dill pickle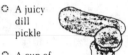

○ A cup of pasta tossed with fresh tomatoes and basil

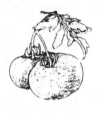

○ A cup of beans cooked in Sloppy Joe sauce served on toast

○ An English muffin spread with tomato sauce and mushrooms and baked until hot — to make a mini cheese-less pizza

○ A frozen banana

○ A cup of herb tea stirred with a cinnamon stick

○ Four breadsticks

○ Four ounces of fruit juice mixed with four ounces of club soda to make a fruit juice spritzer

○ Six melba rounds dotted with strawberry jam

○ One-half cup of split pea soup with four non-fat crackers

○ One Dole frozen Fruit and Juice bar

○ Twenty frozen grapes

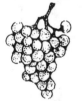

○ Raw vegetables dipped in fat-free dressing

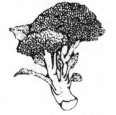

○ One fresh ear of corn lightly sprinkled with salt

○ A skewer of mushrooms grilled over the coals until lightly browned

○ A steaming baked potato stuffed with hot vegetables

○ Three ginger snaps

○ One slice of toast sprinkled with cinnamon and sugar

○ A homemade oat bran muffin spread with raspberry jam

○ One fruit-kabob — assorted melon balls and fruit chunks on a skewer

Figure 10–2 Nutrition education handout for older adults as prepared by the Gerontological Nutrition Dietetic Practice Group of the American Dietetic Association. The handout describes snacks with less than 1 gram of fat. Courtesy of the Physicians Committee for Responsible Medicine, Washington, DC.

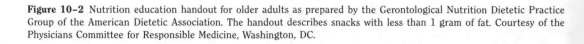

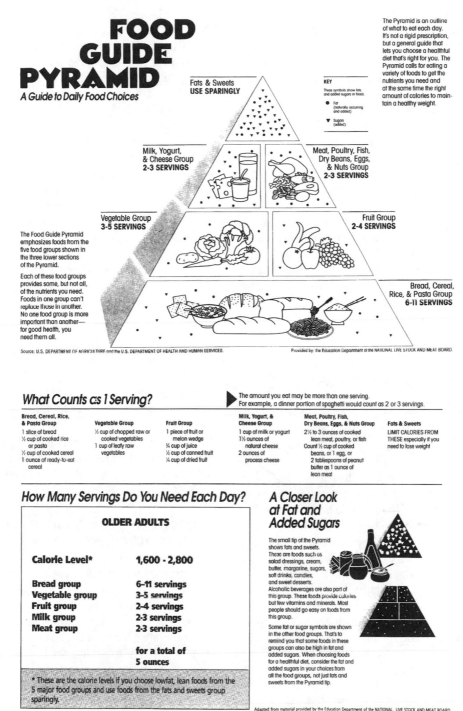

Figure 10–3 Nutrition education handout for older adults as prepared by the Gerontological Nutrition Dietetic Practice Group of the American Dietetic Association. The handout reinforces older adult food choices using the Food Guide Pyramid. *Source:* Reprinted from Gerontological Nutrition Dietetic Practice Group, American Dietetic Association. *GN Newsletter,* Winter 1992, pp. 17–18.

food is maintained at or below 45°F throughout the meal service period or until delivered to the homebound participant.[79]

Systematic temperature checks of food are taken and recorded daily at several points; at the end of production, at delivery, at serving time for congregate sites, and at the point of packaging for home-delivered foods. Temperatures are taken no less than one time per week per route prior to handing the food to the recipient.

For food safety and reduced chance of foodborne illness, holding time between the completion of cooking and beginning of food service at the congregate site is not to exceed two hours. For home-delivered meals, the holding time between the completion of cooking and delivery of the last meal is not to exceed two hours. Frozen, home-delivered meals may exceed the two-hour time limit when the food is maintained at 32°F or less and in a frozen state until delivery[79] (see Chapter 6 for more detail on food safety).

Effect of Home-Delivered Meals

Two important questions about the home-delivered meal programs in the United States have been posed recently: (1) Does the program serve those who are currently most needy? (2) Does the meal program reduce the need for higher levels of care?[83] Roe stated that the rationale for serving home-delivered meals has generally been based on non-nutritional criteria (e.g., a warm meal, contact with a deliverer, improved quality of life, alleviation of distress and food insecurity among the disabled) and that the indices of benefit are rarely quantitative.

Assessment of older adults' needs for food assistance have been based on anecdotal reports by elderly of the number of times they go without food, the type of discharge diet order from the hospital, living status, and advanced age.[84-86] The assessment method has been haphazard, and no generally accepted system of assessment has been defined.

A 1984 survey conducted by the Texas Department of Aging reported that dependence on a meal served by a community agency was higher among the homebound than among those who obtained meals at congregate sites. The need was greater in geographic areas of poverty and among minority groups.[87] However, another study showed that in geographic areas that contained a large minority population, programs were the least innovative and fewer meals were provided during the week.[88]

Studies have shown that meal recipients have fewer hospitalizations and a better meal quality; however, among minority groups, those who receive meals are more likely than nonminority elders to have several hospitalizations due to lack of management of their diabetes and hypertension.[89,90] Recommendations that have been made regarding home-delivered meals are as follows[83]:

- Make provisions for weekends and evenings.
- Focus on special diets (e.g., individuals with diabetes).
- Reduce the amount of fat in the meals.
- Ensure good sources of folate, since this is often lacking in the food prepared or selected by older adults.
- Conduct research to determine if the home meals program reduces hospital costs and institutionalization.
- Determine if meal program deficiencies are due to lack of innovation, lack of case management, or unequal access to health care.

HEALTHY LIFE FOR SENIORS—A CHOICE OR AN OUTCOME?

Future cohorts of older people may be healthier and more independent well into their 80s and 90s. Fries suggests healthier lifestyles and better health care during youth and middle years will promote maximum life span in future years. Future cohorts may have fewer debilitating illnesses and may experience "compressed morbidity"—only a few years of major illness in very old age. Older adults of the future may die a "natural death"—death due to the natural wearing out of all organ systems by approximately age 100.[91] This change could significantly affect health services, employment, and leisure activities for future generations of elderly Americans. An increase in short-stay convalescent centers and home health services may occur.

In 1989, Verbrugge analyzed the National Health Interview Survey from 1958 to 1985 and reported that successive cohorts of middle-aged and older persons reported more morbidity in terms of short-term disability and days of restricted activity than previous cohorts. Morbidity rates increased over a 27-year interval for heart disease, cancer, diabetes, hypertension, and non-life-threatening diseases like arthritis. Mortality rates did not change.[92]

It is likely that earlier diagnosis and better secondary and tertiary prevention and clinical care, including high-tech screening and treatment, will promote survival from major illnesses. Recent cohorts of older adults experience more chronic conditions than previous cohorts, but gradual changes in health habits such as less smoking, less consumption of alcohol and saturated fats, increased exercise, and decreased loneliness—especially at mealtime (see Exhibit 10-3)—may improve the well-being of future elders. Popular physical activities among senior adults are outlined in Table 10-6. Healthier lifestyles for people currently in their 20s and 30s will give them more years without illness and may result in fewer chronic health problems when they reach old age.[92]

Exhibit 10-3 Ideas To Combat Eating Alone among Older Adults

- Plan meals as special events once or twice a week. Set the table, light candles, play music, or eat when a television show or sports event that you and your friends like is on.
- Invite friends over for meals, bring a part of the meal to a friend's house, or trade portions of "planned leftovers" for an early evening meal two or three nights a week.
- Eat out once a week or so. Many restaurants have lower prices and smaller portions at lunchtime for seniors. Some may offer reduced prices for older adults.
- Plan a daytime outing once a week with a friend. Go to lunch and visit a museum or attend an afternoon concert or theater performance.
- Visit or join a senior center for lunch; participate in meals offered by your local agency on aging.
- Form a gourmet club with others who eat alone.
- Participate in a church or community service club. Volunteer to participate in social functions.
- Choose a nonprofit health organization to support as a volunteer and give time during mealtime.

Info Line

The National Institutes of Health and the National Cancer Institute have an information service at 1-800-4-CANCER (1-800-422-6237). This service gives older adults information about various screening and treatment programs. Spanish-speaking staff are available. The mailing address is Office of Cancer Communications, National Cancer Institute, Building 31, Room 10A24, Bethesda, MD 20892.

Crimmins studied National Health Interview Survey cohorts from 1969 to 1981 and reported greater limited activity for males up to age 74 and females up to age 72.[93] This contrasted with Palmore who studied 45-to-64 year olds and reported no change in days of restricted activity but some decline in the number of days of bed disability.[94]

Schneider and Brody suggest that the average period of decreased livelihood will increase, since the number of very old people having multiple chronic illnesses will increase and some diseases will begin in old age.[95] Rice and Feldman propose that there will be people who achieve advanced old age while still in very good health.[96] At the same time, another group of equally old people will experience extended morbidity.

The concept of "active" versus "dependent" life expectancy has arisen.[97] The end point of "active" life expectancy is defined as the loss of independence and the need to rely on others for most activities of family living.[97] Life expectancy has increased beyond 65 years, but about one-fourth of those additional years will require dependent living.[98] A 65-year-old woman in 1990 had approximately 18.6 years of life remaining, with 12.6 years in active life expectancy and 6.0 years in dependency. A 65-year-old man could live

Table 10–6 Popular Exercises for Senior Adults with Benefits and Energy Expenditure

Exercise	Energy Expenditure	Benefits	Locations
Swimming	90 calories in 20 minutes	Increases heart rate; good source of exercise for people with arthritis or other joint problems; provides a daily dose of vitamin D if outdoors.	Local YMCA and colleges have pools for swimming classes and aqua aerobics.
Walking	148 calories in 20 minutes	Increases heart rate; burns calories; is a way to relax and socialize with friends; is a weight-bearing exercise, which is good for bone and muscle development; provides a daily dose of vitamin D from the sunlight.	An adult can walk just about anywhere. Some fun places to walk are the park, the school track, the shopping mall, or around the neighborhood.
Dancing	98 calories in 20 minutes	Is a weight-bearing exercise, fun, and a way to meet new friends and socialize.	Local colleges and YMCA often have dance classes.
Bowling	84 calories in 20 minutes	Is a way to socialize while having fun, a weight-bearing exercise, and a form of friendly competition with friends.	Local bowling lanes have leagues that an individual can join.

Source: Adapted from Evans WJ. Exercise, Nutrition and Aging. *J Nutr.* 1992;122:796–801.

14.4 more years with 2.4 years in a dependent state. Some gerontologists suggest that a deficit in the active life expectancy of 1.0 to 2.5 years will occur for poor older adults compared with those who are not impoverished. Kane, Ouslander, and Abrass describe this as a growing bimodal distribution of older people, with one group healthier and free of disease and another, larger group of elders surviving diseases but living with compressed morbidity.[99] Many erroneous prejudices exist that form a barrier to the older adult's and society's enjoyment of elder life. This is called *ageism*.[100]

One important goal of health planners and practitioners is to approach a rectangular survival curve. Advances in medicine, public hygiene, and health have increased the percentage of people surviving into their 70s and 80s. Ideally all people would survive to a maximum life span and create a "rectangular curve" (see Chapter 1 , Figure 1-4). Support organizations for seniors are listed in Appendix 10–C.

NUTRITION SCREENING INITIATIVE

The broadest multidisciplinary effort ever initiated in the United States to encourage the incorporation of nutrition screening, assessment, and care of elders into a health care system is called the Nutrition Screening Initiative. The initiative responds to the 1988 Surgeon General's Workshop on Health Promotion and Aging and the *Healthy People 2000* objectives for increased interdisciplinary collaboration assessing nutritional status and providing nutrition intervention.[101,102] Focusing on an initial five-year period, the American Dietetic Association, the American

Academy of Family Physicians, and the National Council on the Aging joined with 35 key health, aging, and medical organizations and professionals to form a coalition for the initiative.[103] If older persons are at risk of poor nutrition, screening can identify the problem(s) and possible primary, secondary, and tertiary interventions. The major risk factors of poor nutritional status are inappropriate food intake, poverty, social isolation, dependency/disability, acute/chronic diseases or conditions, chronic medication use, and advanced age (80 and above). Table 10–7 identifies major and minor indicators of poor nutritional status. The screening process can likewise build professional collaboration to expand programs on a community level.

Screening can be administered at three levels using instruments developed by the Nutrition Screening Initiative: the "Determine Your Nutritional Health" checklist, Level I Screen for seniors, and Level II Screen for seniors (see Appendix 10-D). The checklist has two elements[104,105]:

1. a self-assessment using a series of statements to which elders respond

2. a mnemonic device (the word DETER-MINE) that provides basic education on nutritional risk factors

The checklist is a public-awareness instrument. It can be administered by any level of health care professional or self-administered. By summing the checklist, older adults receive a nutritional score that ranges from no risk, to moderate risk, to high nutritional risk.

The Level I Screen is a basic nutrition screen designed for social service and health professionals to identify older Americans who may need medical or nutritional attention. This instrument can identify individuals who may be good candidates for meal assistance such as home or congregate meal programs or nutrition therapy and education.[103]

The Level II Screen provides more specific diagnostic information on nutritional status. It is designed for health and medical professionals to use with older adults who have a potentially serious medical or nutritional problem. This instrument contains a detailed history of weight change and laboratory and clinical indicators of protein and calorie malnutrition, obesity, and other dis-

---

Table 10–7 Major and Minor Indicators of Poor Nutritional Status of Older Adults

Major Indicators	Minor Indicators
Weight loss	Alcoholism
Under-/overweight	Cognitive impairment
Low serum albumin	Chronic renal insufficiency
Change in functional status	Multiple concurrent medications
Inappropriate food intake	Malabsorption syndromes
Mid-arm muscle circumference less than 10th percentile	Anorexia, nausea, dysphagia
Triceps skinfold less than 10th percentile or greater than 95th percentile	Change in bowel habit
Obesity	Fatigue, apathy, memory loss
Nutrition-related disorders	Poor oral/dental status, dehydration
• Osteoporosis	Poorly healing wounds
• Osteomalacia	Loss of subcutaneous fat and/or muscle mass
• Folate deficiency	Fluid retention
• B_{12} deficiency	Reduced iron, ascorbic acid, zinc

Source: Adapted from Nutrition Screening Initiative p. 2.

orders. Specific health and social service professionals are easily identified to save time and money and to reduce confusion. To promote monitoring of nutritional status, a few of the items in the checklist can be repeated when the Level I and Level II Screens are administered.

The Nutrition Screening Initiative convened an intervention roundtable to identify practical ways to prevent and to treat nutritionally related problems. Health care professionals who work with older adults in any of six key areas (social services, oral health, mental health, medication use, nutrition education and counseling, and nutrition support) can choose among a variety of interventions. A manual entitled *Implementing Nutrition Screening and Intervention Strategies* provides a step-by-step process to develop and refine programs for nutrition screening and intervention.[106] The programs can evolve in community-based care, acute and long-term care, and outpatient or ambulatory care settings. An algorithm that identifies the flow from the checklist to interventions in different types of health care is provided in Figure 10–4.[104]

Info Line

For more information and to obtain materials, contact The Nutrition Screening Initiative, 2626 Pennsylvania Avenue NW, Suite 301, Washington, DC 20037. Telephone: (202) 625-1662.

The Nutrition Screening Initiative was used in addition to 14 demographic questions to survey 11,891 older adults in Indiana in 1994. Congregate meal service provided 65% of the respondents ($N = 7670$), and home-delivered meals included 36% ($N = 4223$). Respondents were 70% female and 27% male, with missing data on 3% of the respondents; 85% were white and not of Hispanic origin, and 8% were African American.[107]

The residential location of respondents reflected 72% who lived independently in their home or apartment and 21% who lived in a retirement complex. Of the respondents, 38% resided in a town with a population of 10,000 to 50,000, 30% lived in a rural setting of less than 10,000 people, 6% lived on a farm, 13% resided in a suburb or central city with more than 50,000 people, and 13% did not complete the information.

Of the respondents, 69% were 75 to 106 years old, and 31% were 60 to 74 years old. Over one-half (55%) were widowed; 27% were married; and 60% lived alone. Thirty-two percent had completed high school; an additional 12% had complete some or all of college; and 17% had completed a minimum of an 8th grade education. Of the respondents, 68% owned and used a microwave oven. Fifty-seven percent stated that the noon meal received from the congregate or home delivery was their main meal of the day; 59% described the meal as well-balanced and healthy.

Responses from the "Determine Your Nutritional Health" checklist revealed that 53% eat alone most of the time, and 52% take three or more different prescribed or over-the-counter drugs daily. Thirty-five percent state that they have an illness or condition that makes them change the kind and/or amount of food they eat. The compilation of responses to the checklist showed 37% were at no nutritional risk, 30% were at moderate risk, and 33% were at high nutritional risk.[107]

A similar assessment was conducted among Medicare beneficiaries 70 years and older in New England. A 14-item checklist provided information. Of the respondents, 24% were at high nutritional risk. Of these, 56% reported their health as fair or poor; 38% had dietary patterns with less than 75% of the RDAs for three or more nutrients.[108] Various Nutrition Screening Initiative activities throughout the United State are listed in Table 10–8.

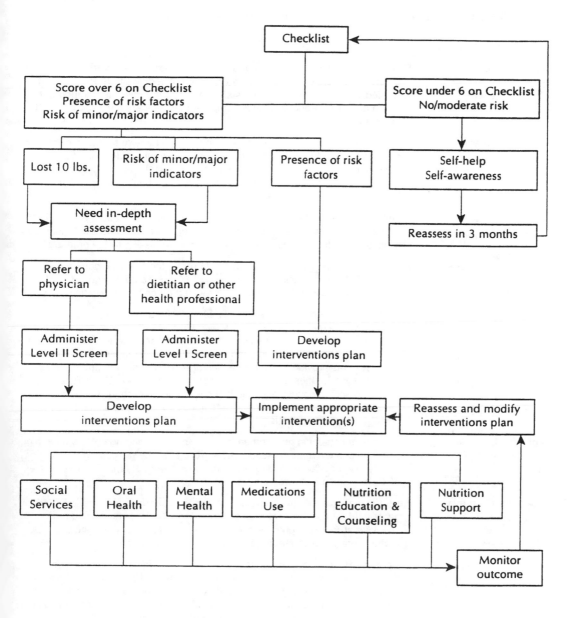

Figure 10-4 Flow of nutrition screening data from checklist to outcome. *Source:* Nutrition Screening Initiative. *Report of Nutrition Screening I: Toward a Common View.* Washington, DC: Nutrition Screening Initiative, 1991.

Table 10–8 Community-Based Nutrition Screening Initiative Activities in the United States

City and State	Activity
Washington, DC	Dietitians at Howard University conduct nutrition assessments at the Downtown Cluster Day Care Center through a College of Allied Health Sciences grant. Trained volunteers and day care staff administer the checklist through both group and one-to-one sessions. Completed screens are reviewed by an RD for referrals.
Merrillville, Indiana	Following a pilot project suggested by the Visiting Nurse Association home care agency dietitian, approval was gained for agency-wide adoption of checklist screening and intervention for all patients, not just the elderly. All new admissions are screened, and the checklist is readministered every six months.
Denver, Colorado	A dietitian-social worker team working with the Veterans Affairs Medical Center home care program uses NSI materials to collaborate and conduct a nutrition assessment within two weeks of the patient's admission to the program.
Flowood, Mississippi	From 849 checklists administered by the contract food service company drivers, 54% of the senior participants were found to be at high risk for malnutrition. Training for drivers was provided by company dietitians.
Lubbock, Texas	A total of 300 rural older adults were evaluated with a modified checklist and level I and II screens. University graduate students were used to assist dietitians in administering the screening tools at congregate meal sites, local churches, community centers, and homes of the older individuals. Immediate feedback was provided about potential for moderate or high nutritional risk, as well as information about eating according to the Food Guide Pyramid. A follow-up screening was held within three months, which included anthropometric measures, the Mini-Mental State Examination, and the Geriatric Depression Scale.
Monterey, California	Second-year screening revealed an increase in the percentage of clients at high risk. The percentage increased to 40% from 29% the previous year. The new survey also showed that for those seniors who were at high risk, total scores of 10 to 15 points showed up more often.
Ridgecrest, California	Health career students from a local high school were used to assist the nutrition consultant for the Senior Citizen Nutrition Program in administering the checklist at three congregate nutrition sites. A follow-up screening was held at the center for those receiving moderate or high risk scores.
Boston, Massachusetts	Deaconess Hospital began an ElderCare program in fall 1991 for inpatients only; it has expanded to include an outpatient assessment component where consultations are arranged for patients with identified nutrition problems. The "Determine Your Nutritional Health" checklist is being used for screening in the radiation therapy clinic and as a part of Pre-Admission Testing Clinic procedures.
Arlington, Virginia	The checklist has been incorporated into a specific screening form that is administered to all patients who are over 80 years old or those with an admission diagnosis of pneumonia, cardiovascular accident, hip fracture, or AIDS, or those who have been in the hospital for more than seven days. Information added to the checklist questions included height, weight history, albumin level, total lymphocyte count, nutrition-related diagnoses, and diet history.

Source: Adapted from "In the Field," *GN Newsletter*. Spring, 1994, p. 12.

Info Line

Nutrition Screening Initiative—Older American's Prayer

The Nutrition Screening Initiative and the Nutrition Institute of Louisiana at Methodist Hospital are my advocates, I shall not starve;

They consider me at risk for poor nutrition status if I suddenly lie down in green pastures or alternative settings;

They screen me and intervene to assure that I receive appropriate foods and waters;

They restoreth my depleted nutrients, activity, independence and dignity;

They guideth me in straight dietary paths for the sake of prevention of illness, dependence and disability;

Yea, though I swim, jog or walk, even with assistive devices, through the valley of the shadow of ignorance and inadequate reimbursement, I will fear no evil, for they art with me;

Their component organizations, individuals and staff, they comfort me;

They preparest a table, meal or artificial nutrition support before me despite limited resources;

They have anointed my head and other parts of my body, with moderate amounts of unsaturated oils;

If my cup runneth over, they will adjust my calorie and fluid needs;

Surely goodness and mercy shall follow me all the days of my life because through their interventions, I will optimize my independence and execute a living will while I am still competent;

And I shall dwell in various environments, but preferably at home, enjoying a good quality of life, until my final residence when I shall dwell in the house of the Lord forever.

Source: Reprinted from Older American's Prayer. Albert Barrocas, M.D., F.A.C.S. 1991 in memory of Bess Handmacher and the Nutrition Screening Initiative.

NATIONAL INSTITUTES OF HEALTH RESEARCH AMONG POSTMENOPAUSAL WOMEN

Several research initiatives are directed specifically toward women in the later adult years. Major research programs during the later 1990s include the following.[109]

Postmenopausal Estrogen/Progestin Interventions

Postmenopausal Estrogen/Progestin Interventions (PEPI) were begun in 1987 and continued until 1995. The effects of various postmenopausal estrogen-replacement therapies on risk factors for osteoporosis and selected cardiovascular risk factors (e.g., HDL cholesterol, systolic blood pressure, fibrinogen, and insulin) are being evaluated. The study population comprises women, ages 45 to 64, of all ethnic groups and with or without a uterus.

Participants were randomized to one of five treatment arms. Intervention drugs are Premarin, Provera, micronized progesterone, placebo, or a combination of these agents. PEPI has completed the follow-up phase, and data analysis will continue through 1996.[110]

Women's Health Trial: Feasibility Study in Minority Populations

The Women's Health Trial (WHT), which began in September 1991, is to evaluate the feasibility of recruiting women of different socioeconomic status and minority groups and determining if they can reach and practice a modified fat-eating pattern. Approximately 2,250 postmenopausal women, ages 50 to 69, who have an eating pattern of about 38% or more of total calories from fat at the beginning are randomized to a control group (40% of the women) or to the dietary intervention group (60% of the women). The aim is to reduce total fat to 20% of calories; reduce saturated fat and dietary cholesterol intakes; and increase intake of fruits, vegetables, and grains. WHT is the feasibility study for one arm of the NIH Women's Health Initiative (see Chapter 9). Three clinical centers are involved: one enrolls at least 50% African-American women, one enrolls at least 50% Hispanic women, and one reflects the US female population in general.

Cardiovascular Health Study

The Cardiovascular Health Study was started in 1988 with a study population of men and women 65 years and older. The purpose is to determine the degree to which known risk factors predict coronary heart disease (CHD) and stroke among older adults. The study will identify the predictors of mortality and functional impairments in CHD or stroke by following seniors for six years until the year 2000.

Initial data analysis shows: (1) postmenopausal estrogen use is associated with thinner carotid walls, which may lower cardiovascular risk; (2) major electrocardiographic abnormalities are common in this age group for both women and men, irrespective of heart disease history; (3) total cholesterol levels and cholesterol/HDL cholesterol ratios were lower and HDL cholesterol levels were higher than expected; (4) isolated systolic hypertension was associated with various indicators of subclinical cardiovascular disease in both women and men; and (5) there is a potential underestimation of the prevalence of cardiovascular disease among older adults.

Randomized Trial of Low-Dose Aspirin in Female Nurses (Women's Health Study)

The Women's Health Study began in 1991 to study 41,600 postmenopausal female nurses 45 years and older, who had no previous history of heart disease or contraindications to aspirin. The purpose is to evaluate the effect of low-dose aspi-

rin and the antioxidants beta-carotene and vitamin E in the primary prevention of heart disease in postmenopausal women. Aspirin has been efficacious in preventing and reducing vascular disease in men, and this study will investigate use of low-dose aspirin and antioxidants in reducing vascular risk among women.

Trial of Antioxidant Therapy of Cardiovascular Disease in Women

Complementing the Women's Health Study, the Trial of Antioxidant Therapy of Cardiovascular Disease in Women began in May 1993. The purpose is to study the effects of antioxidant therapy on the cardiovascular health of women who have a prior history of disease. About 8,000 high-risk, postmenopausal female nurses, 45 years and older, will be randomized to one of three antioxidants (beta-carotene, vitamin C, or vitamin E) and followed until 1998.

Systolic Hypertension in the Elderly Program

The Systolic Hypertension in the Elderly Program began in 1984 to determine the effect of long-term use of antihypertensive therapy on isolated systolic hypertension. Approximately 4,736 men and women 60 years and over (57% women and 14% African-American men and women) compose the study sample. Results to date show a 36% decline in stroke, a 27% reduction in CHD, and a 32% reduction in all cardiovascular disease events.

Women's Health Initiative

Currently in the early recruitment stage, the Women's Health Initiative is an "umbrella" research effort of the National Institutes of Health. The study population comprises approximately 160,000 postmenopausal women, ages 50 to 79. This collaborative study has two goals: (1) to evaluate the effectiveness of specific, untested preventive approaches to cancer, heart disease, and osteopathic fractures; and (2) to evaluate

Exhibit 10-4 *Healthy People 2000* Objectives for Older Adults

---

2.3   Reduce overweight to a prevalence of no more than 20% among people aged 20 and older and no more than 15% among adolescents aged 12 through 19.

2.5   Reduce dietary fat intake to an average of 30% of calories or less and average saturated fat intake to less than 10% of calories among people aged 2 and older.

2.6   Increase complex carbohydrate and fiber-containing foods in the diets of adults to 5 or more daily servings for vegetables (including legumes) and fruits, and to 6 or more daily servings for grain products.

2.7   Increase to at least 50% the proportion of overweight people aged 12 and older who have adopted sound dietary practices combined with regular physical activity to attain an appropriate body weight.

2.9   Decrease salt and sodium intake so at least 65% of home meal preparers prepare foods without adding salt, at least 80% of people avoid using salt at the table, and at least 40% of adults regularly purchase foods modified or lower in sodium.

2.13   Increase to at least 85% the proportion of people aged 18 and older who use food labels to make nutritious food selections.

2.18   Increase to at least 80% the receipt of home food services by people aged 65 and older who have difficulty in preparing their own meals or are otherwise in need of home-delivered meals. (Baseline data available in 1991.)

2.21   Increase to at least 75% the proportion of primary care providers who provide nutrition assessment, counseling, and referral to qualified nutritionists or dietitians.

8.1   Increase years of healthy life to at least 65 years. (Baseline: An estimated 62 years in 1980.)

Special Population Targets		
Years of Healthy Life	*1980 Baseline*	*2000 Target*
8.1a Blacks	56	60
8.1b Hispanics	62	65
8.1c People aged 65 and older	12*	14*

*Years of healthy life remaining at age 65.

8.8   Increase to at least 90% the proportion of people aged 65 and older who had the opportunity to participate during the preceding year in at least one organized health promotion program through a senior center, lifecare facility, or other community-based setting that serves older adults. (Baseline data available in 1992.)

13.4   Reduce to no more than 20% the proportion of people aged 65 and older who have lost all of their natural teeth. (Baseline: 36% in 1986.)

Special Population Target		
Complete Tooth Loss Prevalence	*1986 Baseline*	*2000 Target*
13.4a Low-income people (annual family income <$15,000)	46%	25%

17.1 and 21.1   Increase years of healthy life to at least 65 years. (Baseline: An estimated 62 years in 1980)

Special Population Targets		
Years of Healthy Life	*1980 Baseline*	*2000 Target*
17.1a Blacks	56	60
17.1b Hispanics	62	65
17.1c People aged 65 and older	12*	14*

*Years of healthy life remaining at age 65.

continues

Exhibit 10-4 continued

> *Note:* Years of healthy life (also referred to as quality-adjusted life years) is a summary measure of health that combines mortality (quantity of life) and morbidity and disability (quality of life) into a single measure. For people aged 65 and older, active life-expectancy, a related summary measure, also will be tracked.

17.3   Reduce to no more than 90 per 1,000 people the proportion of all people aged 65 and older who have difficulty in performing two or more personal care activities, thereby preserving independence. (Baseline: 111 per 1,000 in 1984–85.)

Special Population Target		
Difficulty Performing Self-Care Activities (per 1,000)	*1984–85 Baseline*	*2000 Target*
17.3a People aged 85 and older	371	325

> *Note:* Personal care activities are bathing, dressing, using the toilet, getting in and out of bed or chair, and eating.

Source: Reprinted with permission from *Healthy People 2000: National Health Promotion and Disease Prevention Objectives.* Washington, DC: US Department of Health and Human Services; 1991. DHHS (PHS) Publication 91-50212.

strategies at the community level to achieve healthful behaviors (see Chapter 9).

HEALTHY PEOPLE 2000 ACTIONS

In the HP2K objectives, attention has been given to improving the quality of life and reducing any disparity in care among older adults of different ethnic groups (see Exhibit 10-4). Community nutrition professionals have several avenues to develop and to implement programs for senior adults.

REFERENCES

1. Riley MW, Riley J. Longevity and social structure: The potential of the added years. In: Pifer A, Bronte L, eds. *Our Aging Society: Paradox and Promise.* New York, NY: WW Norton; 1986:53–77.

2. Perry D. The links of aging research to disease prevention. *Nutr Rev.* 1994;52(8):S48.

3. Lawton MP, Nahemow L. Ecology and the aging process. In: Eisdorfer C, Lawton MP, eds. *Psychology of Adult Development and Aging.* Washington, DC: American Psychological Association; 1973:619–674.

4. Hooyman NR, Kiyak HA. *Social Gerontology—A Multidisciplinary Perspective.* 3rd ed. Boston, Mass: Allyn & Bacon, Inc; 1993.

5. Social Security Administration, US Department of Health and Human Services. *Social Security Bulletin: Annual Statistical Supplement.* Washington, DC: US Government Printing Office; 1990.

6. American Association of Retired Persons. *A Profile of Older Americans 1990.* Washington, DC: American Association of Retired Persons; 1990.

7. Rosenwaike IA. A demographic portrait of the oldest old. *Milbank Memorial Fund Q: Health and Society.* 1985;63:187–205.

8. US Bureau of the Census. *Marital Status and Living Arrangements. Current Population Reports.* Washington, DC: US Department of Commerce; March 1990. Series P-20, no. 1450.

9. Sullivan DH, Martin WE, Flaxman N, et al. Oral health problems and involuntary weight loss in a population of frail elderly. *J Am Geriatr Soc.* 1993;41:725–731.

10. Wong ND, Wilson PWF, Kannel WB. Serum cholesterol as a prognostic factor after myocardial infarction: The Framingham Study. *Ann Intern Med.* 1991;115:687–698.

11. Evans WJ, Meredith CN. Exercise and nutrition in the elderly. In: Munro HN, Danford DE, eds. *Nutrition, Aging and the Elderly.* New York, NY: Plenum Publishing Corporation; 1989:89.

12. Keller HH. Malnutrition in institutionalized elderly: How and why? *J Am Geriatr Soc.* 1993;41:1212–1218.

13. Warner HR, Butler RN, Sprott RL, et al, eds. *Modern Biological Theories of Aging.* New York, NY: Raven Press; 1987.

14. Schneider EL, Reed JD. Life extension. *N Engl J Med.* 1985;313:1159–1168.

15. Institute of Medicine. *Extending Life, Enhancing Life: A National Research Agenda on Aging.* Washington, DC: National Academy Press; 1992.

16. Finch CE. *Longevity, Senescence and the Genome.* Chicago, Ill: University of Chicago Press; 1991.

17. McCormick AM, Campisi J. Cellular aging and senescence. *Current Opinion in Cell Biol.* 1991;3:230–234.

18. Goldstein S. Replicative senescence: The human fibroblast comes of age. *Science.* 1990;249:1129–1133.

19. Hayflick L, Moorhead PS. The serial cultivation of human diploid cell strains. *Experimental Cell Research.* 1961;25:585–621.

20. Harman D. The free radical theory of aging. In: Warner HR, Butler RN, Sprott, RL, et al, eds. *Modern Biological Theories of Aging.* New York, NY: Raven Press; 1987.

21. Shock NW, Greulich RG, Andres RA, et al. *Normal Human Aging: The Baltimore Longitudinal Study of Aging.* Washington, DC: US Government Printing Office; 1984.

22. National Institutes of Health. National Institute on Aging. *In Search of the Secrets of Aging.* Bethesda, Md: National Institutes of Health; May 1993:1–35. NIH publication No. 93-2756.

23. National Research Council, Commission on Life Sciences, Food and Nutrition Board. *Recommended Dietary Allowances.* 10th ed. Washington, DC: National Academy Press; 1989.

24. Soldo B, Agree E. America's elderly. *Population Bulletin.* 1988;43:1–46.

25. US Bureau of the Census. *Projections of the Population of the US by Age, Sex and Race: 1988–2080.* Washington, DC: US Department of Commerce; 1989. Current Population Reports. Series P-25, no. 1018.

26. Torres-Gil F. Hispanics: A special challenge. In: Pifer A, Bronte L, eds. *Our Aging Society.* New York, NY: WW Norton; 1986.

27. Lopez-Aqueres W, Kemp B, Plopper M, et al. Health needs of the Hispanic elderly. *J Am Geriatr Soc.* 1984;32:191–198.

28. US Bureau of the Census. *Age, Sex, Race and Hispanic Origin Information from the 1990 Census.* Washington, DC: US Department of Commerce; 1991.

29. Lacayo C. Hispanics. In: Palmore E, ed. *Handbook on the Aged in the United States.* Westport, Conn: Greenwood Press; 1984.

30. US Senate Special Committee on Aging. *Developments in Aging: 1989,* Vol. 1. Washington, DC: US Government Printing Office; 1990.

31. US Bureau of the Census. *State Population and Household Estimates with Age, Sex and Components of Change: 1981–1988.* Washington, DC: US Department of Commerce; 1989. Current Population Reports. Special Studies Series P-25, no. 1044.

32. Longino CF, Biggar JC, Flynn CB, et al. The retirement migration project. Final report to the National Institute on Aging. University of Miami; 1984.

33. Rudman D, Feller AG. Protein-calorie undernutrition in the nursing home. *J Am Geriatr Soc.* 1989;37:173–178.

34. Baker H, Frank O, Thind IS, et al. Vitamin profiles in elderly persons living at home or in nursing homes, versus profile in healthy young subjects. *J Am Geriatr Soc.* 1979;27:444–450.

35. Abbasi AA, Rudman D. Undernutrition in the nursing home: Prevalence, consequences, causes and prevention. *Nutr Rev.* 1994;52(4):119.

36. Stiedemann M, Jansen C, Harrill I. Nutritional status of elderly men and women. *J Am Diet Assoc.* 1978;73:132–139.

37. Phillips P. Grip strength, mental performance and nutritional status as indicators of mortality risk among female geriatric patients. *Age and Aging.* 1986;15:53–56.

38. Katz IR, Beaton-Wimmer P, Parmelle P, et al. Failure to thrive in the elderly: Exploration of the concept and delineation of psychiatric components. *J Geriatr Psychiatry.* 1993;6:161–169.

39. Verdery RB, Goldberg AP. Hypercholesterolemia as a predictor of death: A prospective study of 224 nursing home residents. *J Gerontol.* 1991;46:M84–90.

40. Goldberg AF, Mattson DE, Rudman D. The relationship of growth to alveolar ridge atrophy in an older male nursing home population. *Special Care in Dentistry.* 1988; 8:184–186.

41. Veis SI, Logemann JA. Swallowing disorders in persons with cerebrovascular accident. *Arch Phys Med Rehabil.* 1985;66:372–375.

42. Palmer ED. Dysphagia in parkinsonism. *JAMA.* 1974;229:1349.

43. Cheah KC, Beard OW. Psychiatric findings in the population of a geriatric evaluation unit; implications. *J Am Geriatr Soc.* 1980;28:153–156.

44. Rovner BW, Kafonek S, Filipp L, et al. Prevalence of mental illness in a community nursing home. *Am J Psychiatry.* 1986;143:1446–1449.

45. Winograd CH, Brown EM. Aggressive oral refeeding in hospitalized patients. *Am J Clin Nutr.* 1990;52:967–968.

46. Anthony PS, Ireton-Jones CS. Dietitians in home care: A new challenge. *Support Line.* 1994;16(6):1-5.

47. Howard L, Heaphey L, Timchalk M. A review of the current national status of home parenteral and enteral nutrition from the provider and the consumer perspective. *J Parenteral and Enteral Nutr.* 1986;10:416-424.

48. Collopy B, Dubler N, Zuckerman C. The ethics of home care: Autonomy and accommodation. *Hastings Center Report.* March/April 1990:20(2);1-16S.

49. Regenstein M. Reimbursement for nutrition support. *Nutr in Clin Prac.* 1989;4:194-202.

50. Pfeil LA, Katz PR, Davis PJ. Water metabolism. In: Morley JE, Glick Z, Rubenstein LZ, eds. *Geriatric Nutrition.* New York, NY: Raven Press; 1990:193-202.

51. Crowe MJ, Forsling ML, Rolls BJ, et al. Altered water excretion in healthy elderly men. *Age and Aging.* 1987;16:285-293.

52. Chernoff R. Thirst and fluid requirements. *Nutr Rev.* 1994;52(8):(II)S3-S5.

53. Fanelli MT, Stevenhagen KJ. Characterizing consumption patterns by food frequency methodologies: Core foods and variety of foods in diets of older Americans. *J Am Diet Assoc.* 1985;85:1570-1576.

54. Brown EL. Factors influencing food choices and intake. *Geriatrics.* 1976;31:89-92.

55. Rolls BJ. Appetite and satiety in the elderly. *Nutr Rev.* 1994;52(8):(II)S9-S10.

56. Rolls BJ, McDermott TM. Effects of age on sensory specific satiety. *Am J Clin Nutr.* 1991;54:988-996.

57. Schiffman S. Changes in taste and smell: Drug interactions and food preferences. *Nutr Rev.* 1994;52(8):(II)S11-S14.

58. Hamilton EMN, Whitney EN, Sizer FS. *Nutrition Concepts and Controversies.* 5th ed. Whitney EN, Sizer FS, eds. New York, NY: West Publishing Company; 1991.

59. Krumholz HM, Seeman TE, Merrill SS, et al. Lack of association between cholesterol and coronary heart disease mortality and morbidity and all-cause mortality in persons older than 70 years. *JAMA.* 1994;272:1335-1340.

60. Wolfsen CR, Barker JC, Mitteness LS. Constipation in the daily lives of frail elderly. *Arch Fam Med.* 1993;2: 853-858.

61. Rosenbloom CA, Whittington FJ. The effects of bereavement on eating behaviors and nutrient intakes in elderly widowed persons. *J Gerontol.* 1993;48:223S-229S.

62. Butler RN. Senile dementia of the Alzheimer type (SDAT). In: Abrams WB, Berkow B, eds. *The Merck Manual of Geriatrics.* Rahway, NJ: Merck Sharp & Dohme Research Laboratories; 1990:933-937.

63. Claggett SM. Nutritional factors relevant to Alzheimer's disease. *J Am Diet Assoc.* 1989;89:392-396.

64. National Institute on Aging. *Alzheimer's Disease Costs the Nation an Estimated 90 Billion Dollars per Year.* Washington, DC: US Department of Health and Human Services; 1993. NIH publication 93-3409.

65. Huey E. *Nutritional Assessment of Patients with Alzheimer's Disease in Three Stages of the Disease.* Long Beach, Calif: California State University Long Beach; 1995. Thesis.

66. Katzman R. Medical progress—Alzheimer's disease. *N Engl J Med.* 1986;312:964-971.

67. McKhann G, Drachman D, Folstein M, et al. Clinical diagnosis of Alzheimer's disease: Report of the NINCDS-ADRDA work group under the auspices of Department of Health and Human Services Task Force on Alzheimer's disease. *Neurology.* 1984;34:939-944.

68. Gray GE. Nutrition and dementia. *J Am Diet Assoc.* 1989;849:1795-1802.

69. Wolf-Klein GP, Silverston FA, Levy AP. Nutritional patterns and weight change in Alzheimer patients. *International Psychogeriatrics.* 1992;4(10):103-118.

70. Breteler MB, Claus JJ, Duijn CM, et al. Epidemiology of Alzheimer's disease. *Epidemiological Reviews.* 1992; 14:59-82.

71. Litchford MD, Wakefield LM. Nutrient intakes and energy expenditures of residents with senile dementia of the Alzheimer's type. *J Am Diet Assoc.* 1987;87:211-213.

72. Singh S, Mulley GP, Losowsky MS. Why are Alzheimer patients thin? *Age and Aging.* 1988;17:21-28.

73. Egbert AM. "The Dwindles": Failure to thrive in older patients. *Postgrad Med.* 1993;94:199-212.

74. Bendich A, Butterworth CE, eds. *Micronutrients in Health and in Disease Prevention.* New York, NY: Marcel Dekker Inc; 1991.

75. Young VR. Amino acids and proteins in relation to the nutrition of elderly people, *Age and Aging.* 1990;19: S10-S24.

76. Committee on Diet and Health, Food and Nutrition Board, Commission on Life Sciences, National Research Council. *Diet and Health: Implications for Reducing Chronic Disease Risk.* Washington, DC: National Academy Press; 1989.

77. Blumberg JB. Considerations of the Recommended Dietary Allowances for older adults. *Clin Appl Nutr.* 1991;1: 18-19.

78. Blumberg J. Nutrient requirements of the healthy elderly—Should there be specific RDAs? *Nutr Rev.* 1994;52(8):(II)S15-S18.

79. Older Americans Act Title IIIC. US Congress, 1965.

80. Gerontological Nutrition Dietetic Practice Group. American Dietetic Association. Chicago, Ill. 1994.

81. US Department of Agriculture/US Department of Health and Human Services. *Nutrition and Your Health: Dietary Guidelines for Americans.* 2nd ed. Washington, DC: US Government Printing Office; 1985. HG-232.

82. *The California Daily Food Guide.* Sacramento, Calif: California Department of Health and Human Services and California Department of Education; 1990.

83. Roe D. Development and current status of home-delivered meals program in the United States: Are the right elderly served? *Nutr Rev.* 1994;52(1):30–33.

84. Food Research and Action Center. *A National Survey of Nutritional Risk among the Elderly.* Washington, DC: Food Research and Action Center; 1987.

85. Bernard MA, Rombeau JL. Nutritional support for the elderly patient. *Nutrition, Aging and Health.* New York, NY: Alan R. Liss; 1989;229–258.

86. Lowe BF. Future directions for community-based long-term care research. *Milbank Q.* 1988;66:552–571.

87. Hunger and Nutrition Research Project. *Hunger among the Elderly: Myth or Reality.* Texas Department of Aging. Final report. 1984.

88. Balsam AL, Rogers BL. *Service Innovations in the Elderly Nutrition Program. AARP Report.* Boston, Mass: Tufts University; July 1988.

89. Roe DA, HoSang G. Supplemental Nutrition Assistance Program (SNAP). Final Report, August 1988.

90. Roe DA. Supplemental Nutrition Assistance Program (SNAP). Final Report, October 1989.

91. Fries JF. Aging, natural death, and the compression of morbidity. *N Engl J Med.* 1980;303:130–135.

92. Verbrugge L. Recent, present and future health of American adults. *Ann Rev Public Health.* 1989;10:333–361.

93. Crimmins EM. Evidence on the compression of morbidity. *Gerontologica Perspecta.* 1987;1:45–49.

94. Palmore EB. Trends in the health of the aged. *Gerontologist.* 1986;26:298–302.

95. Schneider EL, Brody JA. Aging, natural death, and the compression of morbidity: Another view. *N Engl J Med.* 1983;309:854–856.

96. Rice DP, Feldman JJ. Living longer in the United States: Demographic changes and health needs of the elderly. *Milbank Fund Memorial Quarterly: Health and Society.* 1983;61:362–396.

97. Katz S, Branch LG, Granson MH, et al. Active life expectancy. *N Engl J Med.* 1983;309:1218–1224.

98. Manton KG, Stallard E. Cross-sectional estimates of active life expectancy for the US elderly and oldest-old populations. *J Gerontology.* 1991;46:S170–182.

99. Kane RL, Ouslander JG, Abrass IB. *Essentials of Clinical Geriatrics.* 2nd ed. New York, NY: McGraw Hill; 1989.

100. Butler RN. Ageism: Another form of bigotry. *Gerontologist.* 1969;9:243–246.

101. *Surgeon General's Workshop on Health Promotion and Aging.* Washington, DC: US Government Printing Office; 1988. No. 1988-201-875/83669.

102. US Department of Health and Human Services, Public Health Service. *Healthy People 2000. National Health Promotion and Disease Prevention Objectives.* Boston, Mass: Jones and Bartlett Publishers; 1992.

103. Nutrition Screening Initiative. *Report of Nutrition Screening I: Toward a Common View.* Washington, DC: Nutrition Screening Initiative; 1991.

104. Nutrition Screening Initiative. *Nutrition Screening Manual for Professionals Caring for Older Americans.* Washington, DC: Nutrition Screening Initiative; 1991.

105. Nutrition Screening Initiative. *Nutrition Interventions Manual for Professionals Caring for Older Americans.* Washington, DC: Greer, Margolis, Mitchell, Grunwald & Associates, Inc; 1992.

106. Nutrition Screening Initiative. *Implementing Nutrition Screening and Intervention Strategies.* Washington, DC: Nutrition Screening Initiative, 1993.

107. Eigenbrod J, Spangler AA. The Nutrition Screening Initiative Survey of Elderly Nutrition Program Participants in Indiana. Presented at Indiana Dietetic Association Annual Meeting; November 1994; Nappanee, Ind.

108. Posner BM, Jette AM, Smith KW, et al. Nutrition and health risks in the elderly: The nutrition screening initiative. *Am J Public Health.* 1993;83:972–978.

109. National Institutes of Health. *Heart Memo.* Bethesda, Md: National Institutes of Health; 1994.

110. The writing group for the PEPI Trial. Effects of estrogen and estrogen/progestin regimens on heart disease risk factors in postmenopausal women. *JAMA.* 1995;273:199–208.

Appendix 10-A

RDAs for Persons 51 Years Old and Above

Nutrient	Female	Male
Energy, calories		
51–75 years	1,800 (1,400–2,200)	2,400 (2,000–2,800)
75⁺ years	1,600 (1,200–2,000)	2,050 (1,650–2,450)
Protein, grams	50	63
Vitamins		
A, mcg RE	800	1,000
D, mcg	5	5
E, mg a-TE	8	10
K, mcg	65	80
C, mg	60	60
Thiamin, mg	1.0	1.2
Riboflavin, mg	1.2	1.4
Niacin, mg	13	15
B_6, mg	1.6	2.0
Folate, mcg	180	200
B_{12}, mcg	2.0	2.0
Minerals		
Calcium, mg	800	800
Phosphorus, mg	800	800
Magnesium, mg	280	350
Iron, mg	10	10
Zinc, mg	12	15
Iodine, mcg	150	150
Selenium, mcg	55	70

Source: Adapted from National Research Council, Commission on Life Sciences, Food and Nutrition Board. *Recommended Dietary Allowances*, Tenth Edition. Washington, DC: National Academy Press, 1989.

Appendix 10-B

Nutritionally Adequate Meal Pattern for Older Adults

A nutritionally adequate meal pattern can be planned by seniors if they know how many servings they need each day:

Component	Amount
Energy Level*	1,600–2,800
Bread group	6–11 servings
Vegetable group	3–5 servings
Fruit group	2–4 servings
Milk group	2–3 servings
Meat group	2–3 servings for a total of 5 ounces

*These are the energy levels if you choose low-fat, lean foods from the five major food groups and use foods from the fats and sweets group sparingly. Generally, women should choose the lower energy levels and men the upper level or sedentary men and women choose the lower level and active men and women the upper level.

Source: US Department of Agriculture and the US Department of Health and Human Services.

Appendix 10-C

Agencies and Organizations That Provide Assistance for Elders on Topics of Nutrition and Health

- Administration on Aging
  330 Independent Avenue, SW
  Washington, DC 20201
  (202) 619-0724
  US government agency that provides information on health and aging programs, offered through state and area agencies on aging.

- Alzheimer's Association
  919 N Michigan Avenue, Suite 1000
  Chicago, IL 60611
  (312) 335-8700
  (800) 272-3900 toll-free hotline
  Offers a hotline that provides information and assistance for families coping with Alzheimer's disease.

- American Association of Retired Persons
  1909 K Street, NW
  Washington, DC 20049
  (202) 434-2277
  Membership organization for people over age 50, offering publications and volunteer programs on a variety of economic, social, and health issues.

- American Dietetic Association
  216 West Jackson Boulevard
  Suite 800
  Chicago, IL 60606
  (312) 899-0040
  Professional organization that offers assistance in locating registered dietitians in communities.

- American Geriatrics Society
  770 Lexington Avenue
  Suite 300
  New York, NY 10021
  (212) 308-1414

Professional organization of physicians with geriatric training, offering assistance in locating a doctor in your community with special training in treating older adults.

- Arthritis Foundation
  1314 Spring Street, NW
  Atlanta, GA 30309
  (404) 872-7100
  Provides information and programs on arthritis, including treatment options and self-help materials for those with arthritis and their families.

- Food and Drug Administration
  Office of Consumer Affairs
  5600 Fishers Lane, HFE 88
  Rockville, MD 20857
  (301) 443-3170
  US government agency that provides information and literature about the safety of food additives, drugs, and medical devices.

- Human Nutrition Information Service
  USDA
  6505 Belcrest Road
  Hyattsville, MD 20782
  (301) 436-5724
  US government agency that provides information on using the Dietary Guidelines and the Food Guide Pyramid and preparing foods.

- National Cancer Institute
  Office of Cancer Communications
  Building 31, Room 10A24
  9000 Rockville Pike
  Bethesda, MD 20892
  (800) 422-6237 toll-free hotline
  US government agency that provides information on cancer prevention and treatment.

- National Heart, Lung, and Blood Institute
Information Office
Building 31, Room 4A21
9000 Rockville Pike
Bethesda, MD 20892
(301) 496-4236
US government agency that conducts research and provides information about heart, lung, and blood diseases.

- National Institute on Aging
Public Information Office
Federal Building, Room 6C12
9000 Rockville Pike
Bethesda, MD 20892
(301) 496-1752

US government agency that provides information on health and other issues of interest to older people.

- Office of Disease Prevention and Health Promotion
National Health Information Center
PO Box 1133
Washington, DC 20013-1133
(800) 336-4797
US government agency that operates a clearinghouse and hotline to provide health information and referrals.

Appendix 10-D

Nutrition Screening Initiative Assessment Instruments

The "Determine Your Nutritional Health" checklist of the Nutrition Screening Initiative can be administered by any level of health care professional. Level I Screen for seniors can be administered by health and social service professionals to identify those in need of food assistance and nutrition therapy. Level II Screen for seniors contains specific diagnostic questions that health and medical professionals can use to identify seniors at high nutritional risk.

Exhibit 10–D1 Determine Your Nutritional Health Checklist

The Warning Signs of poor nutritional health are often overlooked. Use this checklist to find out if you or someone you know is at nutritional risk.

DETERMINE YOUR NUTRITIONAL HEALTH

Read the statements below. Circle the number in the yes column for those that apply to you or someone you know. For each yes answer, score the number in the box. Total your nutritional score.

	YES
I have an illness or condition that made me change the kind and/or amount of food I eat.	2
I eat fewer than 2 meals per day.	3
I eat few fruits or vegetables, or milk products.	2
I have 3 or more drinks of beer, liquor, or wine almost every day.	2
I have tooth or mouth problems that make it hard for me to eat.	2
I don't always have enough money to buy the food I need.	4
I eat alone most of the time.	1
I take 3 or more different prescribed or over-the-counter drugs a day.	1
Without wanting to, I have lost or gained 10 pounds in the last 6 months.	2
I am not always physically able to shop, cook and/or feed myself.	2
TOTAL	

Total Your Nutritional Score. If it's —

0-2   **Good!** Recheck your nutritional score in 6 months.

3-5   **You are at moderate nutritional risk.** See what can be done to improve your eating habits and lifestyle. Your office on aging, senior nutrition program. senior citizens center or health department can help. Recheck your nutritional score in 3 months.

6 or more   **You are at high nutritional risk.** Bring this checklist the next time you see your doctor. dietitian or other qualified health or social service professional. Talk with them about any problems you may have. Ask for help to improve your nutritional health.

These materials developed and distributed by the Nutrition Screening Initiative, a project of:

 AMERICAN ACADEMY OF FAMILY PHYSICIANS

 THE AMERICAN DIETETIC ASSOCIATION

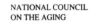 NATIONAL COUNCIL ON THE AGING

Remember that warning signs suggest risk, but do not represent diagnosis of any condition. Turn the page to learn more about the Warning Signs of poor nutritional health.

continues

Exhibit 10–D1 continued

> **The Nutrition Checklist is based on the Warning Signs described below.**
> **Use the word DETERMINE to remind you of the Warning Signs.**

DISEASE

Any disease, illness or chronic condition which causes you to change the way you eat, or makes it hard for you to eat, puts your nutritional health at risk. Four out of five adults have chronic diseases that are affected by diet. Confusion or memory loss that keeps getting worse is estimated to affect one out of five or more of older adults. This can make it hard to remember what, when or if you've eaten. Feeling sad or depressed, which happens to about one in eight older adults, can cause big changes in appetite, digestion, energy level, weight and well-being.

EATING POORLY

Eating too little and eating too much both lead to poor health. Eating the same foods day after day or not eating fruit, vegetables, and milk products daily will also cause poor nutritional health. One in five adults skip meals daily. Only 13% of adults eat the minimum amount of fruit and vegetables needed. One in four older adults drink too much alcohol. Many health problems become worse if you drink more than one or two alcoholic beverages per day.

TOOTH LOSS/MOUTH PAIN

A healthy mouth, teeth and gums are needed to eat. Missing, loose or rotten teeth or dentures which don't fit well or cause mouth sores make it hard to eat.

ECONOMIC HARDSHIP

As many as 40% of older Americans have incomes of less than $6,000 per year. Having less—or choosing to spend less—than $25–30 per week for food makes it very hard to get the foods you need to stay healthy.

REDUCED SOCIAL CONTACT

One-third of all older people live alone. Being with people daily has a positive effect on morale, well-being and eating.

MULTIPLE MEDICINES

Many older Americans must take medicines for health problems. Almost half of older Americans take multiple medicines daily. Growing old may change the way we respond to drugs. The more medicines you take, the greater the chance for side effects such as increased or decreased appetite, change in taste, constipation, weakness, drowsiness, diarhea, nausea, and others. Vitamins or minerals when taken in large doses act like drugs and can cause harm. Alert your doctor to everything you take.

INVOLUNTARY WEIGHT LOSS/GAIN

Losing or gaining a lot of weight when you are not trying to do so is an important warning sign that must not be ignored. Being overweight or underweight also increases your chance of poor health.

NEEDS ASSISTANCE IN SELF CARE

Although most older people are able to eat, one out of every five have trouble walking, shopping, buying and cooking food, especially as they get older.

ELDER YEARS ABOVE AGE 80

Most older people lead full and productive lives. But as age increases, risk of frailty and health problems increase. Checking your nutritional health regularly makes good sense.

 The Nutrition Screening Initiative, 2626 Pennsylvania Avenue, NW, Suite 301, Washington, DC 20037
The Nutrition Screening Initiative is funded in part by a grant from Ross Laboratories, a division of Abbott Laboratories.   **A5944/MARCH 1992**

Source: Reprinted from Nutrition Screening Initiative. *Report of Nutrition Screening I: Toward a Common View.* Washington, DC: Nutrition Screening Initiative, 1991.

Exhibit 10–D2 Level I Screen for Seniors

Level 1 Screen

Body Weight

Measure height to the nearest inch and weight to the nearest pound. Record the values below and mark them on the Body Mass Index (BMI) scale to the right. Then use a straight edge (ruler) to connect the two points and circle the spot where this straight line crosses the center line (body mass index). Record the number below.

Healthy older adults should have a BMI between 24 and 27.

Height (in):_____
Weight (lbs):_____
Body Mass Index:_____
(number from center column)

Check any boxes that are true for the individual:

❏ Has lost or gained 10 pounds (or more) in the past 6 months.

❏ Body mass index <24

❏ Body mass index >27

For the remaining sections, please ask the individual which of the statements (if any) is true for him or her and place a check by each that applies.

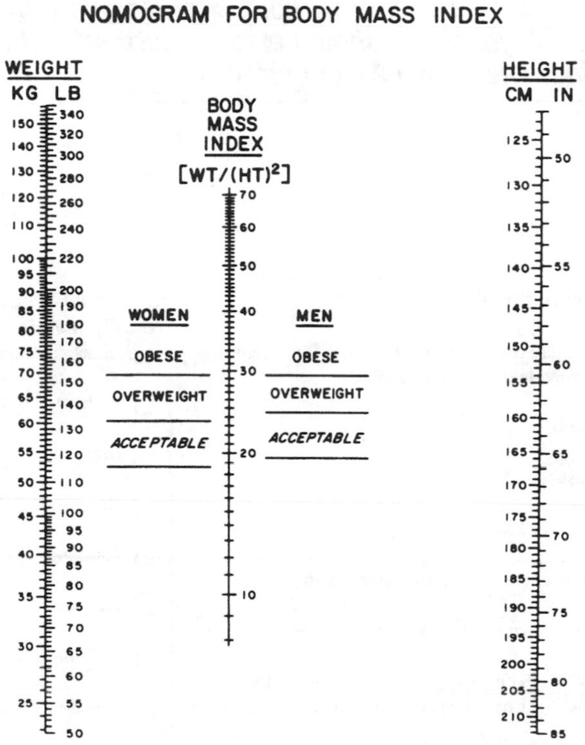

NOMOGRAM FOR BODY MASS INDEX

WEIGHT
KG LB

BODY MASS INDEX
$[WT/(HT)^2]$

WOMEN
OBESE
OVERWEIGHT
ACCEPTABLE

MEN
OBESE
OVERWEIGHT
ACCEPTABLE

HEIGHT
CM IN

Source: Copyright © 1978, George A. Bray, MD.

LEVEL I SCREEN

Name :

Date:

Eating Habits

❏ Does not have enough food to eat each day

❏ Usually eats alone

❏ Does not eat anything on one or more days each month

❏ Has poor appetite

❏ Is on a special diet

❏ Eats vegetables two or fewer times daily

❏ Eats milk or milk products once or not at all daily

❏ Eats fruit or drinks fruit juice once or not at all daily

❏ Eats breads, cereals, pasta, rice, or other grains five or fewer times daily

❏ Has difficulty chewing or swallowing

❏ Has more than one alcoholic drink per day (if woman); more than two drinks per day (if man)

❏ Has pain in mouth, teeth, or gums

continues

Exhibit 10-D2 continued

A physician should be contacted if the individual has gained or lost 10 pounds unexpectedly or without intending to during the past 6 months. A physician should also be notified if the individual's body mass index is above 27 or below 24.

Living Environment

☐ Lives on an income of less than $6000 per year (per individual in the household)

☐ Lives alone

☐ Is housebound

☐ Is concerned about home security

☐ Lives in a home with inadequate heating or cooling

☐ Does not have a stove and/or refrigerator

☐ Is unable or prefers not to spend money on food (<$25-30 per person spent on food each week)

Functional Status

Usually or always needs assistance with (check each that apply):

☐ Bathing

☐ Dressing

☐ Grooming

☐ Toileting

☐ Eating

☐ Walking or moving about

☐ Traveling (outside the home)

☐ Preparing food

☐ Shopping for food or other necessities

If you have checked one or more statements on this screen, the individual you have interviewed may be at risk for poor nutritional status. Please refer this individual to the appropriate health care or social service professional in your area. For example, a dietitian should be contacted for problems with selecting, preparing, or eating a healthy diet, or a dentist if the individual experiences pain or difficulty when chewing or swallowing. Those individuals whose income, lifestyle, or functional status may endanger their nutritional and overall health should be referred to available community services: home-delivered meals, congregate meal programs, transportation services, counseling services (alcohol abuse, depression, bereavement, etc.), home health care agencies, day care programs, etc.

Please repeat this screen at least once each year--sooner if the individual has a major change in his or her health, income, immediate family (e.g., spouse dies), or functional status.

These materials developed by the Nutrition Screening Initiative.

Source: Nutrition Screening Initiative. *Report of Nutrition Screening I: Toward a Common View.* Washington, DC: Nutrition Screening Initiative, 1991.

Exhibit 10–D3 Level II Screen

Level II Screen

Complete the following screen by interviewing the patient directly and/or by referring to the patient chart. If you do not routinely perform all of the described tests or ask all of the listed questions, please consider including them but do not be concerned if the entire screen is not completed. Please try to conduct a minimal screen on as many older patients as possible, and please try to collect serial measurements, which are extremely valuable in monitoring nutritional status. Please refer to the manual for additional information.

Anthropometrics

Measure height to the nearest inch and weight to the nearest pound. Record the values below and mark them on the Body Mass Index (BMI) scale to the right. Then use a straight edge (paper, ruler) to connect the two points and circle the spot where this straight line crosses the center line (body mass index). Record the number below; healthy older adults should have a BMI between 24 and 27; check the appropriate box to flag an abnormally high or low value.

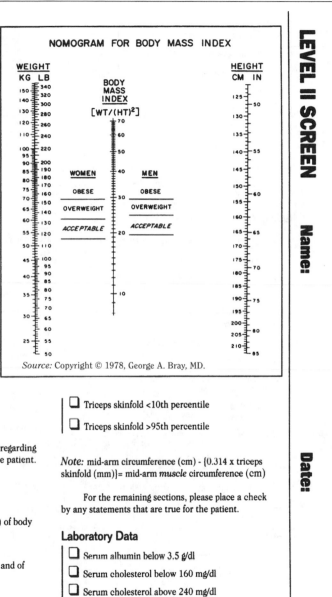

Source: Copyright © 1978, George A. Bray, MD.

Height (in):_____
Weight (lbs):_____
Body Mass Index
(weight/height^2):_____

Please place a check by any statement regarding BMI and recent weight loss that is true for the patient.

☐ Body mass index <24

☐ Body mass index >27

☐ Has lost or gained 10 pounds (or more) of body weight in the past 6 months

Record the measurement of mid-arm circumference to the nearest 0.1 centimeter and of triceps skinfold to the nearest 2 millimeters.

Mid-Arm Circumference (cm):_____
Triceps Skinfold (mm):_____
Mid-Arm Muscle Circumference (cm):_____

Refer to the table and check any abnormal values:

☐ Mid-arm muscle circumference <10th percentile

☐ Triceps skinfold <10th percentile

☐ Triceps skinfold >95th percentile

Note: mid-arm circumference (cm) - {0.314 x triceps skinfold (mm)}= mid-arm *muscle* circumference (cm)

For the remaining sections, please place a check by any statements that are true for the patient.

Laboratory Data

☐ Serum albumin below 3.5 g/dl

☐ Serum cholesterol below 160 mg/dl

☐ Serum cholesterol above 240 mg/dl

Drug Use

☐ Three or more prescription drugs, OTC medications, and/or vitamin/mineral supplements daily

continues

Exhibit 10–D3 continued

Clinical Features

Presence of (check each that apply):

☐ Problems with mouth, teeth, or gums

☐ Difficulty chewing

☐ Difficulty swallowing

☐ Angular stomatitis

☐ Glossitis

☐ History of bone pain

☐ History of bone fractures

☐ Skin changes (dry, loose, nonspecific lesions, edema)

Percentile	Men		Women	
	55-65 y	65-75 y	55-65 y	65-75 y
Arm circumference (cm)				
10th	27.3	26.3	25.7	25.2
50th	31.7	30.7	30.3	29.9
95th	36.9	35.5	38.5	37.3
Arm muscle circumference (cm)				
10th	24.5	23.5	19.6	19.5
50th	27.8	26.8	22.5	22.5
95th	32.0	30.6	28.0	27.9
Triceps skinfold (mm)				
10th	6	6	16	14
50th	11	11	25	24
95th	22	22	38	36

From: Frisancho AR. *New norms of upper limb fat and muscle areas for assessment of nutritional status.* Am J Clin Nutr 1981; 34:2540-2545. © 1981 American Society for Clinical Nutrition.

Eating Habits

☐ Does not have enough food to eat each day

☐ Usually eats alone

☐ Does not eat anything on one or more days each month

☐ Has poor appetite

☐ Is on a special diet

☐ Eats vegetables two or fewer times daily

☐ Eats milk or milk products once or not at all daily

☐ Eats fruit or drinks fruit juice once or not at all daily

☐ Eats breads, cereals, pasta, rice, or other grains five or fewer times daily

☐ Has more than one alcoholic drink per day (if woman); more than two drinks per day (if man)

Living Environment

☐ Lives on an income of less than $6000 per year (per individual in the household)

☐ Lives alone

☐ Is housebound

☐ Is concerned about home security

☐ Lives in a home with inadequate heating or cooling

☐ Does not have a stove and/or refrigerator

☐ Is unable or prefers not to spend money on food (<$25-30 per person spent on food each week)

Functional Status

Usually or always needs assistance with (check each that apply):

☐ Bathing

☐ Dressing

☐ Grooming

☐ Toileting

☐ Eating

☐ Walking or moving about

☐ Traveling (outside the home)

☐ Preparing food

☐ Shopping for food or other necessities

Mental/Cognitive Status

☐ Clinical evidence of impairment, e.g. Folstein<26

☐ Clinical evidence of depressive illness, e.g. Beck Depression Inventory>15, Geriatric Depression Scale>5

Patients in whom you have identified one or more major indicator (see pg 2) of poor nutritional status require immediate medical attention; if minor indicators are found, ensure that they are known to a health professional or to the patient's own physician. Patients who display risk factors (see pg 2) of poor nutritional status should be referred to the appropriate health care or social service professional (dietitian, nurse, dentist, case manager, etc.).

These materials developed by the Nutrition Screening Initiative.

Source: Nutrition Screening Initiative. *Report of Nutrition Screening I: Toward a Common View.* Washington, DC: Nutrition Screening Initiative, 1991.

Part III

Secondary and Tertiary Prevention— Managing Disease and Avoiding Complications

11

Coronary Heart Disease

Learning Objectives

- Discuss the epidemiology of cardiovascular heart disease in the United States.
- Define the role of nutrition in the etiology, prevention, and treatment of cardiovascular heart disease.
- Identify the *Healthy People 2000* objectives for cardiovascular heart disease.
- Describe how community nutritionists can be actively involved in primary, secondary, and tertiary care of coronary heart disease in the United States.
- List the major food components that increase or decrease coronary heart disease.

High Definition Nutrition

Arteriosclerosis—a group of diseases characterized by thickening and loss of elasticity of arterial walls.

Atherosclerosis—a common form of arteriosclerosis with plaques forming within the intima of medium and large arteries.

Casein—the principal protein of milk; the basis of curd and cheese.

Dyslipidemia—abnormal blood lipids or fats; the most common form is hypercholesterolemia.

Endogenous—developing or originating within the organism.

Exogenous—developing or originating outside the organism.

Protein—any one of a group of complex organic nitrogenous compounds widely distributed in plants (i.e., vegetable protein) and animals (i.e., animal protein).

Thrombosis—the formation or presence of a blood clot within a blood vessel during life.

Vitamin A toxicity—intake of at least 100,000 IU per day for 10 years.

Vitamin D toxicity—chronic intake of at least 6,000 IU per day.

AN OVERVIEW OF CORONARY HEART DISEASE

Coronary heart disease (CHD) is the result of atherosclerosis or hardening of arteries due to the development of lipid-laden, calcified plaques in the arterial wall. The integrity of the arteries and the flow of blood are reduced. If this occurs in the coronary arteries, a myocardial infarction or sudden death can result; strokes result from atherosclerosis in the cerebral arteries. CHD remains the number 1 cause of death in the United States, killing over 500,000 individuals annually. About one million people have angina pectoris, and 1,250,000 experience a myocardial infarction each year.[1]

In 1986 age-adjusted mortality rates from CHD, mortality rates for black men were about 8% lower than for white men; rates for black women were almost 20% higher than for white women. Hispanic men and women have CHD mortality rates that are 5 to 15% below those of non-Hispanics. Asian/Pacific Islanders appear to have the lowest risk of early death, but subgroups vary. Native Hawaiians have higher death rates from cardiovascular and other chronic diseases. Heart disease is a significant contributor to mortality from any cause among Native Americans.[1]

A number of risk factors have been linked to the development of CHD and the rate of its development, including genetic predisposition, sex, age, elevated serum total cholesterol, cigarette smoking, elevated blood pressure, obesity, and physical inactivity. Hyperlipidemia is the major risk factor for CHD. Hyperlipidemia results from an overproduction of cholesterol, triglyceride, and very-low-density lipoprotein (VLDL) by the liver, and the defective removal of lipids and lipoproteins by the liver—that is, an altered removal of low-density lipoprotein (LDL), the chief transport modality for cholesterol, by the LDL receptor in the liver. Diet has a direct impact on serum total cholesterol level. Specifically, high-fat eating patterns have been linked to CHD, and the link has been reinforced by international human and animal experiments.[1]

The pathophysiology of atherosclerosis is directly related to levels of total serum cholesterol, LDL, VLDL, and remnant particles; it is inversely associated with high-density lipoproteins (HDL) (see Table 11–1).[2] High CHD rates occur among individuals who have elevated blood cholesterol levels (greater than 240 mg/dL or 6.21 mmol/L). However, many CHD cases are diagnosed in individuals who have a serum total cholesterol

less than 240 mg/dL. The average cholesterol level for US adults is 210 mg/dL; it is estimated that 55% of U.S. adults have a serum total cholesterol of at least 200 mg/dL.[1]

Stabilization and reversibility of atherosclerotic coronary lesions have been demonstrated. During the past 30 years, several clinical trials have shown that not only can CHD be prevented, but that life expectancy can be increased. Important trials include the following:

- The multicenter Lipid Research Coronary Primary Prevention Trial—a randomized trial with middle-aged men assigned to cholestyramine or placebo; both groups followed a moderate, low-cholesterol diet.
- The Cholesterol-Lowering Atherosclerosis Study—a randomized, placebo-controlled trial with drug and diet.
- The Leiden Study—a noncontrol group trial of men with stable angina prescribed a low-cholesterol, high-polyunsaturated fat, vegetarian diet.
- The Oslo Trial—a diet and smoking intervention of normotensive men with elevated cholesterol levels.
- The Cardiff, Wales Trial—a test of a high-fish diet.
- The Lifestyle Heart Trial in San Francisco—a less than 10% fat, high-fiber diet with stress management for men and women.
- The Helsinki Heart Study—a double-blind, placebo-controlled trial of two mental hospital populations.

Table 11–1 Relative Ranking of Atherogenicity of Lipoproteins

Lipoproteins	Atherogenicity Ranking
Chylomicrons	0
VLDL (triglyceride and cholesterol)	2+
Remnants (IDL) of VLDL and chylomicrons (triglyceride and cholesterol)	3+
LDL (cholesterol), including IDL, lipoprotein-a, LDL I–IV	4+
HDL, including HDL_2, HDL_3	–4

Source: Data from Connor, W.E., Hypolipidemic Effects of Dietary Omega-3 Fatty Acids in Normal and Hyperlipidemic Humans: Effects and Mechanisms, *Health Effects of Polyunsaturated Fatty Acids in Seafoods,* by A. Simopoulos, R.R. Kifer, and R.E. Martin, eds., pp. 173–210, Academic Press, © 1986.

Thrombosis is the major complication of atherosclerosis. If it were not present, the atherosclerosis would be far less serious. Lifelong dietary habits can either promote or prevent thrombosis by affecting coagulation and platelets. Dietary fat and cholesterol serve as precursors for prostaglandins. Saturated fat and cholesterol suppress the LDL receptor, resulting in increased LDL levels. In addition, saturated fat is thrombogenic (tending to produce blood clots within blood vessels). Polyunsaturated vegetable oils contain omega-6 fatty acids, which lower plasma LDL levels; monounsaturated vegetable fats have less saturated fat and can lower LDL; and omega-3 fatty acids from fish decrease plasma LDL and VLDL and lower cholesterol and triglyceride levels.[2] Stearic acid is a saturated fatty acid and especially potent in raising the LDL level of blood.

After a fatty meal, particles and remnants circulate in the plasma. The Stypven time, analogous to the prothrombin time or the time required to coagulate the blood, is greatly accelerated due to the fat; fibrinolysis is lessened. Levels of lipoprotein-a (Lp-a) increase, and Lp-a binds to fibrin and prevents plasmin from dissolving clots that occur naturally. Lp-a is high in cholesterol and may promote atherosclerosis. Fatty acids are also released when lipoprotein lipase acts on triglyceride-rich remnants after chylomicron breakdown. The released fatty acids also become atherogenic.[2]

Ketogenic, low-calorie diets (which convert protein residue to ketone bodies) may promote thrombosis in overweight coronary patients due to the resulting high plasma-free fatty acid levels and reduced prostacyclin concentrations. Obese hypertriglyceridemic patients have increased levels of activated factor VII, which is highly associated with thrombosis.

Saturated fatty acid (SFA) intake expressed as the percentage of total energy has repeatedly shown a strong correlation with CHD mortality rates across multiple countries.[3] When graphing the percentage of total energy from saturated fat against CHD, the slope is nearly two and one-half times steeper than the slope of serum cholesterol and CHD. A study of Japanese migrants to Hawaii and San Francisco demonstrates the positive effect of dietary fat composition on CHD

rates.[4] However, within a population it has been difficult to observe and to document a significant effect of exogenous saturated fat intake on CHD. Various dietary components that influence plasma lipid and lipoprotein levels have been identified[5] (see Table 11-2).

A 10 to 20% reduction of plasma total cholesterol occurs in concert with dietary saturated fatty acids and cholesterol at $\leq$7% of energy and $\leq$200 mg per day, respectively. Increasing soluble fiber can accentuate the loss, with an additional reduction up to 10% in plasma total cholesterol.[5]

The current recommendation is that SFA should contribute less than 10% of total energy,[6] and less than 7% for the treatment of elevated plasma total cholesterol and LDL cholesterol levels.[7] The US eating pattern contains about 13% of energy from SFA and about 7% of energy from omega-6 fatty acids.[8] The literature is extensive regarding the role of food composition and eating habits on lipid levels.

A 1970 study of about 12,000 men in 18 populations from seven countries (Finland, Greece, Italy, Japan, The Netherlands, the United States, and Yugoslavia) opened our eyes to the food-lipid association. The percentage of energy from SFA was highly correlated with the five-year CHD incidence rate and with serum cholesterol concentration. Among the groups, 80% of the serum cholesterol variability was explained by SFA intake.[3] When the Framingham Study[9] could not confirm these results, several reasons were given[10]:

- the homogeneity of the dietary pattern within a population
- a large intra-individual variation from day to day in the fat composition of food intake
- genetic and metabolic heterogeneity within a population
- unrefined dietary assessment methods
- confounding variables

Diets with less saturated fat tend to lower the plasma total cholesterol[11-14] (see Table 11-3). SFAs are found in animal fat, coconut fat, and palm and palm kernel oils. Omega-6 fatty acids are hypocholesterolemic. They are found mainly in vegetable oils.

Table 11–2 Major Dietary Components or Conditions and Their Effect on Plasma Total Cholesterol and LDL Cholesterol

Effect	Component
Lowers total cholesterol and LDL cholesterol levels	Omega-6 fatty acids Monounsaturated fatty acids Soluble fiber Carbohydrate Vegetarianism Alcohol
Raises total cholesterol and LDL cholesterol levels	Saturated fatty acids Cholesterol Overweight/obesity
Unknown (being studied)	Coffee Omega-3 fatty acids* Protein

*Omega-3 fatty acids are hypotriglyceridemic and hypocholesterolemic. For individuals with hypertriglyceridemia, omega-3 fatty acids elevate LDL cholesterol levels.

Source: Adapted from Kris-Etherton, P.M., Krummel, D., Russel, M.E., et al., The Effect of Diet on Plasma, Lipids, Lipoproteins, and Coronary Heart Disease. *Journal of the American Dietetic Association,* Vol. 88, p. 1373, with permission of the American Dietetic Association, © 1988.

Table 11–3 Sources and Effect of Dietary Fatty Acids on Plasma Lipids

Fatty Acids		Common Sources	Major Effect on Plasma Lipids
Saturated			
C12:0	(lauric)	Coconut, palm kernel oil	Increases plasma total cholesterol
C14:0	(myristic)	Coconut	Increases plasma total cholesterol
C16:0	(palmitic)	Palm oil, beef	Increases plasma total cholesterol
C18:0	(stearic)	Cocoa butter, beef	Decreases plasma total cholesterol, has no effect, or raises it less than expected
Monounsaturated			
C18:1	(oleic)	Oil, beef, olive oil, rapeseed	Decreases plasma total cholesterol[25]
Polyunsaturated			
Omega-6			
C18:2	(linoleic)	Corn oil, cottonseed oil, soybean oil, sunflower oil	Decreases plasma total cholesterol[18,26]
Omega-3			
C20:5	Eicosapentaenoic	Atlantic and king mackerel, Atlantic and Pacific herring (sardines), lake trout, chinook salmon, albacore tuna, Atlantic and sockeye salmon, bluefish, pink and chum salmon, Atlantic halibut, coho salmon, marine lipids (cod liver oil and omega-3 fatty acid supplements)	Decreases plasma triglycerides, variable LDL cholesterol, and HDL cholesterol effects[27]
C22:6	Docosahexaenoic		

Note: References cited in this table are included with end-of-chapter references.

Source: Adapted from Kris-Etherton, P.M., Krummel, D., Russel, M.E., et al., The Effect of Diet on Plasma, Lipids, Lipoproteins, and Coronary Heart Disease. *Journal of the American Dietetic Association,* Vol. 88, p. 1373, with permission of the American Dietetic Association, © 1988.

The quantities of SFA, omega-6 fatty acids, and cholesterol are important determinants of blood lipid level. The effect of the quality and quantity of fat on blood cholesterol when exogenous cholesterol is modified is seen in the Keys[15] and Hegsted[16] predictive equations.[17] Two predictive equations were developed to determine the magnitude of change in plasma total cholesterol when there are changes in the fatty acid composition of an individual's eating pattern.[15,16] Keys (Minnesota) equation is as follows:

$$\triangle \text{ CHOL} = 1.35 \ (2 \ \triangle S - \triangle P) + 1.52 \ \triangle Z$$

Hegsted (Harvard) equation is as follows:

$$\triangle \text{ CHOL} = 2.16 \ \triangle S - 1.65 \ \triangle P + 0.0677 \ \triangle C - 0.53,$$

Where $\triangle$ CHOL = estimated change in serum cholesterol in mg/dL;
$\triangle S$ = change in percentage of daily calories from saturated fat;
$\triangle P$ = change in percentage of daily calories from polyunsaturated fat;
$\triangle Z$ = change in the square root of daily dietary cholesterol in mg/1,000 kcal; and $\triangle C$ = change in dietary cholesterol in mg/day.

Both equations predict a twofold plasma cholesterol-raising effect of SFA that is approximately twice the cholesterol-lowering effect of omega-6 fatty acids. The effect of dietary fat on serum cholesterol is a function of the expression 2S – P.[18]

LIPID RESPONSE TO DIETARY CHANGE

Cocoa butter is comprised of the SFA stearic acid (C18:0). In dietary manipulation studies it has either decreased,[19] not affected,[20] or increased[15] plasma total cholesterol.

When stearic acid replaces palmitic acid, it can lower cholesterol,[21] but different SFAs evoke different responses (e.g., stearic acid is hypocholesterolemic (lowers blood cholesterol) compared with palmitic acid but hypercholesterolemic (raises blood cholesterol) compared with linoleic acid). For this reason, health care providers must consider individual food selections when promoting a less than 10% SFA intake.[6] Foods rich in

stearic acid may be hypocholesterolemic rather than hypercholesterolemic.

The extent of the plasma lipid response is related to an individual's baseline plasma lipid level. The response of plasma lipid levels to various amounts of SFA, monounsaturated fatty acid (MFA), and omega-6 fatty acids when total fat and cholesterol are modified is outlined in Table 11-4.[11-14,22-25]

Cholesterol-lowering responses have ranged from +4% to –17%, with a mean level of –11%. LDL and plasma total cholesterol levels tend to decline when lipid-lowering foods are consumed; HDL levels have decreased in some studies.

In an Australian study of 163 men and 66 women, 16 to 80 years old, adipose tissue level of linoleic acid was positively associated with coronary artery disease (CAD). Platelet linoleic acid levels had a positive association with CAD; and by controlling for possible confounding factors, the platelet concentration of eicosapentaenoic acid (i.e., omega-3) had an inverse association with CAD for men, whereas the docosapentaenoic acid concentration had an inverse association with CAD for women.[26]

This study contradicts several population, cross-sectional, and case-control studies that have shown an inverse association between CHD and linoleic acid concentration of adipose tissue.[27-30] Speculation is that the linoleic acid increases the risk of new atherosclerotic lesions,[31] but further research is warranted.

Saturated fatty acids consistently raise plasma total cholesterol, and omega-6 fatty acids lower it. Their effects differ, as saturated fatty acids are twice as powerful as omega-6 fatty acids. A 1% increase in the SFA intake increases plasma total cholesterol by 2.7 mg/dL. A 1% increase in omega-6 fatty acids results in a 1.4 mg/dL reduction in total cholesterol.[15]

Fish oil can lower plasma triglyceride, but intake must be about 90 to 120 grams for an effect. This amount is abnormally high for average individuals to consume. A realistic eating pattern would contain two to three fish meals a week as a healthy, preventive approach.[32]

Studies of West Greenland Eskimos and Caucasian Danes show great contrast in eating and in health outcome.[33,34] Total fat intake was simi-

Table 11–4 Plasma Lipid Response to Modified Fat Diets Made of Whole Foods

Fat Content	N	Mean Initial Plasma Cholesterol (mg/dL)	Span (weeks)	SFA (%kcal)	PUFA (%kcal)	MFA (%kcal)	Chol (mg/day)	2S - P	Total-C	LDL-C	HDL-C
<30% kcal from fat											
Grundy[11]	38	230	6	6.9	6.4	5.9	250	7.4	-13	-19	-10
Snook[22]	11*	250	4	6.7	6.7	6.7	100	6.7	-7	-9	-30
Grundy[23]	9	210	8	10	10	10***	250	10	-17	-23	NE
30% kcal											
Mensink[12]	48	195	5	6.7	5.2	9.3**	390	8.2	-8	—	-17
Kuusi[24]	38	250	12	10	4	7	350	16	-10	-11	-11
30% kcal											
Grundy[11]	11*	250	4	4	4	28	100	0	-13	-18	-7
Grundy[23]	9	210	8	10	17	13	250	3	-17	-24	-13
Weisweiler[25]	15	210	12	12	12	12***	250	12	-15	-19	NE
30% kcal											
Weisweiler[13]	22	219	6	10	10	12k	400	10	-12	-9	NE
Schwandt[14]	30	204	12	18	13	6**k	370	23	+4	-3	NE

NE = no effect.
*Formula used, not whole food.
**Low-fat and high-fat diets had different 2S - P dietary factors.
*** Low-fat and high-fat diets had similar 2S - P dietary factors.
kHigh-fat diets with different 2S - P dietary factors.

Source: Adapted from Kris-Etherton, P.M., Krummel, D., Russel, M.E., et al., The Effect of Diet on Plasma, Lipids, Lipoproteins, and Coronary Heart Disease, *Journal of the American Dietetic Association,* Vol. 88, p. 1373, with permission of the American Dietetic Association, © 1988.

lar, but the Danes consumed about twice as much SFA and omega-6 fatty acids as the Eskimos. The age-adjusted mortality from myocardial infarction for Greenland Eskimos was about 10% of the mortality for Danes. For the Eskimos, plasma total cholesterol, triglycerides, LDL, and VLDL levels were lower and HDL levels were higher. Eskimos consume about 5 to 10 g/day of omega-3 fatty acids by eating fish, seal, walrus, and whale.[33,34]

Omega-3 fatty acids reduce triglyceride levels and may lower cholesterol level.[35] The effect is dose-related.[36] Fish oil may also serve other roles (for example, it may lessen the hyper-cholesterolemic effect of dietary cholesterol, reduce platelet aggregation and blood clotting, lessen inflammation, and reduce the viscosity of blood by improving the oxygen supply to tissues and narrowed vessels).[32,37,38]

Fish oil containing omega-3 fatty acids alters platelet function. Using the fish oil diet, a 14% decrease in platelet adhesiveness and a four-minute increase in bleeding time has been observed.[39] These changes are due to prostaglandins, which are made from essential fatty acids.

A decreased production of thromboxane A2 and increased synthesis of prostacyclins are responsible for the antithrombic action of the omega-3 fatty acids. Fish oil stops the formation of the atherosclerotic plaque by reducing cellular growth factors and the adhesion of macrophages to the endothelium. Fish oils also promote the endothelial-derived relaxing factor and inhibit the synthesis of interleukin-1-alpha from monocytes. Recurrent stenosis after coronary angioplasty was less in patients who were given fish oil before the procedure.[39] Fish oil decreases blood viscosity, which is a thrombosis-inducing factor, and it reduces fat level in the blood after a fatty meal. The omega-3 fatty acids in fish and fish oil prevent two important aspects of CHD:

the lipid-rich atherosclerotic plaque and thrombosis. Incorporating fish and fish oil into the low-cholesterol, low-saturated-fat diet is essential to achieve maximal beneficial effects.[39]

A daily intake of 90 to 120 grams of fish oil tends to create a positive lipid profile with lower plasma triglycerides and total cholesterol levels. A 30% to 71% lowering of plasma triglycerides using capsules in hypercholesterolemic and hypertriglyceridemic patients was reported. Patients took 20 MaxEPA (Advanced Medical Nutrition, Hayward, California) capsules (1 gram each with 0.18 grams eicosapentaenoic acid and 0.12 grams docosapentaenoic acid per capsule) daily for two years.[39]

Strong warnings have been issued against the routine continuous use of fish oil supplements.[40] Concerns include safety, proper dosages, length of treatment, and the side effects of long-term use. At a level of 30 to 40 mL cod liver oil per day, risk of vitamin A and D toxicity can occur. Vitamin A toxicity is known to occur in some persons who ingest as little as 100,000 IU per day for about 10 years or 200,000 IU per day for five years. Other side effects include increased bleeding, alteration of impaired immune function,[41] and potential intake of environmental toxins. Individuals with normal plasma lipid levels should not use fish oil supplements since their role as a CHD preventive therapy is not clear.[5]

When monounsaturated fatty acids such as those provided by olive and peanut oil are substituted for SFA, lower plasma total cholesterol and LDL cholesterol levels without lower HDL levels are reported.[11,42,43] A level of 10 to 15% of calories from MFA is recommended.[6,8,43] A three-week eating pattern that was 38% of calories from fat, 10% from SFA, 25% from MFA (mainly olive oil), and 4% from omega-6 fatty acids lowered plasma apolipoprotein by 7.4% more.[44] This suggests that an eating pattern with the fat mainly of MFA may be one of the most effective lipid-lowering patterns.

Considering the various lipid responses to fatty acid composition of the eating pattern, current findings strongly suggest that health care providers use percentage of energy from SFA, MFA, polyunsaturated fatty acids (PUFA) and omega-6 fatty acids and not use a polyunsaturated to saturated fatty acid ratio when making eating pattern recommendations. This provides a more accurate description of the healthful amounts of the various fatty acids.[45] This approach allows individuals to learn about the various sources of fat and their effects, as well as how to apply this information to individual eating patterns.[45]

THE ROLE OF TOTAL FAT

Even though fat composition has a major influence on blood lipids, total fat intake has influenced the CHD morbidity and mortality in three different populations.[46] Plasma lipids respond the same to a low-fat diet[11] and a high-fat diet[25] when saturated and polyunsaturated fat composition are the same.[7]

The total amount of fat may be more influential than nutritionists once thought. A significant correlation between total fat intake and the percent of body fat was reported for 155 moderately overweight, middle-aged men.[47] The hypothesis is that first, a high-fat diet may contribute to obesity; second, exogenous fat is stored in body fat more efficiently than carbohydrate; and third, the outcome is an increased CHD risk.[48] Studies show that women who follow a 15 to 20% fat eating pattern consume 11% fewer calories than women who have 45 to 50% of their total calories from fat, and they experience a 15% energy surplus.[49]

THE ROLE OF DIETARY CHOLESTEROL

Exogenous cholesterol increases plasma total cholesterol and lipoprotein cholesterol levels. Cholesterol-rich chylomicron and VLDL remnants may be atherogenic and increase as cholesterol is ingested.[50] Total daily cholesterol intake should not exceed 300 mg/day.[6] Plasma cholesterol response is greatest with changes in cholesterol intake below 500 mg/day.

The first report of a correlation between dietary cholesterol and plasma cholesterol levels ($r = 0.90$) involved a study of the Tarahumara Indians.[51] This Mexican population was unacculturated and inhabited the Sierra Madre Occidental Mountains. At the same time in US cross-sectional studies, a lack of association between cholesterol intakes and plasma cholesterol levels was consistently reported when intakes were between 200 and 1,500 mg per day.[52,53] Reasons given then and now for the lack of significant correlation are[50]:

- the large day-to-day variation in the plasma cholesterol level
- an inadequate number of 24-hour recalls to estimate dietary cholesterol accurately
- a similar or narrow range of dietary cholesterol intake
- inappropriate end points
- undefined independent variables affecting blood cholesterol

Two major studies, the Western Electric Study and the Lipid Research Clinics Coronary Primary Prevention Trial, reported a significant association between exogenous cholesterol change and changes in plasma total cholesterol.[54,55] Observations from the Western Electric Study involved a 25-year follow up and reported a positive and independent association between dietary cholesterol and risk of CHD death.[56]

In other studies, participants were assigned to regimens that either added a specified number of eggs each day to their usual eating pattern or involved eating a prepared meal.[57] The dietary manipulations involved one or more of the following:

- varying amounts of dietary cholesterol
- different time periods for the experimental diet
- men only, women only, or men and women combined
- various ages of individuals
- different baseline blood cholesterol levels
- alteration of the quantity and quality of fat
- crossover and double-blind research designs
- various numbers of blood cholesterol samples due to –5% to +10% change in level[57] per day for an individual

Plasma cholesterol responds to dietary cholesterol. The response to cholesterol intake between 0 and 500 mg/day can be termed as linear or curvilinear.[50] Most individuals compensate for different exogenous cholesterol levels and show no serum cholesterol change. Other individuals are sensitive to changes in cholesterol intake.

In one study, 80% of the participants responded to dietary change and the response was predictable.[58] For 20%, the plasma response was either much higher or much lower than expected. It appears that about one-half of individuals have a predictable or greater than anticipated cholesterol response; 16% have less than one-half of the predicted response.[59]

THE ROLE OF TRANS FATTY ACIDS

Health-conscious consumers have recently become concerned with trans fatty acids, which appear naturally in the fat of beef, butter, milk, and lamb.[60] Commercially prepared, partially hydrogenated margarines and solid cooking oils are also high in trans fatty acids.

Trans fatty acids are produced during the hydrogenation of vegetable oils. This process adds hydrogen to unsaturated fatty acids in the oil and modifies the fat by changing it from a liquid to a soft or solid state. Partially hydrogenated vegetable oils are used to replace naturally solid, saturate-rich fats, such as lard and beef tallow. They are used in margarines, baked foods, and in commercial frying, where vegetable oils cannot be used. Margarines made in the United States are comprised of 0 to 30% trans fatty acids; stick margarines have more trans fatty acids than soft, tub margarines. The main sources of trans fatty acids in the US eating pattern are stick margarine, shortening, commercial frying fats, and high-fat baked goods.[60]

Clinical trial data show that at high levels, trans fatty acids resemble saturated fatty acids and raise serum LDL cholesterol and modestly lower HDL levels. Trans fatty acids do not reduce HDL cholesterol when ingested at current average levels.

The US population currently consumes about 12 to 14% of total energy from saturated fatty acids, and about 2 to 4% from trans fatty acids. This is an average 8 to 13 grams of trans fatty acids per day.[60]

In the Netherlands, consumption of trans fatty acids is approximately twice that of US residents, yet no adverse effects on heart disease have been attributed to their ingestion. Dutch, US and Australian researchers have shown that trans fatty acids have far more moderate effects on blood cholesterol levels than saturated fatty acids. A recent US Department of Agriculture (USDA) study involving healthy persons who consumed an average amount of trans fatty acids did not report a lower HDL level among the treatment group. Consuming twice the level of trans fatty acids reduced HDL levels by 2.8%.[60]

Mortality from CHD has declined in the United States during the past 20 years. At the same time, there has been a change from consuming highly saturated animal fats to eating more unsaturated vegetable oils and margarines, which contain no cholesterol but have the essential fatty acid, linoleic acid, and the antioxidant, vitamin E.[60]

Partially hydrogenated vegetable fats and oils can be used to replace saturated animal fats in foods, replace saturate-rich frying, and substitute for saturated baking fats. Totally liquid vegetable oils are often unsuitable for fried and baked products because they form oxidation products during frying and do not perform well in baked foods. Partially hydrogenated vegetable oils, which can be used in baked products, decrease the saturated fatty acid intake and maintain the quality of commercially baked goods.

Data from the Nurses' Health Study of 87,000 women were evaluated for the association of trans fatty acid content of foods on plasma LDL cholesterol. Dietary data were obtained from a semiquantitative food frequency with 61 foods. Women were followed for eight years; within that time, 431 new cases of CHD were documented. During the analysis of the data, the age and the total energy intake of the women were controlled. A direct association appeared between trans fatty acid intake and CHD risk, and a relative risk of 1.50 resulted when comparing the highest with the lowest quintile of trans fatty acid intake. Multivitamin use; saturated and monounsaturated fat; linoleic acid; dietary cholesterol; fiber; and vitamin E, C, and A intakes did not enhance or dilute the association. By analyzing data only for women with a consistent margarine intake for one decade, a relative risk of 1.67 was noted. Further, a significant association was reported between higher risk for CHD and intakes of major food sources of trans fatty acids. This means that as intake of margarine, cookies, cake, and white bread increased, the risk of CHD increased.[61]

THE ROLE OF CARBOHYDRATE

The complement of a low-fat eating pattern is a high-dietary-carbohydrate (CHO) pattern. An eating pattern with approximately 80% of calories from CHO (i.e., a very-high-CHO and very-low-fat diet), which is markedly different from the typical American eating pattern, decreases plasma total cholesterol, LDL, and HDL.[62,63] An eating pattern with 50% to 65% of calories from CHO has also significantly lowered plasma lipids.[64]

There is no clear consensus about the temporal response of plasma triglycerides to dietary CHO. An increased consumption of simple CHOs may create a greater plasma triglyceride response than that observed for complex CHOs.[65] Factors affecting the plasma lipid response to increased dietary CHOs include the following:

- the rate at which dietary CHO is increased
- the fiber content of the eating pattern
- the type of carbohydrate
- initial plasma lipid, lipoprotein, glucose, and insulin status of the individual.

These issues need to be investigated in well-controlled experiments.

THE ROLE OF FIBER

Soluble fiber has a beneficial effect on plasma lipid levels by binding cholesterol and bile acids in the small intestine and carrying them into the colon for elimination. Plasma total cholesterol and LDL cholesterol are lowered, and HDL cholesterol is either unchanged or raised when soluble fiber is added to the eating pattern (see Table 11-5). Current recommendations are to increase dietary fiber intake to 20 to 25 g/day

Table 11-5 Plasma Lipid Change with Various Dietary Fibers

Type of Fiber	Hyperlipidemic Participant	Food	Dry Weight (g/day)	% Change Tot-C	LDL-C	HDL-C	Triglyceride
Soluble							
Pectin	No	Fruits	31	-13	NR	—	—
	No		40–50	-13	NR	NR	—
	Yes			-13	NR	NR	—
Guar	No	Oats	20	-13	NR	—	—
	Yes		13	-13	-15	—	-13
Legumes	Yes	Beans	115	-19	-24	-12	—
	Yes		140	-7	—	—	-25
Oats	Yes	Oatmeal	100	-13	-14	—	—
	Yes		100	-19	-23	-5	—
Insoluble							
Cellulose	No	Wheat	15	—	—	—	—
Lignin	No	Vegetables	12	—	—	—	—

NR = not reported.

Source: Adapted from Kris-Etherton, P.M., Krummel, D., Russel, M.E., et al., The Effect of Diet on Plasma, Lipids, Lipoproteins, and Coronary Heart Disease, *Journal of the American Dietetic Association,* Vol. 88, p. 1373, with permission of the American Dietetic Association, © 1988.

and not to exceed 40 to 50 g/day.[66] This includes oats, legumes, pectin, psyllium, and selected gums.

A long-term, longitudinal study of healthy, middle-aged men in England reported that energy and fiber consumption have a significant association with the incidence of CHD.[67] A lower incidence of CHD was noted for men who ate high-fiber cereals and abundant calories. Men who developed clinically significant heart disease (N = 45) consumed 6.7 grams dietary fiber per day from cereals, not fruits, vegetables, and nuts. Men who developed clinical CHD during the study (N = 292) had an average daily fiber intake of 8.9 grams. In the Zutphen Study, CHD mortality was about four times higher for men in the lowest quintile of dietary fiber intake than for those in the highest quintile.[68]

Pectin and guar gum have each reduced plasma total cholesterol by 10% or more.[69-71] Ten grams per day of psyllium hydrophilic mucilloid has lowered serum total cholesterol by 15% and LDL by 20% in hypercholesterolemic men.[72] Five to 11 grams of soluble fiber for six weeks has demonstrated an additional 5.6 to 6.5 mg/dL lowering of plasma total cholesterol after the effect of

a moderate cholesterol-lowering eating pattern.[73] The addition of one cup of hot oat bran cereal and five oat bran muffins daily (47 grams dietary fiber) created a significant plasma lipid response[74]; however, the study methods were questionable. In addition, the practicality of the regimen is a concern. Pectin is sticky, difficult to add to foods, and attaches to the oral mucosa for hours. A possible alternative is eating apples; the pectin in two to eight apples a day can have a hypocholesterolemic effect.[75]

High fiber only from fruits and vegetables that provide 42 grams per day did not decrease plasma total cholesterol in one study,[76] whereas small amounts of legumes and especially beans effectively lower both plasma total cholesterol and triglycerides. When an eating pattern high in fiber from citrus pectin (28 grams) is ingested, a significant reduction in plasma total cholesterol by 13 mg/dL has been observed. Eating patterns very high in both CHO (72% of kcal) and fiber (74 grams per day) have lowered fasting plasma triglycerides in hypertriglyceridemic individuals with diabetes.[77] Some dietary fibers bind bile acids, increase fecal bile acid, enhance steroid excretion, and decrease lipid and sterol absorption.[70]

In a double-blind, placebo-controlled trial with men and women 21 to 70 years old with primary hypercholesterolemia (i.e., total serum cholesterol greater than 220 mg/L), 37 followed a high-fat diet and 81 consumed a low-fat diet. Participants were randomly assigned to take either 5.1 grams of psyllium or a placebo two times daily. The total cholesterol levels of participants on psyllium and on either the low- or high-fat diet declined 10 to 15 mg/dL, and cholesterol values decreased by 11 to 13 mg/dL.[78] The importance of this trial is that psyllium was shown to have an independent effect and may be a substitute for drug therapy among primary hypercholesterolemic individuals.

THE ROLE OF PROTEIN

Epidemiological studies have shown that animal protein in an eating pattern is positively correlated ($r = 0.78$) and the vegetable protein is negatively correlated ($r = -0.40$) with CHD mortality rates.[51] In human studies, when animal protein is replaced with soybean protein, there is either a small hypolipidemic effect or no effect.[79-81] Several studies conducted with hypercholesterolemic patients have reported that soy protein lowers serum total cholesterol more effectively than casein.[82]

THE ROLE OF DIETARY IRON

A fairly new hypothesis being explored regards the role of high iron status as a risk for heart disease. There are limited data to suggest that iron is a pro-oxidant and may have an etiological role in cardiovascular disease. The rationale is that oxidation of LDL contributes to arterial plaque formation and that oxidation has an immediate role in damaging tissue during and immediately following heart attack and stroke.[83-86] The pros of this hypothesis are as follows:

- Iron protects premenopausal women due to loss of iron during menstrual bleeding.
- Postmenopausal estrogen therapy may cause intermittent bleeding resulting in a lowering of body iron stores.

- Aspirin protects an individual because it causes gastrointestinal blood and iron loss.
- Coronary risk reduction may be linked to exercise because exercise increases runner's anemia.
- The low mortality from CHD in developing countries may be due to high rates of iron-deficiency anemia.

Epidemiologic studies that have supported the hypothesis address several points. (1) One study examined a cohort of 1,931 men in Finland with 51 experiencing a myocardial infarct during the three-year follow up. If serum ferritin was equal to or greater than 200 micrograms/L, the men had a 2.2-fold increased risk of infarct. Exogenous iron intake had a positive association with the risk of infarct; a 5% increase in risk occurred for each 1 mg increase in iron intake.[87] (2) An 11-country study found that CHD mortality rates were associated with the liver iron-serum cholesterol product in men and in men and women combined.[88]

The cons of this hypothesis are as follows:

- Hormones are primarily responsible for the changes in women with menopause.
- Exercise primarily influences cardiovascular fitness.
- Geographic differences in CHD are due to lifestyle differences (e.g., smoking, energy intake, and expenditure).
- Iron status cannot account for the trends in CHD mortality.

Studies that have not supported the iron and CHD hypothesis are as follows:

- US study of 45,720 men, for whom 880 were diagnosed with CHD in the four-year follow-up period and no associations were noted between iron and CHD risk[89]
- US study with 238 experimental and 238 control males, showing that men with high ferritin levels did not have a higher risk of infarct[90]
- US study of 171 older men and 406 older women reporting no significant difference in serum ferritin levels for those with and without coronary artery disease[91]

- US study with 1,827 Caucasian men and 2,410 Caucasian women for whom 489 had an infarct and 900 developed CHD in the 16-year follow up. (For women only, serum iron was inversely linked to infarct, but total iron-binding capacity, transferrin saturation and exogenous iron were not associated with infarct for men or women. Serum iron and transferrin saturation did have an inverse association with CHD for men and woman.)[92]

THE ROLE OF COFFEE

The United States has experienced a surge in coffee consumption during the 1990s. In 1989 there were about 200 specialty coffee outlets in the United States, compared to 4,500 in 1994. In addition, there are numerous opportunities to request or purchase coffee in every restaurant, fast food facility, gasoline station, bank, and grocery store. America's fondness for coffee includes espresso, latte, mocha, and cappuccino.[93]

Info Line

Cappuccino is coffee made with espresso, a minimal amount of steamed milk, and a large foam cap made from a few ounces of milk. It is named because of the cap of foam on top, which resembles the hooded robe of the Capuchin friars or Roman Catholic monks. It provides 51–130 mg caffeine per serving. *Espresso*, derived from the same bean as coffee but brewed with less water, provides 30–57 mg caffeine per serving. *Latte*, a basic espresso with steamed milk and often a dollop of frothed milk on top, provides 51–130 mg caffeine per serving. *Mocha* is generally espresso with a small amount of steamed milk, 1 to 2 ounces of mocha or chocolate syrup, and sometimes a dollop of frothed milk. It provides 57–130 mg caffeine per serving.

Findings regarding coffee consumption and plasma lipid levels are not consistent.[5] Both an

association and a causal relationship have been noted. The recommended range of intake varies from one to two cups per day to nine or fewer cups per day.

In Norway, the Tromso Heart Study reported coffee consumption as a major determinant of total serum cholesterol level.[94] Coffee intake was correlated with total serum cholesterol level in the 14,667 men and women—even after adjustment for age, logarithm of body-mass index, leisure-time physical activity, cigarette smoking, and alcohol consumption.

Serum total cholesterol was 31 mg/dL higher in men who drank more than nine cups per day compared with men who drank less than one cup per day. A corresponding increase of 26 mg/dL was noted for women. HDL cholesterol was higher in both men and women who drank one to four cups than for individuals who drank less than one cup per day. At five or more cups per day, HDL cholesterol was lower for women, but this was not true for men. In effect, each cup of coffee raised serum total cholesterol by 1.6 mg/dL in men and 1.3 mg/dL in women.[95]

In a prospective study of 1,130 medical students followed for 19 to 35 years, heavy coffee drinkers (five or more cups per day) had two to three times greater risk for CHD, even after adjustment for age, smoking, blood pressure, and baseline serum cholesterol.[96] In two studies, abstinence from coffee for four to five weeks created a greater than 10% decrease in plasma total cholesterol.[97,98]

Haffner et al[95] opened a new avenue of speculation by reporting that the regression coefficients in the multiple regression analyses were more significant when coffee rather than caffeine was the independent variable. This implicates components in coffee other than caffeine. To provide conclusive data on the effects of coffee, decaffeinated coffee, and caffeine on plasma lipid levels, further clinical investigations are recommended.[99]

THE ROLE OF ALCOHOL

Epidemiological and clinical studies have reported a protective effect of moderate alcohol consumption (i.e., 7 to 14 ounces of alcohol per week) on the incidence of CHD, and an additional beneficial effect of alcohol on HDL cholesterol levels.

Cross-sectional data of 4,855 male and female participants in the Lipid Research Clinics Program Prevalence Study showed a significant association between alcohol consumption and HDL cholesterol levels ($r = 0.21$ for men and 0.25 for women).[100] Men, aged 50 to 69 years, with the highest alcohol consumption (42 to 85 grams per day) had an HDL cholesterol level of 55 mg/dL, which reflected levels of young women; nondrinkers had 42 mg/dL level. In addition, alcohol consumption explained 4% to 6% of the total variance in HDL cholesterol.

A small amount of alcohol (i.e., one drink a day) may protect against CHD, because it affects the subfractions HDL_2 and HDL_3 and may be an anticlotting factor. Three weeks of abstinence decreased total HDL and HDL_3. Both increased when alcohol intake resumed.[101] Other researchers have reported that about 9 grams of alcohol per day for a month can raise HDL cholesterol by 7%, primarily due to an increase in HDL_2.[102]

Alcohol increases plasma triglyceride levels. It is associated with hypertension, alcoholic hepatitis, and cirrhosis. Certain cancers, fetal alcohol syndrome, psychosocial problems, and serious accidents are linked to habitual alcohol intake. Increasing alcohol intake to favorably change HDL cholesterol and hence lower CHD risk appears inappropriate. If one drinks, moderation of alcohol intake is recommended.[100]

VEGETARIANISM

A vegetarian diet that is low in total fat, SFA, and cholesterol, and high in fiber, has been shown to promote a favorable plasma lipoprotein profile.[103,104] Plasma lipid and lipoprotein levels of 73 men and 43 women on a vegetarian eating pattern were lower when compared with omnivores (i.e., total cholesterol, 126 and 184; LDL cholesterol, 73 and 118; VLDL cholesterol, 12 and 17; and HDL cholesterol, 42 and 49).[105] The lower HDL cholesterol level among vegetarians is reflected in a lower HDL_2 cholesterol level.[106]

Further research is needed to identify the factor(s) creating plasma lipid variations between vegetarians and omnivores. Plasma total cholesterol, LDL cholesterol, and HDL cholesterol all decline when omnivores follow a vegetarian eating pattern (i.e., 13%, 15%, and 10%, respectively). Apolipoprotein A-1 removal rate is accelerated for vegetarians and persons who consume low-fat, high-CHO foods.[107,108] LDL production rate is lower for vegetarians.[108] A higher linoleic acid and lower arachidonic acid concentration in platelets is reported for vegans and lacto-ovo-vegetarians compared with omnivores.[109]

THE ROLE OF ANTIOXIDANTS

Antioxidants, including vitamin E, beta-carotene, and vitamin C, donate electrons to electron-seeking compounds. They stop oxidizing agents from breaking double bonds of fatty acids and prevent the alteration of DNA by electron-seeking substances. Data connecting antioxidants to a reduced risk of CHD are limited, but the Nurse's Health Study and the Health Professionals Follow-Up Study report a decreased risk of CHD for men and women with higher vitamin E intakes.

The Nurse's Health Study enrolled 87,000 women, 34 to 59 years old, in 1976 and followed them for eight years. The sample reported 552 cases of documented CHD during the follow up. The relative risk of CHD for women with the highest vitamin E intake, 2.8 IU per day, was 0.66 (95% CI of 0.50–0.87). Women with more than two years of vitamin E supplementation had a relative risk of 0.59 (95% CI of 0.38–0.91). Interestingly, dietary sources of vitamin E, multivitamin supplement users, and vitamin C intake were not linked to reduced risk.[110,111]

The Health Professionals Follow-Up Study analyzed the association of CHD risk and vitamin E intake. In 1986, 51,529 men 40 to 75 years old with no CHD were enrolled; the study reported 667 new CHD cases four years later. A significant trend of lower CHD risk with higher vitamin E intakes was noted ($p = 0.003$). Men who consumed 60 or more IU each day had a relative risk of 0.64, compared to men who ingested 7.5 IU a day. Men who took 100 IU per day of vitamin E had a relative risk of 0.63 (95% CI of 0.47–0.84).[112]

These two studies suggest that men and women who take vitamin E supplementation may have a lower CHD risk. However, the new US Nutrition Labeling Education Act (see Chapter 2) recommends an increased intake of fruits and vegetables rather than vitamin supplementation. The National Academy of Science's Food and Nutrition Board is considering revisions of the Recommended Dietary Allowances to include potential supplementation for nutrients that demonstrate preventive effects on chronic diseases (see Chapter 2).

Traditional reliance on whole foods is being challenged in the scientific community, which seems reasonable. What does not appear reasonable is the decision by the free enterprise system to market megavitamin doses when research data are not consistent and have not reached a consensus.

THE NATIONAL CHOLESTEROL EDUCATION PROGRAM

In 1984, the National Institutes of Health (NIH) Consensus Development Conference on Lowering Blood Cholesterol to Prevent Heart Disease recommended creating and implementing a national cholesterol education program. The National Cholesterol Education Program (NCEP) began in 1985 with the goal to reduce the prevalence of elevated blood cholesterol in the United States and contribute to the reduction of CHD morbidity and mortality. The NCEP has issued several reports, including the Adult Treatment Panel I and II guidelines, the Population Strategies Panel report, and the report of the Panel on Blood Cholesterol Levels in Children and Adolescents.

1988 Cholesterol Guidelines—Adult Treatment Panel I

With the first report of the Adult Treatment Panel (ATP I), an LDL-cholesterol level of 160 mg/dL or higher placed an individual at high risk for CHD.[7] A level of 130 to 159 mg/dL was clas-

sified as a borderline value, with less than 130 mg/dL considered desirable. A triglyceride level greater than 250 mg/dL was considered elevated. Other major risk factors for CHD included male sex, cigarette smoking, hypertension, diabetes mellitus, family history of premature myocardial infarction or sudden death, an HDL-cholesterol level below 35 mg/dL and confirmed by repeated measurement, history of occlusive peripheral vascular disease or cerebrovascular disease, and severe obesity more than 30% above ideal body weight).[7,113] The goals of treatment were to reduce LDL below 160 mg/dL or below 130 mg/dL in the presence of CHD or two or more CHD risk factors.

Secondary causes of dyslipidemia were to be identified and corrected if possible. The causes of elevated LDL levels were identified as hypothyroidism, diabetes mellitus, nephrotic syndrome, obstructive liver disease, progestins, and anabolic steroids. Causes of decreased HDL levels included hypertriglyceridemia, obesity, diabetes mellitus, cigarette smoking, sedentary lifestyle, beta-blockers, progestins, and anabolic steroids. Factors causing hypertriglyceridemia included obesity, diabetes mellitus, sedentary lifestyle, alcohol intake, renal insufficiency, estrogens, and beta blockers.[7]

The ATP I report stated that modification of diet and increased exercise level were the cornerstone of therapy of patients with dyslipidemia. In the Step 1 diet, dietary fat was restricted to less than 30% of total energy. Dietary saturated fat was restricted to less than 10% total energy, cholesterol to less than 300 mg/dL, and calories were restricted in overweight individuals. All individuals at risk were to be referred to a registered dietitian for an initial assessment of their present eating pattern, instruction, and follow up.[7]

If the minimal goals of therapy were not achieved by three months, the Step 2 diet was to be adopted, which restricted saturated fats to less than 7% of total energy and cholesterol to less than 200 mg/day. Medical nutrition therapy was to continue for at least six months prior to considering medication, unless the patient had established CHD or pancreatitis. If medical nutrition therapy was not effective in reaching target

LDL-cholesterol values, or if CHD or pancreatitis was established, then drug therapy was to be considered as an adjunct to diet. At the time of ATP I, the use of severe dietary fat restriction rather than an increase in monounsaturated fat to lower LDL-cholesterol levels was being evaluated. Currently, lowering saturated fat by replacing it with complex carbohydrates is preferred because this is less calorically dense and promotes weight loss.[7]

1990 Expert Panel on Population Strategies for Blood Cholesterol Reduction

In 1990 epidemiological, clinical, and experimental evidence clearly demonstrated that the likelihood that a person will develop or die from CHD is directly related to the level of blood cholesterol.[1] Data from the 361,662 men screened for the Multiple Risk Factor Intervention Trial demonstrate a continuous association, with risk increasing as cholesterol increases (see Figure 11–1).

In the 1990 report, approaches to lowering blood cholesterol were redefined. People with high blood cholesterol levels of 240 mg/dL (6.21 mmol/L) or above have high CHD rates. However, an even larger number of cases of CHD occurs in Americans with blood cholesterol levels below 240 mg/dL, reflecting both the large number of people in this group (75% of the population) and the fact that individuals with mildly to moderately elevated blood cholesterol levels (and/or other risk factors) have an increased risk of CHD. The average cholesterol level for the adult US population in 1990 was about 210 mg/dL. Approximately 55% of US adults had cholesterol levels at or above 200 mg/dL.[1]

For these reasons, two kinds of strategies are recommended: (1) a patient-based strategy, which seeks to help those who have a high risk of CHD because of their high blood cholesterol level, and (2) a population-based strategy, which seeks to reach all Americans. The population approach aims to promote the adoption of eating patterns that will help to lower the blood cholesterol level of individuals and to reduce the average cholesterol level throughout the population.

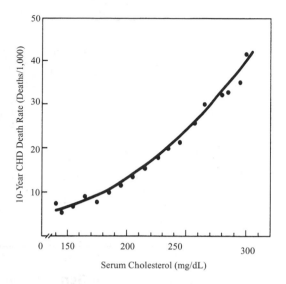

From 361,662 Men Screened for MRFIT Program

Figure 11–1 The relationship between serum cholesterol level and coronary heart disease mortality. There is an increase in mortality with increasing serum total cholesterol level. *Source:* Reprinted from *Report of the Expert Panel on Population Strategies for Blood Cholesterol Reduction* by the National Cholesterol Education Program, p. 7, U.S. Department of Health and Human Services, Public Health Service, NIH Publication No. 90-3046, November 1990.

When both approaches are used, the effects are synergistic.[1]

Figures 11–2 through 11–5 illustrate conceptually the anticipated effects of these two approaches, both separately and combined. The result of implementing the population strategy should be an approximate reduction of 10% or more in the average blood cholesterol level of the US population. This should lead to an approximate reduction of 20% or more in CHD and, consequently, to significant improvement in the health and quality of life of Americans.

The panel recommends the following average nutrient intakes for healthy Americans[1]:

- less than 10% of total calories from saturated fatty acids
- an average of 30% or less of total calories from all fat
- dietary energy levels needed to reach or maintain a desirable body weight
- less than 300 mg of cholesterol per day

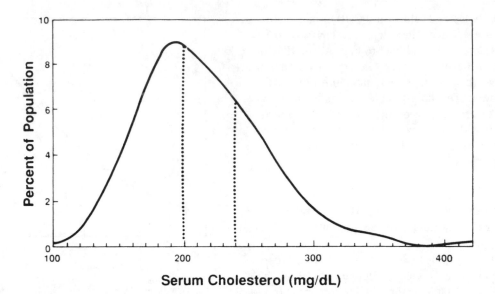

Figure 11-2 Population distribution of serum cholesterol values. The borderline and high cutoff levels are shown as dotted lines to indicate the proportions of the population above or below 200 or 240 mg/dL (i.e., 5.17 or 5.21 mmol/L). *Source:* Reprinted from *Report of the Expert Panel on Population Strategies for Blood Cholesterol Reduction* by the National Cholesterol Education Program, p. 10, U.S. Department of Health and Human Services, Public Health Service, NIH Publication No. 90-3046, November 1990.

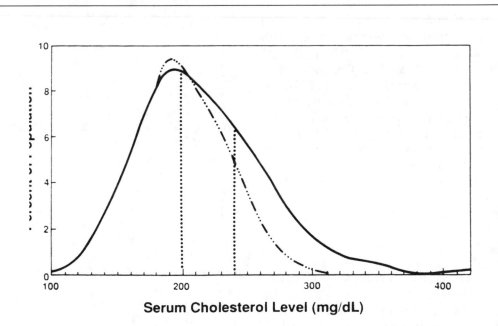

Figure 11-3 Expected shift in population distribution of serum cholesterol values with widespread application of Adult Treatment Panel guidelines. The dotted-dashed line represents an estimate of the effect of treating many people with elevated cholesterol levels. *Source:* Reprinted from *Report of the Expert Panel on Population Strategies for Blood Cholesterol Reduction* by the National Cholesterol Education Program, p. 10, U.S. Department of Health and Human Services, Public Health Service, NIH Publication No. 90-3046, November 1990.

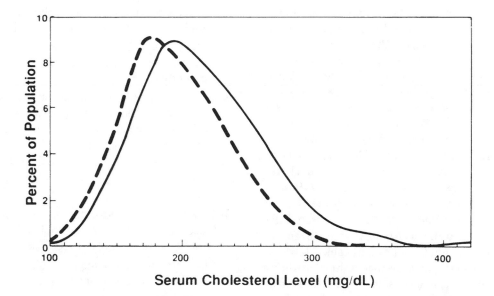

Figure 11-4 Expected shift in population distribution of serum cholesterol values if the recommendations of the Expert Panel on Population Strategies for Blood Cholesterol Production result in a 10% decrease in blood cholesterol of Americans. The dashed line shows the effect of the recommendations. *Source:* Reprinted from *Report of the Expert Panel on Population Strategies for Blood Cholesterol Reduction* by the National Cholesterol Education Program, p. 10, U.S. Department of Health and Human Services, Public Health Service, NIH Publication No. 90-3046, November 1990.

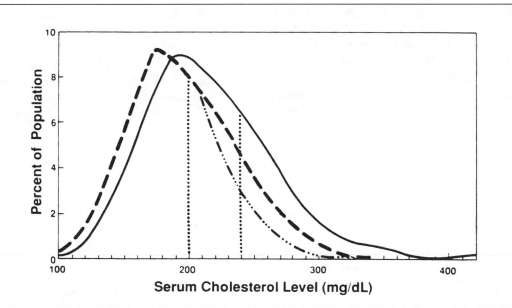

Figure 11-5 Anticipated combined effects of the recommendations of the Adult Treatment Panel (dotted-dashed line) and the Expert Panel on Population Strategies for Blood Cholesterol Reduction (dashed line). *Source:* Reprinted from *Report of the Expert Panel on Population Strategies for Blood Cholesterol Reduction* by the National Cholesterol Education Program, p. 10, U.S. Department of Health and Human Services, Public Health Service, NIH Publication No. 90-3046, November 1990.

These recommendations are generally appropriate for all segments of the population. However, new data suggest that serum cholesterol may not be predictive for women 65 years of age and older. As healthy infants join the eating patterns of others in their family, usually at about two years of age or older, a low-fat eating pattern is currently recommended but still controversial. The panel's recommendations are consistent with those of the National Research Council's *Diet and Health*,[114] the American Heart Association's *Dietary Treatment of Hypercholesterolemia*,[115] as well as with the *Dietary Guidelines for Americans*.[116] A comparison of the recommended nutrient intakes with current intakes for US adults is shown in Table 11-6.

The panel recommends that healthy Americans select, prepare, and consume foods that contain lower amounts of saturated fatty acids, total fat, and cholesterol. Specific practices can help Americans lower blood cholesterol levels. These eating patterns are fully compatible with cultural and ethnic considerations and with personal preferences for good food[1]:

- Eat a greater quantity and variety of fruits, vegetables, breads, cereals, and legumes.
- Eat more low-fat dairy products, such as skim or low-fat milk and skim or low-fat milk products, in place of high-fat milk products.
- Eat moderate amounts (e.g., about 6 ounces per day, cooked) of trimmed, lean red meat, poultry without skin, or fish, in place of foods high in saturated fatty acids.
- Eat egg yolks only in moderation. Egg whites do not contain cholesterol, and they can be eaten often.
- Use oils, margarines, and shortenings with vegetable oils that contain primarily unsaturated fatty acids instead of saturated or partially hydrogenated fatty acids.
- Read food labels. Choose foods with lower amounts or proportions of fat and/or saturated fatty acids.
- Choose prepared baked goods that have been made with unsaturated vegetable oils and, at most, small amounts of egg yolk.
- Choose "convenience foods" guided by low saturated fatty acid, total fat, and cholesterol content and cost.
- When preparing foods, keep use of fats to a minimum, use smaller amounts of ingredients high in saturated fatty acids, and use low-fat alternatives.
- In restaurants and fast-food outlets, select menu items that are low in saturated fatty acids, total fat, and cholesterol, as well as cooked foods that are baked, boiled, or broiled without fat.
- Recognize that no single food or supplement (e.g., fish oil supplements or dietary fiber) is the answer to achieving a desirable blood cholesterol level, and that a habitual pattern

Table 11-6 Recommended versus Current Fat Intake of US Population

Dietary Component	Recommended 1990*	Current (Adults) 1993
Saturated fatty acids	<10% of total calories	13% of total calories
Total fat	Average 30% or less**	36–37%
Polyunsaturated	Up to 10%	7%
Monounsaturated	Remaining fat calories	14%
Cholesterol	<300 mg a day	304 mg/435 mg (women/men)

*National Cholesterol Education Program.
**Total fat calories (30% or less) = saturated + polyunsaturated + monounsaturated.

Source: Reprinted from *Report of the Expert Panel on Population Strategies for Blood Cholesterol Reduction* by the National Cholesterol Education Program, U.S. Department of Health and Human Services, Public Health Service, NIH Publication No. 90-3046, November 1990.

of eating that is consistently low in saturated fatty acids, total fat, and cholesterol is recommended.

1993 Cholesterol Guidelines—Adult Treatment Panel II

The National Cholesterol Education Program (NCEP) issued the Second Report of the Expert Panel on Detection, Evaluation, and Treatment of High Blood Cholesterol in Adults (ATP II) five years after the first report.[117] ATP II classified blood cholesterol levels for adults as desirable, borderline, and high (see Table 11–7).

The ATP II report focuses on the clinical approach to lowering cholesterol. It offers guidelines to identify and treat people who need professional help to lower their blood cholesterol levels. In the ATP II report, high levels of LDL cholesterol are the primary target of cholesterol-lowering therapy. Medical nutrition therapy is the first line of secondary treatment to lower high blood cholesterol. Drug therapy is reserved for only high-risk patients. These themes continued from the first report.

The ATP II report makes new recommendations in three important areas: cholesterol-lowering treatment in relation to CHD risk status, including age; HDL cholesterol; and an expanded approach to medical nutrition therapy[117] (see Table 11–8). The updated report recommends:

- more aggressive treatment of patients with CHD or other atherosclerotic diseases

- consideration of a person's age, as well as sex, in choosing therapy
- determination of HDL-cholesterol level, together with total cholesterol, as part of initial testing
- greater emphasis on physical activity and weight loss in combination with dietary therapy as the first line of treatment of high blood cholesterol
- delay of drug treatment in most young adult men and premenopausal women with high levels of LDL cholesterol but an otherwise low risk for CHD

The ATP II report lists the ages at which a patient's risk of CHD is strong enough to warrant more aggressive treatment. These ages are 45 years and older for men and 55 years and older for women. Women who have undergone premature menopause and receive no estrogen-replacement therapy would need more aggressive treatment at an earlier age.

Positive risk factors for CHD that were also identified in the ATP I report are family history of CHD at an early age, smoking cigarettes, hypertension, a low HDL cholesterol (below 35 mg/dL), and diabetes. A high HDL cholesterol (60 mg/dL or greater) is considered a "negative risk factor," because it lowers the risk for CHD.

The ATP II report stresses that the risk of CHD increases with age. The report recommends lowering high blood cholesterol among healthy elderly persons and postmenopausal women. Treatment would rely primarily on dietary therapy. The

Table 11–7 Blood Cholesterol Levels for Adults, NCEP Adult Treatment Panel II

Level	Category
<200 mg/dL (5.17 mmol/L)	Desirable blood cholesterol
200–239 mg/dL (5.17–6.18 mmol/L)	Borderline-high blood cholesterol
>240 mg/dL (6.21 mmol/L)	High blood cholesterol

Source: Data from Adult Treatment Panel, NIH, Second Report of the Expert Panel on Detection, Evaluation, and Treatment of High Blood Cholesterol in Adults, *Journal of the American Medical Association,* Vol. 269, American Medical Association, 1993.

Table 11–8 Cholesterol and Triglyceride Goals To Prevent and Treat Coronary Heart Disease

Group or Factor Risk	Triglyceride (mg/dL)	Cholesterol (mg/dL)	LDL (mg/dL)	HDL (mg/dL)
Children and young adults	<140	below 180	below 110	—
Adults 20–45	<140	below 200	below 120	—
Adults above 45 years	<140	below 220	below 130	—
Men	—	—	—	≥40
Women	—	—	—	≥50

Source: Reprinted from Adult Treatment Panel, NIH, Second Report of the Expert Panel on Detection, Evaluation, and Treatment of High Blood Cholesterol in Adults, *Journal of the American Medical Association,* Vol. 269, American Medical Association, 1993.

report recommends that drug therapy not be used with these patients unless CHD risk is high.

The ATP II report notes that clinical trials have not yet answered the question of whether lowering high blood cholesterol with drugs also reduces total mortality. Clinical trials have not been large enough to evaluate this question. Caution is recommended in the use of drug treatment in patients without CHD, except for high-risk patients. Reliance is placed on dietary therapy, until large clinical trials have provided an answer about total mortality.[117]

The report concludes that prevention and treatment of high blood cholesterol can be cost-effective if diet is used as the mainstay of therapy and drugs are reserved for high-risk patients. Prevention of CHD through lowering cholesterol could substantially reduce the country's annual cost from CHD in medical treatments and lost wages—a cost currently between $50 billion and $100 billion.

Additional NCEP Activities

Additional activities for NCEP include the following:

- to combine clinical and public health strategies to help reduce blood cholesterol levels among high-risk individuals and the general population
- to disseminate the NCEP reports and patient education brochures widely to more than 41 organizations representing a diverse group

of health professionals from the public and private sectors
- to encourage all health professionals to use the ATP II guidelines to identify and to target coronary patients and others at high risk of CHD for aggressive therapy. Many of these individuals are not receiving cholesterol-lowering treatment, and they will account for nearly half of all future heart attacks.[117]

LOWERING CHOLESTEROL LEVELS

Data from the third National Health and Nutrition Examination Survey (NHANES) show that the average blood cholesterol levels in the United States dropped significantly in the last 12 years.[118] There has been a substantial reduction in the proportion of adults with high blood cholesterol.

Between the NHANES II (1976–1980) and the first phase of the NHANES III (1988–1991), the average cholesterol level among adults ages 20 to 74 declined from 213 to 205 mg/dL (see Figure 11-6). Mean cholesterol levels decreased in men and women, in African Americans and whites, and in all age groups.

This significant 12-year drop in cholesterol levels is part of a trend that has occurred over the past 35 years. This drop has coincided with declining blood pressure levels and smoking rates and a 54% decrease in mortality from CHD.[118] Decreases in high blood cholesterol, smoking, and high blood pressure have made a major contribution to the decline in CHD deaths. Lifestyle improvements and better

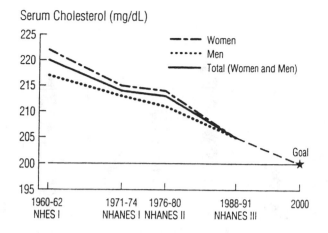

Figure 11-6 Trends in age-adjusted mean serum total cholesterol. *Source:* Data from CDC, NCHS, NHES I; NHANES I, NHANES II, NHANES III (Phase 1, 1988–91).

diagnosis and treatment of CHD have also contributed.

The decline in overall cholesterol levels occurred because of declining LDL levels. The mean LDL level dropped from 136 to 128 mg/dL. The decline in LDL levels may be due to changes in the consumption of saturated fat and dietary cholesterol, use of lipid-lowering drugs, hormone use, or changes in the prevalence of other factors such as obesity or physical activity. As the dietary intake and other data from the NHANES III become available, these issues will be examined further.[118]

The decline in average cholesterol levels is accompanied by a shift in distribution of cholesterol values among the entire population. The proportion of the population with high blood cholesterol levels, 240 mg/dL and above, dropped from 26% to 20% (see Figure 11-7). The proportion with borderline-high total cholesterol levels, 200 to 239 mg/dL, has not changed significantly (30% to 31%). There has been a substantial increase from 44% to 49% in the proportion of the population with desirable cholesterol levels below 200 mg/dL. There has also been a decline in the proportion of the population who need dietary therapy (36% to 29%).[118]

It appears that public health programs designed to reduce serum cholesterol levels are proving successful. Combined public health and

clinical strategies recommended by the NCEP and many cooperating organizations have made a substantial contribution to the decline in cholesterol levels as a whole and to the decline in the percentage of individuals with especially high levels.

The NCEP recommends two strategies for lowering the cholesterol levels of Americans. One is a clinical strategy, which detects and treats individuals at high risk of coronary heart disease. The second is a public health strategy, which attempts to shift the cholesterol levels of the entire population to a lower range through dietary changes.[117]

Applying the ATP II definitions of treatment to the NHANES III data, the percentage of adults over age 20 who would be candidates for dietary therapy is estimated to be 29% (Figure 11-8). This is a decline from 36% derived by the application of the ATP II definitions to the NHANES II.

Among the new recommendations of the ATP II guidelines is a greater emphasis on physical activity and weight loss in combination with medical nutrition therapy as the secondary prevention approach for high blood cholesterol. ATP II guidelines single out patients with existing CHD for especially aggressive therapy to lower their cholesterol levels. About 32% of men and 27% of women are candidates for dietary therapy. Of 52 million adults (29%) who would require di-

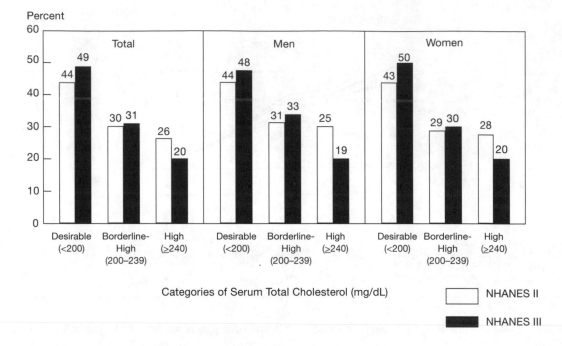

Figure 11-7 Percent distribution of serum total cholesterol values for US adults (20-74 years) by sex for NHANES II and NHANES III. *Source:* Data from NHANES II (1976-80), NHANES III (Phase 1, 1988-91).

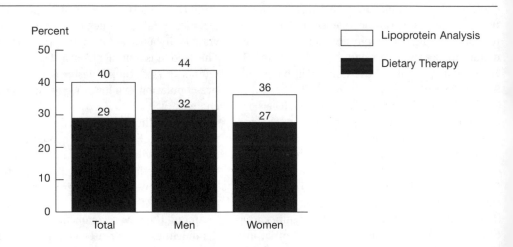

Figure 11-8 Percent of US adults who require lipoprotein analysis and dietary therapy. *Source:* Reprinted from NHLBI Data Fact Sheet and Declining Serum Cholesterol Levels Among U.S. Adults, *Journal of the American Medical Association,* Vol. 269, American Medical Association, 1993.

etary therapy, 11 million people already have CHD.[119]

The ATP II recommendations reserve drug therapy for patients at high risk for coronary heart disease and only after unsuccessful dietary therapy. In contrast to the 29% of adults who would require medical nutrition therapy, the analysis of the NHANES III data indicates that about 7% of all adults, or 12.7 million Americans, might require cholesterol-lowering drug treatment. Of those patients who are candidates for drug therapy, about 4 million would be patients with CHD.

The goal to reduce the mean serum cholesterol level of US adults to below 200 mg/dL—as stated in *Healthy People 2000: National Health Promotion and Disease Prevention Objectives*[119]—appears to be attainable. Another *Healthy People 2000* objective, to reduce the prevalence of high blood cholesterol to no more than 20% of adults, essentially has been achieved. However, 52 million US adults still need medical nutrition therapy as a secondary prevention for high blood cholesterol. There remains a huge challenge.[117]

Drug therapy remains a common treatment for hyperlipidemia. In patients with isolated LDL levels of ≥160 mg/dL in the presence of CHD or two or more CHD risk factors, drug therapy is recommended. LDL levels of ≥190 mg/dL, regardless of risk factors, also require drug therapy if an appropriate trial of medical nutrition therapy fails to bring results. The goal of therapy is to lower LDL to <130 mg/dL in high-risk individuals and to <160 mg/dL in other individuals.

Some clinicians have found that to lower LDL levels by more than 15%, medications must include one of the following: bile acid binding resins (cholestyramine and colestipol), nicotinic acid, and the HMG CoA reductase inhibitors (lovastatin, pravastatin, and simvastatin).[9] In asymptomatic patients over 45 years of age, resins may be preferred. If the individual is unwilling or unable to take resins, or target values are not achieved, then nicotinic acid could be used. If the individual is unwilling or unable to take nicotinic acid or target values are not achieved, then an HMG CoA reductase inhibitor can be used. Combinations of resins and nicotinic acid, or resins and an HMG CoA reductase inhibitor,

are also very effective if target values cannot be achieved with a single agent. In individuals with established heart disease, an HMG CoA reductase inhibitor is the drug of choice because of compliance issues.

For individuals with combined elevations of LDL and triglyceride, nicotinic acid is preferred. If nicotinic acid is contraindicated, or the individual is unwilling or unable to take this agent, or target values are not achieved, then an HMG CoA reductase inhibitor can be used. Combinations of bile acid binding resin and nicotinic acid, resin and gemfibrozil, or resin and an HMG CoA reductase inhibitor can also be used. If heart disease is diagnosed, then an HMG CoA reductase inhibitor is preferred and compliance is usually good.

Individuals with severe hypertriglyceridemia (greater than 1,000 mg/dL) are treated with diet, exercise, and weight reduction. If diabetes is present, glucose control is important. If triglyceride levels remain greater than 1,000 mg/dL, then gemfibrozil can be prescribed to lower triglyceride levels to less than 500 mg/dL and to reduce the risk of recurrent pancreatitis. Other medications that can be used include fish-oil capsules and, in nondiabetic participants, nicotinic acid.

Drug therapy is not recommended for the treatment of HDL deficiency, moderate hypertriglyceridemia in combination with HDL deficiency, or hypertriglyceridemia alone. Modifying lifestyle, as previously mentioned, and attempting to correct secondary causes are important. While prospective studies support the view that raising HDL cholesterol levels is beneficial in reducing CHD, no prospective primary or secondary trial has been conducted with individuals who have HDL deficiency.[8-10] Individuals with coronary artery disease (CAD) frequently have decreased HDL cholesterol levels.[111] For isolated hypertriglyceridemia, even less information is available. Elevated triglyceride levels have not been clearly shown to be a risk factor for CAD, nor has lowering triglyceride levels clearly been shown to reduce CAD risk.

For individuals with established CHD, efforts should be made to optimize the lipid profile, specifically to lower LDL levels to below 100 mg/

dL, lower triglyceride levels to below 200 mg/dL, and increase HDL levels to above 40 mg/dL. These goals are often difficult to achieve without combination drug therapy. Medications that can be used include HMG CoA reductase inhibitors, gemfibrozil, or nicotinic acid. The combinations of nicotinic acid and resins, HMG CoA reductase inhibitors and resins, or gemfibrozil and resins, can be used. Some combinations are not well tolerated. The combination of HMG CoA reductase inhibitor and gemfibrozil is currently not recommended because of the potential for myositis. For individuals without CHD but with two or more CHD risk factors, especially when decreased HDL levels are present, the goal is to lower LDL levels to below 130 mg/dL, to raise HDL levels to above 40 mg/dL, and to keep triglyceride levels below 200 mg/dL, using both medical nutrition and drug therapy. For other patients, efforts should be made to keep the LDL level below 160 mg/dL with medical nutrition therapy and, if necessary, with the addition of pharmacologic therapy.[113]

Results from the 12-year follow up of 316,099 men who were 35 to 57 years of age when screened for participation in the Multiple Risk Factor Intervention Trial give detailed and precise determination of associations of serum cholesterol, blood pressure, and cigarette smoking to risk of death from CHD.[120] A strong incremental association with coronary death was observed for serum total cholesterol at levels above 180 mg/dL. At high levels, a 10 mg/dL lower level of serum cholesterol was associated with 10% lower risk of coronary death. Strong incremental associations with coronary death were observed for cigarette smoking, systolic blood pressure at levels above 110 mm Hg, and diastolic pressure at levels above 70 mm Hg. The age-adjusted coronary death rate for a nonsmoker with systolic blood pressure below 118 mm Hg and serum cholesterol below 182 mg/dL was 3.1 deaths per 10,000 person-years. In contrast, the corresponding rate for a smoker with systolic blood pressure of at least 142 mm Hg and serum cholesterol of at least 245 mg/dL was 20 times higher or 62.6 deaths per 10,000 person-years. These results support the inference that the great majority of coronary deaths in middle-aged men could be prevented if cigarette smoking were eliminated and if blood pressure and serum cholesterol were maintained at optimal levels by hygienic means from youth through adulthood.

PREVENTION OF CHD

Can a lifelong low-fat eating pattern exert beneficial effects on CHD rates beyond an influence on blood cholesterol? New approaches to cholesterol reduction are needed, and a few are outlined below.

Worksite Intervention

In Ohio, 80 upper-management male employees participated in a company-sponsored, comprehensive physical exam. The 70 participants who had a triglyceride level above 5.17 mmol/L, (mg% cholesterol) were invited to participate in a nutrition education program. The study was nonrandomized, with 33 men in the intervention and 37 in the control group. All participants completed three-day dietary records before and after the nutrition education program. The intervention included a year-long program of individualized instruction, group sessions, and telephone follow up. Participants in the intervention group decreased their intakes of energy, cholesterol, and percentage of energy from total fat and protein. Carbohydrate and dietary fiber intakes increased. Significant decreases in plasma total cholesterol (from 6.15 ± 0.17 mmol/L to 5.43 ± 0.16 mmol/L), triglycerides (from 1.68 ± 0.87 mmol/L to 1.49 ± 0.67 mmol/L), body weight (from 86 ± 2.3 kg to 81 ± 1.6 kg), and body fat (from 24% ± 3.5% to 21% ± 3.5%) were observed for the intervention group. This worksite intervention suggests that primary prevention programs can decrease risk factors associated with coronary heart disease.[121]

Parent-Child Tutorial Program

During a nutrition education intervention pilot study, 44 children from 4 to 10 years of age were identified as having plasma LDL cholesterol levels between the 90th and 99th percentiles. They were randomized to either a parent-child tutorial program or a usual-care setting. The tutorial program was home-based and included a picture book and an audiotaped story complemented by activities and a guide for parents. Knowledge of health-promoting foods, food records, and biochemical measures were obtained at baseline, three-month, and six-month observation points. At the six-month follow up, significant increases in knowledge were reported, cholesterol intake increased for the control children but decreased for the treatment children, and both groups experienced a 10% decline in the average LDL cholesterol levels.[122]

Lifestyle Heart Trial

The Lifestyle Heart Trial was conducted in San Francisco with 41 middle-aged men randomized to either an 8% fat, vegetarian eating regimen or a control group. Stress management, moderate aerobic exercise, and smoking cessation were included in the experimental arm. Annual coronary angiograms demonstrated regression of coronary lesions in the experimental group and progression among the controls. Changes in total cholesterol and LDL cholesterol levels from baseline to one year for treatment and control groups were: experimental— 225 to 171 mg/dL total cholesterol and 151 to 95 mg/dL LDL; control— 244 to 231 mg/dL total cholesterol and 167 to 157 LDL.[123]

Garlic Consumption

Several alternative therapies have emerged in the CHD prevention arena. One approach has been the use of garlic for reducing total serum cholesterol when it is above 200 mg/dL. When combining data from five studies, a statistically significant treatment effect was noted. The mean difference in cholesterol change for the treatment compared to the placebo group was a decrease of 23 mg/dL. It appears that individuals with a total serum cholesterol over 200 mg/dL can lower their blood cholesterol by 9% by consuming one-half to one clove of garlic per day for four to six months.[124]

Modified Eating Behavior

Research on the role of dietary factors in the etiology of CHD has prompted the American Heart Association, the National Cholesterol Education Program, and others to recommend changes from the current American diet to a diet lower in saturated fats and cholesterol. Changing people's eating habits, however, is not an easy task and involves more than making dietary prescriptions. Inducing a person to change eating behavior is not simply determined by "what is good for him or her," but affected by a variety of psychological factors.[125]

It has been suggested that lowering plasma cholesterol by either dietary change or medication may result in elevated levels of depression and/or aggressive hostility, one component of Type A behavior.[126] Accordingly, depression could increase the likelihood for suicide, and aggressive hostility could elevate the risk of dying from other violent episodes. If this hypothesis is correct, one should expect increases in depression and aggressive hostility among those who change their diet to reduce plasma cholesterol levels.

Contrary to the above hypothesis, data gathered from the Family Heart Study indicate that those who improved their diet and reduced their plasma cholesterol levels showed reductions in depression and aggressive hostility[125] (see Table 11–9). These results are consistent with predictions derived from the psychological theory of self-efficacy.[127]

Intervention studies have verified the importance of modified eating behavior in reducing coronary risk. Interventions to reduce coronary risk may be most beneficial for Type A, coronary-prone individuals, especially after they are convinced that their own behavior can influence their health status. Participation in cholesterol-lowering programs is not associated with reduced psychological well-being. Improvements in diet appear to be associated with reductions in depression and aggressive hostility, as well as with lowered plasma cholesterol levels. Overall, psycho-

Table 11–9 Diet and Depression, Hostility, and Plasma Cholesterol Levels

Variable	Typical American Diet (N = 140)			Low-Fat, High Complex Carbohydrate Diet (N = 165)			P Value
	Mean	SE	95% CI	Mean	SE	95% CI	
Depression*	-1.1	1.2	(-3.4 to 1.2)	-4.0	0.9	(-5.8 to -2.2)	0.04
Hostility*	-0.9	1.1	(-3.1 to 1.3)	-4.2	0.9	(-6.0 to -2.4)	0.03
Plasma cholesterol	+1.7	0.9	(0.0 to 3.5)	-1.0	0.8	(-2.6 to 0.6)	0.02

Notes:
*A negative score reflects improvement.
SE = standard error; CI = confidence internal

Source: Adapted from Weidner G, Connor SL, Hollis JF, Connor WE. Improvements in Hostility and Depression in Relation to Dietary Change and Cholesterol-Lowering: The Family Heart Study. *Annals of Internal Medicine.* 1992;117:820–823.

logical factors are powerful predictors of health outcomes and appear to be influenced by health behaviors.

THE EFFECTS OF SERUM TOTAL CHOLESTEROL REDUCTION ON MORTALITY FROM NONCARDIOVASCULAR CAUSES

At a time when high serum total cholesterol has been shown to have a positive association with cardiovascular disease, cancer, and all-cause mortality, some researchers have questioned lowering serum cholesterol.[128-131] Some data suggest that a low serum cholesterol may increase mortality from noncardiovascular causes.

The Multiple Risk Factor Intervention Trial (MRFIT) observed an excess number of deaths among men with low serum cholesterol levels.[132] Of men with a serum total cholesterol below 160 mg/dL, 6% had a higher death rate from lung cancer, suicide, chronic obstructive lung disease, hepatic cirrhosis, alcohol dependence, liver cancer, lymphatic and hematopoietic cancers, or hypertension-induced intracerebral hemorrhage.[120] Of consideration is whether these diseases contributed to a lowered serum total cholesterol, rather than the low cholesterol inducing the diseases and mortality. Community-based intervention studies—such as MRFIT, the Oslo, and World Health Organization and European Collaborative trials—used strategies to change eating behavior

and reported fewer CHD events and lower CHD mortality and all-cause mortality.[120,133,134]

Can Eating Pattern Influence Risk of All-Cause Mortality?

The preferred eating pattern is one which contains a wide variety of foods. Kant and colleagues[118] analyzed the relation between dietary variety and all-cause mortality using the NHANES I Epidemiologic Follow-Up Study, 1982 to 1987 database. The study sample included 4,160 men and 6,264 women between 25 to 74 years of age at baseline in 1971 to 1975. Total intake of five major food groups was assessed by assigning the presence of the food group in a 24-hour recall a score of 1 and following with an additional 1 for each of the different five food groups consumed.[118]

The results showed that 25% of the participants had a food group score of less than 4; about 5% had a score below 3. Fruit, dairy, and vegetable groups were the food groups most frequently missed by the study participants. More men than women had a lower score. Income and education both had a positive association with the score. For women, body mass index was inversely associated with the score. Compared with women, men who smoked had lower scores.

For both men and women, there was an inverse association between the age-adjusted risk of all-cause mortality and the food group score. When potential confounders were controlled, the relative risk for men consuming two or fewer food groups was 1.5; the relative risk for women was 1.4.[118] This data analysis suggests that a food group analysis can be linked with total mortality and, specifically, lack of variety accompanies increased risk of death.

Several concerns have been raised about these data. First, use of one 24-hour food record limits the representativeness of individual intake. The large sample size might minimize this effect. Second, accuracy of the amount of food reported as eaten and the consistent assignment of what constitutes a serving in any one of the five food groups is assumed, but not known. Third, changes in eating behaviors for health promotion in the general population between 1971 and 1975 were probably much less than the changes individuals made in the 1980s. The extent of dietary behavioral change in this cohort during the latency period was not known. Fourth, it is not known whether an improvement in food quality (i.e., eating patterns that have balance, variety, or moderation) can lower all-cause mortality including CHD deaths.

THE CURRENT CHALLENGE

Powerful medical nutrition and drug therapies are now available to achieve both intensive plasma lipid lowering and an antithrombotic effect. Both are important for the management of every individual at risk or with overt CHD. Not only is an improved understanding of the atherosclerotic process needed, but also it is necessary to understand the role of healthy eating on longer life among low- versus high-risk individuals. The Lipid Research Clinic Trial demonstrated that, for every 1% lowering of the plasma cholesterol concentration, there was a 2% reduction in CHD events. The challenge continues to be to implement therapies to lower plasma cholesterol level in the US population.

NCEP RECOMMENDATIONS FOR HEALTH PARTNERS

The National Cholesterol Education Program endorses the following recommendations:

- Health professionals should both practice and advocate recommended eating patterns. They should ensure that education of future health professionals includes appropriate nutrition education. Health professionals should work with industry, government, voluntary groups, and health care agencies to facilitate adoption of the recommended eating patterns.[1]

- The food industry, food and animal scientists, and food technologists should increase efforts to design, modify, prepare, promote, label, and distribute good-tasting, safe foods that are lower in saturated fatty acids, total fat, and cholesterol.

- Government agencies should provide consistent, coordinated nutrition statements and policies emphasizing low-saturated fatty acid, low-fat, and low-cholesterol eating patterns; expand and standardize food labeling requirements to identify clearly the content of saturated fatty acids, total fat, cholesterol, and total calories; and take other steps to improve the consumer comprehension necessary to achieve the recommended eating patterns.

- Education at all levels should incorporate curricula that emphasize the background, benefits, and methods of achieving eating patterns that are lower in saturated fatty acids, total fat, and cholesterol. This recommendation includes elementary through high schools, vocational programs (especially in culinary arts), colleges, universities, and health professional schools.

- Measurement of blood cholesterol, followed by appropriate education and counseling, is best initiated in the health care setting; but in specific circumstances and especially for selected segments of hard-to-reach population groups, public screening for blood cholesterol, when carried out with high-quality standards, is appropriate.

- Research and surveillance must be ongoing to develop new information concerning diet, blood lipids, and CHD; the development of better databases concerning food composition, food consumption patterns, illness rates, food product development, and nutrition education and communication is critical.

Info Line

The American Heart Association is a national voluntary health organization whose mission is to reduce death and disability from cardiovascular disease and stroke. Affiliates are organized by city and county throughout the United States. Professional subunits focus on cardiovascular education and research topics (e.g., epidemiology, high blood pressure, and arteriosclerosis). The national office is located at 7272 Greenville Avenue, Dallas, Texas 75231-4596.

Implementation of these recommendations will promote adoption of eating patterns that will help most Americans lower their levels of blood cholesterol and their risk of CHD.

DIETARY FAT AND CHOLESTEROL ASSESSMENT INSTRUMENTS

Several dietary fat and cholesterol assessment instruments are available. A few are described below:

- Fat/Cholesterol Avoidance Scale—a seven-item, self-administered scale allows individuals to report their food selection and preparation practices. Scores can be used to assess and/or group individuals into those with heart-healthy versus unhealthy eating.[135,136]

- A Cholesterol-Saturated Fat Index (CSI)—calculated as follows:

$$CSI = (1.01 \times g \text{ saturated fat}) + (0.05 \times mg \text{ cholesterol})$$

A low CSI indicates low saturated fat and/or cholesterol content or hypocholesterolemic and low atherogenic potential, respectively. For example, a typical 2,000 kcal American eating pattern with 40% fat, 14% or 31 g saturated fat, and 400 mg cholesterol, has a CSI of 51.[137]

- The Block Fat Screen—a self-administered frequency tool that requires about four minutes. Foods are based on a medium portion and reflect high fat content. An average fat intake can be calculated to group individuals into low- or high-fat consumers.[138]

- The New American Eating Pattern—an approach to eating that involves a gradual modification of current habits through careful, programmed changes in high-fat, high-cholesterol, low-complex carbohydrate, and high-salt diet. The program is people-friendly and based on beneficial experiences of 233 families. Changes in eating pattern are directed by three phases and self-assessment to gauge achievement of goals.[139]

- The Eating Pattern Assessment Tool—a self-administered instrument divided into two sections (one that assesses intake of food characterized by high fat and cholesterol and another that contains lower-fat food groupings as an alternate). The instrument is designed to assess overall fat and cholesterol intake and the frequency of such intakes and to educate about fat-containing foods with educational messages.[140]

HEALTHY PEOPLE 2000 ACTIONS

Reducing dietary fat, increasing complex carbohydrate and fiber-containing foods, lowering obesity, and monitoring blood cholesterol levels are the focus of HP2K objectives to lower CHD deaths. Community nutrition professionals can integrate numerous community-based and high-risk approaches into their programs to address the number one cause of death in the United States[141] (see Exhibits 11–1 and 11–2).

Exhibit 11-1 *Healthy People 2000* Health Status Objectives Targeting Coronary Heart Disease

---

2.1   Reduce coronary heart disease deaths to no more than 100 per 100,000 people. (Age-adjusted baseline:
and 15.1 135 per 100,000 in 1987.)

Special Population Target

Coronary Deaths (per 100,000)	1987 Baseline	2000 Target
2.1a Blacks	163	115
and 15.1a		

2.5   Reduce dietary fat intake to an average of 30% of calories or less and average saturated fat intake to <10%
          of calories among people aged 2 and older. (Baseline: 36% of calories from total fat and 13% from saturated
          fat for people aged 20 through 74 in 1976–80; 36% and 13% for women aged 19 through 50 in 1985.)

2.6   Increase complex carbohydrate and fiber-containing foods in the diets of adults to 5+ daily servings for
          vegetables (including legumes) and fruits, and to 6 or more daily servings for grain products. (Baseline: 2½
          servings of vegetables and fruits and 3 servings of grain products for women aged 19 through 50 in 1985.)

2.7   Increase to at least 50% the proportion of overweight people aged 12 and older who have adopted sound
          dietary practices combined with regular physical activity to attain an appropriate body weight. (Baseline:
          30% of overweight women and 25% of overweight men for people aged 18 and older in 1985.)

15.6   Reduce the mean serum cholesterol level among adults to no more than 200 mg/dL. (Baseline: 213 mg/dL
          among people aged 20 through 74 in 1976–80, 211 mg/dL for men and 215 mg/dL for women.)

15.7   Reduce the prevalence of blood cholesterol levels of 240 mg/dL or greater to no more than 20% among
          adults. (Baseline: 27% for people aged 20 through 74 in 1976–80, 29% for women and 25% for men.)

15.8   Increase to at least 60% the proportion of adults with high blood cholesterol who are aware of their
          condition and are taking action to reduce their blood cholesterol to recommended levels. (Baseline: 11% of
          all people aged 18 and older, and thus an estimated 30% of people with high blood cholesterol, were aware
          that their blood cholesterol level was high in 1988.)

15.9   Reduce dietary fat intake to an average of 30% of calories or less and average saturated fat intake to less
          than 10% of calories among people age 2 and older. (Baseline: 36% of calories from total fat and 13% from
          saturated fat for people aged 20 through 74 in 1976–80; 36% and 13% for women aged 19 through 50 in
          1985.)

Source: Reprinted from *Healthy People 2000: National Health Promotion and Disease Prevention Objectives,* U.S. Department of
Health and Human Services, Public Health Service, Publication No. 91-50212, 1991.

Exhibit 11-2 Model Nutrition Objective for Reduced Risk Reduction

---

By 19___, the chronic disease risk factor ___*___ among (target population) will be reduced from _____% to
_____ %.

*Obesity; hypertension; elevated serum cholesterol; poor physical fitness; excess intake of dietary fat, cholesterol, sodium, alcohol,
and sugar; inadequate intake of dietary fiber, fruits and vegetables, and calcium.

Source: Adapted from *Model State Nutrition Objectives,* The Association of State and Territorial Public Health Nutrition Directors,
1988.

REFERENCES

1. National Cholesterol Education Program. *Report of the Expert Panel on Population Strategies for Blood Cholesterol Reduction.* Bethesda, Md: US Department of Health and Human Services; 1990. NIH publication 90-3046.

2. Connor WE. Hypolipidemic effects of dietary omega-3 fatty acids in normal and hyperlipidemic humans: Effects and mechanisms. In: Simopoulos A, Kifer RR, Martin RE, eds. *Health Effects of Polyunsaturated Fatty Acids in Seafoods.* New York, NY: Academic Press; 1986:173-210.

3. Keys A. Coronary heart disease in seven countries. *Circulation.* 1970;41:1.

4. McGee D, Reed D, Yano K, et al. Ten-year incidence of coronary heart disease in the Honolulu Heart Program: Relationship to nutrient intake. *Am J Epidemiol.* 1984;119:667-676.

5. Kris-Etherton PM, Krummel D, Russel ME, et al. The effect of diet on plasma, lipids, lipoproteins, and coronary heart disease. *J Am Diet Assoc.* 1988;88:1373.

6. The Nutrition Committee, American Heart Association. Dietary guidelines for healthy American adults. *Circulation.* 1988;77:721A.

7. National Cholesterol Education Program. Report of the National Cholesterol Education Program Expert Panel on detection, evaluation and treatment of high blood cholesterol in adults. *Arch Intern Med.* 1988;148:36.

8. National Research Council. *Designing Foods: Animal Product Options in the Market Place.* Washington, DC: National Academy Press; 1988.

9. Castelli WP, Garrison RJ, Wilson PWF, et al. Incidence of coronary heart disease and lipoprotein cholesterol levels: The Framingham Study. *JAMA.* 1986;256:2835.

10. Samuel P, McNamara DJ, Shapiro J. The role of diet in the etiology and treatment of atherosclerosis. *Ann Rev Med.* 1983;34:179.

11. Grundy SM. Comparison of monounsaturated fatty acids and carbohydrates for lowering plasma cholesterol. *N Engl J Med.* 1986;314:745.

12. Mensink RP, Katan MB. Effect of monounsaturated fatty acids versus complex carbohydrates on high density lipoproteins in healthy men and women. *Lancet.* 1987;1:122.

13. Weisweiler P, Janetschek P, Schwandt P. Influence of polyunsaturated fats and fat restriction on serum lipoproteins in humans. *Metabolism.* 1985;34:83.

14. Schwandt P, Janetschek P, Weisweiler P. High density lipoproteins unaffected by dietary fat modification. *Atherosclerosis.* 1982;44:9.

15. Keys A, Anderson JT, Grande F. Serum cholesterol response to changes in the diet. IV. Particular saturated fatty acids in the diet. *Metabolism.* 1965;14:776.

16. Hegsted DM, McGandy RB, Meyers ML, et al. Quantitative effects of dietary fat on serum cholesterol in man. *Am J Clin Nutr.* 1965;17:281.

17. Bronsgeest-Schoute DC, Hautvast JGAJ, Hermus RJJ. Dependence of the effects of dietary cholesterol and experimental conditions on serum lipids in man. *Am J Clin Nutr.* 1979;32:2183.

18. Anderson JT, Grande F, Keys A. Cholesterol-lowering diets. *J Am Diet Assoc.* 1973;62:133.

19. Connor WE, Witiak DT, Stone DB, et al. Cholesterol balance and fecal neutral steroid and bile acid excretion in normal men fed dietary fats of different fatty acid composition. *J Clin Invest.* 1969;48:1363-1375.

20. Grande F, Anderson JT, Keys A. Comparison of effects of palmitic and stearic acids in the diet on serum cholesterol in man. *Am J Clin Nutr.* 1970;23:1184.

21. Bonanome A, Grundy SM. Effect of dietary stearic acid on plasma cholesterol and lipoprotein levels. *N Engl J Med.* 1988;318:1244.

22. Snook JT, DeLany JP, Vivian VM. Effect of moderate to very low fat defined formula diets on serum lipids in healthy subjects. *Lipids.* 1985;20:808.

23. Grundy SM, Nix D, Whelan MF, et al. Comparison of three cholesterol-lowering diets in normolipemic men. *JAMA.* 1986;256:2351.

24. Kuusi T, Ehnholm C, Huttunen J, et al. Concentration and composition of serum lipoproteins during a low-fat diet at two levels of polyunsaturated fat. *J Lipid Res.* 1985;26:360.

25. Weisweiler P, Drosner M, Janetschek P, et al. Changes in very low and low density lipoproteins with dietary fat modifications. *Atherosclerosis.* 1983;49:325.

26. Hodgson JM, Wahlquist MR, Boxall JA, et al. Can linoleic acid contribute to coronary artery disease? *Am J Clin Nutr.* 1993;58:228-234.

27. Logan RL, Thomson M, Riemersma RA, et al. Risk factors for ischaemic heart-disease in normal men aged 40– Edinburgh-Stockholm Study. *Lancet.* 1978;1:949-954.

28. Riemersma RA, Wood DA, Butler S, et al. Linoleic acid content in adipose tissue and coronary heart disease. *Br Med J.* 1986;292:1423-1427.

29. Wood DA, Riemersma RA, Butler S, et al. Adipose tissue and platelet fatty acids and coronary heart disease in Scottish men. *Lancet.* 1984;2:117-121.

30. Wood DA, Riemersma RA, Butler S. Linoleic and eicosapentaenoic acids in adipose tissue and platelets and risk of coronary heart disease. *Lancet.* 1987;1:177-183.

31. Blankenhorn DH, Johnson RL, Mack WJ. The influence of diet on the appearance of new lesions in human coronary arteries. *JAMA.* 1990;263:1646-1652.

32. National Dairy Council. Nutrition and health effects of unsaturated fatty acids. *Dairy Council Dig.* 1988;59:1.

33. Dyerberg J. Linolenate-derived polyunsaturated fatty acids and prevention of atherosclerosis. *Nutr Rev.* 1986;44:125.

34. Bang HO, Dyerberg J, Hjorne N. The composition of food consumed by Greenland Eskimos. *Acta Med Scand.* 1976;200:69.

35. Herold PM, Kinsella JE. Fish oil consumption and decreased risk of cardiovascular disease: A comparison of findings from animal and human feeding trials. *Am J Clin Nutr.* 1986;43:566.

36. Simons LA, Hichie JB, Balasubramaniam S. On the effects of dietary omega-3 fatty acids (MaxEPA) on plasma lipids and lipoproteins in patients with hyperlipidemia. *Atherosclerosis.* 1985;54:75.

37. Nestel PJ. Fish oil attenuates the cholesterol induced rise in lipoprotein cholesterol. *Am J Clin Nutr.* 1986;43:752.

38. Leaf A, Weber PC. Cardiovascular effects of omega-3 fatty acids. *N Engl J Med.* 1988;318:549.

39. Saynor R, Verel D, Gillott T. The long-term effect of dietary supplementation with fish lipid concentrate on serum lipids, bleeding time, platelets and angina. *Atherosclerosis.* 1984;50:3.

40. Omega-3 fatty acids: Eat fish, or fish oils? *CNI Weekly.* 1987;17:6.

41. Simopoulos AP, Salem N. Purslane: A terrestrial source of omega-3 fatty acids. *N Engl J Med.* 1986;315:833.

42. Mattson FH, Grundy SM. Comparison of effects of dietary saturated, monounsaturated, and polyunsaturated fatty acids on plasma lipids and lipoproteins in man. *J Lipid Res.* 1985;26:194.

43. Grundy SM, Bonanome A. Workshop on monounsaturated fatty acids. *Arteriosclerosis.* 1987;7:644.

44. Baggio G, Pagan A, Muraca M, et al. Olive oil-enriched diet: Effect on serum lipoprotein levels and biliary cholesterol saturation. *Am J Clin Nutr.* 1988;47:960.

45. Nichaman MZ, Hamm P. Low-fat, high-carbohydrate diets and plasma cholesterol. *Am J Clin Nutr.* 1987;45:1155.

46. Gordon T, Kagan A, Garcia-Palmieri M, et al. Diet and its relation to coronary heart disease and death in three populations. *Circulation.* 1981;63:500.

47. Dreon DM, Frey-Hewitt B, Ellsworth N, et al. Dietary fat: Carbohydrate ratio and obesity in middle-aged men. *Am J Clin Nutr.* 1988;47:995.

48. Acheson KJ, Flatt JP, Jequier E. Glycogen synthesis versus lipogenesis after a 500 g carbohydrate meal in man. *Metabolism.* 1982;31:1234.

49. Lissner L, Levitsky DA, Stupp BJ, et al. Dietary fat and the regulation of energy intake in human subjects. *Am J Clin Nutr.* 1987;46:886.

50. Grundy SM, Barrett-Connor E, Rudel LL, et al. Workshop on the impact of dietary cholesterol on plasma lipoproteins and atherogenesis. *Arteriosclerosis.* 1988;8:95.

51. Connor WE, Cerqueira MT, Connor R, et al. The plasma lipids, lipoproteins, and diet of the Tarahumara Indians of Mexico. *Am J Clin Nutr.* 1978;31:1131.

52. *The Framingham Study—An Epidemiological Investigation of Cardiovascular Diseases. Sec. 24. The Framingham Diet Study.* Washington, DC: US Department of Health, Education and Welfare; 1970.

53. Gordon T, Fisher M, Ernst N, et al. Relation of diet to LDL cholesterol, VLDL cholesterol, and plasma total cholesterol and triglycerides in white adults: The Lipid Research Clinics Prevalence Study. *Arteriosclerosis.* 1982;2:502.

54. Shekelle RB, Shryock AM, Paul O. Diet, serum cholesterol, and death from coronary heart disease: The Western Electric Study. *N Engl J Med.* 1981;304:65.

55. Gordon DJ, Salz KM, Roggenkamp KJ, et al. Dietary determinants of plasma cholesterol change in the recruitment phase of the Lipid Research Clinics Coronary Primary Prevention Trial. *Arteriosclerosis.* 1982;2:537.

56. Shekelle R, Stamler J. Dietary cholesterol and risk of death in middle-aged men. *CVD Newsletter.* 1988;43:168. Abstract.

57. Hegsted DM, Nicolosi RJ. Individual variation in serum cholesterol levels. *Proc Natl Acad Sci USA.* 1987;84:6259.

58. Jacobs DR, Anderson JT, Hannan P, et al. Variability in individual serum cholesterol response to change in diet. *Arteriosclerosis.* 1983;3:349.

59. Katan MB, Beynen AC, De Vries JHM. Existence of constant hypo- and hyper-responders to dietary cholesterol in man. *Am J Epidemiol.* 1986;123:221.

60. Food and Nutrition Science Alliance: The American Dietetic Association (ADA), American Institute of Nutrition (AIN), The American Society for Clinical Nutrition, Inc. (ASCN), Institute of Food Technologists (IFT). *Statement on Trans Fatty Acids.* Chicago, Ill: Food and Nutrition Science Alliance; 1994.

61. Willett WC, Stampfer MJ, Manson JE, et al. Intake of trans fatty acids and risk of coronary heart disease among women. *Lancet.* 1993;341:581–585.

62. Keys A, Fidanza F, Scardi V, et al. Studies on serum cholesterol and other characteristics of clinically healthy men in Naples. *Arch Intern Med.* 1954;93:328.

63. Keys A, Kimura N, Bronte-Stewart B, et al. Lessons from serum cholesterol studies in Japan, Hawaii, and Los Angeles. *Ann Intern Med.* 1958;48:83.

64. Hallfrisch J, West S, Fisher C, et al. Modification of the United States' diet to effect changes in blood lipids and lipoprotein distribution. *Atherosclerosis.* 1985;57:179.

65. Glinsmann WH, Irausquin H, Park YK. Evaluation of health aspects of sugar contained in carbohydrate sweeteners. Report of Sugars Task Force, 1986. *J Nutr.* 1986;116(Suppl):55.

66. Floch MH, Maryniuk MD, Bryant C, et al. Practical aspects of implementing increased dietary fiber intake. *Nutr Today*. 1986;21:27.

67. Morris JN, Marr JW, Clayton DG. Diet and heart: A postscript. *Br Med J*. 1977;2:1307–1314.

68. Kromhout D, Bosschieter EB, DeLezenne Coulander C. Dietary fibre and 10-year mortality from coronary heart disease, cancer, and all causes. The Zutphen Study. *Lancet*. 1982;1:518.

69. Jenkins DJA, Reynolds D, Leeds AR, et al. Hypocholesterolemic action of dietary fiber unrelated to fecal bulking effect. *Am J Clin Nutr*. 1979;32:2430.

70. Miettinen TA, Tarpila S. Effects of pectin on serum cholesterol, fecal bile acids, and bilary lipids in normolipidemic and hyperlipidemic individuals. *Clin Chim Acta*. 1977;70:471.

71. Jenkins DJA, Reynolds D, Slavin B, et al. Dietary fiber and blood lipids: Treatment of hypercholesterolemia with guar crisp bread. *Am J Clin Nutr*. 1980;33:575.

72. Anderson JW, Zettwoch N, Feldman T, et al. Cholesterol-lowering effects of psyllium hydrophilic mucilloid for hypercholesterolemic men. *Arch Intern Med*. 1988;148:292.

73. Van Horn LV, Liu K, Parker D, et al. Serum lipid response to oat product intake with a fat-modified diet. *J Am Diet Assoc*. 1986;86:759.

74. Anderson JW, Story L, Sieling B, et al. Hypocholesterolemic effects of oat-bran or bran intake for hypercholesterolemic men. *Am J Clin Nutr*. 1984;40:1146.

75. Truswell AS. Effects of different types of dietary fiber on plasma lipids. In Heaton KW, ed. *Dietary Fiber: Current Developments of Importance to Health*. London, England: Libbey and Co; 1978.

76. Stasse-Wolthuis M, Albers HFF, Van Jeveren JGC, et al. Influence of dietary fiber from vegetables and fruits, bran or citrus pectin on serum lipids, fecal lipids and caloric function. *Am J Clin Nutr*. 1980;33:1745.

77. Anderson JW, Chen WL. Plant fiber, carbohydrate and lipid metabolism. *Am J Clin Nutr*. 1979;32:346.

78. Sprecher DL, Harris BV, Goldberg AC, et al. Efficacy of psyllium in reducing serum cholesterol levels in hypercholesterolemic patients on high or low-fat diets. *Ann Intern Med*. 1993;119:545–554.

79. Van Raaij JM, Katan MB, Hautvast JG, et al. Effects of casein versus soy protein diets on serum cholesterol and lipoproteins in young healthy volunteers. *Am J Clin Nutr*. 1981;34:1261.

80. Carroll KK, Giovannetti PM, Huff MW, et al. Hypocholesterolemic effect of substituting soybean protein for animal protein in the diet of healthy young women. *Am J Clin Nutr*. 1978;31:1312.

81. Sacks FM, Breslow JL, Wood PG, et al. Lack of an effect of dairy protein (casein) and soy protein on plasma cholesterol of strict vegetarians: An experiment and a critical review. *J Lipid Res*. 1983;24:1012.

82. Carroll KK. Hypercholesterolemia and atherosclerosis: Effects of dietary protein. *Fed Proc*. 1982;41:2792.

83. Langseth L. Is high iron status a risk for heart disease? *Food and Nutr News*. 1994;66(3):17–19.

84. Steinberg D, Parthasarthy S, Carew TE, et al. Beyond cholesterol: Modifications of low-density lipoprotein that increase its atherogenicity. *N Engl J Med*. 1989;320:915–924.

85. Luc G, Fruchart JC. Oxidation of lipoproteins and atherosclerosis. *Am J Clin Nutr*. 1991;53:206S–209S.

86. Goldhaber JI, Weiss JN. Oxygen free radicals and cardiac reperfusion abnormalities. *Hypertension*. 1992;20:118–127.

87. Salonen JT, Nyyssonen K, Korpela H, et al. High stored iron levels are associated with excess risk of myocardial infarction in eastern Finnish men. *Circulation*. 1992;86:803–811.

88. Lauffer RB. Iron stores and the international variation in mortality from coronary artery disease. *Med Hypothesis*. 1991;35:96–102.

89. Rimm EB, Ascherio A, Stampfer MJ, et al. Dietary iron intake and risk of coronary disease among men. *Circulation*. 1993;87:692.

90. Stampfer MJ, Grodstein F, Rosenberg I, et al. A prospective study of plasma ferritin and risk of myocardial infarction in US physicians. *Circulation*. 1993;87:688.

91. Aronow WS. Serum ferritin is not a risk factor for coronary artery disease in men and women aged ≥62 years. *Am J Cardiol*. 1993;72:347–348.

92. Cooper RS, Liao Y. Iron stores and coronary heart disease: Negative findings in the HANES I Epidemiologic Follow-up Study. *Circulation*. 1993;87:686.

93. Specialty Coffee Association of America, Long Beach, Calif; 1994.

94. Thelle DS, Arnesen E, Forde OH. The Tromso Heart Study. *N Engl J Med*. 1983;308:1454.

95. Haffner SM, Knapp JA, Stern MP, et al. Coffee consumption, diet and lipids, *Am J Epidemiol*. 1985;122:1.

96. Lacroix AZ, Mead LA, Liang KY, et al. Coffee consumption and the incidence of coronary heart disease. *N Engl J Med*. 1986;315:977.

97. Forde OH, Knutsen SF, Arnesen E, et al. The Tromso Heart Study: Coffee consumption and serum lipid concentrations in men with hypercholesterolemia: A randomized intervention study. *Br Med J*. 1985;290:893.

98. Arnesen E, Forde OH, Thelle DS. Coffee and serum cholesterol. *Br Med J*. 1984;288:1960.

99. Leonard-Green TK, Watson RR. Caffeine and health risk. *J Am Diet Assoc*. 1988;88:370. Authors' reply to letter.

100. Ernst N, Fisher M, Smith W, et al. The association of plasma high density lipoprotein cholesterol with dietary intake and alcohol consumption. The Lipid Research Clinics Program Prevalence Study. *Circulation*. 1980;62(Suppl IV):41.

101. Haskell WL, Camargo C, Williams PT, et al. The effect of cessation and resumption of moderate alcohol intake on high-density-lipoprotein subfractions. *N Engl J Med.* 1984; 310:805.

102. Burr ML, Fehily AM, Butland BK, et al. Alcohol and high-density-lipoprotein cholesterol: A randomized controlled trial. *Br J Nutr.* 1986;56:81.

103. Gear JS, Mann JI, Thorogood M, et al. Biochemical and hematological variables in vegetarians. *Br Med J.* 1980;280:1415.

104. Burslem J, Schonfeld G, Howald MA, et al. Plasma apoprotein and lipoprotein lipid levels in vegetarians. *Metabolism.* 1978;27:711.

105. Sacks FM, Castelli WP, Donner A, et al. Plasma lipids and lipoproteins in vegetarians and controls. *N Engl J Med.* 1975;292:1148.

106. Lock DR, Varhol A, Grimes S, et al. Apo A-I/Apo A-II ratios in plasma of vegetarians. *Metabolism.* 1983;32:1142.

107. Nestel PJ, Billington T, Smith B. Low density and high density lipoprotein kinetics and sterol balance in vegetarians. *Metabolism.* 1981;30:941.

108. Blum CB, Levy RI, Eisenberg S, et al. High density lipoprotein metabolism in man. *J Clin Invest.* 1977;60:795.

109. Fisher M, Levine P, Weiner B, et al. The effect of vegetarian diets on plasma lipids and platelet levels. *Arch Intern Med.* 1986;146:1193.

110. Dugan L. Antioxidants in the prevention of coronary heart disease. *Scan Pulse.* 1994;13(3):1-2.

111. Stampfer MJ, Hennekens CH, Manson JE, et al. Vitamin E consumption and the risk of coronary disease in women. *N Eng J Med.* 1993;328:1444-1449.

112. Rimm EB, Stampfer MJ, Ascherio A, et al. Vitamin E consumption and the risk of coronary disease in men. *N Engl J Med.* 1993;328:1450-1456.

113. Shaefer, EJ. Hyperlipoproteinemia. In: Rakel RD, ed. *Conn's Current Therapy 1991.* Philadelphia, Pa: WB Saunders; 1991:515-522.

114. National Research Council. *Diet and Health: Implications for Reducing Chronic Disease Risk.* Washington, DC: National Academy Press; 1989.

115. American Heart Association. *Dietary Treatment of Hypercholesterolemia. A Handbook for Counselors.* Dallas, Tex: American Heart Association; 1988.

116. US Department of Agriculture/US Department of Health and Human Services. *Nutrition and Your Health: Dietary Guidelines for Americans.* 2nd ed. Washington, DC: US Government Printing Office; 1985. HG-232.

117. National Cholesterol Education Program. Second Report of the Expert Panel on Detection, Evaluation, and Treatment of High Blood Cholesterol in Adults. Summary Report. *JAMA.* 1993;269(23):3015-3023.

118. Kant AK, Schatzkin A, Harris TB, et al. Dietary Diversity and Subsequent Mortality in the First National Health and Nutrition Examination Survey Epidemiologic Follow-Up Study. *Am J Clin Nutr.* 1993;57:434-440.

119. *Healthy People 2000: National Health Promotion and Disease Prevention Objectives.* Washington, DC: US Department of Health and Human Services; 1991. DHHS (PHS) publication 91-50212.

120. Neaton JD, Wentworth D. Serum cholesterol, blood pressure, cigarette smoking, and death from coronary heart disease. *Arch Intern Med.* 1992;152:56-64.

121. Baer JT. Improved plasma cholesterol levels in men after a nutrition education program at the worksite. *J Am Diet Assoc.* 1993;93:658-663.

122. Stallings VA, Cortner JA, Shannon BM, et al. Preliminary report of a home-based education program for dietary treatment of hypercholesterolemia in children. *Am J Health Promot.* 1993;8:106-108.

123. Ornish D, Brown SE, Scherwitz LW, et al. Can lifestyle changes reverse coronary heart disease? *Lancet.* 1990;336:129-133.

124. Warshafsky S, Kamer RS, Sivak SL, Effect of garlic on total serum cholesterol: A meta-analysis. *Ann Intern Med.* 1993;119:599-605.

125. Weidner G, Connor SL, Hollis JF, et al. Improvements in hostility and depression in relation to dietary change and cholesterol-lowering: The Family Heart Study. *Ann Intern Med.* 1992;117:820-823.

126. Muldoon MF, Manuch SB, Matthews KA. Lowering cholesterol concentrations and mortality: A quantitative review of primary prevention trials. *Br Med J.* 1990;301: 309-314.

127. Bandura A. *Social Foundations of Thought and Action: A Social Cognitive Theory.* Englewoood Cliffs, NJ: Prentice Hall; 1986.

128. WHO Expert Committee on the Prevention of Coronary Heart Disease. *Prevention of Coronary Heart Disease.* Geneva, Switzerland: World Health Organization; 1982. Technical report series no. 678.

129. Klag MJ, Ford DE, Mead LA, et al. Serum cholesterol in young men and subsequent cardiovascular disease. *N Engl J Med.* 1993;328:313-318.

130. Stamler J. Established major coronary risk factors. In: Marmot M, Elliott P, eds. *Coronary Heart Disease Epidemiology: From Aetiology to Public Health.* New York: Oxford University Press; 1992:35-66.

131. Stamler J, Stamler R, Brown WV, et al. Serum cholesterol: Doing the right thing. *Circulation.* 1993;88: 1954-1960.

132. Hulley SB, Walsh JMB, Newman TB. Health policy on blood cholesterol—time to change directions. *Circulation.* 1992;86(3):1026-1029.

133. Holme I, Hjermann I, Helgeland A, et al. The Oslo Study: Diet and anti-smoking advice. *Prev Med.* 1985;14:279.

134. World Health Organization European Collaborative Group: European Collaborative Trial of Multifactorial Prevention of Coronary Heart Disease: Final Report. *Lancet.* 1986;1:869–872.

135. Knapp JA, Hazuda HP, Haffner SM, et al. A saturated fat/cholesterol avoidance scale: Sex and ethnic differences in a biethnic population. *J Am Diet Assoc.* 1988;2: 172–177.

136. Frank GC, Zive M, Nelson J, et al. Fat and cholesterol avoidance among Mexican American and Anglo preschool children and parents. *J Am Diet Assoc.* 1991;8:954–961.

137. Connor SL, Artaud-Wild SM, Classick-Kohn CJ, et al. The cholesterol/saturated-fat index: An indication of the

hypercholesterolemic and atherogenic potential of food. *Lancet.* 1986;1:1229–1232.

138. Block G, Clifford C, Naughton MD, et al. A brief dietary screen for high fat intake. *J Nutr Ed.* 1989;199–207.

139. Connor SL, Connor WE. *The New American Diet.* New York, NJ: Simon & Schuster; 1986.

140. Peters JR, Quiter ES, Brekke ML, et al. The Eating Pattern Assessment Tool: A simple instrument for assessing dietary fat and cholesterol intake. *J Am Diet Assoc.* 1994;94(9):1008–1022.

141. Kaufman M. *Nutrition in Public Health—A Handbook for Developing Programs and Services.* Gaithersburg, Md: Aspen Publishers, Inc; 1990:570.

12

Cancer

Learning Objectives

- Discuss the epidemiology of cancer in the United States.
- Define the role of nutrition in the etiology, prevention, and treatment of cancer.
- Identify the *Healthy People 2000* objectives for cancer.
- Describe how community nutritionists can be actively involved in a cancer control network in the United States.
- List the major food sources or food components and how they protect the body and reduce cancer risk.
- Identify the basic elements of a healthy eating pattern for primary and secondary prevention of cancer.

High Definition Nutrition

Antioxidants—vitamins C and E and beta-carotene, which neutralize free radicals and other reactive chemicals and terminate harmful chemical reactions.

Carcinogenesis—the process of promoting cancer.

Conjugated linoleic acid—a natural component in animal food, especially dairy products, which has a cancer-preventing effect.

Lignin—a phenol similar in structure to estrogen that is hypothesized to decrease estrogen exposure and cancer risk.

Meta-analysis—aggregate analysis of similar studies to determine consistency of results.

Phytoestrogens—plant estrogens that may prevent binding of endogenous estrogens to the estrogen receptor.

SEER—the National Cancer Institute's Surveillance, Epidemiology, and End Results data registry that tracks cancer incidence, patient survival, and mortality.

The epidemiology of cancer shows that cancer is not an inevitable outcome of aging. Cancer is related to metabolic stresses linked to individual lifestyles. Variables that define lifestyle are tobacco and alcohol use, food intake, leisure time activity, occupational and environmental exposure, family cohesion, and personality.[1]

Epidemiologic and experimental studies have yielded data to answer many questions about cancer incidence and the role of eating patterns. Epidemiologic data come from ecologic correlations, cohort studies, case-control studies, and metabolic epidemiologic studies. Experimental studies, likewise, give strong support for a diet-cancer link. Data from metabolic studies focus largely on the colon cancer and bile acid metabolite association, breast and estrogen relation, and prostate and androgen association.

A key element in cancer epidemiology is the role of nutrition. Nutrition is thought to affect many different cancers because it appears to be a cofactor to chemical carcinogenesis.[1] Biomarkers may be very important in nutritional carcinogenesis, because tests of a cancer-to-diet hypothesis in homogeneous populations are inconclusive. Some researchers believe that nutritional carcinogenesis may best be studied by comparing the food intakes of diverse populations and by focusing more on biomarkers. If research uses specific biomarkers, the pathogenesis of a cancer may be clarified, and then further exploration with preventive strategies may be possible.[1]

INCIDENCE

Cancer incidence increases with age, and most cases affect adults at the middle of their adult life or older. For children aged 1 through 14, cancer causes more deaths in the United States than any other disease. More than 8 million US residents living today have a history of cancer. Of these, 5 million were diagnosed more than five years ago; because these individuals are still living, they are considered cured or having no evidence of disease. Their life expectancy is the same as a person who was never diagnosed with cancer.[2-4]

Each year about 1,208,000 new cancer cases are diagnosed. In a given year, about 538,000 individuals will die of cancer—which is more than 1,400 people per day. A startling 20% of all deaths in the United States are from cancer, and the increase in cancer mortality has been steady during the past half century. The age-adjusted rate in 1990 was 174 per 100,000. Lung cancer accounts for the greatest increase in cancer mortality; removing lung cancer deaths from cancer mortality would create a decline of 14% for the period from 1950 to 1990.[2]

In 1985, approximately 910,000 Americans developed cancer, and 462,000 Americans died of the disease. The 1994 estimates were that 632,000 men and 576,000 women would be diagnosed with cancer during that year, and 538,000 deaths would occur (see Exhibit 12-1).

Long-term survival from cancer has increased for each decade since 1900. Fewer than 20% of individuals diagnosed with cancer in 1930 survived five years. This contrasts with 25%, 33%, and 40% in 1940, 1960, and 1994, respectively. This represents a savings in lives of 85,000 per year from 1960 to 1994. A relative five-year survival rate of 53% is seen for all cancers and is commonly used to measure the success of early detection, treatment, and follow up.[2]

Psychosocial and behavioral research demonstrate that lifestyle and environmental factors influence an individual's general health and chances of developing cancer, and also that lifestyle influences an individual's ability to cope with cancer and cancer treatment. Behavioral modification can assist with the management of cancer side effects (e.g., pain, nausea, and vomiting), as well the ability to handle stress during treatment and recovery.[2]

Several cancers are linked to eating behavior risk factors:

- Colon and rectum cancer are linked to high-fat and/or low-fiber food intake.
- Breast cancer is linked to variations in fat intake.
- Prostate cancer may be linked to dietary fat.
- Pancreatic cancer is linked to high fat intake.
- Oral cancer is linked to excess use of chewing tobacco and alcohol-containing mouthwash before and after eating.

ETHNIC DIFFERENCES

The projected number of new cancers diagnosed in the United States in 1994 is 1,208,000; 120,000 will be among African Americans and 35,000 among other ethnic groups. Cancer incidence is 6% higher for African Americans than for whites. Mortality is likewise higher for African Americans than whites (230 compared with 170 per 100,000 in 1990). A comparison of the number of cancer deaths for various ethnic groups is given in Exhibit 12-2.

African Americans have significantly higher incidence and mortality rates for cancer of the

Exhibit 12-1 Leading Sites of Cancer Incidence and Death—1994 Estimates

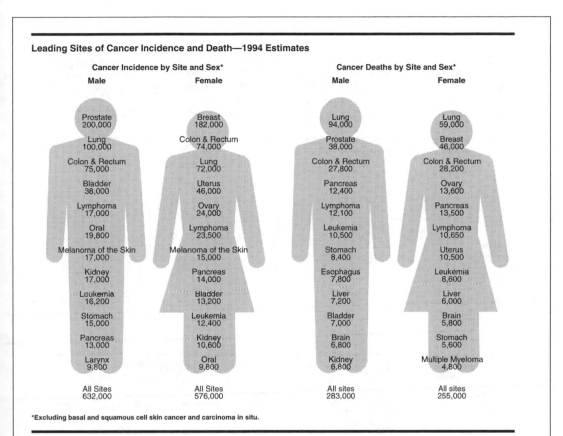

Leading Sites of Cancer Incidence and Death—1994 Estimates

Cancer Incidence by Site and Sex*

Male

Prostate	200,000
Lung	100,000
Colon & Rectum	75,000
Bladder	38,000
Lymphoma	17,000
Oral	19,800
Melanoma of the Skin	17,000
Kidney	17,000
Leukemia	16,200
Stomach	15,000
Pancreas	13,000
Larynx	9,800
All Sites	632,000

Female

Breast	182,000
Colon & Rectum	74,000
Lung	72,000
Uterus	46,000
Ovary	24,000
Lymphoma	23,500
Melanoma of the Skin	15,000
Pancreas	14,000
Bladder	13,200
Leukemia	12,400
Kidney	10,600
Oral	9,800
All Sites	576,000

Cancer Deaths by Site and Sex*

Male

Lung	94,000
Prostate	38,000
Colon & Rectum	27,800
Pancreas	12,400
Lymphoma	12,100
Leukemia	10,500
Stomach	8,400
Esophagus	7,800
Liver	7,200
Bladder	7,000
Brain	6,800
Kidney	6,800
All sites	283,000

Female

Lung	59,000
Breast	46,000
Colon & Rectum	28,200
Ovary	13,600
Pancreas	13,500
Lymphoma	10,650
Uterus	10,500
Leukemia	8,600
Liver	6,000
Brain	5,800
Stomach	5,600
Multiple Myeloma	4,800
All sites	255,000

*Excluding basal and squamous cell skin cancer and carcinoma in situ.

Percentage of Population (Probability) Developing Invasive Cancers at Certain Ages

		Birth to 39	40 to 59	60 to 79	Ever (Birth to Death)
All sites	Male	1.68 (1 in 60)	7.51 (1 in 13)	32.27 (1 in 3)	42.52 (1 in 2)
	Female	1.91 (1 in 52)	9.29 (1 in 11)	23.06 (1 in 4)	38.88 (1 in 3)
Breast	Female	0.45 (1 in 222)	3.78 (1 in 26)	6.78 (1 in 15)	12.20 (1 in 8)
Colon & rectum	Male	0.06 (1 in 1,667)	0.91 (1 in 110)	4.45 (1 in 22)	6.12 (1 in 16)
	Female	0.05 (1 in 2,000)	0.73 (1 in 137)	3.34 (1 in 30)	5.96 (1 in 17)
Prostate	Male	Less than 1 in 10,000	0.78 (1 in 128)	10.71 (1 in 9)	13.05 (1 in 8)
Lung	Male	0.04 (1 in 2,500)	1.60 (1 in 63)	6.69 (1 in 15)	8.43 (1 in 12)
	Female	0.03 (1 in 3,333)	1.07 (1 in 93)	3.49 (1 in 29)	5.02 (1 in 20)

Note: This chart shows the risks of being diagnosed with the most common cancers over certain age intervals. These risks are calculated for persons free of the specified cancer at the beginning of the age interval. Risk estimates do not assume all persons live to the end of the age interval or to any fixed age. Risk estimates are presented to give an approximate measure of the burden of cancer to society. Measures are based on population level rates and do not take into account individual behaviors and risk factors. For example, lung cancer is rare among nonsmokers or persons not heavily exposed to environmental tobacco smoke, so the risk for a nonsmoking man getting lung cancer in his lifetime is much lower than 8.4%, and it is much higher for a smoker. It is clear that the risk of developing cancer increases with age. For prostate cancer, the risk before age 60 is very low, but between 60 and 80, 1 in 9 men will be diagnosed with prostate cancer.

Source: American Cancer Society, *Cancer Facts and Figures—1994.*

Exhibit 12-2 Number of Cancer Deaths for Black, American Indian, Chinese, Japanese, and Hispanic Persons, United States, 1990

The most requested graphics in *Cancer Facts & Figures—1994* have been assembled in a format that makes it easier for you to reproduce them. If you need additional copies of this packet, contact the American Cancer Society's National Media Office at 212-382-2169. Please note: all graphic materials should credit the American Cancer Society.

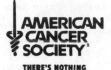

THERE'S NOTHING MIGHTIER THAN THE SWORD

Five-Year Relative Survival Rates by Stage at Diagnosis*

Site	All Stages %	Local %	Regional %	Distant %
Oral	53	78	42	19
Colon-rectum	58	89	58	6
Pancreas	3	8	4	2
Lung	13	46	13	1
Melanoma	84	92	55	14
Female breast	79	93	72	18
Cervix uteri	67	90	52	13
Corpus uteri	83	94	69	27
Ovary	39	88	36	17
Prostate	77	92	82	28
Bladder	79	91	46	9
Kidney	55	86	57	10

*Adjusted for normal life expectancy. This chart based on cases diagnosed in 1983-87, followed through 1990.

Number of Cancer Deaths for Black, American Indian, Chinese, Japanese, and Hispanic Persons, United States, 1990

Cancer Site	Black Males	Black Females	American Indian	Chinese	Japanese	Hispanic*
All sites	31,995	25,082	1,275	1,527	1,122	14,003
Oral cavity	1,000	311	23	60	23	232
Esophagus	1,433	541	19	45	32	233
Stomach	1,341	917	67	117	132	811
Colon & rectum	2,898	3,169	117	166	168	1,414
Liver & other biliary	757	615	68	168	66	769
Pancreas	1,442	1,581	52	65	77	795
Lung (male)	10,632	—	205	238	148	1,824
Lung (female)	—	4,512	117	145	75	787
Melanoma of skin	51	55	9	2	3	89
Breast (female)	—	4,659	89	88	79	1,246
Cervix uteri	—	972	47	22	12	296
Other uterus	—	899	12	15	14	168
Ovary	—	975	34	29	22	385
Prostate	5,181	—	59	42	56	728
Bladder	466	381	9	21	12	210
Kidney	563	382	39	12	14	355
Brain & CNS†	372	319	21	35	14	376
Lymphoma	747	573	50	47	42	688
Leukemia	854	737	52	47	27	735
Multiple myeloma	745	708	39	15	6	273

*Persons classified as of Hispanic origin on death certificates may be of any race. Hispanic origin reporting, however, may be incomplete on death certificates in some states. These numbers are believed to include over 90% of cancer deaths in Hispanics in 1990.

†CNS = Central nervous system.

Source: Reprinted from *Cancer Facts & Figures—1994*, p. 18, with permission of the American Cancer Society, © 1994.

esophagus, uterine, cervix, stomach, liver, prostate, larynx, and multiple myeloma. The five-year survival rate is lower, which may be in part due to late diagnosis. Many of these cancer sites have screening tests available, which strengthens the argument for early detection and timely treatment. Hispanics and Native Americans also have lifestyle and cultural differences that influence participation in screening and prevention activities. Values and belief systems and socioeconomic factors including access to care are important influential factors in overall diagnosis and survival.[2]

MONITORING

The best end point for cancer intervention should be reduction in the incidence of cancer.[1] Surveillance, Epidemiology, and End Results (SEER) data registries show changes in incidence and mortality for specific cancers and changes in trends. SEER is the major component of the National Cancer Institute's system for tracking cancer incidence, patient survival, and mortality. It consists of 11 population-based cancer registries covering 12% of the nation's population. National surveillance and monitoring must continue to acknowledge the successful reduction of any cancers that appear preventable.[3,4]

CANCER CONTROL OBJECTIVES

The National Cancer Institute (NCI) has established a set of quantified objectives to be used in charting a course to significantly reduce the US cancer mortality rate. A reduction in the mortality rate of 25% to 50% from the 1980 level is possible through full and rapid application of existing knowledge of cancer prevention, screening and detection, and state-of-the-art treatment methods. The NCI has set a goal of a 50% reduction in the cancer mortality rate by the year 2000. Achievement of this goal depends on a reduction in smoking by 50% from 1980 levels, the adoption of prudent eating pattern and screening measures, and accelerated and widespread appli-

cation of gains in state-of-the-art cancer treatment methods.[4]

A set of specific cancer control objectives has been chosen to help guide the nation's cancer control program toward this overall goal. Linked to the objectives is a set of cancer control indicators that NCI uses to measure progress toward achievement of the objectives (see Table 12–1). These objectives can be adjusted to reflect specific regional cancer rates and cancer control problems. They can direct the development of and serve as objectives for regional cancer control efforts across the United States.[4]

Much of cancer incidence can be prevented through changes in smoking and diet. The scientific evidence for smoking as a cancer cause has been recognized for over 20 years. The evidence for diet has emerged over the past decade and has progressed to the extent that recommendations for dietary change are widespread.[4]

Smoking

About 30% of all cancer deaths (over 130,000 deaths per year) are related to smoking. Approximately 54 million Americans—about one in every three adults—smoke cigarettes daily, and those who smoke two or more packs daily have lung cancer mortality rates 20 times higher than nonsmokers. Since 1953, lung cancer rates have increased 172% among men and 256% among women (see Exhibit 12–3). Lung cancer exceeds breast cancer as the leading cause of cancer death among women in all states in the United States. Cigarette smoking is further associated with cancers of the larynx, head and neck, esophagus, bladder, kidney, pancreas, and stomach. These facts are tempered, however, by the knowledge that cancer risk returns to near normal within 10 years after stopping smoking for all smoking-induced cancers, except for lung cancer, which requires about 15 years for risk to return to normal.[4]

Progress has been made in reducing the percentage of adult smokers since the 1964 Surgeon General's report on smoking and health. In 1965, 52% of men were smokers; in 1983, the figure

Table 12–1 Cancer Surveillance Indicators

Indicator	Measure	Source
Mortality	Deaths per 100,000 persons	National Center for Health Statistics mortality data
Incidence	Cases per 100,000 persons	SEER*; other population-based registries
Survival	Relative survival by cancer site	SEER; other registries, either population- or hospital-based
Smoking	Percentage of adults and children who smoke; time since quitting	National Health Interview Survey; Current Population Survey
Diet	Percent obesity; percent fat and fiber in the diet	National Health and Nutrition Examination Survey; US Department of Agriculture Survey
Occupation	Percent exposed; percent screened in workplace	National Health Interview Survey; Current Population Survey; other population surveys
Screening	Percentage of eligible persons screened	National Health Interview Survey; Current Population Survey; other population surveys
Treatment	Distribution by cancer stage of diagnosis; percentage of cancer patients treated via multidisciplinary approaches; cancer patient survival	SEER; population-based, hospital-based, or Cancer Center-based registry; Medicare Data System; Directory of Medical Specialties
Knowledge, attitudes, and beliefs	Percent population/ethnic groups with particular knowledge and beliefs about cancer	Supplement to National Health Interview Survey; independent population surveys
Costs	Indirect/direct	Medicare Data System; National Medical Care Utilization and Expenditure Survey; surveys of medical insurance

*SEER: Surveillance, Epidemiology, and End Results Program.

Source: Data from the American Cancer Society, 1994.

was 34.8%. In 1965, 34.2% of women were smokers; in 1983, the figure was 29.5%, which represented a decrease, but not as great a decrease as for men. However, smoking and the use of smokeless tobacco (chewing tobacco) continues to be a severe problem for our youth. More than 100,000 youths age 12 and under are habitual smokers, and nearly 4,000 youths begin smoking every day.

These figures present both a promise—that declines are possible—and a challenge—to reinforce and accelerate the decline into a consistent trend in smoking reduction, and to stop smoking and other tobacco use among our nation's youth.[4] An additional challenge is to provide strategies to assist individuals who stop smoking from gaining weight. Smoking and chewing tobacco are habits some individuals use to curb their appetite and to maintain their body weight.[5]

Dietary Components

Doll and Peto conducted an extensive review of cancer causes and estimated that 35% of can-

Exhibit 12-3 Cancer Deaths Rates by Site, Males and Females, United States, 1930–1990

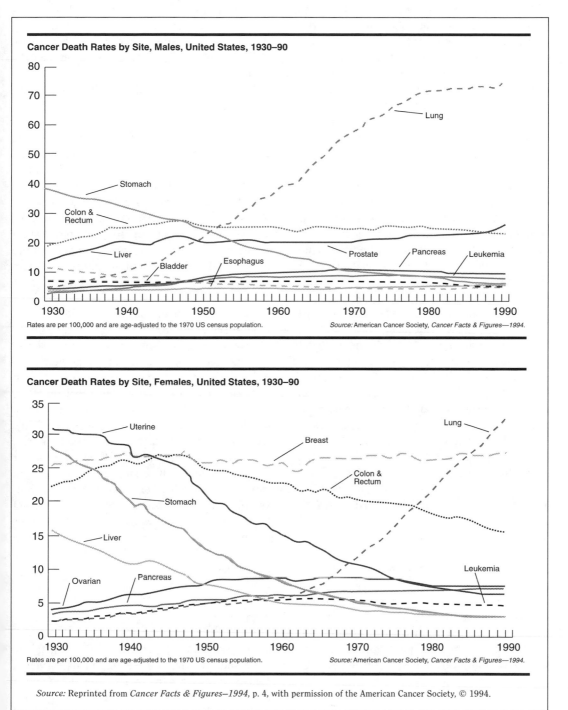

Cancer Death Rates by Site, Males, United States, 1930–90

Rates are per 100,000 and are age-adjusted to the 1970 US census population.

Source: American Cancer Society, *Cancer Facts & Figures—1994.*

Cancer Death Rates by Site, Females, United States, 1930–90

Rates are per 100,000 and are age-adjusted to the 1970 US census population.

Source: American Cancer Society, *Cancer Facts & Figures—1994.*

Source: Reprinted from *Cancer Facts & Figures–1994*, p. 4, with permission of the American Cancer Society, © 1994.

cer deaths may be related to dietary components, with the possible range of effect being 10 to 70%. A midrange estimate of 35% would mean that about 150,000 lives could be saved annually through dietary changes. These estimates cannot be considered definitive. Research to test the effectiveness of dietary interventions to reduce cancer incidence and mortality for particular cancer sites is currently underway. Even the most conservative estimates represent a potentially significant impact on cancer mortality.[6]

Certain changes in eating behavior are prudent because they will reduce cancer incidence. Limiting the consumption of fat to 30% of total calories and eating fruits, vegetables, and whole-grain cereal products daily will lower the risk of cancer.[7] The NCI concurs, and recommends a diet low in fat and high in fiber-rich foods. In 1984, an NIH Consensus Conference on cholesterol and heart disease noted that an eating pattern low in fat might reduce heart disease and lower the risk of cancer simultaneously.[4]

The NCI estimates that a minimum of 30,000 lives could be saved in the year 2000 based on modification of dietary factors. Current clinical trials show positive results of reducing the incidence of cancer by changing eating pattern or using chemopreventive agents. Current research in chemoprevention, diet, and nutrition suggests that 35% of all cancers could possibly be prevented by modifying diet and nutrition.[4]

ADVANCES IN CANCER SCREENING AND TREATMENT

Community nutrition professionals may find that primary and secondary prevention of all cancers must involve a more aggressive approach toward eating behavior. Likewise, understanding the screening and detection approaches recommended for several major cancers, even if there is no known dietary link, equips professionals with skills to communicate more effectively with their clients.[4]

Screening

Statistics indicate that, for most cancers, detection and treatment of early-stage disease pro-vides a much greater chance of patient survival than detection and treatment at later stages of the disease. Consequently, cancer mortality for breast and cervical cancer can be greatly reduced through aggressive screening (see Exhibit 12–4).

Breast cancer accounts for about 18% of all cancer deaths among women, and recent data show that the age-adjusted incidence and mortality from breast cancer in women has not changed during the past decade. Results from a long-term clinical study of over 60,000 women enrolled in the Health Insurance Plan of New York show that breast cancer mortality is reduced 30% in women over age 50 who are screened for breast cancer by mammography and physical examination.[8] A study from Sweden duplicates the 30% mortality reduction found in the Health Insurance Plan study.[9] The fact that breast cancer mortality for women over 50 has not decreased indicates that women may not be taking advantage of screening. An American Cancer Society survey reports that only 15% of women over 50 reported receiving an annual mammogram.

Cervical cancer screening has long been known to be effective. Use of the Papanicolaou (Pap) smear can reduce the risk of mortality from invasive cervical cancer by as much as 75%.[10] This fact, coupled with current screening figures, yields the estimate that use of the Pap smear for screening could reduce mortality from cervical cancer in the United States by at least 25%. Surveys indicate that, at most, 79% of women aged 20 to 39 and 57% of women aged 40 to 70 for whom the risk of cervical cancer is great follow recommended guidelines on screening for cervical cancer.

Treatment

The most recent figures from NCI's SEER Program indicate that the likelihood of surviving cancer for at least five years from the point of detection, compared with the survival of the general population, is over 49% for cases diagnosed in 1976 through 1981, compared to 48% for cases diagnosed in 1973 through 1975, and an estimated 38% for cases diagnosed in 1960 to 1963.[3]

Exhibit 12-4 Summary of American Cancer Society Recommendations for the Early Detection of Cancer in Asymptomatic People

Summary of American Cancer Society Recommendations For the Early Detection of Cancer in Asymptomatic People

Test or Procedure	Population		
	Sex	Age	Frequency
Sigmoidoscopy, preferably flexible	M & F	50 and over	Every 3-5 years
Fecal Occult Blood Test	M & F	50 and over	Every year
Digital Rectal Examination	M & F	40 and over	Every year
Prostate Exam*	M	50 and over	Every year
Pap Test	F	All women who are, or who have been, sexually active, or have reached age 18, should have an annual Pap test and pelvic examination. After a woman has had three or more consecutive satisfactory normal annual examinations, the Pap test may be performed less frequently at the discretion of her physician.	
Pelvic Examination	F	18-40 Over 40	Every 1-3 years with Pap test Every year
Endometrial Tissue Sample	F	At menopause, if at high risk**	At menopause and there-after at the discretion of the physician
Breast Self-Examination	F	20 and over	Every month
Breast Clinical Examination	F	20-40 Over 40	Every 3 years Every year
Mammography***	F	40-49 50 and over	Every 1-2 years Every year
Health Counseling and Cancer Checkup****	M & F M & F	Over 20 Over 40	Every 3 years Every year

*Annual digital rectal examination and prostate-specific antigen should be performed on men 50 years and older. If either is abnormal, further evaluation should be considered.
**History of infertility, obesity, failure to ovulate, abnormal uterine bleeding, or unopposed estrogen or tamoxifen therapy.
***Screening mammography should begin by age 40.
****To include examination for cancers of the thyroid, testicles, prostate, ovaries, lymph nodes, oral region, and skin.

Source: Reprinted from *Cancer Facts & Figures—1994*, p. 11, with permission of the American Cancer Society, © 1994.

If lung cancer is removed from the most recent figure, the chances of surviving cancer for at least five years, which for most cancer sites indicates a cure, is 56%. The figures show a steady gain in survival rates, and for some cancers the gains have been dramatic. In 1960, only 40% of patients survived Hodgkin's disease for more than five years; the latest SEER figures show the rate to be 74%, an increase attributable to improvements in radiation and chemotherapy.

Survival from testicular cancer has increased from 76% in 1973 to 1975 to 87% among patients diagnosed between 1977 and 1981, because of significant advances in treatment. An NIH Cancer Center Development Panel concluded that mortality can be reduced through adjuvant postsurgical therapies of chemotherapy in premenopausal women and hormonal or tamoxifen therapy in postmenopausal women. In both cases, the treatments are recommended for women with positive lymph node involvement, and treatments are recommended for postmenopausal women with positive estrogen receptors.[4]

The increased survival rate for many specific sites is small, but a steady trend toward an overall increase in cancer survival during past decades is apparent. Analysis of data from the NCI SEER Program indicates the rate of increase in the overall cancer survival rate is about 0.5% annually. The primary reasons for this steady improvement are gains in treatment efficacy and/or earlier detection. For other sites, such as prostate cancer, the increased survival is not fully understood. These improved survival rates may be influenced strongly by the increased detection of asymptomatic disease that might otherwise have remained undiagnosed or by improved attention to eating and exercise patterns. Another avenue for medical nutrition therapy for nutrition professionals is tertiary prevention, such as assisting cancer patients during treatments and helping to reduce symptoms. Table 12–2 outlines nutrition-related problems and recommended treatments that comprise the majority of tertiary treatment.[11]

Dissemination and application of existing state-of-the-art cancer therapy can significantly increase national cancer survival rates. When current survival figures from the SEER Program are compared with estimated survival from state-of-the-art treatments, the differences in survival translate into a 15% reduction in the cancer mortality rate. In addition to the gains in survival reasonably expected with aggressive application of state-of-the-art cancer treatment, further advances in research are confirmed. If trends in improved survival are also taken into account and estimated through the year 2000, then the reduction in mortality from increased application of state-of-the-art treatment could reach 25%.

PATTERNS OF CANCER OCCURRENCE

The prospect of surviving cancer is not the same for all Americans. Survival rates can potentially be improved through application of state-of-the-art primary, secondary, and tertiary treatment. Survival differences have been observed for different ethnic groups and, most importantly, for different socioeconomic groups. Patients with lower socioeconomic status (SES) characteristics have lower survival rates for the cancer sites studied to date. If differences in survival by SES are related to access to the health care system early in the disease or access to state-of-the-art treatment, then the potential for mortality reduction would be even greater than now projected.[4]

Estimates of survival by race show that blacks have a lower chance of surviving cancer. Five-year analyses show that much of the difference can be explained by socioeconomic status. On the whole, both black and white Americans with low incomes have a poorer prognosis from cancer than those whose incomes are above the median.[12] A challenge facing the health care community is to develop systems that enable professionals to practice state-of-the-art technology and allow patients to have access to state-of-the-art treatment and screening. With the current proposals for health care reform, neither condition is ensured.

Other evidence of differential survival among population groups has been demonstrated over the past 15 to 20 years. For example, Mormons and Seventh Day Adventists have cancer death rates far below the general population. Mortality from colorectal cancer among Californian Mor-

Table 12–2   Managing Cancer Symptoms—Common Nutritional Problems and Recommended Medical Nutrition Therapy

Nutrition Related Problems	*Recommended Treatment*
Stomatitis/esophagitis	• Eat foods at room temperature or cold foods. • Eat soft, moist, and tender foods. • Use a straw for liquids. • Avoid mouth irritants (citrus, spicy, salty, or rough foods). • Practice good oral hygiene. • Use oral anesthetics. • Use nutritional supplements.
Anorexia	• Relax at mealtime. • Stay active. • Eat nutrient-dense foods. • When hungry, eat small, frequent meals and snacks. • Vary eating places. • Use nutritional supplements consistently but sparingly.
Nausea	• Keep lips moistened. • Use sugarless hard candies, gum, and popsicles. • Moisten foods with gravies. • Avoid nutrient-dense foods like margarine, juices. • Try saliva substitutes. • Avoid fluids with meals. • Eat small, but frequent meals slowly. • Eat bland, dry foods. • Avoid fried, spicy-hot, very sweet, and very tart foods. • Drink plenty of fluids. • Avoid foods with strong odors. • Eat foods at room temperature or cooler. • Avoid favorite foods to prevent nausea.
Constipation	• Drink plenty of fluids. • Include high-fiber foods such as raw fresh fruits and vegetables, bran, whole grains, and legumes. • Keep active. • Try a hot beverage one-half hour before usual time for a bowel movement. • Only use medication per doctor's order.
Weight gain	• Do NOT go on a diet. Evaluate cause of weight gain. • Use behavior modification techniques. • Avoid high-fat, high-sugar foods in excess. • Keep active.
Dysphagia	• Eat finely chopped foods. • Swallow food and follow with a fluid.

Source: Adapted from National Cancer Institute. *Eating Tips: Tips and Recipes for Better Cancer Treatment.* NIH Publication. 1994.

mons is only 70% and 78% of the general white population for men and women, respectively. Their incidence of cancers of the lung, larynx, tongue, gums and mouth, esophagus, and bladder is 55% lower than for the US population.[13]

In addition, there are geographic differences in cancer mortality rates adjusted for age and sex differences. About 10% of US counties have less than 71% of the average national rate. In these counties, using age-adjusted mortality rates from 1950 to 1969, the mortality for breast cancer in women is 13.4 deaths per 100,000 compared with 25.5 deaths per 100,000 women in the United States. Mortality in these counties for lung cancer in men is 17.5 deaths per 100,000 persons, compared with 38.0 deaths per 100,000 in the United States.[14]

As noted earlier, many US ethnic minorities have a worse cancer experience than US whites. The exceptions to this are certain segments of the US Asian population, who have better overall cancer survival rates and better survival rates for certain cancer sites than whites. Addressing the cancer needs of minorities is critical to achieve a 50% lower cancer mortality by the year 2000. Ethnic-specific cancer incidence, mortality excess, and poorer survival experience require aggressive and long-term "catch-up" efforts to achieve the overall goal.

The most extensive cancer data available on US minorities are for blacks. Blacks have greater age-adjusted incidence and mortality rates from many cancers and lower survival rates than whites for all but 3 of 25 primary cancer sites.[15] Table 12–3 gives a summary of cancer differences between blacks and whites arrayed in four groups: sites for which blacks have higher incidence, higher mortality, lower survival, and higher survival than whites.

Blacks experience high rates of smoking-related cancers. Many of these cancers (lung, esophagus, and pancreatic cancers) have high fatality rates in all population groups. This suggests the need to control these illnesses through primary prevention rather than through treatment—the intervention being the prevention and cessation of tobacco use. Cancers with poorer survival for blacks compared to whites include some cancers with lower incidence in blacks (bladder and uterus cancer).

The cancer survival differences between blacks and whites are not completely understood. Socioeconomic factors influence the survival differences, and there is a greater proportion of blacks than whites at low socioeconomic levels.[15] Socioeconomic status is associated with a variety of factors, including host factors—immune and nutritional status/function—that influence cancer

Table 12–3 A Comparison of Cancer Incidence, Mortality, and Survival: US African Americans and Caucasians

	Occurrence for African Americans		
Higher Incidence	*Higher Mortality*	*Lower Survival*	*Higher Survival*
Esophagus	Esophagus	Rectum	Brain
Stomach	Stomach	Breast	Ovary
Pancreas	Pancreas	Corpus uterus	Stomach
Larynx	Larynx	Testis	
Male lung	Male lung	Bladder	
Cervix	Cervix		
Prostate	Corpus uterus		
Multiple myeloma	Prostate		
	Multiple myeloma		

Source: Adapted from *Cancer Control Objectives*, National Cancer Institute, 1993.

development and response to treatment. Furthermore, unequal distribution of health facilities and trained health personnel may result in poor access to cancer screening, detection, and treatment among certain segments of the population. Socioeconomic status also affects educational attainment and, thus, occupation. Occupation may affect exposure rates to occupational carcinogens. For example, studies of cancer risk in the steel and rubber industries show that black employees work in the most hazardous work sites, including those with toxic/carcinogen exposures.[16]

A possible factor in surviving cancer is an individual's general health status. Low-income persons tend to have poorer health and a shorter life expectancy than affluent persons. Therefore, community nutrition efforts aimed at improving general health status address improved cancer survival.[16]

STRENGTH OF THE CANCER CONTROL NETWORK

The ability to effect a reduction in cancer mortality depends in part on the existence and application of a number of resources, including the following:

- the means to provide information on prevention, screening, and treatment to the public and to health care professionals, including community nutrition professionals
- a system of providing patients access to state-of-the-art cancer prevention and treatment
- a mechanism for maintaining continued research progress and for fostering new research
- a cancer control network with organizational and personnel capabilities for a variety of cancer interventions

A network of cancer research centers has been developed, although some of the areas of the country remain underserved. Programs are being developed and evaluated to increase the pace of clinical research and to bring the benefits of clinical research to communities (e.g., the Community Clinical Oncology Program and the Cooperative Group Treatment Outreach Program). Physician Data Query, a computerized information system on cancer treatment, has been introduced and is available to clinicians through the National Library of Medicine or through commercial information systems. The capability to monitor progress in cancer control has been increased through the expansion of the SEER Program, which tracks cancer incidence and mortality in 12% of the US population. The Cancer Information System maintains a nationwide, toll-free telephone network for immediate answers to cancer-related questions from cancer patients, their families, the general public, and health professionals.

Actions and coordination of multiple actions are necessary to decrease cancer mortality before the year 2000. The overall goal is to reduce the projected cancer mortality rate by 50%. Predictions are that a 7% to 10% reduction in cancer mortality rate can be realized if dietary fat is lowered to less than 25% of total calories and dietary fiber is increased to 20 to 30 grams per day. A concerted effort with specific action plans at the local, state, and professional level have been recommended as follows[4]:

- *National Cancer Institute*—to guide and support basic and applied research in screening, diagnosis, treatment, and public education; to provide information and technical assistance to other agencies and organizations interested in conducting cancer control activities; and to conduct public and professional education programs.
- *Other federal agencies*—to sponsor appropriate research and data collection; to publicize information nationally; to offer technical assistance to program planners; and to promote appropriate regulatory measures.
- *State agencies*—to integrate cancer control techniques into state health care delivery and health promotion programs; to develop survey and surveillance capabilities; to collaborate on an interstate basis in forming coalitions and implementing programs; to coordinate program planning among various

state agencies (e.g., agriculture, environmental protection, health, aging); and to develop policies that promote cancer prevention.

- *Local government*—to promote primary prevention through health education in schools; to develop local health promotion programs and coalitions; to provide technical assistance to community organizations that are planning health promotion programs; to cooperate with state and federal agencies to provide survey data or capability; and to offer screening programs through local health clinics.

- *Private industry*—to offer health promotion and worksite wellness programs and screening programs to employees; to collaborate with employee groups to promote worksite health promotion programs; to monitor employee use of measures to prevent exposure to carcinogens in the workplace; to offer onsite food options consistent with cancer prevention; and to develop insurance policies that reward risk-avoidance behavior.

- *Professional organizations*—to incorporate cancer control knowledge into basic training curricula and continuing education; to increase the number of questions about cancer prevention and control on licensure examinations; to include more articles in journals about cancer control and the role of the health professional; to counsel patients about prevention steps they can take for themselves; and to provide assistance to other organizations and agencies developing cancer control programs.

- *Voluntary organizations*—to increase offerings of health education and screening programs at the community level; to form coalitions for cancer control; and to collaborate with federal agencies in disseminating health information and materials nationally.

- *The media*—to increase coverage about cancer causes, prevention, and control, especially about tobacco and dietary components; to communicate more closely with scientists and health professionals; and to enhance their understanding of research methods and implications for technology transfer.

Info Line

The American Cancer Society is the nationwide, community-based voluntary health organization dedicated to eliminating cancer as a major health problem by preventing cancer, saving lives from cancer, and diminishing suffering from cancer through research, education, and services. Affiliates are set up at the local and regional level and listed in the white pages of the telephone book.

March 15–April 15 is National Cancer Control Month. Contact American Cancer Society, 1599 Clifton Road NE, Atlanta, GA 30329-4251; 800/ACS-2345.

SURVEILLANCE ACTIONS

An NCI Surveillance Working Group formulated a set of actions to track the progress of cancer control and included indicators that measure progress toward specific health and eating behavior objectives (i.e., percent fat, fiber, and obesity). The actions are as follows:

- Identify sources of baseline information for indicators.
- Establish cooperative working arrangements for data collection.
- Monitor and report annually on changes in the indicators through the year 2000.
- Detail progress toward the objectives every five years (2000, 2005, and 2010).

DIETARY MODIFICATION—BREAST AND COLON CANCER INCIDENCE

Breast Cancer

For US women, breast cancer has the highest incidence and, after lung cancer, the second highest mortality. Approximately one out of every nine women will develop breast cancer during her life.

In 1991, about 175,000 cases of breast cancer were diagnosed, and approximately 44,500 deaths occurred. Breast cancer incidence has increased about 2% per year since the early 1970s, and mortality rates have remained fairly stable over the past 50 years.

International correlation studies show a linear relationship between breast cancer and total dietary fat availability and fat consumption. Studies of individuals who migrated from areas with diets low in animal fat and protein to areas with a more typical "Western" diet show higher cancer rates among the migrants when compared with incidence in the country of origin (e.g., migration from Japan to Hawaii and from Italy to Australia). International correlation studies also show a strong positive association of per capita fat consumption with breast cancer incidence and mortality rates. Breast cancer is more common in countries with high average consumption of total and saturated fat, protein (particularly animal protein), and total calories. For example, breast cancer incidence is more than five times higher in the United States than in Japan.[3,8,17]

Persons migrating from areas with low rates of fat consumption to areas with high rates acquire the higher cancer rates of their adopted country; for example, Japanese migrants to Hawaii and Italian migrants to Australia experience higher rates of breast cancer, suggesting that environmental factors are important. Although consistent evidence from animal studies supports a positive association between increased dietary fat intake and increased risk of breast cancer, analytical epidemiologic studies of individuals including both case-control and cohort studies have produced inconsistent results. This may be partly due to the known difficulty of quantifying individual dietary intake.

Colorectal Cancer

Colorectal cancer is the third leading cause of cancer deaths in US women, and the incidence is second only to that of breast cancer. Approximately 78,500 new cases were diagnosed in 1991, and approximately 31,000 deaths from colorectal cancer occurred. Epidemiologic and animal stud-ies conducted over the past few decades have established a strong link between dietary factors and colorectal cancer. Various dietary constituents have been implicated, including fat, excess calories, and reduced dietary fiber.[3,8,17]

In observational studies, the link between dietary fat and colorectal cancer is inconsistent. The large Nurses' Health Study showed a positive correlation between total fat intake and colon cancer risk. High intake of fruits and vegetables have been consistently related to lower risk of colon cancer, whereas the consumption of cereal grain products has been either unrelated or associated with lower risk of colon cancer. The majority of analytic epidemiological studies that have had reasonable capability assessing dietary fiber have generally shown a protective effect of fiber. A worksheet to aid individuals in evaluating their fiber intake is presented in Table 12-4.[16,17] Later in this chapter, fiber research studies are discussed.

ESTROGEN, FIBER, AND CANCER

Exposure to estrogens is associated with increased risk of estrogen-dependent cancers such as cancers of the breast, endometrium, and prostate.[18] Scientific data suggest that diet may influence risk of estrogen-dependent cancers by altering estrogen exposure. Obesity may increase estrogen levels, and vegetarian diets may decrease estrogen levels. The mechanisms by which diet influences estrogen levels relate to estrogen synthesis and metabolism.

Estrogens originate in the ovary, adipose and muscle tissue, and liver. Estradiol produced in the ovary is the primary circulating estrogen in premenopausal women. Estrone, produced mainly in adipose and muscle tissue, is the primary estrogen in postmenopausal women. Higher levels of estrone-sulfate and 16-hydroxylated estrogens were noted in breast cancer patients than in controls.[18]

Factors that alter the levels of sex hormone-binding globulin (SHBG) may influence estrogen availability, and factors that influence enterohepatic circulation of estrogens may affect estrogen excretion and alter plasma levels. Plant

Table 12–4 How To Rate Your Fiber Intake

Food	Serving Size	Usual Number of Servings per Day	Grams of Fiber per Serving	Fiber Intake
Beans: Pinto, red, lima, navy, black-eyed	½ cup	_____	3	_____
Broccoli	1 cup	_____	3	_____
Brown rice	¾ cup	_____	3	_____
Carrots	¾ cup	_____	2	_____
Green peas	½ cup	_____	4	_____
Lentils	½ cup	_____	8	_____
Pears	1 small	_____	3	_____
Strawberries/blueberries	1 cup	_____	3–4	_____
Wheat bran cereals	1 cup	_____	5–10	_____
Wheat bran muffins and breads	1 muffin/slice	_____	2	_____

Your Average Daily Fiber Intake _____

Rating (count the number of servings of food you ate):

- 2 or fewer—try adding a few more. It's easy!
- 3–5—You're on your way to better health!
- 6 or more servings—you're doing fine. Keep it up!

Source: Adapted from *Nutrition Fact Sheet: Focus on Fiber* by the National Center for Nutrition and Dietetics with permission of the American Dietetic Association, © 1994.

---

estrogens (phytoestrogens) may prevent binding of endogenous estrogens to the estrogen receptor.[18]

Weight reduction, anorexia nervosa, and starvation lower estrogen levels and increase SHBG. Vegetarian diets are associated with a low incidence of cancers of the breast, endometrium, and prostate.[19] Vegetarian diets reduce estrogen exposure by: (1) decreasing enterohepatic circulation of plasma estrogen with concomitant increases in fecal and decreased plasma and urinary estrogens; (2) decreasing estradiol availability by increasing SHBG; (3) decreasing hepatic estrogen sulfation with subsequent decreased plasma estrone-sulfate levels[20]; and (4) altering estrogen metabolism.[19]

Isoflavone Phytoestrogens

One of the most important classes of dietary compounds known to influence estrogen expo-

sure is the phytoestrogens, plant compounds that possess weak estrogenic activity (see Figure 12–1).[20-22] Phytoestrogens inhibit estrogen synthesis, blocking the actions of potent estrogens, interfering with estrogen receptor replenishment, and increasing SHBG synthesis.

Phytoestrogens include isoflavones, and daidzein and genistein are the two most common ones. Phytoestrogens have been shown to act as antiestrogens (see Table 12–5). They bind to the estrogen receptor and prevent more potent compounds from binding and exerting their effects. They contain phytochemicals that are known or believed to block specific pathways that lead to the development of breast cancer (see Figure 12–2).[23]

Soybeans and other legumes are the primary food sources of daidzein and genistein in humans[24] and may be a contributing factor for low incidence of breast and prostate cancer in Japanese women and men.[25] Dietary soy has been shown to be inversely associated with breast can-

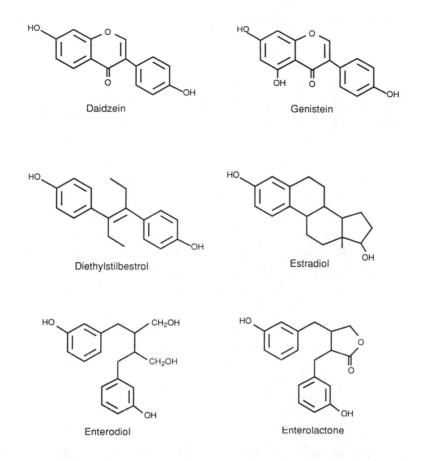

Figure 12-1 Comparison of the structures of selected isoflavone phytoestrogens (daidzein and genistein), lignins (enterodiol and enterolactone), and estrogens (diethylstilbestrol and estradiol). *Source:* Reprinted from Kurzer, M.S. Diet, Estrogen and Cancer. *Contemporary Nutrition.* 1992;17(7):1-2.

cer risk in Singapore.[26] Animal studies have shown that dietary soy decreases mammary tumor development in rats[27] and reduces precancerous changes in a prostatic cancer model for mice.[28]

Lignins

Lignins are heterocyclic phenols similar in structure to estrogens and isoflavones that are hypothesized to decrease estrogen exposure and cancer risk. Lignins are abundant in seeds, especially flax seed, in the form of a glycoside[29] that is converted into mammalian lignins—

enterolactone and enterodiol—and excreted in the urine.

Enterolactone, the most important animal lignin, may have antiestrogenic properties. Postmenopausal women with breast cancer, as compared with omnivorous and vegetarian controls, excrete lower amounts of urinary lignins.[30] Enterolactone and enterodiol are excreted in significantly lower amounts in urine of nonvegetarians as compared to vegetarians.[30]

Enterolactone and other lignin metabolites have been shown to inhibit in vitro estrogen synthesis.[31] They also have been shown to bind the

Table 12–5 14 Major Plant Phytochemicals with Cancer-Protective Properties

	Sulfides	Phytates	Flavonoids	Glucarates	Carotenoids	Coumarins	Monoterpenes	Triterpenes	Lignins	Phenolic acids	Indoles	Isothiocyanates	Phthalides	Polyacetylenes
Garlic	*						*	*		*				
Green tea			*	*		*				*				
Soybeans		*	*		*	*		*	*	*				
Cereal grains		*	*	*	*	*		*		*				
Cruciferous	*		*	*	*	*	*	*		*	*	*		
Umbelliferous			*		*	*	*	*		*			*	*
Citrus			*	*	*	*	*	*		*				
Solanaceous			*	*	*	*	*	*		*				
Cucurbitaceous			*		*	*	*	*						
Licorice root			*			*		*		*				
Flax seed			*			*			*	*				

Source: Reprinted from Caragay, A.B., Cancer Preventive Foods and Ingredients, *Food Technology*, April 1992, pp. 65–68, with permission of the Institute of Food Technologists, © 1992.

estrogen receptor[32] and to inhibit estradiol stimulated breast cancer cell growth in vitro.[33]

Flax seed is the most concentrated food source of lignin precursors.[29] When expressed per 100 grams net weight, flax seed consumption results in an average 100-fold greater total lignin production than consumption of other oil seeds, cereals, and legumes. Fruit and vegetable consumption results in very low lignin production. These foods, however, may contribute significantly to lignin production when consumed in amounts greater than normally consumed.[22]

The link between a high-fiber eating pattern and health promotion has been suggested for many years.[34] Burkitt's report in 1969 heightened the interest.[35] Some researchers report that specific foods high in dietary fiber—such as fruits, vegetables, and grains—protect against degenerative disease.[34,36,37] Approximately 45% of total dietary fiber intake in the United States is from fruits and vegetables; grains provide 25% of fiber.[38] All other foods provide the remaining 30%.

Adlercreutz[32] has suggested that phytoestrogens or lignins, not dietary fiber, protect against Western diseases. The link connecting colon and breast cancer to diet in epidemiologic studies is that certain populations consume small amounts of specific fiber-rich foods, especially grain, that contain lignins, which are precursors to mammalian lignins. Phytoestrogens and lignins are thought to be anticarcinogenic, antiproliferative, and antihormonal.[39] Thus, a diet high in fiber increases fecal bulk and is speculated to influence estrogen metabolism in a favorable direction, giving protection against both colon and breast cancer. Since lignins are associated with high-fiber foods—such as grains, certain berries, and seeds—it is difficult to distinguish the protective properties of phytoestrogens or lignins from dietary fiber.[40]

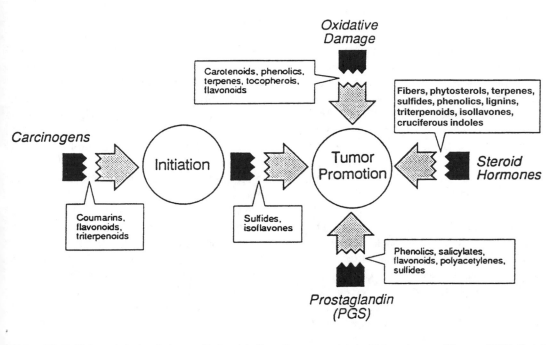

Figure 12-2 Dietary phytochemicals can affect metabolic pathways associated with breast cancer (Pierson, 1992). Certain phytochemicals are known or believed to block specific pathways that lead to the development of breast cancer. *Source:* Reprinted from Caragay, A.B., Cancer Preventive Foods and Ingredients, *Food Technology*, April 1992, pp. 65–68, with permission of the Institute of Food Technologists, © 1992.

Large Bowel Cancer and Fiber

Correlation studies that compare national colorectal cancer incidence or mortality rates with estimates of national dietary fiber consumption suggest that fiber intake may protect against colon cancer.[41] Case-control studies[41,42] support the protective role of dietary fiber in colorectal cancer. A recent case-control study in Argentina reports that dietary fiber is highly protective against colon cancer.[43]

Different fiber sources were associated with varying risks of colon and rectal cancer in a western New York population.[44] Patients with pathologically confirmed, single, primary cancers of the colon and rectum, as well as age-, sex-, and neighborhood-matched controls were interviewed regarding usual quantity and frequency of consumption of foods. For colon cancer, risk decreased with intake of grain fiber for both females and males and with intake of fruit/vegetable fiber for males only. For rectal cancer,

fruit/vegetable fiber intake was associated with decreased risk, whereas grain fiber was not. This study suggests that different fibers have different protective effects on cancer risk, which may also vary by gender.[44]

A prospective study of colon cancer risk among women reports no association between dietary fiber intake and colon cancer.[45] Low intake of fiber from fruits may contribute to colon cancer risk, but not statistically independent of meat intake. Colon cancer risk reduction has been reported in a prospective study where individuals had a more frequent consumption of vegetables and high-fiber grains.[46] Human observational studies and animal experiments suggest that calcium may decrease the risk of colorectal cancer, possibly because increased formation of the calcium salt of bile acids decreases promotion of cancer. The vitamin D and calcium supplementation trial in the Women's Health Initiative will answer questions regarding the effect of supplementation on colorectal cancer (see Chapter 9).

Breast Cancer and Fiber

Fat and fiber content of one's eating pattern are generally inversely related, and it is difficult to separate their independent effects. International comparisons show an inverse correlation between breast cancer death rates and consumption of fiber-rich foods.[44] An exception is Finland, where intake of both fat and fiber is high and the breast cancer mortality rate is low. Data suggest that the high level of fiber in the rural Finnish diet can modify the breast cancer risk associated with a high-fat diet.[47]

A meta-analysis of 12 case-control studies of dietary factors and risk of breast cancer found that high dietary fiber intake was associated with a reduced breast cancer risk.[48] Graham et al[49] found that the risk of breast cancer was lowest in those who reported the highest intakes of dietary fiber. Willett et al[50] found no indication of a protective effect of fiber consumption on breast cancer incidence in a prospective cohort of 89,494 women in the Nurses' Health Study who were 34 to 59 years of age and were followed for eight years. These authors suggest that the relationship between dietary fiber and breast cancer risk warrants further research since they could not exclude the possibility that specific fractions of dietary fiber may protect against breast cancer.

Dietary fiber increases intestinal transit rate and bulk and thereby dilutes intestinal constituents that may promote carcinogenesis.[36,41,51] Lampe et al[52,53] found that different dietary fibers have different effects on bowel function and that these differences vary between men and women. Kashtan et al[54] studied colonic fermentation and markers of colorectal cancer risk in patients with polyps. They found no significant differences between oat bran, a more fermentable fiber, and wheat bran, a less fermentable fiber, on putative risk factors for colon cancer.

Lipkin and colleagues[55,56] suggest that proliferation rates of epithelial cells that line colorectal mucosa crypts are related to risk of colorectal cancer, with proliferation rates highest in colon cancer patients and lowest in noncancer patients. Intermediate rates occur for patients with familiar polyposis. DeCosse et al[57] found that a daily dietary supplement of 22.5 grams of wheat bran fiber significantly reduced the number of adenomatous polyps in the low sigmoid colon and rectum of patients with familial polyposis. Alberts et al[58] studied the effects of wheat bran fiber on rectal epithelial cell proliferation in patients with resection for colorectal cancers. They found that the wheat bran fiber supplement inhibited DNA synthesis and rectal mucosa cell proliferation in this high-risk group, suggesting that fiber could be used as a chemopreventive agent for colorectal cancer.

Few studies have examined the effects of dietary fiber on hormone metabolism while holding fat content of the eating pattern constant. Rose et al[59] found that when wheat bran was added to the usual eating pattern of premenopausal women, it significantly reduced serum estrogen concentrations, while neither corn bran nor oat bran had the same effect. High-fiber intakes may diminish the extent to which unconjugated estrogens undergo intestinal absorption. Dietary fiber intake was increased from about 15 grams per day to 30 grams per day in this study, an increase similar to that recommended by the National Cancer Institute. Rose believes an increase in dietary fiber intake to about 30 grams per day can favorably modify breast cancer risk by reducing circulating estrogens.[60]

ANIMAL STUDIES

Cohen et al[61] reported that rats fed a diet supplemented with wheat bran developed significantly fewer mammary tumors than rats on diets not supplemented with wheat bran. Boffa et al[62] found that fiber-free and 20% high-fiber diets were associated with hyperproliferation, a risk factor for colon cancer. They suggest that moderate amounts of fiber, 5% and 10% in their animal model, may have protective effects on cell proliferation, differentiation, and carcinogenesis, while fiber-free diets and diets supplemented with too much fiber have the potential to promote colon carcinogenesis. Increasing current intake of dietary fiber to 20 to 35 grams per day from a variety of food sources, including vegetables, legumes, and grains, appears prudent and necessary.[63]

CONJUGATED LINOLEIC ACIDS

A recent area of investigation has been the role of conjugated linoleic acid (CLA) in the inhibition of uncontrolled cell growth or neoplasia.[64] Linoleic fatty acid is essential for tumor growth.[65] However, it can be modified to yield protective properties. When linoleic acid is heated, the double bonds migrate from the cis 9 and 12 positions to the cis or trans 9 and 11 or 10 and 12 positions. The biologically active form appears to be the 9-cis, 11-trans isomer.[66]

In 1991, Ip et al demonstrated that a test diet with 1.0% or 1.5% CLA reduced tumor incidence by 42% and 50%, and reduced tumor multiplicity by 56% and 59%, respectively.[67] In related research, a daily 0.5 gram dose of CLA for 22 weeks not only lowered plasma total and low-density lipoprotein (LDL) cholesterol by 13% and 17%, respectively, but also reduced the severity of atherosclerosis in rabbits.[68,69]

CLA is found naturally in animal foods, especially dairy products. The proposed cancer-preventing effect occurs at a level slightly above the estimated daily US consumption.[70] The concern is to balance an intake that provides protection with one that does not exceed the 30% total fat intake.

THE NEED FOR A CONTROLLED TRIAL OF A LOW-FAT EATING PATTERN

Many different types of epidemiologic studies have addressed the hypothesis that dietary intakes of fat, grains, fruits, and vegetables are related to the incidence of breast and colorectal cancers. Animal experiments are important for demonstrating plausible biological mechanisms and for confirming or explaining the results of epidemiological studies, but the results cannot on their own be extrapolated to humans. If a marker for disease exists, then clinical metabolic studies may be performed to test the effect of dietary modifications on the marker. No such marker currently exists for breast or colorectal cancer.

Studies correlating international data on incidence of disease with food disappearance data and migrant studies provide useful evidence for these hypotheses. However, this information is not entirely reliable, because the studies do not link dietary habits with disease incidence at the individual level. They also cannot adequately control for confounding factors that may influence the disease rate.

Case-control studies overcome some of these problems but suffer from possible biases in the selection of cases and controls, differential recall of dietary intake by cases and controls, and nondifferential error in the measurement of dietary intake. Prospective cohort studies avoid selection and recall biases but still rely upon food questionnaires that are known to involve substantial measurement error. These problems are compounded by the narrow range of intakes of the populations typically entering a case-control or cohort study.

The role of antioxidant vitamins C and E and beta-carotene in cancer prevention is of considerable interest. These nutrients neutralize free radicals and other reactive chemicals and terminate the harmful chemical reactions.

Beta-carotene, the most common plant source of vitamin A, is a food colorant. The rich yellow, orange, and red pigment of fruits and vegetables is due to its presence. However, beta-carotene has another unique property. Beta-carotene, vitamin C, and vitamin E all assist the body to resist unstable chemicals that damage cells.

More than 100 population-based studies showed a strong association between lowered risk of chronic diseases (e.g., heart disease and cancer) and the high daily intake of antioxidant vitamins. Such studies are still being conducted. However, health authorities in the United States have become proactive and recommend a minimum of five fruits and vegetables a day and the use of whole-grain products as a means of achieving the Recommended Dietary Allowances (RDAs) for the antioxidants.[71] Good food sources of vitamin C, vitamin, E, and beta-carotene are outlined in Table 12–6.[72] Americans average about 1.5 mg of beta-carotene per day, which is only 25 to 30% of the RDA.[73,74]

WORKSITE INTERVENTION

Preventive efforts have taken the form of organized intervention at the job site. The many benefits include having the support of management for employee wellness; using the physical environment for instruction including exercise rooms, cafeterias, walking areas, and meeting rooms; scheduling classes conveniently before, during, and after work; using the group dynamics of the employees to form classes and to develop healthy competition if needed.

The Treatwell Intervention

Primary prevention efforts involving worksite interventions often include separate treatment and control groups.[75,76] In the Treatwell Intervention in Massachusetts, 1,762 employees repre-

sented eight control and five intervention companies. Eligibility criteria for participation were:

- company size (200–2,000 employees)
- presence of a cafeteria with a kitchen in which to implement the cafeteria-based intervention
- an annual employee turnover rate of less than 25%
- fewer than 25% of employees working rotating shifts, part-time, or off-site
- company stability, defined as having no plans for geographic relocation or major layoffs during the intervention period

The purpose of the intervention was to reduce fat consumption and increase consumption of fiber in the eating patterns of the intervention group using food-focused messages (see Table 12–7). The secondary effect of the dietary changes on other nutrients was evaluated. Each participant completed a health-habits questionnaire before and after the 15-month intervention. In addition, the nutrient and energy intakes were determined from the Wil-

---

Table 12–6 Food Sources of Vitamin C, Vitamin E, and Beta-carotene

Nutrient	Good Food Sources
Vitamin C	Vegetables such as asparagus, broccoli, brussels sprouts, cauliflower, cabbage, green peppers, kale, snow peas, and sweet potatoes Fruits such as cantaloupes, grapefruits, honeydew melons, oranges, tangerines, and strawberries
Vitamin E	Almonds, hazelnuts Peanut butter Salad/vegetable oils Sunflower seeds Wheat germ
Beta-carotene	Dark, green leafy vegetables such as collard greens, kale, mustard greens, peppers, spinach, turnip greens, and Swiss chard Yellow-orange vegetables such as carrots, pumpkins, sweet potatoes, and winter squash Yellow-orange fruits such as apricots, cantaloupes, mangoes, papayas, and peaches

Source: Adapted from Food Sources of Vitamin C, E, and Beta Carotene, American Cancer Society brochure.

Table 12–7   Eating Pattern Messages Linked to Food Items in the Treadwell Food Frequency
Questionnaire (FFQ)

Message	*FFQ Items[1]*
Trim fat.	
• Choose fish.	• Fish
• Choose skinned turkey or chicken.	• Ratio of chicken and turkey without skin to chicken and turkey with skin
• Choose lean red meat.	• Red meat
	• Hamburger fat score
– Keep to 6 oz. or less (cooked) a day.	• Unable to quantify
• Choose low-fat dairy products.	• Ratio of skin and low-fat to whole milk
– skim, 1%, or 2% milk	
– low-fat yogurt, cheese, and ice milk	• Unable to quantify
• Use half the amount of fat or oil you normally use.	
– in cooking or baking	• Fats and oils added in cooking
– as spreads	• Margarine and butter
Add fiber.	
• Eat at least one serving of a high-fiber cereal every day.	• Proportion of cold cereal eaters who consumed low- and high-fiber cereals at baseline and at follow up
• Eat at least one serving of fruit per meal and for snacks.	• All fruit
• Eat at least one serving of vegetables at lunch and dinner.	• All vegetables
• Eat at least one of these foods at each meal:	
– whole-grain bread	• Dark and whole-grain bread
– rice or pasta	• Rice and pasta
– potato	• Potatoes, mashed or baked
– dried beans, peas, or lentils	• Beans or lentils, dried

[1]Food items derived from the FFQ that are related to the eating pattern messages, or derivations based on one or more FFQ responses.

Source: Reprinted from Hunt, M.K. et al., Impact of Worksite Cancer Prevention Program on Eating Patterns of Workers, *Journal of the Society for Nutrition Education*, Vol. 25, No. 5, pp. 236–243, with permission of the Society for Nutrition Education, © 1993.

lett semiquantitative food frequency questionnaire.[77]

Participants in the intervention group decreased their use of margarine and butter as spreads (p <0.01) and increased their intake of vegetables (p <0.02) significantly more than did workers in control companies.

The greatest change in nutrient content occurred for nontargeted dietary components. Specifically, significantly greater increases were observed for vitamin A and beta-carotene. Marginally significant increases were noted for vitamin B_6, moderate decreases were seen for saturated and monounsaturated fats, and small increases were noted for polyunsaturated fats.[75] This observation is important, because analysis of the total nutrient intake beyond the targeted nutrients is warranted. Healthy eating refers to the total composition of an eating pattern, not just the fat or sodium content.

Of equal importance is the choice of research instruments when trying to assess nutrient composition in a large study group. The Willett food frequency questionnaire is useful when ranking individuals into percentiles of intake and to identify outliers for specific dietary components. Frequencies in general should not be used to estimate the mean nutrient intake of an individual or a group.

Women's Intervention Nutrition Study

The purpose of the Women's Intervention Nutrition Study (WINS) was to evaluate the feasibility of integrating dietary fat intake reduction into adjuvant treatment strategies for postmenopausal women with breast cancer by determining the degree of adherence to such a dietary program.[78] WINS was a step-by-step, individualized approach to reduce total fat intake and fat components (see Table 12–8). It was based on behavioral and social learning theory about dietary behavioral change (see Table 12–9).[79,80]

The primary end point was group dietary fat intake using four-day food records and unannounced 24-hour telephone recalls. Fasting blood for lipid analysis was obtained at baseline and at 3, 6, 12, 18, and 24 months. Anthropometric data collection included body weight, height, and waist

and hip circumference taken at baseline and at three-month intervals.

Changes in mean intake of energy, total fat, and percentage of energy from fat calculated from four-day food record data show total fat and percent energy derived from fat significantly different between the two dietary groups ($p < 0.001$). The percentage of energy from fat determined three months' postrandomization was lower (19.5% versus 22.2% when the target was 15%).[78]

The low-fat eating plan in the dietary intervention group did not involve changes in total energy intake. This group had reduced body weights compared with the weights seen in the dietary control group at all observation points. The body weight difference was 3.26 kg 18 months after randomization (1.46 ± 5.01 kg weight loss versus 1.80 ± 6.34 kg weight gain, for intervention and control group patients, respectively, $p < 0.001$).[78]

This study demonstrated that significant dietary fat intake reduction can be achieved during breast cancer treatment and maintained for at least two years by patients in a multicenter

Table 12–8   Changes in Eating Pattern Composition from Baseline to Six Months for Treatment and Control Participants, WINS Study

	Daily Intake by Dietary Group				
	Intervention (N = 96)			Control (N = 100)	
Nutrient	Baseline	6 Months		Baseline	6 Months
Total energy, kcal	1,755 ± 447	1,466 ± 395		1,731 ± 395	1,544 ± 369
Protein, g	73 ± 20	70 ± 19		75 ± 18	68 ± 16
Carbohydrate, g	218 ± 65	223 ± 72		212 ± 57	195 ± 57
Fiber, g	17.4 ± 5.7	18.4 ± 6.7		16.9 ± 6.2	16.6 ± 6.4
Fat total, g	66 ± 23	33 ± 14*		66 ± 20	56 ± 20
Calories from	11.3 ± 4.5	6.8 ± 3.0*		11.4 ± 4.2	10.2 ± 4.3
Total fat, %	33.4 ± 6.0	20.5 ± 6.2*		34.3 ± 5.6	32.1 ± 7.3
Monounsaturated fats, %	12.3 ± 4.1	7.6 ± 4.1*		11.7 ± 3.5	12.4 ± 5.1
Polyunsaturated fats, %	6.6 ± 2.8	4.6 ± 2.7*		6.7 ± 2.9	6.7 ± 3.1
Linoleic acid (c18:2)	12.8 ± 6.1	6.4 ± 3.4*		12.1 ± 4.7	10.7 ± 5.1

Note: values are mean ± SD.
*Difference from baseline to 6 months is for intervention versus control group ($p < 0.001$).

Source: Reprinted from Buzzard, I.M., Asp, E.H., Chlebowski, R.T., et al., Diet Intervention Methods to Reduce Fat Intake: Nutrient and Food Group Composition of Self-Selected Low-Fat Diets, Journal of the American Dietetic Association, Vol. 90, pp. 42–49, with permission of the American Dietetic Association, © 1990.

Table 12–9 The Women's Intervention Nutrition Study Dietary Intervention Protocol for Low-Fat Eating

Step	Content
1	Teaching basic concepts about low-fat and high-fat foods, recipe modification, and food preparation methods via four biweekly visits, eight monthly, and two bimonthly visits
2	Establishing an individualized, daily fat-gram goal (initially, 20% energy as fat, then 15% energy as fat); monitoring with a food diary and the following tools: • fat-gram counter • brand-name guide • keeping score booklet
3	Setting individual long- and short-term goals for eating behaviors

Source: Data from Buzzard, I.M., Asp, E.H., Chlebowski, R.T., et al., Diet Intervention Methods to Reduce Fat Intake: Nutrient and Food Group Composition of Self-Selected Low-Fat Diets, *Journal of the American Dietetic Association*, Vol. 90, pp. 42–49, American Dietetic Association, © 1990.

study. Feasibility of the fat modification was established. A definitive trial is now needed to test the hypothesis that a program of dietary fat intake reduction that complements systemic adjuvant therapy can reduce disease recurrence and increase survival duration of postmenopausal women with localized breast cancer.[78]

This fat intake reduction program could be broadly implemented by registered dietitians at the hospital and community level. The approximate cost of instruction for the low-fat eating plan is projected to be about $375 to $400. This is based on current professional charges for five hours of a registered dietitian's service and reflects the percentage of effort required in the WINS Study. Costs associated with breast cancer management, including costs for local therapy to the diseased breast, are approximately $10,000. Tamoxifen for five years plus chemotherapy would cost $15,000.[81] A program for dietary fat intake reduction costing $375 represents less than a 2% increase in the $25,000 cost associated with current management of early-stage breast cancer.[55]

The Women's Health Initiative

The randomized, controlled clinical trial component of Women's Health Initiative (WHI) will enroll approximately 63,000 postmenopausal women 50 to 79 years of age at 40 clinical centers. This trial has three interventions, and women can enroll in one or more of the intervention components. The first will evaluate the effect of a low-fat dietary pattern on prevention of breast and colon cancer and coronary heart disease. The second will examine the effect of hormonal-replacement therapy on prevention of coronary heart disease and osteoporotic fractures. The third will evaluate the effect of calcium and vitamin D supplementation on prevention of osteoporotic fractures and colon cancer (see Chapter 9).

Women who are ineligible or unwilling to participate in the trial will be offered the opportunity to enroll in a concurrent, long-term observational study that will delineate new risk factors and biological markers for diseases in women. It is expected that about 100,000 women will join this part of the study. Thus, a total of approximately 163,000 women will be studied over time.[82] The broad geographic distribution of the clinical centers allows recruitment in medically underserved areas and targets minority populations to obtain a cross-section of the US population.[82]

The WHI Community Prevention Study of strategies to enhance adoption of healthful behaviors will evaluate how the many behaviors of proven value to women's health can be widely adopted. This aspect of WHI will mobilize community resources to enhance adoption of these behaviors through education, removal of barriers, and improvement of social supports. The behaviors to be targeted are derived from the national goals described in *Healthy People 2000*. Special emphasis will be focused on minorities, the medically underserved, and socioeconomically disadvantaged populations, as these groups have received too little attention and have lagged in adoption of preventive behaviors.[59]

ADOPTION OF INSTRUMENTS USED IN CARDIOVASCULAR RESEARCH

In clinical trials and community-based interventions that focus on cancer, many of the instruments previously used in cardiovascular research are adopted (e.g., the Block Fat Screen described in the Chapter 11 and the Willett Semi-Quantitative Food Frequency questionnaire briefly described below).

The Willett Semi-Quantitative Food Frequency instrument is a dietary assessment instrument based on the principle that the average eating pattern over weeks, months, or years is preferred to a recall or record of foods eaten for a short period of time (e.g., one to seven days). It consists of a food list of about 60 to 100 foods and a five- to seven-item frequency response component. It can be either self-administered or administered in a one-to-one interview. Foods included are eaten fairly often by a majority of individuals, provide nutrients or dietary components of interest (e.g., vitamin C or cholesterol), or allow the investigator to discriminate or rank individuals on intake. Guidelines for development of a food frequency questionnaire and testing the reproducibility and validity of the instrument are available.[83]

HEALTHY PEOPLE 2000 ACTIONS

Several HP2K objectives are directed toward cancer risk reduction using dietary behavior modification (see Exhibit 12–5). Dietary fat, fiber, complex carbohydrate, and total energy intakes are the major focus. Community nutrition professionals can blend these objectives with national cancer control objectives to direct their programs and to target high-risk subgroups in the population (see Exhibit 12–6).

Exhibit 12–5 *Healthy People 2000* Objectives for Cancer Control

2.2	Reverse the rise in cancer deaths to achieve a rate of no more than 130 per 100,000 people. (Age-adjusted baseline: 133 per 100,000 in 1987.)
2.5	Reduce dietary fat intake to an average of 30% of calories or less and average saturated fat intake less than 10% of calories among people aged 2 and older. (Baseline: 36% of calories from total fat and 13% from saturated fat for people aged 20 through 74 in 1976–80; 36% and 13% for women aged 19 through 50 in 1985.)
2.6	Increase complex carbohydrate and fiber-containing foods in the diets of adults to 5+ daily servings for vegetables (including legumes) and fruits, and to 6+ daily servings for grain products. (Baseline: 2½ servings of vegetables and fruits and 3 servings of grain products for women aged 19 through 50 in 1985.)
2.7	Increase to at least 50% the proportion of overweight people aged 12+ who have adopted sound dietary practices combined with regular physical activity to attain an appropriate body weight. (Baseline: 30% of overweight women and 25% of overweight men for people aged 18 and older in 1985.)
16.1	Reverse the rise in cancer deaths to achieve a rate of no more than 130 per 100,000 people. (Age-adjusted baseline: 133 per 100,000 in 1987.)
16.7	Reduce dietary fat intake to an average of 30% of calories or less and average saturated fat intake less than 10% of calories among people aged 2 and older. (Baseline: 36% of calories from total fat and 13% from saturated fat for people aged 20 through 74 in 1976–80; 36% and 13% for women aged 19 through 50 in 1985.)

Source: Adapted from *Healthy People 2000: National Health Promotion and Disease Prevention Objectives*, U.S. Department of Health and Human Services, Public Health Service, Publication No. 91-50212, 1991.

Exhibit 12-6 Model Nutrition Objective for Reduced Risk Reduction

By 19____, the chronic disease risk factor _____*_____ among (target population) will be reduced from _____% to _____%.

*Obesity; hypertension; elevated serum cholesterol; poor physical fitness; excess intake of dietary fat, cholesterol, sodium, alcohol, or sugar; inadequate intake of dietary fiber, fruits and vegetables, or calcium.

Source: Adapted from *Model State Nutrition Objectives*, The Association of State and Territorial Public Health Nutrition Directors, 1988.

REFERENCES

1. Wynder EL. Metabolic epidemiology and the causes of cancer, presented at UCLA Extension conference, Nutritional Medicine in Medical Practice; Santa Monica, Calif: January 22-23, 1993.

2. American Cancer Society. *Cancer Facts and Figures.* Atlanta, Ga: American Cancer Society; 1994.

3. National Cancer Institute. *Surveillance, Evaluation and End Result Data.* Bethesda, Md: National Cancer Institute; 1994.

4. National Cancer Institute. *Cancer Control Objectives for the Nation.* Bethesda, Md: National Cancer Institute; 1993.

5. Ogden J, Fox P. Examination of the use of smoking for weight control in restrained and unrestrained eaters. *Int J of Eating Disorders.* 1994;16:177-185.

6. Doll R, Peto R. The causes of cancer: Quantitative estimates of available risks of cancer in the United States today. *J Natl Cancer Inst.* 1981;66:1191-1308.

7. National Research Council. *Diet and Health: Implications for Reducing Chronic Disease Risk.* Washington, DC: National Academy Press; 1989.

8. Shapiro S, Venet W, Strax P, et al. *Periodic Screening for Breast Cancer. The Health Insurance Plan Project and Its Sequelae, 1963-1986.* Baltimore, Md: Johns Hopkins University Press; 1988.

9. Tabar L, Faqerberg CJ, Gad A, et al. Reduction in mortality from breast cancer after mass screening with mammography: Randomized trial from the breast cancer screening working group of the Swedish National Board of Health and Welfare. *Lancet.* 1985;1(8433):829-832.

10. Stenkvist B, Bergshrome R, Eklund G, et al. Papanicolaou smear screening & cervical cancer: What can you expect? *JAMA.* 1984;252:1423-1426.

11. National Cancer Institute. *Eating Tips: Tips and Recipes for Better Cancer Treatment.* Bethesda, Md: National Institutes of Health; 1994.

12. Pollack ES. Tracking cancer trends: Incidence and survival. *Hospital Practice.* 1984;19(8):99-102, 105-108, 111-112.

13. Mills PK, Beeson WL, Phillips RL, et al. Cohort study of diet, lifestyle, and prostate cancer in Adventist men. *Cancer.* 1989;64:598-604.

14. Enstrom JE, Kamin LE. Smoking cessation among California physicians: An example of cancer control progress. *Clin and Biol Res.* 1984;156:255-264.

15. Hunter CP, Redmond CK, Chen VW, et al. Breast cancer: Factors associated with stage at diagnosis in black and white women, black/white cancer survival study group. *J Natl Cancer Inst.* 1993;85:1129-1137.

16. Public Health Service. *Occupational Hazard Rates among Black Employees.* Bethesda, Md: US Department of Health and Human Services; 1985.

17. National Center for Nutrition and Dietetics. *Nutrition Fact Sheet: Focus on Fiber.* Chicago, Ill: American Dietetic Association; 1994.

18. Kurzer MS. Diet, estrogen and cancer. *Contemporary Nutr.* 1992;17(7):1-2.

19. Adlercreutz H. Western diet and Western diseases: Some hormonal and biochemical mechanisms and associations. *Scan J Clin Lab Invest.* 1990;50(Suppl):3-23.

20. Woods MN, Gorbach SL, Longcope C, et al. Low-fat, high-fiber diet and serum estrone sulfate in premenopausal women. *Am J Clin Nutr.* 1989;49:1179-1183.

21. Setchell KDR, Adlercreutz H. Mammalian lignins and phyto-oestrogens: Recent studies on their formation, metabolism and biological role in health and disease. In: Rowland IR, ed. *Role of the Gut Flora in Toxicity and Cancer.* London, England: Academic Press; 1988:316-345.

22. Messina M, Barnes S. The role of soy products in reducing risk of cancer. *J Natl Cancer Inst.* 1991;83:541-547.

23. Caragay AB. Cancer preventive foods and ingredients. *Food Technol.* April 1992;46:65-68.

24. Gustafson DR, Kurzer MS. Flavonoid inhibition of aromatase enzyme activity (AA) in human adipose stromal cells (ASC). *Fed Proc.* 1991;5(5):A931.

25. Adlercreutz H, Honjo H, Higashi A, et al. Urinary excretion of lignins and isoflavonoid phytoestrogens in Japanese

men and women consuming a traditional Japanese diet. *Am J Clin Nutr.* 1991;54:1093-1100.

26. Lee HP, Gourley L, Duffy SW, et al. Dietary effects on breast-cancer risk in Singapore. *Lancet.* 1991;337:1197-2000.

27. Messina M, Messina VJ. Increasing use of soyfoods and their potential role in cancer prevention. *J Am Diet Assoc.* 1991;91:836-840.

28. Makela S, Pylkkanen L, Santti R, et al. Role of plant estrogen and estrogen-related altered growth of the mouse prostate. In: *Effects of Food on the Immune and Hormonal Systems.* Schwerzenbach, Switzerland: Swiss Federal Institute of Technology and University of Zurich; 1991:135-139.

29. Thompson LU, Robb P, Serraino M, et al. Mammalian lignin production from various foods *Nutr Cancer.* 1991;16:43-52.

30. Adlercreutz H, Heikkinen R, Woods M, et al. Excretion of the lignins enterolactone and enterodiol and of equol in omnivorous and vegetarian postmenopausal women and in women with breast cancer. *Lancet.* 1982;1:1295-1299.

31. Adlercreutz H, Bannwart C, Wahala K, et al. Inhibition of human aromatase by mammal lignins and isoflavonoid phytoestrogens. *J Steroid Biochem Molec Biol.* 1993;44:147-153.

32. Adlercreutz H, Mousavi Y, Clark J, et al. Dietary phytoestrogens and cancer: In vitro and in vivo studies. *J Steroid Biochem Molec Biol.* 1992,41.331-337.

33. Mousavi Y, Adlercreutz H. Enterolactone and estradiol inhibit each other's proliferative effect on MCF-7 breast cancer cells in culture. *J Steroid Biochem Molec Biol.* 1992;41:615-619.

34. Potter JD. Reconciling the epidemiology, physiology, and molecular biology of colon cancer. *JAMA.* 1992;268:157-177.

35. Burkitt DP, Walker AR, Painter NS. Effects of dietary fiber on stools and the transit times, and its role in the causation of disease. *Lancet.* 1972;2(792):1408-1412.

36. Klurfeld DM. Dietary fiber-mediated mechanisms in carcinogenesis. *Cancer Res.* 1992;5:2055S-2059S.

37. Block G, Patterson B, Subar A. Fruit, vegetables, and cancer prevention: A review of the epidemiological evidence. *Nutr Cancer.* 1992;18:1-29.

38. Block G, Lanza E. Dietary fiber sources in the United States by demographic group. *J Natl Cancer Inst.* 1987;79:83-91.

39. Thompson LU. *Contemporary Nutrition.* Minneapolis, Minn: General Mills Inc; 1992.

40. Slavin JL. Dietary fiber and cancer update. *Contemporary Nutr.* 1992;17(8):1-2.

41. Bingham SA. Mechanisms and experimental and epidemiological evidence relating dietary fiber (non-starch polysaccharides) and starch to protection against large bowel cancer. *Proc Nutr Soc.* 1990;49:153-171.

42. Willett W. The search for the causes of breast and colon cancer. *Nature.* 1989;338:389-394.

43. Iscovich JM, Abbe KA, Castelleto R, et al. Colon cancer in Argentina: II. Risk from fiber, fat, and nutrients. *Int J Cancer.* 1992;51:858-861.

44. Freudenheim JF, Graham S, Horvath PJ, et al. Risks associated with source of fiber and fiber components in cancer of the colon and rectum. *Cancer Res.* 1990;50:3295-3300.

45. Willett WC, Stampfer MJ, Colditz GA, et al. Relation of meat, fat, and fiber intake to the risk of colon cancer in a prospective study among women. *N Engl J Med.* 1990;33:1664-1672.

46. Thun MJ, Calle EE, Namboodini MM, et al. Risk factors for fatal colon cancer in a large prospective study. *J Natl Cancer Inst.* 1992;84:1491-1500.

47. Rose DP. Dietary fiber, phytoestrogens, and breast cancer. *Nutrition.* 1992;8:47-51.

48. Howe GR, Hirohata T, Hislop TG, et al. Dietary factors and risk of breast cancer: Combined analysis of 12 case-control studies. *J Natl Cancer Inst.* 1990;82:561-569.

49. Graham S, Hellmann R, Marshall J, et al. Nutritional epidemiology of postmenopausal breast cancer in western New York. *Am J Epidemiol.* 1991;134:552-566.

50. Willett WC, Hunter DJ, Stampfer MJ, et al. Dietary fat and fiber in relation to risk of breast cancer: An 8-year fol low-up. *JAMA.* 1992;268:2037-2044.

51. Eastwood MA. The physiological effect of dietary fiber: An update. *Annual Rev Nutr.* 1992;12:19-35.

52. Lampe JW, Fredstrom SB, Slavin JL, et al. Sex differences in colonic function: A randomized trial. *Gut.* 1993;34:531-536.

53. Lampe JW, Slavin JL, Melcher EA, et al. Effects of cereal and vegetable fiber feeding on potential risk factors for colon cancer. *Cancer Epid Biomarkers Prevention.* 1992;1:207-211.

54. Kashtan H, Stern HS, Jenkins DJ, et al. Colonic fermentation and markers of colorectal-cancer risk. *Am J Clin Nutr.* 1992;55:723-728.

55. Lipkin M, Enker WE, Winawer SJ. Tritiated-thymidine labeling of rectal epithelial cells in "non-prep" biopsies of individuals at increased risk for colonic neoplasia. *Cancer Lett.* 1987;37:153-161.

56. Terpstra OT, van Blankenstein M, Dees J, et al. Abnormal pattern of cell proliferation in the entire colonic mucosa of patients with colon adenoma or cancer. *Gastroenterology.* 1987;92:704-708.

57. DeCosse JJ, Miller HH, Lesser ML. Effect of wheat fiber and vitamins C and E on rectal polyps in patients with familiar adenomatous polyposis. *J Natl Cancer Inst.* 1989;81:1290-1297.

58. Alberts DS, Einspahr J, Rees-McGee S, et al. Effects of dietary wheat bran fiber on rectal epithelial cell prolifera-

tion in patients with resection for colorectal cancers. *J Natl Cancer Inst.* 1990;8:1280-1285.

59. Rose DP, Goldman M, Connolly JM, et al. High fiber diet reduces serum estrogen concentration in premenopausal women. *Am J Clin Nutr.* 1991;54:520-525.

60. Rose DP. Plasma estrogens, diet, and breast cancer. *Nutrition.* 1990;7:139-140.

61. Cohen LA, Kendall ME, Zang E, et al. Modulation of N-nitromethylurea-induced mammary tumor promotion by dietary fiber and fat. *J Natl Cancer Inst.* 1991;83:496-501.

62. Boffa LC, Lupton JR, Mariani MR, et al. Modulation of colonic epithelial cell proliferation, histone acetylation, and luminal short chain fatty acids by variation of dietary fiber (wheat bran) in rats. *Cancer Res.* 1992;52:5906-5912.

63. Pilch SM. *Physiological Effects and Health Consequences of Dietary Fiber.* Bethesda, Md: Life Sciences Research Office, Federation of American Societies for Experimental Biology; 1987:149-157.

64. Ha YL, Grimm NK, Pariza MW. Anticarcinogens from fried ground beef: Heat altered derivatives of linoleic acid. *Carcinogenesis.* 1987;8:1881-1887.

65. Ip C, Carter CA, Ip MM. Requirement of essential fatty acid for mammary tumorigenesis in the rat. *Cancer Res.* 1985;45:1997-2001.

66. Kritchevsky D. Diet and cancer, conjugated linoleic acid in food: Scientists study its role as inhibitor of cancer-causing substances. *Food and Nutr News.* 1994;66(3):22-23.

67. Ip C, Chin SF, Scimeca JA, et al. Mammary cancer prevention by conjugated dienoic derivative of linoleic acid. *Cancer Res.* 1991;51:6118-6124.

68. Lee KN, Kritchevsky D, Pariza MW. Conjugated linoleic acid and atherosclerosis in rabbits. *Atheroscler.* 1994;108(1):19-25.

69. Nicolosi RJ, Courtemanche KV, Laitinen L, et al. Effect of feeding diets enriched in conjugated linoleic acid on lipoproteins and aortic atherogenesis in hamsters. *Circulation.* 1993;88(Suppl):2458.

70. Ip C, Singh M, Thompson HJ, et al. Conjugated linoleic acid suppresses mammary carcinogenesis and proliferation activity of the mammary gland in the rat. *Cancer Res.* 1994;54:1212-1215.

71. National Cancer Institute. *5-A-Day Initiative.* Bethesda, Md: National Cancer Institute; 1992.

72. American Cancer Society. *Food sources of Vitamin C, E, and Beta Carotene.* Public information brochure. Date unknown.

73. Human Nutrition Information Service. *Nationwide Food Consumption Survey: Continuing Survey of Food Intakes by Individuals. Women 19-50 Years and Children 1-5 Years, 1 Day, 1985.* Washington, DC: US Department of Agriculture; 1985:102.

74. Patterson BH, Block G, Rosenberger WF, et al. Fruit and vegetables in the American diet: Data from the NHANES II survey. *Am J Public Health.* 1990;80:1443-1449.

75. Hunt MK, Hebert JR, Sorensen G, et al. Impact of worksite cancer prevention program on eating patterns of workers. *J Soc Nutr Ed.* 1993;25:236-243.

76. Hebert JR, Harris DR, Sorensen G, et al. A work-site nutrition intervention: Its effects on the consumption of cancer-related nutrients. *Am J Public Health.* 1993;83: 391-394.

77. Willett WC, Reynolds RD, Cottnell-Hoehner S, et al. Validation of a semi-quantitative food frequency questionnaire: Comparison with a 1-year diet record. *J Am Diet Assoc.* 1987;87:43-47.

78. Chlebowski RT, Blackburn GL, Buzzard IM, et al. Adherence to a dietary fat intake reduction program in post menopausal women receiving therapy for early breast cancer. *J Clin Oncology.* 1993;11:2072-2080.

79. Buzzard IM, Asp EH, Chlebowski RT, et al. Diet intervention methods to reduce fat intake: Nutrient and food group composition of self-selected low-fat diets. *J Am Diet Assoc.* 1990;90:42-49.

80. Chlebowski RT, Nixon DW, Blackburn GL, et al. A breast cancer nutrition adjuvant study (NAS): Protocol design and initial patient adherence. *Breast Cancer Res Treat.* 1987;10:21-29.

81. Eddy DM. Screening for breast cancer. *Ann Intern Med.* 1989;111:389-399.

82. National Institutes of Health. *Women's Health Initiative.* Bethesda, Md: National Institutes of Health; 1994.

83. Willett W. *Nutritional Epidemiology.* New York, NY: Oxford University Press; 1990:69-126.

13

Diabetes Mellitus

Learning Objectives

- Identify the warning signs of insulin-dependent and non-insulin-dependent diabetes mellitus.
- Compare prevalence of diabetes mellitus among different ethnic groups.
- Identify risk factors for developing diabetes and its complications.
- Identify how medical nutrition therapy can reduce cardiovascular disease risks and other complications.

High Definition Nutrition

Complications—both insulin-dependent and non-insulin-dependent diabetes may precipitate tissue-damaging complications. Microvascular complications affect small blood vessels in three organ systems: retinopathy (the eyes), nephropathy (the kidneys), and neuropathy (the nerves).

Glycemic index (GI)—the area under the postprandial glucose curve for a particular food. It is expressed as a percentage of the response compared to a reference food such as white bread when the carbohydrate content is the same for both foods. The index is not popular and not widely used by medical professionals, but the public is sensitized to the concept.

HbA1c or glycated hemoglobin—describes glucose control over a three-month period by measuring the amount of glucose that becomes incorporated into hemoglobin. Hemoglobin is the blood protein molecule that transports oxygen to body tissues. A high percentage of HbA1c indicates poor control, whereas a low percentage ($\leq$6%) indicates good control.

Insulin-dependent diabetes mellitus—insulin-dependent diabetes mellitus (IDDM) or Type I diabetes commonly develops in people under 30 years of age. Insulin is required; without insulin, life-threatening diabetic ketoacidosis called diabetic coma occurs. IDDM accounts for 5 to 10% of all cases of diabetes.

Non-insulin-dependent diabetes mellitus—non-insulin-dependent diabetes (NIDDM) or Type II diabetes is the most common form of diabetes (90 to 95% of all cases). It generally begins in middle age but can occur earlier or later. Individuals are instructed to follow a modified eating and exercise pattern and placed on oral hypoglycemic drugs (e.g., biguanides or sulfonylureas); many receive insulin.

Tight control—a phrase that indicates blood glucose levels equal to a standard.

OVERVIEW OF DIABETES MELLITUS

Diabetes mellitus affects 14 million Americans, nearly 1 in every 20 people, creating over 500,000 new cases each year. The frightening fact is that only about 50% of diabetes cases are thought to be diagnosed. Early detection is the challenge. Distinct differences are noted for the incidence of diabetes among ethnic groups (see Table 13-1). Figure 13-1 illustrates the age-specific prevalence by ethnicity, sex, and age in the United States from 1988 to 1990. Diabetes is neither a "mild" disease nor a "curable" disease. Insulin is crucial to the daily survival of about a million people, but it is not a cure. People with diabetes are at risk for serious health complications.[1]

The complications are macrovascular and/or microvascular. Macrovascular complications are due to atherosclerosis of large blood vessels. The result is reduced blood flow to tissues. Complications include angina, heart attacks, strokes, and amputations. Smoking, high blood pressure, and abnormal blood lipid levels are additional risk factors, with complications including heart disease, stroke, kidney disease, blindness, nerve damage, and severe infection leading to gangrene and foot and leg amputations[1] (see Table 13-2). Microvascular complications lead to visual loss,

Table 13-1   Diabetes Rates by Ethnicity, United States

Ethnic Group	Rate
Caucasians	1 in 20
African Americans	1 in 10
Asian Americans	1 in 8
Latinos	1 in 7
Native Americans	1 in 4

Source: Data from American Diabetes Association, 1993.

kidney failure, and multiple neurological symptoms. Some patients experience pain, burning, and loss of sensation in their lower limbs as a neurological complication.

An individual with diabetes cannot uptake glucose from the blood into energy for cellular use. High levels of glucose in the blood and urine result. Individuals with diabetes have a genetic tendency to develop the disease, but the environment also has an impact.

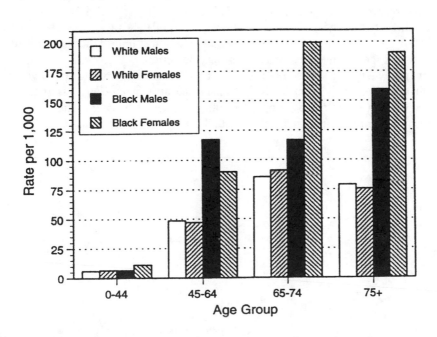

Figure 13-1 US average age-specific prevalence of diabetes by race, sex, and age, 1988-1990. *Source:* Reprinted from *Diabetes Surveillance, 1993*, p. 17, U.S. Department of Health and Human Services, Public Health Service, Centers for Disease Control and Prevention, 1993.

Table 13–2 Percentage of Complications from Diabetes Mellitus per Year, United States

Complications	Insulin Dependent	Non-Insulin Dependent*
Retinopathy		
• Proliferative	25%	10%
Nephropathy	34%	19%
Neuropathy		
• Autonomic	20–40%	20–40%
• Male impotence	35–75%	35–75%

*The total number of complications are greater for NIDDM due to the greater prevalence of cases.

Source: Data from the American Diabetes Association, 1994.

In normal metabolism, glucose is absorbed from the digestive tract, transported by the blood to the body's cells, and assisted by insulin to enter the cells. The cells either use the glucose for immediate energy or store it. Insulin is a hormone produced by the pancreas. Individuals with diabetes may lack sufficient insulin, have a defect in insulin function, or have decreased receptors on cells. Body cells are then unable to use the glucose, which increases in the blood and spills into the urine. To prevent complications, blood glucose levels must be kept near a normal range.[1]

There are two main types of diabetes with distinctly different warning signs (see Table 13–3). Insulin-dependent diabetes mellitus (IDDM) occurs most often in children and young adults and requires treatment with insulin injec-tions that is coordinated with dietary and physical activity habits. This form of diabetes was previously called juvenile-onset diabetes or Type I. Approximately 5% of all cases are IDDM. Non-insulin-dependent diabetes mellitus (NIDDM) or Type II diabetes occurs most often in adults over 40, especially the obese. This type has previously been called adult-onset diabetes. The adults most at risk for diabetes are those who are overweight; over 40; have a family history of diabetes; or are of black, Hispanic, or Native American descent.[1] Approximately 95% of all diabetes cases are NIDDM. The most important public health goal is early detection.

Type I diabetes may result from a genetically transmitted autoimmune process that destroys insulin-producing beta cells of the pancreas,[2] but not all carriers develop the disease. In some indi-

Table 13–3 The Warning Signs of Diabetes

IDDM	NIDDM
Rapid onset	Gradual onset
Frequent urination	Any of the insulin-dependent symptoms
Excessive thirst	Unrecognized symptoms
Extreme hunger	Recurring or hard-to-heal skin, gum, or bladder
Dramatic weight loss	infections
Irritability	Fatigue
Weakness and fatigue	Blurred vision
Nausea and vomiting	Tingling or numbness in hands or feet
	Itching

Source: Adapted from *Who We Are, What We Do*, p. 1, with permission of the American Diabetes Association, © 1988.

viduals, the process interacts with the early consumption of cow's milk.[3-7]

The American Academy of Pediatrics Committee on Nutrition reexamined their 1983 position paper in light of current research.[8] The low iron concentration and bioavailability of cow's milk and the possibility of blood loss motivated the committee to recommend exclusion of whole cow's milk during the first year of life to decrease the incidence of iron-deficiency anemia. The preferred food during the first year of life is breast milk. When breastfeeding is discontinued, iron-fortified infant formula rather than cow's milk is the best substitute throughout the first year of life.[2]

Diabetes, in fact, is sometimes considered an accelerated model of aging. Not only do its complications mimic the physiologic changes that can accompany old age, but its victims have shorter-than-average life expectancies.

RECOMMENDED EATING PATTERN FOR PATIENTS WITH NIDDM

NIDDM is a heterogeneous disorder demonstrated by insulin resistance and abnormalities in insulin secretion.[9,10] A clear genetic susceptibility for NIDDM exists, but environmental factors play a major role. Diet, physical fitness, and obesity affect insulin resistance.[9,11-13] Obesity is a major predisposing factor and found in approximately 80% of people who develop NIDDM.[14]

Medical nutrition therapy goals for NIDDM patients are[15]:

- to implement self-management training
- to achieve physiologic blood glucose levels with self-monitoring
- to maintain desirable plasma lipids
- to attain and maintain a reasonable body weight

The rationale is to reduce microvascular complication (i.e., neuropathy, nephropathy, and retinopathy) and to retard the atherosclerotic macrovascular disease. The development of microvascular complications is linked to lack of glycemic control,[16] whereas atherosclerosis is associated with risk factors of NIDDM (e.g., obesity, dyslipidemia, hyperinsulinemia, hypertension, platelet dysfunction, and other metabolic abnormalities unique to diabetes).[1]

Physical activity, oral hypoglycemic agents (e.g., metformin, a biguanide), and eating behavior are the focus to prevent macrovascular complications. This is important, because deaths from cardiovascular disease occur two to three times more often in diabetics compared to nondiabetics and represent the major cause of death in patients with NIDDM.[17,18] Biochemical indicators of diabetes control are outlined in Table 13-4. Hypertriglyceridemia and hypercholesterolemia are more common among individuals with diabetes than in the general population. They are major risk factors for coronary heart disease (CHD) in persons with diabetes.[19] At any level of serum cholesterol, mortality from CHD is three to five times greater among persons with diabetes compared to persons who are not diabetic.[19]

An optimal eating pattern for NIDDM patients is moderate in protein (12 to 20%) and moderate in carbohydrate and fat. There is no restriction in mono- or disaccharides if total energy intake promotes a reasonable body weight.[20] This type of eating pattern demonstrates that glycemic control can occur with a varied eating pattern. If serum cholesterol levels are elevated, individuals should have eating patterns low in both total and saturated fat.[19-23] Monounsaturated fatty acids do not appear to provide an added benefit. The American Diabetes Association recommends increasing the fiber content of foods to prevent colorectal cancer and views the general alcohol recommendation of one alcoholic beverage a day as acceptable.[24,25] The key is to customize the eating pattern for acceptance and glycemic control.

Blood sugar may vary in its response to different foods, but the glycemic index (GI) is not used widely. High carbohydrate diets may adversely effect glycemic control, raise very-low-density lipoprotein (VLDL) and triglyceride levels, and reduce high-density lipoprotein (HDL) cholesterol levels.[26,27] Foods with low GI values produce low postprandial glycemic levels. Most grain products, breads, and cereals have a high GI. Legumes in-

Table 13-4 Biochemical Indices and Values for Evaluation of Diabetes Mellitus Control

Biochemical Index	Normal*	Acceptable	Fair	Poor
Fasting plasma glucose	115	140	200	>200 mg/dL
Postprandial plasma glucose	140	175	235	>235 mg/dL
Glycosylated (glycated) hemoglobin	6	8	10	>10%
Fasting plasma cholesterol	200	225	250	>250 mg/dL
Fasting plasma triglyceride	150	175	200	>200 mg/dL

*Adjust for normal values of laboratory; increase limits for elderly patients.

Source: Adapted from Diabetes Care, Vol. 16, No. 2, pp. 106–112, with permission of the American Diabetes Association, © 1993.

cluding beans, peas, and lentils; pastas; and whole grains like oats, barley, and corn; and raw fruits have a low GI. Total and soluble dietary fiber content of food and the form of starch granules influence the GI. White pasta and some legumes are either less accessible or inhibit the activity of digestive enzymes.[28]

Monounsaturated fat may not increase and may even lower low-density lipoprotein (LDL) cholesterol levels.[29-31] LDL cholesterol levels may not change, VLDL and triglyceride levels may decline, and HDL cholesterol levels may increase when more than 50% of the food energy is from fat and about 35% is from carbohydrate compared to a 60% or higher carbohydrate eating pattern. Other studies have shown that if high-carbohydrate diets are primarily refined and also high in dietary fiber, then adverse effects on glycemic control, VLDL, and triglycerides may not occur.[22,24,26,32,33]

Weight loss lowers insulin resistance and improves glucose use.[34] The Prospective Diabetes Study in the United Kingdom[35] evaluated the response of 3,044 new NIDDM patients to dietary modification. Overweight or obese patients followed a three-month, low-calorie diet that had 30% of calories from fat. Of the patients, 16% with a 13% reduction in body weight experienced a near normal fasting plasma glucose due to the weight loss.

Twenty urban, free-living, obese native Hawaiians received a high-fiber, 7% fat, and 78% carbohydrate diet.[36] They could eat when and as much as they wanted. An automatic decline in energy intake of about 1,000 kcal per day occurred three

months later. In addition, a significant mean weight loss of 17 pounds with a range of 4.4 to 33 pounds was observed. Fasting serum glucose declined from 160 mg/dL to 122 mg/dL. Hypoglycemia was common for several women, warranting a change in medications. Significantly lower fasting serum triglycerides, total cholesterol, LDL cholesterol, and systolic and diastolic blood pressures were also reported.

Ten overweight NIDDM patients living in Derby, Western Australia, were returned to a seven-week hunter-gatherer existence.[37] All experienced a reduction in dietary fat from 40% of calories to 13% of calories. Physical activity increased, and an average weight loss of 17.6 pounds occurred. Fasting plasma glucose concentrations declined from 207 mg/dL to 118 mg/dL, and a significant reduction in fasting plasma insulin and triglycerides occurred.

One can identify the optimal carbohydrate-containing foods for persons with diabetes by using the postprandial glycemic effect of foods.[38] In one 12-week crossover study, high- and low-GI diets were compared.[39] Glycemic control improved for individuals on the low-GI diet compared with those on the high-GI diet. The low-GI diet produced a lower eight-hour plasma glucose profile, less glycosuria, and a significantly lower glycosylated hemoglobin level (i.e., 7.0 ± 0.3% versus 7.9 ± 0.5%).[37]

A few studies have compared eating pattern with meal frequency. Smaller, frequent meals can reduce postprandial insulin secretion and enhance peripheral tissue insulin sensitivity.[40,41] A one-day evaluation among 11 NIDDM patients showed that "nibblers" who consumed food with hourly snacks had significant reductions in mean blood glucose, serum insulin, and C-peptide concentration during a 9.5-hour study period when compared with those who ate three meals and one snack.[42] This suggests that eating over a longer period ("grazing") and consuming foods that are slowly absorbed (foods high in soluble fiber) or that have a low GI can be beneficial.

Secondary and tertiary prevention in the form of nutrition counseling that leads to self-management may lower additional medical cost for individuals with diabetes. Two examples of nutrition intervention and the reported savings due to the intervention are described in Exhibit 13–1.

THE DIABETES CONTROL AND COMPLICATIONS TRIAL

The Diabetes Control and Complications Trial was a multicenter, randomized clinical trial designed to compare intensive with conventional diabetes therapy and the effects on the development and progression of the early vascular and neurologic complications of IDDM.[43-45]

A total of 1,441 patients 13 to 39 years old were recruited at 29 centers from 1983 through 1989. In June 1993, after an average follow up of 6.5 years (range 3 to 9 years), the independent data monitoring committee[46] determined that the study results warranted terminating the trial.

Conventional therapy (*N* = 143 patients) consisted of one or two daily injections of insulin that contained mixed, intermediate, and rapid-acting insulins; daily self-monitoring of urine or blood glucose; and extensive education about a tailored eating pattern and exercise.[43,47] The goals of conventional therapy included the absence of symptoms attributable to glycosuria or hyperglycemia; the absence of ketonuria; the maintenance of normal growth, development, and reasonable body weight; and freedom from severe or frequent hypoglycemia.

Intensive therapy (*N* = 77 patients) included the administration of insulin three or more times daily by injection or an external pump. The pump dosage was adjusted according to the results of self-monitoring of blood glucose performed at least four times per day, dietary intake (see Table 13–5), and anticipated exercise. The goals of the intensive therapy were as follows:

- preprandial blood glucose concentrations between 70 and 120 mg per deciliter (i.e., 3.9 to 6.7 mmol per liter)
- postprandial concentrations of less than 180 mg per deciliter (i.e., 10 mmol per liter)
- a weekly 3 AM measurement of greater than 65 mg per deciliter (i.e., 3.6 mmol per liter)
- HbA1c monthly measurement within the normal range (e.g., less than 6.05%)[44]

Adherence and effectiveness were reflected in the substantial difference over time between the HbA1c values of the intensive therapy group and those of the conventional therapy group. A statistically significant difference in the average HbA1c value was maintained after baseline between the intensive therapy and conventional therapy groups in both cohorts (p <0.001).

After five years, the cumulative incidence of retinopathy in the intensive therapy group was approximately 50% less than in the conventional therapy group. After an average of six years of follow up, retinopathy developed in 23 patients in the intensive therapy group and 91 patients in the conventional therapy group. Intensive therapy lowered the adjusted mean risk of retinopathy by 76%, with a 95% confidence interval of 62% to 85%.

During the study period, intensive therapy reduced the average risk of retinopathy progression by 54% (95% confidence interval of 39% to 66%). Intensive therapy reduced hypercholesterolemia by 34%, defined as a serum concentration of low-density lipoprotein cholesterol greater than 160 mg per deciliter or 4.14 mmol per liter (95% confidence interval of 7% to 54%, p = 0.02). When all major cardiovascular and peripheral vascular events were combined, intensive therapy reduced the risk of macrovascular disease by 41%. This was 0.5 events per 100 patient-years, from 0.8 events (95% confidence interval of 10% to 68%).[44]

Exhibit 13-1 Cost-Savings Examples of Secondary Prevention in Diabetes

---

EXAMPLE 1

Site:	Physician office, Springfield, Illinois
Patient:	46-year-old male with NIDDM, hyperlipidemia, and obesity; diet only.
RD Intervention:	Comprehensive diabetes education (8 hours in group sessions) and 6 follow-up visits (individualized)
Health Outcome:	Lost 46.8 lbs. Reduced fasting blood sugar from 165 to 86 mg/dL; hemoglobin A1C reduced from 7.0 to 4.6%. Cholesterol reduced from 280 to 142 mg/dL. Triglycerides reduced from 250 to 80 mg/dL. Risk of heart disease and diabetes complications reduced. Blood pressure reduced to 164/98 mm Hg. Symptoms disappeared.

Cost Savings (based on 5 years):

Oral hypoglycemic agent	$ 780.00
Cholesterol-lowering medication	3720.00
Liver function tests to monitor side effects of hypocholesterolemic medication	224.00
Hypertension medication	1740.00
Total	$6464.00

RD Intervention Cost: −245.00
Intervention Benefit (Cost Savings): $6219.00
(Compiled by Anne Daly, RD, MS, CDE)

EXAMPLE 2

Site:	Teaching Hospital Clinic, Boston, Massachusetts
Patient:	43-year-old woman with gestational diabetes. Referred to RD/CDE for nutrition assessment and management of diabetes and pregnancy. Strong family history of NIDDM—both parents, several aunts and uncles. Initial glycohemoglobin 6.4%. Glucose Tolerance Test Fasting = 100 mg/dL, 1 hr = 231 mg/dL, 2 hr = 146 mg/dL, 3 hr = 164 mg/dL.
RD Intervention:	Comprehensive assessment and treatment plan with an individualized 1800-calorie meal plan, reinforce instruction in self-monitoring blood glucose (SMBG), and ketone testing. Brief follow-up visit to assess weight gain and SMBG results.
Health Outcome:	Vaginal delivery (induced at 38 weeks due to ruptured membranes) resulting in normal weight baby boy 6 pounds, 10 ounces. Apgar score of 9, without respiratory distress and normal blood sugars.
Cost Savings:	Avoided C-section delivery of macrosomic baby (C-section 6-day stay $7,230 − vaginal delivery 3-day stay $4,095) = $3,135
RD Intervention Cost:	RD/CDE comprehensive appointment ($55) + RD/CDE follow up appointment ($25) = −80
Cost Savings:	$3,055

Source: Reprinted from DCE Cost-Savings Data Collection, *On the Cutting Edge*, Winter 1993, p. 22, with permission of the American Dietetic Association, © 1993.

Table 13–5 Dietary Guidelines Used in the Diabetes Control and Complications Trial

Dietary Component	Guideline
Energy	To achieve and maintain 90% to 120% of reasonable body weight and/or provide for normal growth and development
Carbohydrate	50% of total daily energy intake; 45% to 55% is the acceptable range. Simple sugars should contribute no more than 25% of energy from carbohydrate
Fat	30% of total energy intake with upper acceptable limit of 35%
Cholesterol	Intake of no more than 600 mg/day. Amended in July 1988 to be consistent with the National Cholesterol Education Program Step 1 guidelines (i.e., intake of cholesterol <300 mg/day; total fat <30% of total energy; saturated fatty acids <10% of total energy; polyunsaturated fatty acids up to 10% of total energy; monounsaturated fatty acids 10% to 15% of total energy)
Polyunsaturated to saturated fat ratio	One is desirable; 0.8 is the acceptable lower limit.
Fiber	Encouraged without use of pharmacologic fiber supplements
Alcohol	In moderation
Protein	10% to 25% of total daily energy intake but no less than 0.8 g/kg for adults, 0.84 g/kg for persons aged 15 to 18 years, and 1.0 g/kg for persons aged 11 to 14 years

Source: Adapted from DCCT. Nutrition Interventions for Intensive Therapy in the Diabetes Control and Complications Trial, *Journal of the American Dietetic Association,* Vol. 93, No. 7, pp. 768–772, with permission of the American Dietetic Association, © 1993.

The incidence of severe hypoglycemia, including multiple episodes in some patients, was approximately three times higher in the intensive therapy group than in the conventional therapy group (p <0.001). In the intensive therapy group, there were 62 hypoglycemic episodes per 100 patient-years in which assistance was required, as compared with 19 such episodes per 100 patient-years in the conventional therapy group. This included 16 and 5 episodes of coma or seizure per 100 patient-years in the respective groups.

There were no deaths, myocardial infarctions, or strokes definitely attributable to hypoglycemia, and no significant differences between groups with regard to the number of major accidents requiring hospitalization (20 in the intensive therapy group and 22 in the conventional therapy group). There were two fatal motor vehicle accidents, one in each group, in which hypoglycemia

may have had a causative role. In addition, a person not involved in the trial was killed in a motor vehicle accident involving a car driven by a patient in the intensive therapy group who was probably hypoglycemia. There were 54 brief hospitalizations to treat severe hypoglycemia in 40 patients in the intensive therapy group, as compared with 36 hospitalizations in 27 patients in the conventional therapy group. This includes 7 and 4 hospitalizations, respectively, to treat hypoglycemia-related injuries.

Weight gain was a problem for individuals who received intensive therapy.[48] There was a 33% increase in the mean adjusted risk of becoming overweight (defined as a body weight more than 120% above the ideal). There were 12.7 cases of excess weight per 100 patient-years in the intensive therapy group, versus 9.3 in the conventional therapy group. At five years, patients who received intensive therapy had gained a mean of 4.6 kg more than patients who received conventional therapy.

The final recommendations from the study were as follows:

- Most individuals with IDDM should be treated with closely monitored intensive regimens, with the goal of maintaining their glycemic status as close to the normal range as safely possible.
- Due to the risk of hypoglycemia, intensive therapy should be implemented with caution, especially in patients with repeated severe hypoglycemia or those unaware of hypoglycemia.
- The risk-benefit ratio with intensive therapy may be less favorable in children under 13 years of age and in patients with advanced complications, such as end-stage renal disease or cardiovascular or cerebrovascular disease.
- Individuals with proliferative or severe nonproliferative retinopathy may be at high risk for accelerated retinopathy after the start of intensive therapy and should be followed closely by their ophthalmologists.[49,50]

The Diabetes Control and Complications Trial did not include individuals with NIDDM. Hyperglycemia is associated with the presence or progression of complications in NIDDM, as it is in IDDM.[51,52] The main conclusions of this trial emphasize the benefits of reducing glycemia in IDDM. However, these conclusions are applicable to individuals with NIDDM. Care should be taken to address age, capabilities, and coexisting diseases when defining the preferred management. Health care professionals should be cautious about the use of therapies other than medical nutrition therapy that are aimed at achieving euglycemia in patients with NIDDM.[45,52]

HYPERTENSION IN DIABETES

People with diabetes are an important and growing subset of the hypertensive population.

Of diabetic complications, 30% to 75% can be attributed to hypertension. The control of hypertension is essential to reduce the likelihood of stroke and coronary heart disease. By controlling hypertension, one can slow the progression of renal failure and potential onset of heart disease.[53]

An optimal blood pressure level has not been identified, but a systolic pressure less than 120 mm Hg and a diastolic pressure less than 80 mm Hg appears advantageous. If neuropathy or micro- or macrovascular complications are present, less than 130/85 mm Hg is considered a normal pressure.

Elevated blood pressure can be reduced with weight loss of 4 to 8 kg minimum, limiting sodium intake to 2,400 mg per day, limiting alcohol intake to no more than two drinks a day, increasing exercise from three to four times a week, and stopping smoking. Alternate approaches include an increase in potassium, calcium, and fish oil, with a decrease in total fat and caffeine intakes. An acute 5 to 15 mm Hg increase in blood pressure is noted 15 minutes after ingestion of 250 mg of caffeine. These alternate approaches to reducing blood pressure vary in effect among individuals, and they remain the focus of continued research.[53]

DIABETES AND DISORDERED EATING

Diabetes may predispose some individuals to aberrant eating patterns. Several physiologic and psychodynamic risk factors are identified, and stages of progression to disordered eating have been described[54] (see Exhibit 13–2). An acute concern for individuals with diabetes who have a disordered eating pattern is ketoacidosis, which results from severe hypoglycemia or hyperglycemia.[55]

The hypoglycemia condition results from food restrictions, delayed meals or snacks, purging to vomit food, frequent use of laxatives or enemas, and excess insulin to hide overeating or binging. Hyperglycemia may be acute or can span several hours. It is strengthened by lack of judgment

Exhibit 13-2 Stages of Progression to Disordered Eating

ABNORMAL EATING

- May or may not eat in response to dysphoria.
- Deliberately "cheats."
- Overeats at meals frequently.

COMPULSIVE EATING

- Loses concept of normal eating.
- Binges at mealtimes.
- Hoards food.
- Has feelings of being denied food that others are allowed.

ADDICTIVE EATING

- Manipulates to obtain food.
- Denies eating.
- Feels guilty about eating.
- Anxious about not having enough food.

EATING DISORDER

- Obsessed with weight and food.
- Has a body-image distortion.
- Binges at meal or nonmeal times.
- Starves.
- Purges to relieve guilt or anxiety or to maintain weight, including skipping insulin.
- Uses food as weapon.

Source: Adapted from Davidow, D.N., and Turner, M., Complications of Coexisting Diabetes Mellitus and Eating Disorders in IDDM, *On the Cutting Edge*, Vol. 15, No. 6, p. 9, with permission of the American Dietetic Association, © 1994.

---

during the stressful period around a binge, inappropriate management of insulin and other medications, and lack of attention to self-care.[56,57] A cluster analysis compiling data from 26 adults with diabetes (12 insulin-dependent and 14 non-insulin-dependent) identified everyday problem situations that cause overeating (see Table 13-6).[57]

Rapid weight gain from fluid retention or insulin edema and efficient use of food energy frequently occurs when blood glucose returns to a normal range. The success in glucose control complicates the management of disordered eating, as the individual may be very anxious about the weight gain and react with a purge or binge.[58] A successful strategy has been flexible insulin administration, which involves allowing the individual to administer an amount of insulin consistent with the amount of food energy consumed. Adjustments are made for premeal blood glucose, exercise plans, and any potential stressors that may occur. Individuals given this liberalization of management should be able to deal honestly with themselves and the amount of food they eat. Individuals with unsuccessful management of eating and diabetes may require counseling with a psychotherapist to curb the binging behavior and regulate their blood glucose levels while taking care of their personal needs.[58]

Table 13–6 Problems That Cause Overeating among Individuals with Diabetes

Situation	Description
Negative emotions	Individual is tempted to overeat to cope with stress and negative emotions.
Resisting temptation	Food, food cues, or cravings are temptations to eat inappropriate foods.
Eating out	Eating at restaurants makes adherence difficult.
Feeling deprived	Individual is tempted to give up trying because of feelings of deprivation.
Time pressure	Time pressure makes eating right or treating reactions very difficult.
Temptation to relapse	Individual considers giving up and no longer trying to eat right.
Planning	Hectic life makes planning what and when to eat difficult.
Competing priorities	Responsibilities and obligations get in the way of eating right.
Social events	Parties, holidays, and socializing are temptations to overeat and make poor food choices.
Family support	Family's behaviors are less than supportive.
Food refusal	People offer inappropriate foods, and it is difficult to refuse without hurting their feelings.
Friends' support	Friends' behaviors are less than supportive.

Source: Adapted from Schlundt, D.G., Emotional Eating, *On the Cutting Edge*, Vol. 15, No. 6, p. 19, with permission of the American Dietetic Association, © 1994.

Info Line

RESOURCES

For a complete, up-to-date list of materials for comprehensive diabetes education, request *Selected Diabetes and Nutrition Education Resources: For the Person with Diabetes* (1994), 80 pages, with a user-friendly index, icons for interpreting the source, and ethnic-specific identifiers. Listings were chosen if they were published between 1989 and 1994, they use the 1989 exchange list, and they are written for individuals who have diabetes and their families. Diabetes Care and Education Practice Group of the American Dietetic Association, 216 W. Jackson Blvd., Suite 800, Chicago, IL 60606-6995.

VIDEOS

Food Guide Pyramid for Persons with Diabetes, National Health Video, Inc., 1994; 16 minutes; $79.95. This video introduces the food pyramid and compares the pyramid to the diabetic exchange lists. Variety, proportion, moderation, and flexibility are addressed. Lower-fat food choices within each group, a brief mention of the importance of label reading, and avoidance of excessive amounts of sodium are given.

How to Read the New Food Label for Persons with Diabetes, National Health Video, Inc., 12021 Wilshire Blvd., Suite 550, Los Angeles, CA 90025. (800) 543-6803. FAX (310) 476-0503. 1994; 13 minutes; $79.95. Points covered include: sugars in foods, serving sizes, nutrients included on the food labels, daily values (DVs), and health claims.

MANAGEMENT STRATEGIES

All people do not follow similar eating patterns, nor do they eat at the same times or places each day. Tastes, cultural differences, and economics influence the eating patterns of individuals with diabetes as much as they influence people without diabetes.

The goal of secondary prevention approaches is to help individuals develop self-management skills. The approaches vary and may evolve around the American Dietetic Association (ADA) exchange list, the USDA Food Guide Pyramid, or counting the total available glucose in foods.[59] Meal planning alternatives need flexibility and ease of understanding. Table 13–7 summarizes various meal-planning approaches, including the degree of complexity and orientation toward glycemic control and weight loss. Medical nutrition therapy was central to the intensive intervention in the Diabetes Control and Complications Trial (DCCT). Post-DCCT recommendations emphasize goals, not rules or regulation; practical and achievable recommendations; and custom-

ized or tailored plans. Benefits for the DCCT intensive-therapy group included neuropathy reduced by 60%; microalbuminuria decreased by 39% for people with no renal disease at baseline and severe albuminuria slowed by over 54%; retinopathy reduced by 76% in primary prevention and by 54% in secondary prevention groups compared with conventional-therapy groups. The current nutrition management strategies for IDDM and NIDDM are presented below.[20,60,61]

IDDM

- If receiving conventional therapy, maintain a consistent timing and amount of food, match insulin with food preferences, disregard fractionated calories using snacks, but synchronize food with insulin.

- Monitor blood glucose and adjust short-acting insulin in relation to the amount of food eaten.

- If multiple injections or the insulin pump is used, integrate insulin with lifestyle (e.g.,

Table 13–7 Characteristics of Various Eating Pattern Strategies

Strategy	Type of Approach*	Degree of Emphasis** Weight Loss/Glycemic Control		Degree of Literacy	Structure	Complexity
US dietary guidelines	a	M	L	L	L	L
Basic four	b	L	L	L	L	L
Personal guidelines	a	M	M	L	M	L
Healthy food choices	a,c	M	M	L	M	L
Food exchange lists	c	M	M–H	M–H	M–H	M–H
High CHO high fiber (HCF)	c	M	M–H	M–H	M–H	M–H
Calorie counting	d	H	L	M	H	M
Total available glucose (TAG)	d	L	H	H	H	H
Point system	d	M	M	M	M	M
Food-choice plan	e	M	M	L	M	L
Individual menus	e	M–H	M–H	L	M	L

*Type of approach corresponding to number is: a = basic nutrition guidelines; b = basic four food groups or food guide pyramid; c = exchange; d = counting approaches; and e = menu planning.
**The degree of emphasis is coded as L = low, M = medium, and H = high.

Source: Adapted from Green, J.A., Diabetes Nutrition Management: A Need for Meal Planning Alternatives, *Diabetes Educator*, Vol. 13, p. 146, with permission of the American Diabetes Association, © 1987.

adjust premeal insulin doses to exercise and food alterations).

- Strive for consistency and optimal blood glucose level.
- Alter dietary composition (i.e., fat, carbohydrate, and protein), based on other risk factors and biochemical measures.
- Recognize that sucrose and fructose have no significant advantage or disadvantage and can be a part of the overall pattern.

NIDDM

- Strive for moderate weight loss of 10 to 20 pounds, with the goal to achieve a "reasonable body weight."
- Space smaller meals and snacks throughout the day to attenuate postmeal hypoglycemia due to impaired insulin secretion.
- Develop an exercise program that can be followed.
- Use a weight-control eating pattern that has either a reduced-calorie (eating 500 fewer kcal/day) or very low-calorie pattern (<800 total kcal/day).
- Dietary composition applies as outlined for IDDM.
- Maintain an intense, ongoing program with contact at one- or two-week intervals.

Additional Strategies

Conducting counseling sessions with individuals with diabetes requires baseline data, an instruction plan with user-friendly materials, and a follow-up strategy. Basic information to be assessed at initial consultations is outlined in Table 13–8.

After the initial one or two visits, a strategy to ensure adherence for a new lifestyle is warranted. It cannot be overemphasized that newly diagnosed individuals with diabetes as well as veterans of the disease need continuous booster sessions. Reinforcement of their positive efforts and realignment of misconceptions and unhealthy practices

are essential to maintain control. Exhibit 13–3 delineates adherence techniques for health care providers.

Info Line

The American Diabetes Association is a nonprofit organization of professionals and volunteers who are concerned with diabetes and its complications. A central theme of diabetes care is to know the causes and strategies to manage high and low blood sugar levels. Spanish and English versions of materials are often available (see Figure 13–2). The association extends to more than 70 countries with over 800 affiliates.

The American Diabetes Association funds meritorious research, publishes the latest scientific findings, and provides services to people with diabetes, their families, health care professionals, and the public. *Diabetes Forecast* is a monthly publication of the American Diabetes Association for the public. It translates research data into layperson's terms and highlights events in the lives of individuals living with diabetes. For more information, contact The American Diabetes Association, Customer Service Department, 1660 Duke Street, Alexandria, VA 22314. Telephone 800-232-3472 or 703-549-1500.

OPPORTUNITIES FOR VOLUNTEERS

A nonprofit organization (e.g., the American Diabetes Association) may be the central resource for diabetes education in a community. The strength of any nonprofit organization depends on the size and enthusiasm of its volunteer force. Family members often become avid volunteers and, in the process, learn how to assist their own family members better. In Los Angeles, the Latino Outreach Programs of the American Diabetes Association provide volunteer opportunities targeted to high-risk groups. For example, volunteers can sign up to assist with the following:

Table 13–8 Baseline and Follow-Up Data To Assist Medical Nutrition Therapy of Diabetes Mellitus

Data	*Component*
Medical/clinical data	Type of diabetes (e.g., IDDM, NIDDM, impaired glucose tolerance, gestational diabetes mellitus) Onset of diabetes Treatment regimen: diet alone, type/amount/schedule of insulin, and oral hypoglycemic agent Medication other than for diabetes Glucose/ketone monitoring methods Health history, including medical problems in addition to diabetes (e.g., allergies, cancer, ulcers) Medical problems associated with diabetes (e.g., renal, hypertension, lipidemia) Family medical history (e.g., other members with diabetes, hypertension, cardio-vascular disease, obesity)
Biochemical data	Blood glucose values: lipids • cholesterol (low- and high-density lipoproteins) • triglycerides Glycated (glycosulated) hemoglobin, blood pressure, proteinuria, creatinine
Anthropometric data	Age, sex, height, weight, frame size, growth rate (children and pregnant women)
Nutrition data	Previous diets or instructions Weight history Use of vitamin/mineral supplements Exercise or activity level Current daily schedule and/or school schedule, workdays/weekends Meal frequency, allergies, and alcohol use Physical factors affecting nutrition • dentation • swallowing problems • sense of smell/taste • diarrhea/constipation Meals away from home
Psychosocial/economic	Patient's expectations and goals Family situation/living situation • who prepares meals • for how many people Financial situation Educational background Employment and/or school schedule • type of job • hours Cooking facilities, food refrigeration, etc. Ethnic or religious considerations

Source: Adapted from *Nutrition Guide for Professionals: Diabetes Education and Meal Planning* by M.A. Powers, ed., p. 10, with permission of the American Diabetes Association and the American Dietetic Association, © 1988.

Exhibit 13-3 Techniques for Encouraging Adherence

- Involve the individual and the primary decision maker as a vital part of the team.
- Establish a supportive working relationship by being nonjudgmental, positive, and helpful.
- Use appropriate language for the individual's understanding.
- Address the individual's concerns.
- Meet his/her expectations.
- Enlist the family and include them in the education process.
- Individualize the medical nutrition therapy to the individual's lifestyle.
- Give feedback on progress: blood glucose, glycosylated hemoglobin, lipid levels, weight.
- Use contingency plans.
- Use relapse prevention therapy.
- Use role-playing scenarios for decision making.
- Schedule frequent follow up.
- Reward adherence to medical regimens.

Source: Adapted from *Nutrition Guide for Professionals: Diabetes Education and Meal Planning* by M.A. Powers, ed., p. 9, with permission of the American Diabetes Association and the American Dietetic Association, © 1988.

- Program Planning Committee–to develop educational activities for patients with diabetes and their families, and publicly represent the American Diabetes Association through participation in community events, health fairs, and media interviews.
- Patient education–to organize and implement monthly patient education programs and seminars.
- Support groups–to facilitate bilingual Latino support groups.
- Youth programs–to organize educational and social programs for Latino children with diabetes and maintain an active youth registry.
- Unidos Contra la Diabetes Health Fair–to plan and implement the annual public education and screening fair, including identification of sponsors, exhibitors, product donations, screening providers, event promotion, and event day logistics.
- Unidos Contra la Diabetes, Una Noche de Honor Fundraising Committee–to participate in the annual testimonial dinner including identifying honorees and soliciting sponsors and auction item donations.

SPECIAL ISSUES IN MANAGING DIABETES

During Childhood and Adolescent

As with adults, a multidisciplinary team approach is recommended (e.g., a physician, a registered dietitian who may be a community nutrition professional, a nurse, and a behavioral specialist trained in pediatric diabetes). A complete nutrition assessment forms the foundation of the eating pattern. It should include the following[15,60,61]:

- Probable reasons for poor weight gain or linear growth should be assessed. Usually these are due to poor glycemic control, inadequate insulin, and overrestriction of food energy. Excessive weight gain may be caused by excessive energy intake, overtreatment of hypoglycemia, overinsulinization, or low activity level.
- The role of parents and caregivers and extent of previous nutrition education should be assessed. Prior food likes and dislikes, lifestyle, and family economics should be determined.

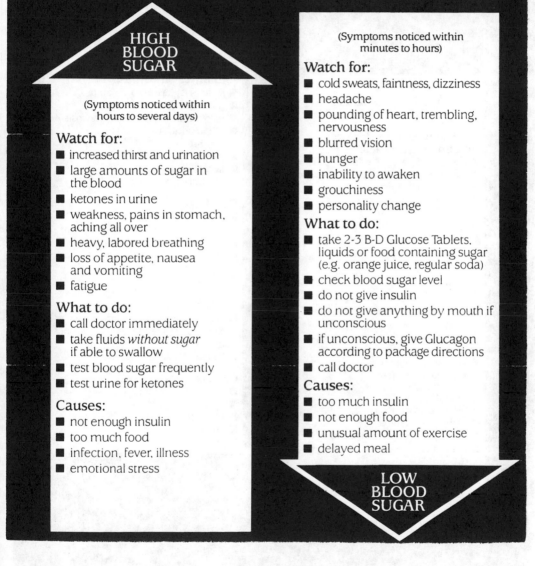

...Know the difference

HIGH BLOOD SUGAR

(Symptoms noticed within hours to several days)

Watch for:
- increased thirst and urination
- large amounts of sugar in the blood
- ketones in urine
- weakness, pains in stomach, aching all over
- heavy, labored breathing
- loss of appetite, nausea and vomiting
- fatigue

What to do:
- call doctor immediately
- take fluids *without sugar* if able to swallow
- test blood sugar frequently
- test urine for ketones

Causes:
- not enough insulin
- too much food
- infection, fever, illness
- emotional stress

(Symptoms noticed within minutes to hours)

Watch for:
- cold sweats, faintness, dizziness
- headache
- pounding of heart, trembling, nervousness
- blurred vision
- hunger
- inability to awaken
- grouchiness
- personality change

What to do:
- take 2-3 B-D Glucose Tablets, liquids or food containing sugar (e.g. orange juice, regular soda)
- check blood sugar level
- do not give insulin
- do not give anything by mouth if unconscious
- if unconscious, give Glucagon according to package directions
- call doctor

Causes:
- too much insulin
- not enough food
- unusual amount of exercise
- delayed meal

LOW BLOOD SUGAR

Figure 13-2 "... Know the difference in high and low blood sugar." Courtesy of Becton Dickinson and Company, Franklin Lakes, New Jersey.

continues

...Conozca la diferencia

**ALTA
CONCENTRACIÓN
DE AZÚCAR
EN LA SANGRE**

(Síntomas que se observan
en el espacío de horas a días)

Estar atento a los siguientes síntomas:
- aumento de la sed y orinar mucho
- gran cantidad de azúcar en la sangre
- cetonas en la orina
- debilidad, dolores estomacales, dolor generalizado
- respiración pesada y dificultosa
- pérdida del apetito, náuseas y vómitos
- fatiga

Qué hacer:
- llamar al médico de inmediato
- si puede tragar, tomar líquidos sin azúcar
- analizar frecuentemente su nivel de azúcar en la sangre
- analizar su orina para determinar si contiene cetonas

Causas:
- insuficiente insulina
- demasiada comida
- infección, fiebre, enfermedad
- tensión emocional

(Síntomas observados
de minutos a horas)

Estar atento a los siguientes síntomas:
- sudor frío, desmayos, mareos
- dolor de cabeza
- palpitaciones, temblores, nerviosismo
- visión borrosa
- hambre
- dificultad en despertarse
- irritabilidad
- cambio de la personalidad

Qué hacer:
- tomar 2-3 Tabletas de Glucosa B-D o ingerir alimentos que contengan azúcar (jugo de naranja, gaseosa)
- comprobar el nivel de azúcar en la sangre
- no administrar insulina
- no administrar nada por la boca si la persona está inconsciente
- si está inconsciente, administrar Glucagon siguiendo las instrucciones del envase
- llamar al médico

Causas:
- demasiada insulina
- insuficiente comida
- ejercicio excesivo
- comida retrasada

**BAJA
CONCENTRACIÓN
DE AZÚCAR
EN LA SANGRE**

Figure 13-2 continued

- A 24-hour recall or food record to reveal a typical day can be computerized to determine total energy, macro- and micronutrient intake, and meal and snack distribution. The child's total eating environment can be reviewed to acquire an accurate picture of the usual eating routine and food sources, including school routine, weekday routine, relationships with siblings and friends, and factors that influence food choices such as self-care skills.

Suggested formula for estimating energy needs of children are outlined in Table 13–9.

During Older Adult Years

Approximately one-half of US individuals with Type II diabetes are over 65 years old. The major reason for glucose intolerance observed among older adults is insulin resistance. Medications to treat comorbidity and polypharmacy in general may complicate diabetes therapy among senior adults. Medications that may increase hyperglycemia include diuretics, glucocorticoids, nicotinic acid, lithium, and other antidepressants. Medications that enhance hypoglycemia are beta-blockers, monoamine oxidase inhibitors, phenylbutazone, large doses of aspirin, and cimetidine. Seniors are at a greater risk from acute illnesses and complications of chronic illnesses. Their recovery from physiologic insults of fractures and acute illness is also slower and impaired when they have diabetes.[20,62] Specific concerns for seniors include the following:

- acute hyperglycemia and dehydration, which can lead to a hyperglycemic hyperosmolar nonketotic syndrome (a very high blood glucose without ketones—i.e., 400 to 2,800 mg/dL); mortality rate is 20% to 40% of patients
- hypoglycemia
- persistent hyperglycemia, which has deleterious effects on the body's defense against infection

During Illness

When illness occurs, glucose levels may rise but individuals must still take insulin. Appetite

---

Table 13–9 Estimating Energy Needs for Children with IDDM

Activity	Method	Formula*
Base energy on nutrition assessment	—	—
Verify energy needs	1	NAS/RDA Guidelines
All children	2	1000 kcal 1st year; +100 kcal/year to age 11;
Girls 11–15 years old		Add 100 kcal or less per year after age 10
>15 years old		Calculate as an adult
Boys 11–15 years old		Add 200 kcal per year after age 10
>15 years old		23 kcal/lb very active; 18 kcal/lb usual; 16 kcal/lb sedentary
	3	1000 kcal for 1st year; add 125 kcal × age for boys, 100 kcal × age for girls, and 20% more kcal for activity

*For toddlers 1–3 years old, use 40 kcal per inch of length.

Source: Adapted from *Maximizing the Role of Nutrition in Diabetes Management* with permission of the American Diabetes Association, © 1994.

often wanes, which restricts food intake. To avoid hypoglycemia, carbohydrates should be replaced during illness. At least 50 grams of carbohydrate should be eaten every 3 to 4 hours (e.g., 2.5 cups of carbonated beverages, three-fourths cup of sherbet, and 3.5 slices of toast). Eight to 12 ounces of liquid should be consumed every hour. Salt foods and beverages are advised if vomiting and diarrhea have occurred, to replace electrolytes.

During Pregnancy

The goal of medical nutrition therapy is to reduce the incidence of birth defects and risk of macrosomia, which can cause a complicated delivery and high-risk nursery care.[63,64]

The prevalence of gestational diabetes mellitus (GDM) varies from 2.5% in Boston to 12.3% in Los Angeles, which is likely due to obesity among Latino women in Los Angeles. This condition is marked by abnormal glucose tolerance during pregnancy, which warrants routine testing of the woman's urine for ketone bodies after a baseline fasting blood glucose. Without monitoring and control, the elevated blood glucose can lead to fetal or infant sickness and potentially death.[65] Infants born to women with gestational diabetes often exceed average birth weights (e.g., over 10 pounds at birth) and may experience increased risk of obesity and impaired glucose tolerance later in life. After delivery, GDM disappears in 90% of cases.[66]

When Post-Exercise, Late-Onset (PEL) Hypoglycemia Occurs

Hypoglycemia can occur 6 to 15 hours after strenuous exercise. This is different from the more immediate type of hypoglycemia that occurs 1 to 2 hours after exercise. PEL can result in stupor, coma, and/or seizures. This can be the result of vigorous swimming for three hours or starting a three mile/day running program. In a two-year prospective case study of 300 persons with IDDM, 48 (16%) had PEL hypoglycemia. Frequent moni-

---

Info Line

Basic recommendations for medical management of gestational diabetes mellitus include the following:

- All pregnant women should be given a 50-g glucose challenge test between 24 and 28 weeks. A 1-hour plasma glucose >140 mg/dL (>7.8 mmol) means referral for a 3-hour 100-g oral glucose tolerance test. If the value is more than 2 standard deviations above the mean, then gestational diabetes mellitus is diagnosed.
- Glucose monitoring is essential in gestational diabetes mellitus to establish when insulin is given.
- A glucose tolerance test between six and eight weeks postpartum is necessary to rule out NIDDM.
- After delivery, women with gestational diabetes mellitus should begin a prevention program focusing on eating and exercise to decrease the 25% to 60% chance she has for developing NIDDM.

Source: Medical Management of Pregnancy Complicated by Diabetes. 2nd Edition. American Diabetes Association, Inc. Alexandria, VA 22314. March, 1995.

---

toring of blood sugar in the evening and overnight is recommended. Food should be added if the person is weak, exhausted, or hungry. Insulin should be reduced.[67,68]

LEGISLATION AND REIMBURSEMENT

A major barrier to quality diabetes care is the nonexistent or limited coverage and reimbursement for diabetes self-management training and medical nutrition therapy.[69] Positioning medical nutrition therapy and diabetes self-management training as secondary prevention with documented cost savings is needed to ensure coverage of the services.

Info Line

Key points regarding health care reform and medical nutrition therapy coverage for individuals with diabetes include the following:

- Medical nutrition therapy is an important component of diabetes care and must be included in the final health care reform bill approved by Congress, because it is cost-effective and medically necessary.
- The 10-year Diabetes Control and Complications Trial, conducted by the National Institutes of Health, found that appropriate metabolic management, including medical nutrition therapy, was effective in reducing the complications of diabetes including eye disease, kidney disease, and nerve damage.
- Inconsistent reimbursement policies by private insurers and Medicare restrict medical nutrition therapy from many patients who, without proper care, develop complications and ultimately incur greater health care costs.
- Benefits language regarding coverage for "medically necessary or appropriate" health professional services should include medical nutrition therapy.

Source: Adapted from Gillespie S. Legislation and Reimbursement: Increasing Access to Medical Nutrition Therapy and Diabetes Self-Management Training. *On the Cutting Edge.* 1993;14(6):1–3; and Wylie-Rosett J. Health Insurance in New York State to Include Diabetes Education and Supplies. *On the Cutting Edge.* 1993;14(6):12.

In July 1993, New York joined Wisconsin and Oregon in including diabetes care as a component of health insurance coverage via State Law A1335/S1014. In New York, every major medical health insurance carrier must include coverage for all diabetes equipment, diabetes supplies, and diabetes self-management education. Services of certified diabetes educators, who may be registered dietitians or registered nurses, are covered. A major challenge was convincing legislators that including coverage of education and supplies would not greatly increase expenditures. Testimony before the Insurance Committee of the General Assembly was strengthened and passage was greatly enhanced with presentation of the results of the Diabetes Control and Complications Trial. Coalitions with other health care providers, consumers, and advocacy organizations were crucial to tip the balance in favor of the legislation.[70]

A CASE FOR PRIMARY PREVENTION OF DIABETES

Can we slow or alter the conversion from a normal glucose tolerance to an impaired glucose tolerance? Longitudinal studies that track this process have not been conducted previously, but there is a growing body of data that points to the role of dietary composition on the incidence of diabetes. The intakes of vegetable fat, potassium, calcium, and magnesium were shown to be inversely associated with the six-year incidence of self-reported diabetes of US nurses ($N = 84,360$).[71] Male Seventh-Day Adventists who had higher meat intake also had an increased death rate due to diabetes.[72] Two short-term studies reported that fish and legume intake were inversely associated and intake of pastries was positively associated with the four-year risk of glucose intolerance.[73] A high-fat intake among individuals with impaired glucose tolerance was significantly associated with the two-year risk of developing NIDDM.[74]

Data from the 30-year follow up of men in the Seven Countries Study showed that, of the 338 men available, 21% had an impaired glucose tolerance. These men had a higher proportion of simple sugars in their eating pattern compared with men with normal glucose tolerance, as well as a higher body mass index. For those with newly diagnosed diabetes, current fat intake and previous intakes of fat, saturated and monounsaturated fatty acids, and cholesterol were higher than intakes of men with no diabetes. Multiple regression analysis identified total fat and saturated

Exhibit 13-4 *Healthy People 2000* Health Status Objectives Targeting Diabetes

2.5   Reduce dietary fat intake to an average of 30% of calories or less and average saturated fat intake to <10% of calories among people aged 2 and older. (Baseline: 36% of calories from total fat and 13% from saturated fat for people aged 20 through 74 in 1976–80; 36% and 13% for women aged 19 through 50 in 1985.)

2.6   Increase complex carbohydrate and fiber-containing foods in the diets of adults to 5+ daily servings for vegetables (including legumes) and fruits, and to 6+ daily servings for grain products. (Baseline: 2½ servings of vegetables and fruits and 3 servings of grain products for women aged 19 through 50 in 1985.)

2.7   Increase to at least 50% the proportion of overweight people aged 12 and older who have adopted sound dietary practices combined with regular physical activity to attain an appropriate body weight. (Baseline: 30% of overweight women and 25% of overweight men for people aged 18 in 1985.)

15.10   Reduce overweight to a prevalence of no more than 20% among people aged 20+ and no more than 15% among adolescents aged 12 through 19. (Baseline: 26% for people aged 20 through 74 in 1976–80, 24% for men and 27% for women; 15% of adolescents aged 12 through 19 in 1976–80.)

Special Population Targets

Overweight Prevalence		*1976–80 Baseline*[*]	*2000 Target*
15.10a	Low-income women aged 20 and older	37%	25%
15.10b	Black women aged 20 and older	44%	30%
15.10c	Hispanic women aged 20 and older		
	Mexican-American women	39%[**]	
	Cuban women	34%[**]	
	Puerto Rican women	37%[**]	
15.10d	American Indians/Alaska Natives	29–75%[***]	30%
15.10e	People with disabilities	36%[$]	25%
15.10f	Women with high blood pressure	50%	41%
15.10g	Men with high blood pressure	39%	35%

[*]Baseline for people aged 20–74.
[**]1982–84 baseline for Hispanics aged 20–74.
[***]1984–88 estimates for different tribes.
[$]1985 baseline for people aged 20–74 who report any limitation in activity due to chronic conditions.

17.9   Reduce diabetes-related deaths to no more than 34 per 100,000 people. (Age-adjusted baseline: 38 per 100,000 in 1986.)

Special Population Targets

Diabetes-Related Deaths (per 100,000)		*1986 Baseline*	*2000 Target*
17.9a	Blacks	65	58
17.9b	American Indians/Alaska Natives	54	48

17.11   Reduce diabetes to an incidence of no more than 2.5 per 1,000 people and a prevalence of no more than 25 per 1,000 people. (Baselines: 2.9 per 1,000 in 1987; 28 per 1,000 in 1987.)

continues

Exhibit 13–4 continued

Special Population Targets

Prevalence of Diabetes (per 1,000)	1982–84 Baseline (20–74 years)	2000 Target
17.11a American Indians/Alaska Natives	69*	62
17.11b Puerto Ricans	55	49
17.11c Mexican Americans	54	49
17.11d Cuban Americans	36	32
17.11e Blacks	36**	32

*1987 baseline for American Indians/Alaska Natives aged 15 and older.
**1987 baseline for blacks of all ages.

Source: Reprinted from *Healthy People 2000: National Health Promotion and Disease Prevention Objectives*, U.S. Department of Health and Human Services, Public Health Service, Publication No. 91-50212, 1991.

Exhibit 13–5 Model Nutrition Objective for Risk Reduction

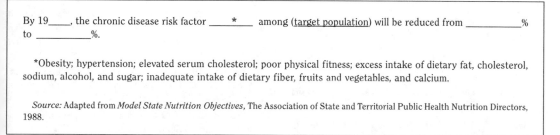

By 19____, the chronic disease risk factor _____*_____ among (target population) will be reduced from _____%
to _____%.

*Obesity; hypertension; elevated serum cholesterol; poor physical fitness; excess intake of dietary fat, cholesterol, sodium, alcohol, and sugar; inadequate intake of dietary fiber, fruits and vegetables, and calcium.

Source: Adapted from *Model State Nutrition Objectives*, The Association of State and Territorial Public Health Nutrition Directors, 1988.

fatty acids as independently and positively associated with two-hour plasma glucose level; the analysis revealed that higher intakes of vitamin C, fish, potatoes, vegetables, and legumes were associated with reduced two-hour plasma glucose levels.[75]

This study creates a new, central theme for diabetes research. Can dietary components predict impaired glucose tolerance and diabetes? The authors of this study hypothesize that the role of dietary factors may differ at different stages of diabetes development. This difference is related to the two-stage process in the development of NIDDM.[76] If the two-step model of NIDDM development is real and food components aid in the process, then we should be able to slow or alter the conversion of glucose tolerance to intoler-

ance with dietary modification. Thus, primary prevention may become a reality.

HEALTHY PEOPLE 2000 ACTIONS

Several HP2K objectives address diabetes mellitus, risk factors of diabetes mellitus, or eating behaviors to improve overall health of Americans predisposed to or diagnosed with diabetes mellitus (see Exhibit 13–4). Targets are defined for blacks, Native Americans, and Hispanics. Kaufman[77] has outlined a model nutrition objective for risk reduction. Community nutrition professionals can use this blueprint to develop diabetes self-management programs (see Exhibit 13–5).

REFERENCES

1. *American Diabetes Association: Who We Are, What We Do.* Alexandria, Va: American Diabetes Association; 1988.

2. Shead NF. Cow's milk, diabetes, and infant feeding. *Nutr Rev.* 1991;51(3):79–81.

3. Savilahti E, Akerblom HK, Tainio V-M, et al. Children with newly diagnosed insulin-dependent diabetes mellitus have increased levels of cow's milk antibodies. *Diabetes Res.* 1988;7:137–140.

4. Yokota A, Yamaguchi Y, Ueda Y, et al. Comparison of islet cell antibodies, islet cell surface antibodies, and anti-bovine serum albumin antibodies in type 1 diabetes. *Diabetes Res Clin Pract.* 1990;9:211–217.

5. Scott FW. Cow milk and insulin-dependent diabetes mellitus: Is there a relationship? *Am J Clin Nutr.* 1990;51:489–491.

6. Martin JM, Trink B, Daneman D, et al. Milk proteins in the etiology of insulin-dependent diabetes mellitus. *Ann Intern Med.* 1991;23:447–452.

7. Virtanen SM, Rasanen L, Aro A, et al. Infant feeding in Finnish children—7 years of age with newly diagnosed IDDM. *Diabetes Care.* 1991;14:415–417.

8. American Academy of Pediatrics, Committee on Nutrition. Statement on cholesterol. *Pediatrics.* 1992;90:469–473.

9. DeFronzo RA, Ferrannini E. Insulin resistance: A multifaceted syndrome responsible for NIDDM, obesity, hypertension, dyslipidemia and atherosclerotic cardiovascular disease. *Diabetes Care.* 1991;14:173–194.

10. Ward WK, Beard JC, Halter JB, et al. Pathophysiology of insulin secretion in non-insulin-dependent diabetes mellitus. *Diabetes Care.* 1984;7:491–502.

11. Lovejob J, DiGirolamo M. Habitual dietary intake and insulin sensitivity in lean and obese adults. *Am J Clin Nutr.* 1992;55:1174–1179.

12. Helmrich SP, Ragland DR, Leung RW, et al. Physical activity and reduced occurrence of non-insulin-dependent diabetes mellitus. *N Eng J Med.* 1991;325:147–152.

13. Toeller M, Greis FA, Dannehl K. Natural history of glucose intolerance in obesity. A ten-year observation. *Int J Obesity.* 1982;6:145–149.

14. Anderson JW. Nutrition management of diabetes mellitus. In: Shils ME, Young VR, eds. *Modern Nutrition in Health and Disease.* 7th ed. New York, NY: Lea and Febiger; 1988.

15. American Dietetic Association. Nutrition recommendations and principles for people with diabetes mellitus. *J Am Diet Assoc.* 1994;94:504–511.

16. Pirart J. Diabetes mellitus and its complication: A prospective study of 4,400 patients observed between 1947 and 1973. *Diabetes Care.* 1978;1:168–188.

17. Anderson JW. Hyperlipidemia and diabetes: Nutrition considerations In: Jovanovic L, Liss AR, eds. *Nutrition and Diabetes.* New York, NY: 1985.

18. Kleinman JC, Donahue RP, Harris MI, et al. Mortality among diabetics in a national sample. *Am J Epidemiol.* 1988;128:389–401.

19. Bierman EL. Atherogenesis in diabetes. *Arteriosclerosis and Thrombosis.* 1992;12:647–656.

20. American Diabetes Association and the Diabetes Care and Education Practice Group of the American Dietetic Association. *Maximizing the Role of Nutrition in Diabetes Management.* Alexandria, Va: American Diabetes Association; 1994.

21. Stone DB, Conner WE. The prolonged effects of a low cholesterol, high carbohydrate diet upon the serum lipids in diabetic patients. *Diabetes.* 1963;12:127–132.

22. Kiehm TG, Anderson JW, Ward K. Beneficial effects of a high carbohydrate, high fiber diet on hyperglycemic diabetic men. *Am J Clin Nutr.* 1976;29:895–899.

23. Barnard RJ, Massey MR, Chern YS, et al. Long term use of a high-complex carbohydrate, high fiber, low fat diet and exercise in the treatment of NIDDM patients. *Diabetes Care.* 1983;6:268–273.

24. O'Dea K, Traianedes K, Ireland P, et al. The effects of diet differing in fat, carbohydrate, and fiber on carbohydrate and lipid metabolism in type II diabetes. *J Am Diet Assoc,* 1989;89:1076–1086.

25. American Diabetes Association. Nutritional recommendations and principles for individuals with diabetes mellitus: 1986. *Diabetes Care.* 1987;10:126–132.

26. Riccardi G, Rivelles A, Dacioni D, et al. Separate influence of dietary carbohydrate and fiber on the metabolic control in diabetes. *Diabetologia.* 1984;26:116–121.

27. Coulston AM, Hollenbeck CB, Swislocki AL, et al. Deleterious effects of high-carbohydrate, sucrose-containing diets in patients with non-insulin-dependent diabetes mellitus. *N Engl J Med.* 1988;319:829–834.

28. Jenkins DJA, Wolever TMS, Taylor RH, et al. Glycemic index of foods: A physiological basis for carbohydrate exchange. *Am J Clin Nutr.* 1981;34:362–366.

29. Garg A, Bonanome A, Grundy SM, et al. Comparison of a high-carbohydrate, sucrose-containing diet in patients with non-insulin-dependent diabetes mellitus. *N Engl J Med.* 1988;319:829–834.

30. Garg A, Grundy SM, Unger RH. Comparison of effects of high and low carbohydrate diets on plasma lipoproteins and insulin sensitivity in patients with mild NIDDM. *Diabetes.* 1992;41:1278–1285.

31. Grundy SM. Comparison of monounsaturated fatty acids and carbohydrates for lowering plasma cholesterol. *N Engl J Med.* 1986;314:745–748.

32. Simpson HCR, Lousley S, Gelkie M, et al. A high carbohydrate leguminous fiber diet improves all aspects of diabetic control. *Lancet.* 1981;1:1–5.

33. Howard BV, Abbott WGH, Swinburn BA. Evaluation of metabolic effects of substitution of complex carbohydrates for saturated fat in individuals with obesity and NIDDM. *Diabetes Care.* 1991;14:786–795.

34. Ravusine E, Bogardus C, Schwartz RS, et al. Thermic effect of infused glucose and insulin in man: Decreased response with increased insulin resistance in obesity and NIDDM. *J Clin Invest.* 1993;72:893–902.

35. UKPDS Group. UK Prospective Diabetes Study 7: Response of fasting plasma glucose to diet therapy in newly presenting type II diabetic patients. *Metabolism.* 1990;39:905–912.

36. Shintani TT. Obesity and cardiovascular risk intervention through the ad libitum feeding of traditional Hawaiian diet. *Am J Clin Nutr.* 1991;153:1647S–1651S.

37. O'Dea K. Marked improvement in carbohydrate and lipid metabolism in diabetic Australian aborigines after temporary reversion to traditional lifestyle. *Diabetes.* 1984;33:596–603.

38. Jenkins DJA, Wolever TMS, Taylor RH, et al. The glycemic response to carbohydrate foods. *Lancet.* 1984;2:388–391.

39. Brand JC, Colaqiuri S, Crossman S, et al. Low-glycemic index foods improve long-term glycemic control in NIDDM. *Diabetes Care.* 1991;14:95–101.

40. Jenkins DJA, Wolever TMS, Vuksan V, et al. Nibbling versus gorging: Metabolic advantages of increased meal frequency. *N Engl J Med.* 1989;321:929–934.

41. Jenkins DJA, Wolever TMS, Ocana AM, et al. Metabolic effects of reducing rate of glucose ingestion by single bolus versus continuous sipping. *Diabetes.* 1990;39:775–781.

42. Jenkins DJA, Ocana A, Jenkins AL, et al. Metabolic advantages of spreading the nutrient load: Effects of increased meal frequency in non-insulin-dependent diabetes. *Am J Clin Nutr.* 1992;55:461–467.

43. Diabetes Control and Complications Trial Research Group. The Diabetes Control and Complications Trial: Design and methodologic considerations for the feasibility phase. *Diabetes.* 1986;35:530–545.

44. Diabetes Control and Complications Trial Research Group. Diabetes Control and Complications Trial: Results of feasibility study. *Diabetes Care.* 1987;10:1–19.

45. Diabetes Control and Complications Trial Research Group. The effect of intensive treatment of diabetes on the development and progression of long-term complications in insulin-dependent diabetes mellitus. *N Engl J Med.* 1993;329:977–986.

46. Siebert C, Clark DM Jr. Operational and policy considerations of data monitoring in clinical trials: The Diabetes Control and Complications Trial experience. *Diabetes Care.* 1993;14:30–44.

47. Diabetes Control and Complications Trial Research Group. *DCCT Manual of Operations.* Springfield, Va: US Department of Commerce; 1993. National Technical Information Service publication 93-183382.

48. Diabetes Control and Complications Trial Research Group. Weight gain associated with intensive therapy in the Diabetes Control and Complications Trial. *Diabetes Care.* 1988;11:567–573.

49. Lawson PM, Champion MC, Canny C, et al. Continuous subcutaneous insulin infusion does not prevent progression of proliferative and preproliferative retinopathy. *Br J Ophthalmol.* 1982;66:762–766.

50. Klein R, Klein BE, Moss SE, et al. The Wisconsin epidemiologic study of diabetic retinopathy. III. Prevalence and risk of diabetic retinopathy when age at diagnosis is 30 or more years. *Arch Ophthalmol.* 1984;102:527–532.

51. Nathan DM, Singer DE, Godine JE, et al. Retinopathy in older type II diabetics: Association with glucose control. *Diabetes.* 1986;35:797–801.

52. American Diabetes Association. Implications of the diabetes control and complications trial. *Diabetes Care.* 1993;16:1517–1520.

53. National High Blood Pressure Education Working Group. Report on hypertension in diabetes. *Hypertension.* 1994;23:145–158.

54. Davidow DN, Turner M. Complications of coexisting diabetes mellitus and eating disorders in IDDM. *On the Cutting Edge.* 1994;15(6):8–10.

55. Marcus MD, Wing RR, Jawad A, et al. Eating disorders symptomatology in a registry-based sample of women with insulin-dependent diabetes mellitus. *Int J Eating Disorders.* 1992;12:425–430.

56. King NL. Overview of eating disorders in diabetes management. *On the Cutting Edge.* 1994;15(6):5–7.

57. Schlundt DG, Pichert JW, Rea MR. Situational obstacles to adherence for adolescents with diabetes. *Diabetes Ed.* 1994;20:207–211.

58. Bossetti BM. Compulsive overeating, obesity and diabetes. *On the Cutting Edge.* 1994;15(6):12–14.

59. Green JA. Diabetes nutrition management: A need for meal planning alternatives. *Diabetes Ed.* 1987;13:146.

60. Diabetes Control and Complications Trial Research Group. Nutrition interventions for intensive therapy in the diabetes control and complications trial. *J Am Diet Assoc.* 1993;93:768–772.

61. American Diabetes Association. Nutrition recommendations and principles for people with diabetes mellitus. *Diabetes Care.* 1994;17:519–522.

62. Avioli LV. Significance of osteoporosis: A growing international health care problem. *Calcif Tissue Int.* 1991;49:S5–S7.

63. Kitzmiller JL, Gavin LA, Gin GD, et al. Preconception care of diabetes: Glycemic control prevents congenital anomalies. *JAMA.* 1991;265:731–736.

64. Jovanovic-Peterson L, Peterson CM, Reed GF, et al. Maternal postprandial glucose levels and infant birth weight: The diabetes in early pregnancy study. *Am J Obstet Gynecol*. 1991;164:103–111.

65. Hamilton EMN, Whitney EN, Sizer FS, eds. *Nutrition–Concepts and Controversies*. 5th ed. New York, NY: West Publishing Company; 1991:413.

66. Green OC, Winter RJ, Depp R, et al. Fuel-mediated teratogenesis: Prospective correlations between anthropometric development in childhood and antepartum maternal metabolism. *Clin Res*. 1987;35:657A.

67. Barnard RJ, Ugianskis EJ, Martin DA, et al. Role of diet and exercise in the management of hyperinsulinemia and associated atherosclerotic risk factors. *Am J Cardiol*. 1992;69:440–444.

68. Goodyear LJ, Smith RJ. *Post Exercise Late Onset Hypoglycemia*. In: *Joslin's Diabetes Mellitus*. Kahn CK and Weir GL, eds. Philadelphia, Pa: Lea and Febiger, 1994; 451–507.

69. Gillespie S. Legislation and reimbursement: Increasing access to medical nutrition therapy and diabetes self-management training. *On the Cutting Edge*. 1993;14(6):1–3.

70. Wylie-Rosett J. Health insurance in New York State to include diabetes education and supplies. *On the Cutting Edge*. 1993;14(6):12.

71. Colditz GA, Manson JE, Stampfer MJ, et al. Diet and risk of clinical diabetes in women. *Am J Clin Nutr*. 1992;55:1018–1023.

72. Snowdon DA, Philips RL. Does a vegetarian diet reduce the occurrence of diabetes? *Am J Public Health*. 1985;75:507–512.

73. Feskens EJM, Bowles CH, Kromhout D. Inverse association between fish intake and risk of glucose intolerance in normoglycemic elderly men and women. *Diabetes Care*. 1991;14:935–941.

74. Marshall JA, Hoag S, Shetterly S, et al. Dietary fat predicts conversion from impaired glucose tolerance to NIDDM: The San Luis Valley Diabetes Study. *Diabetes Care*. 1994;17:50–56.

75. Feskens E, Virtanen SM, Rasanen L, et al. Dietary factors determining diabetes and impaired glucose tolerance. *Diabetes Care*. 1995;18:1104–1112.

76. Saad MF, Knowler WC, Pettitt DJ, et al. A two-step model for the development of non-insulin-dependent diabetes. *Am J Med*. 1991;90:229–235.

77. Kaufman M. *Nutrition in Public Health—A Handbook for Developing Programs and Services*. Gaithersburg, Md: Aspen Publishers, Inc; 1990:570.

Hypertension

Learning Objectives

- Identify the incidence and prevalence of hypertension in the United States.
- List and define the magnitude of influence of dietary components and lifestyle behaviors on blood pressure level.
- Describe major clinical trials and primary prevention studies that use eating behavior change as an intervention.

High Definition Nutrition

Blood pressure—the force that flowing blood exerts against artery walls.
Diastolic blood pressure—blood pressure occurring when the heart relaxes between contractions.
Systolic blood pressure—blood pressure occurring when the heart contracts.

OVERVIEW OF HYPERTENSION

Essential hypertension is a multifactorial condition affecting 60 million adults. Blood pressure regulation is the result of cardiac output and peripheral vascular resistance, which are both influenced by sympathetic outflow and hormones such as angiotensin, insulin, noradrenaline, prostaglandins, kinins, and atrial natriuretic factor.

Stress; extracellular and intracellular cations of sodium, potassium, calcium, and magnesium; and various food components including cations, fats, and alcohol influence cardiac output and peripheral vascular resistance.[1]

Increased energy intake may increase insulin secretion and sympathetic outflow. High energy intakes often accompany high sodium intake, fluid retention, and alteration of intracellular electrolytes. Low sodium intakes may increase angiotensin and noradrenaline, and also cause calcium retention.[1]

Three major nutritional factors are associated with hypertension. These are obesity, high alcohol intake, and high sodium intake.

OBESITY

Epidemiologic studies show an association between obesity and hypertension in a wide variety of socioeconomic, racial, and ethnic groups.[2-5] A strong correlation exists between body weight and blood pressure and between increases in body weight and subsequent development of hypertension.[2,4] Intervention studies show that weight reduction may reduce arterial pressure in overweight, hypertensive patients. A drop in pressure may occur with caloric restriction only, even without reduction in sodium intake and before ideal body weight is achieved. Weight reduction in obese individuals can reduce cardiovascular risk factors, such as hyperlipidemia

---

Info Line

The Joint National Committee on Detection, Evaluation and Treatment of High Blood Pressure Recommendation for Weight Reduction is as follows:

Because of the clear relationship between obesity and blood pressure, all obese hypertensive adults should participate in weight reduction programs, with goal body weight being within 15 percent of desirable weight. Concomitantly, health professionals should vigorously promote weight control, particularly for those at increased risk of becoming hypertensive because of a family history of this condition. These recommendations are made with the clear recognition that weight reduction is difficult to achieve and that the rate of recidivism is high.

Source: Joint National Committee. Report of the Joint National Committee on Detection, Evaluation, and Treatment of High Blood Pressure. *Hypertension.* 1986;8:444–467.

Pacific Islanders) are at a higher risk of hypertension. The National Health and Nutrition Examination Survey II cutoff points for obesity are body mass index greater than 27.8 kg/m^2 for men and 27.3 kg/m^2 for women. Using these cutoff points, the prevalence of excess weight ranges from less than 20% in younger white men to greater than 60% in older African-American women[9,10] (see Chapter 15). With the documented increasing body weight of US youths and adults, the population in general is at a greater risk. Approximately 20 to 30% of hypertension prevalence has been influenced by this trend toward increasing body weight.[3,4]

ALCOHOL

A classic study of alcohol intake among the French military found that those who consumed three liters or more of wine per day had increased chance of being hypertensive.[11] This finding spurred researchers to explore the alcohol and blood pressure hypothesis. Almost all of the 30 or more cross-sectional studies to date have shown a small but significant elevation in blood pressure among individuals who consume three or more drinks per day (i.e., 40 grams of ethanol) compared with nondrinkers. The relationship has persisted after controlling for potentially confounding factors including body mass index, cigarette smoking, and age.[12]

About 5 to 7% of the prevalence of hypertension is assigned to the ingestion of three or more alcoholic drinks per day, which has been noted as a threshold. The prevalence is two times greater in the six-or-more-drinks group than in the two-or-fewer group.[13,14]

Intervention studies demonstrate a short-term pressor effect of alcohol consumption, short-term drops in blood pressure from abstinence or less than one drink per day in heavy drinkers, and normalization of blood pressure in former heavy drinkers who stop drinking.[15] It appears that excess alcohol intake may lead to elevated blood pressure, poor adherence to antihypertensive therapy, and, occasionally, refractory hypertension.[15-17]

and glucose intolerance. Obesity is the strongest risk factor for hypertension. Approximately 50% of women and 39% of men with high blood pressure are overweight. The data are strong and consistent as briefly discussed below.

Many studies have reported a stepwise increase in blood pressure as body weight concomitantly increases. Individuals who are overweight or obese have an increased prevalence and incidence of hypertension compared to individuals who are not overweight or obese.[6,7] In general, an individual who is overweight is at two to six times higher risk of developing hypertension.[4,8]

Since excess weight is common among minority populations, certain groups (i.e., African Americans, Hispanics, Native Americans, and Asian/

SODIUM

Cross-sectional studies show a weak but significant relationship between salt intake and prevalence of hypertension. This weak observation may be due to the lack of standardized blood pressure measurements and sodium intake estimates based upon dietary recall. Primitive, unacculturated societies with sodium intake of less than 50 to 80 mEq/day of sodium have no hypertension and no increase of blood pressure with age. Confounding variables include exercise, lean body mass, societal stress, and potassium intake.[18-20]

Population studies in Western countries have not demonstrated a correlation between habitual salt intake and blood pressure, but the range of sodium intake is limited in Western societies.[21] Intervention studies demonstrate a modest reduction of blood pressure (8 mm Hg systolic and 4 mm Hg diastolic) with sodium intake of less than 100 mEq/day. Sodium restriction may decrease the amount of diuretic and other antihypertensive drugs needed.[19]

The Intersalt study involved over 10,000 adults from 52 countries. Researchers collected 24-hour urine samples and anthropometric measures. Major observations were as follows[22-24]:

- A change of 100 mEq per day in sodium excretion was associated with a change in systolic blood pressure of 2.2 mm Hg.
- A reduction of 100 mEq of sodium intake per day could lower the rise in systolic blood pressure for adults 25 to 55 years old by 9 mm Hg.
- Diastolic blood pressure could be lowered by 4.5 mm Hg.
- Body mass index (BMI) and alcohol intake were predisposing factors for blood pressure elevation.

Research suggests that there is probably a subset of salt-sensitive individuals in whom sodium intake is an important determinant of blood pressure.[25,26] High sodium intake may limit the effectiveness of some antihypertensive drugs. Therefore, sodium restriction to 70 to 100 mEq per day (4 to 5 grams of salt) is recommended for all hypertensive patients.[27]

CALCIUM, POTASSIUM, MAGNESIUM, FAT, AND FIBER

Studies suggest but do not confirm the following[22,23,28-31]:

- Reduced potassium intake may be associated with high blood pressure.
- High potassium intake (greater than 80 mEq or 3 to 4 g/day) has a modest blood-pressure-lowering effect.
- Increased intake of calcium may lower blood pressure in some individuals.
- A within-person or intra-individual relationship exists between dietary magnesium and blood pressure.
- Low intake of saturated fat and high intake of polyunsaturated fat, particularly from fish and fiber, are associated with lower arterial pressure.

Potassium

Potassium supplementation can lower blood pressure. For over 50 years, various mechanisms have been proposed (e.g., a direct natriuretic effect, suppression of the renin-angiotensin and sympathetic nervous systems, baroreceptor function improvement, and less peripheral vascular resistance).[32,33] The first controlled trial to test the effect of potassium supplementation occurred in 1980; this was followed by almost two dozen randomized, controlled trials with crossover designs among normotensive individuals. In addition, clinical trials among hypertensive individuals have been conducted that demonstrate an overall lowering in both systolic and diastolic blood pressure. Potassium's effect on lowering blood pressure may be more powerful among subgroups (e.g., African Americans).

Multicountry studies identify an inverse association between blood pressure and serum, urine, and total body levels and dietary intake of potassium.[23,34] After adjusting for age, sex, body mass index, alcohol intake, and urinary sodium excretion in addition to correcting for a regression to the mean phenomenon, the Intersalt study reported a 2.7 mm Hg reduction in systolic blood pressure for a 60 mmol/24 hour higher excretion of urinary potassium.[23]

The ratio of urinary sodium to potassium is a more powerful factor than the level of potassium alone. The Intersalt study predicted that a reduction of the sodium-to-potassium ratio of 3.1 to 1.0 was associated with a 3.4 mm Hg decrease in the average level of systolic blood pressure.[22] Other studies suggest that a lower intake of dietary potassium among African Americans may be related to the higher prevalence of hypertension in this subgroup.[35]

The evidence about potassium as a beneficial dietary component and the use of potassium supplementation is still developing. Increased potassium intake is recommended as a general preventive approach, primarily for individuals who have normal renal function and who are not taking drugs known to raise serum potassium levels.[27] The drugs could be potassium-sparing diuretics and angiotensin-converting enzyme inhibitors.

Calcium

Increased intake of calcium has been reported to lower blood pressure in some individuals.[36] Some studies suggest that a direct relationship exists between serum calcium concentration and blood pressure.[37] The calcium-blood pressure hypothesis is fueled by more than 30 observational studies reporting an inverse association between calcium intake and either blood pressure level or the prevalence and incidence of hypertension.[31,38-55] The results show a favorable role of calcium and blood pressure for African Americans and women in general, but less influence on white men. Cross-sectional studies have involved samples in Europe, East Asia, South Africa, the Caribbean, and North America, and prospective studies (e.g., the Nurses' Health Study) in the United States.[31,38-40,44-47,52,53,56-59] In the Nurses' Health Study, a significantly lower relative risk of 0.78 for hypertension was associated with dietary calcium intake of 800 mg/day compared with an intake of 400 mg/day.[53] Maternal calcium intake was found to be inversely associated with blood pressure of infants before one year of age.[60]

In more than 25 randomized, clinical trials, most used calcium tablets rather than calcium-rich foods as the intervention. In trials using dietary calcium sources, reductions in both systolic and diastolic blood pressure are noted. However, pooled analysis of trials with normotensive participants suggests an average blood pressure change of -0.99 systolic and -0.54 diastolic (95% confidence interval of -2.20, +0.22 and -1.31, +0.23). The pooling of 23 trials with hypertensive participants suggests an average of -1.48 for systolic (2.40, -0.56) and -0.29 for diastolic pressure (-0.88, +0.30).[54,61-64]

One concern about calcium supplementation is that the risk for developing renal calculi may increase with increased calcium intake. Because the design of many of the calcium supplementation studies and trials did not control for extraneous variables such as sodium intake, other electrolytes, alcohol intake, and exercise, the hypothesis still needs to be tested.

Magnesium

Data regarding magnesium, zinc, and lead are too meager to justify any recommendations. In phase 1 of the Trials of Hypertension Prevention Study, oral supplementation with magnesium resulted in a small lowering of both systolic and diastolic blood pressure (-0.2 and -0.1 mm Hg, respectively). Gastrointestinal upsets were observed among the intervention group, which were deemed unacceptable side effects when the influence of the supplement on blood pressure appears small.[30,65-67]

Fat and Fiber

Contradictory studies suggest that low saturated fat and high polyunsaturated fat intakes are associated with lower arterial blood pressure.[68,69] Increased intake of vegetable proteins and complex carbohydrates as observed among vegetarians in industrialized countries show lower blood pressure levels.[70] Dietary fiber in the form of wheat, wheat bran, pectin, and oat bran have been studied for their hypotensive influence.[71-74] Results are neither strong nor consistent but warrant further exploration.

The large Multiple Risk Factor Intervention Trial (see Chapter 11) with 12,000 participants showed an independent association between systolic blood pressure and saturated fat, exogenous cholesterol per 1,000 kcal, and complex carbohydrate.[75] This observation was not confirmed in studies involving more than 138,000 nurses and healthy male professionals.[28,29]

Observation studies suggest that eating large amounts of fish rich in polyunsaturated omega-3 fatty acids lower rates of coronary artery disease and may lower serum triglycerides, but their role in hypertension control is not known.[69,71,76-78] Evidence is still inadequate to recommend specific dietary changes in fat for hypertension control, even though these changes could potentially lower blood cholesterol and reduce coronary artery disease risk. Further research and exploration of hypotheses linking dietary fat composition amid individuals with different body mass indices and baseline blood pressure levels is needed.

THE EFFECT OF HEALTHY EATING

Healthy eating can improve the efficacy of some pharmacologic agents. Nutritional approaches can be effective as definitive intervention alone but also as adjuncts to pharmacologic therapy. An experimental trial called Trials of Hypertension Prevention was conducted by a collaborative research group. The trial, which involved nonpharmacologic interventions to lower blood pressure, is outlined in Tables 14-1 and 14-2. The sample included 2,182 persons with high normal diastolic blood pressure of 80 to 89 mm Hg. Randomization assignment was one of three lifestyles (weight reduction, sodium reduction, and stress management) and four nu-

Table 14-1 Design of Nonpharmacologic Intervention Trials in Prevention of Hypertension

Study	Sample Size	Demographic Characteristics			Duration of Follow Up Blood Pressure	Intervention
		Mean Age	% Male	% White		
Primary Prevention of Hypertension Trial	201	38	87	82	5 years	Multifactorial (reduced calorie, sodium, and alcohol intake, and increased physical activity)
Hypertension Prevention Trial	252	38	68	80	3 years	Reduced calorie intake
	392	39	62	84		Reduced sodium intake
	255	39	62	82		Reduced calorie and sodium intake
	391	38	63	85		Reduced sodium and increased potassium intake
Trials of Hypertension Prevention	564	43	72	79	18 months	Weight loss (reduced calorie intake and increased physical activity)
	744	43	72	77	18 months	Reduced sodium intake
	562	43	71	84	18 months	Stress management
	471	43	68	85	6 months	Calcium supplementation
	461	43	68	85	6 months	Magnesium supplementation
	351	43	72	87	6 months	Potassium supplementation
	350	43	70	86	6 months	Fish oil supplementation

Source: Adapted from *Working Group Report on Primary Prevention of Hypertension*, p. 10, National High Blood Pressure Education Program, National Institutes of Health, Publication No. 93-2669, May 1993.

Table 14–2 Effect of Nonpharmacologic Interventions on Blood Pressure and Risk of Hypertension in Persons with High Normal Blood Pressure

Study	Average Initial Blood Pressure (mm Hg)		Average Net Change in Blood Pressure (mm Hg)		Effect: Relative Risk of Increased Blood Pressure (95% CI)
	Systolic	Diastolic	Systolic	Diastolic	
Primary Prevention of Hypertension Trial	122.6	82.5	-1.3	-1.02	0.46
Hypertension Prevention Trial	125.0	83.2	-2.4	-1.8	0.77
	123.9	82.8	0.2	0.1	0.79
	124.5	82.9	-1.0	-1.3	0.95
	124.0	82.6	-1.2	-0.7	0.77
Trials of Hypertension Prevention Phase I	124.4	83.8	-2.9	-2.3	0.49/(0.29,0.83)
	125.0	83.8	-1.7	-0.9	0.76/(0.49,1.18)
	124.6	83.7	-0.5	-0.8	1.07/(0.65,1.76)
	125.7	84.0	-0.5	0.2	0.91/(0.43,1.96)
	125.1	83.9	-0.2	-0.1	0.63/(0.27,1.50)
	121.6	80.9	0.1	-0.4	0.87/(0.34,2.21)
	122.7	81.1	-0.2	-0.6	1.11/(0.46,2.67)

Source: Adapted from *Working Group Report on Primary Prevention of Hypertension*, p. 10, National High Blood Pressure Education Program, National Institutes of Health, Publication No. 93-2669, May 1993.

tritional supplementation groups (calcium, magnesium, potassium, and fish oil). After six months, significant decreases in diastolic and systolic blood pressure were noted for the weight reduction and sodium reduction intervention groups. Even with high compliance, neither stress management intervention nor nutritional supplements significantly lowered blood pressure.[30]

The multiple-step intervention program included a "sodium-light" lifestyle intervention (see Exhibit 14–1). Eight group meetings and two one-on-one meetings were held in the first three months. These sessions were followed by less intensive counseling. Positive support was given throughout the study. A total of 327 individuals were assigned to active intervention; 417 were assigned to the control group. An average weight loss of 8.5 pounds and reduction of 2.9 mm Hg and 2.3 mm Hg systolic and diastolic blood pressure were reported after 18 months of inter-

vention. The weight loss alone was associated with a 51% reduction in the incidence of hypertension.[30,79]

The five-year Primary Prevention of Hypertension Trial used a multifactorial intervention with reductions of total energy, sodium, and alcohol intake, and increased physical activity for normotensive individuals. An average 5.9 pounds of weight loss and a reduction of 1.3 mm Hg systolic and 1.2 mm Hg diastolic blood pressure occurred. Individuals involved in the intervention had a 50% lower five-year incidence of hypertension than those who received the usual care.[80]

A third major trial, Hypertension Prevention Trial, demonstrated that energy reduction alone could lower blood pressure and the incidence of hypertension. An average reduction in systolic blood pressure and diastolic blood pressure of 2.4 mm Hg and 1.8 mm Hg, respectively, was experienced by participants who only reduced their total energy intake.[81]

Exhibit 14–1 Sodium-Light Lifestyle Intervention Approach in Phase I of the Trials of Hypertension Prevention

- Intervention objective: To reduce the group average 24-hour urinary sodium excretion to a mean of 80 mmol (1800 mg)
- Nutrition counseling objective: To reduce the individual's 24-hour sodium intake to 60 mmol (1400 mg) without changing other nutrient intakes
- Contact pattern
  - Eight group and two individual counseling sessions over a 3-month period
  - Periodic group meetings and individual telephone or in-person contacts throughout follow-up
- Program content
  - Sodium content of foods
  - Food shopping, label reading, recipe modification, restaurant selections
  - Sodium-specific dietary behavior problem solving
  - Food tasting
  - Take-home packages of low-sodium foods and product samples
  - Local shopping guide for sodium-reduced products
  - Peer support and family involvement
  - Field trips (e.g., to restaurants, supermarkets)
  - Motivational activities
- Adherence monitoring/enhancement
  - Food diaries
  - Attendance
  - Overnight (8-hour) urinary sodium excretion

Source: Reprinted from Kumanyika, S.K., Feasibility and Efficacy of Sodium Reduction in the Trials of Hypertension Prevention, Phase I, *Hypertension*, Vol. 22, pp. 502–512, with permission of the American Heart Association, © 1993.

THE EFFECT OF HYPERTENSION CONTROL

National Health and Nutrition Examination Survey (NHANES) III data collected from 1988 to 1991 show that awareness, treatment, and control of high blood pressure have dramatically improved in the last 20 years. The survey, based on a random sample of US adults, estimates that up to 50 million Americans may have high blood pressure. The situation is improving, because the number of individuals with high blood pressure who know of their condition has increased from 51% in 1971–1972 to 84% in 1988–1991.[82]

The number of Americans who receive medication for high blood pressure has increased significantly over the last 20 years.[83] In 1971–1972, 36% of hypertensive persons took drugs; in 1991, 73% did. The number of hypertensive individuals whose blood pressure was controlled in this time period increased from 44% to 75%.[82]

African-American men are at high risk for high blood pressure, but NHANES III data show a 60% increase in the number of black men whose high blood pressure is under control. African Americans with blood pressure above 140/90 mm Hg have higher rates of awareness, treatment, and control of the high blood pressure than other ethnic groups. However, for hypertensive individuals with blood pressure above 160/95 mm Hg, the rate of treatment and control among blacks is less than among individuals of all other ethnic groups with hypertension.[82]

To guide practitioners, the fifth NIH Joint National Committee on Detection, Evaluation, and Treatment of High Blood Pressure established guidelines for the treatment of elevated blood pressure. The guidelines are based on a classification system (see Table 14–3). Depending on the severity of an individual's high blood pressure, the committee recommends a certain course of action. The recommended treatment begins with changing the patient's lifestyle (i.e., reducing weight, increasing exercise, and limiting salt and alcohol intake). If this course of action does not work, the committee recommends medication.[82]

A corresponding report by the Working Group of the National High Blood Pressure Education Program calls for continuation of the national education program. The campaign educates the general public about high blood pressure, targets high-risk groups such as African-American men, and educates health care providers.[83]

Because about 80% of a person's daily sodium intake is from processed foods, the working group specifically solicits the following[83]:

- food manufacturers to reduce sodium in their products
- supermarkets label shelves to direct customers to low-sodium foods

---

Table 14–3 Hypertension Categories To Classify Blood Pressure Levels of Adults 18 Years and Older

Category	Descriptor	Systolic (mm Hg)	Diastolic (mm Hg)
Normal	Normal	<130	<85
High-normal	High-normal	130–139	85–89
Hypertension*			
Stage 1	Mild	140–159	90–99
Stage 2	Moderate	160–179	100–109
Stage 3	Severe	180–209	110–119
Stage 4	Very severe	≥210	≥120

*Based on readings taken at two or more visits following an initial screening.

Source: Adapted from *The Fifth Report of the Joint National Committee on Detection, Evaluation and Treatment of High Blood Pressure*, p. 4, National High Blood Pressure Education Program, National Heart, Lung and Blood Institute, National Institutes of Health, Publication No. 93-1088, January 1993.

- food service operators to label foods and provide salt substitutes

Preventing strokes means lowering blood pressure or controlling hypertension. The United States has experienced a 37% drop in age-adjusted death rates from stroke or cerebrovascular disease from 1979 to 1992. However, the male-to-female and black-to-white ratios for stroke mortality in 1992 were 1.18 and 1.86. Further, stroke is the third major cause of death in the United States.

Four states with a high incidence of high blood pressure and stroke developed easy-to-read health education materials to explain risk factors for strokes.[84] North Carolina developed materials for low-literacy clients by using focus groups to respond to fourth- and seventh-grade level materials (see Figures 14–1 and 14–2). The focus group participants emphasized the need for simple, direct materials that clearly showed which foods to control and demonstrated the specific ethnic groups being targeted.

HIGH-RISK SUBGROUPS

Hypertension among Older Adults

Hypertension occurs in approximately 60% of non-Hispanic whites, 71% of non-Hispanic blacks, and 61% of Mexican Americans 60 years of older.[82] Systolic hypertension is a known, independent risk factor for coronary heart disease, stroke, and cardiovascular disease. The prevalence of isolated systolic hypertension—defined as systolic blood pressure of 140 mm Hg or greater with diastolic blood pressure less than 90 mm Hg—increases after age 60. The sudden onset of hypertension in older patients suggests the presence of secondary hypertension.

Treating hypertension in older patients is recommended.[85] The Systolic Hypertension in Elder People Study (SHEP) assigned individuals to treatment with a low-dose diuretic, chlorthalidone. If warranted, atenolol or reserpine was added. Individuals who received treatment were compared to those on a placebo who had baseline average systolic blood pressure of 160 mm Hg or greater and diastolic blood pressure greater than 90 mm Hg. The results after an average of 4.5 years clearly favored active treatment. There were 36% fewer fatal and nonfatal strokes and 27% fewer fatal and nonfatal myocardial infarctions in actively treated versus placebo-treated participants. Benefit occurred in all age, race, sex, and blood pressure subgroups. Data from other clinical trials indicate that older patients who have diastolic blood pressure of 90 mm Hg or greater can also benefit from active antihypertensive therapy.

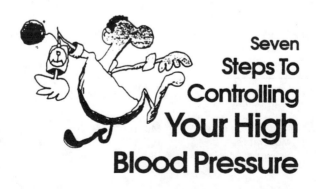

Figure 14–1 "Strike Out Stroke" health education materials developed for low-literacy adults in North Carolina. The materials emphasize control. *Source:* Reprinted from *Info Memo*, Easy-to-Read Materials Produced by Four Stroke Belt Projects, p. 17, National High Blood Pressure Prevention and Control Program, National Heart, Lung, and Blood Institute, 1993.

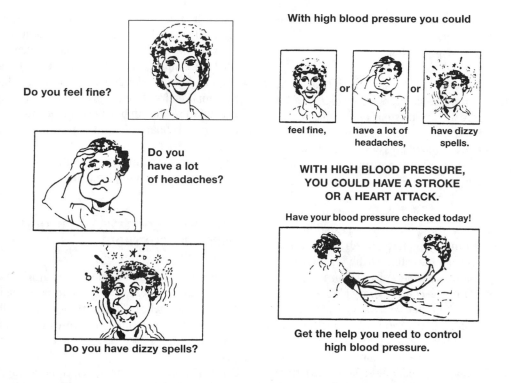

Figure 14-2 "Strike Out Stroke" health education materials developed for low-literacy adults in North Carolina. The materials emphasize the symptoms one can experience and the need to have blood pressure checked frequently. *Source:* Reprinted from *Info Memo*, Easy-to-Read Materials Produced by Four Stroke Belt Projects, p. 17, National High Blood Pressure Prevention and Control Program, National Heart, Lung, and Blood Institute, 1993.

The Working Group Report on Hypertension in the Elderly has issued a report to guide clinicians in their care of elderly, hypertensive patients.[86] The report states that the absolute risk of cardiovascular disease is greater among the elderly but that the benefits of control are also greater. Secondary intervention for elderly hypertensives first addresses lifestyle, focusing on weight control, increased physical activity, and reduction in alcohol and sodium intake. Antihypertensive drug therapy is the second approach, with diuretics and beta-blockers commonly prescribed if lifestyle modification alone does not reduce blood pressure levels.[86]

Hypertension among Individuals with Diabetes Mellitus

Patients with both hypertension and diabetes mellitus are at high risk for cardiovascular complications. The control of hypertension and dyslipidemia and cessation of cigarette smoking can reduce the risk. The blood pressure goal for high-risk individuals is 130/85 mm Hg or less. Lifestyle changes that can improve health outcome include weight reduction among obese individuals with insulin resistance.[87,88]

Hypertension during Pregnancy

Hypertension during pregnancy can create life-threatening outcomes for both mother and fetus. Four diagnostic categories are as follows[89]:

- chronic hypertension
- preeclampsia-eclampsia

- chronic hypertension with superimposed preeclampsia
- transient hypertension

The criteria for diagnosing hypertension in pregnancy are systolic pressure increases of 30 mm Hg or greater and diastolic pressure increases of 15 mm Hg or greater, compared with the mother's average blood pressure before 20 weeks of gestation. If prior blood pressures is not known, 140/90 mm Hg or above is considered abnormal. Chronic hypertension is defined as high blood pressure observed before pregnancy or diagnosed before the 20th week of gestation.

A pregnancy-specific condition called preeclampsia is characterized by an increased blood pressure accompanied by proteinuria, edema, or both. The contemporary phrase is pregnancy-induced hypertension. Occasionally, abnormalities of coagulation and liver function can occur. Preeclampsia may progress rapidly to a convulsive phase called eclampsia. Medical nutrition therapy (e.g., moderate sodium restriction) given along with drug therapy may be effective in reducing complications.[89]

HYPERTENSION DURING CHILDHOOD AND ADOLESCENCE

Studies of a biracial population of children 5 to 14 years old in two communities in Louisiana (the Franklinton and Bogalusa Heart Studies) indicated that height and weight, not age, were the strongest determinants of blood pressure in growing children.[90] Taking nine blood pressures per child in a rigorous, randomized design, registered nurses recorded the resting blood pressures of the children in an unhurried, relaxed atmosphere. Figure 14–3 illustrates the blood pressure levels by age, sex, and community.

Stepwise multiple regression analyses were used to determine variables accounting for the variability of blood pressure. These variables included mood score, community, and previous attendance at an examination. Height accounted for 34% and 30% of the variability in systolic blood

pressure in Bogalusa and Franklinton, respectively. Body mass index explained an additional 5 to 6% of the variability. Other analysis demonstrated a 2.7 mm Hg higher systolic and 1.1 mm Hg higher diastolic blood pressure for black children compared to white children in Franklinton. These data provide supportive evidence that hypertension originates during youth. The exact mechanisms that contribute to the early onset need delineation so primary prevention activities can be developed and implemented.

COMMUNITY PROGRAMS FOR BLOOD PRESSURE CONTROL

Modification of nonpharmacologic or lifestyle factors as primary prevention could potentially reduce the prevalence of hypertension nationally by at least 30% and could reduce the need for antihypertensive drugs in those who are hypertensive.[1]

A primary prevention approach can be complemented by special attempts to lower blood pressure among individuals at high risk of developing hypertension. A high-risk approach targets persons with a high normal blood pressure, a family history of hypertension, and one or more lifestyle factors that predispose them as they age to increases in blood pressure.[30] Achievement of the intervention goals may be constrained by a number of societal barriers. These barriers include a lack of acceptable low-sodium food substitutes and the absence of a national campaign to foster adoption of healthy habits.[91]

Community programs may be an important strategy for primary prevention of hypertension. The Joint National Committee on Detection, Evaluation and Treatment of High Blood Pressure suggests that communities consider the following[82,91]:

- detection, education, and referral for other cardiovascular risk factors
- various strategies to improve adherence:
  1. public, patient, and professional education activities
  2. culturally sensitive approaches

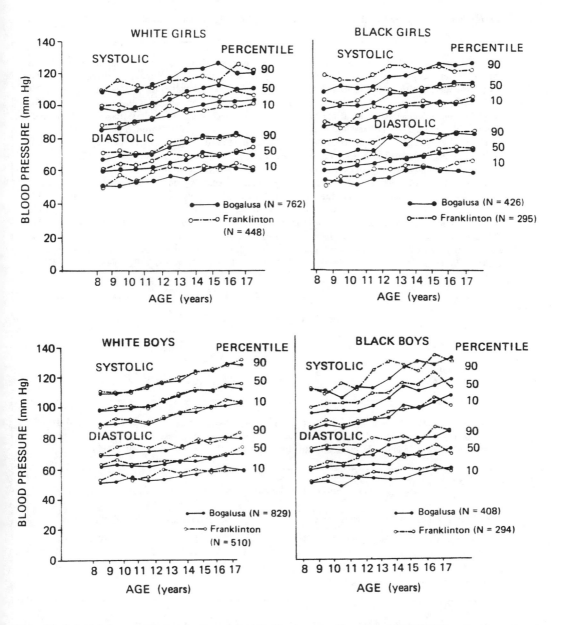

Figure 14-3 Selected percentiles for systolic and diastolic blood pressure for white and black children by age and community, 1978–1979. Levels of diastolic blood pressure for white boys were higher in Franklinton than in Bogalusa (*p* <0.0001). Systolic blood pressure levels for black boys were higher in Franklinton than in Bogalusa (*p* <0.0002). For older girls, systolic levels were higher in Bogalusa than in Franklinton. For younger white girls, diastolic levels were higher in Franklinton than in Bogalusa. For younger black girls, both systolic and diastolic levels were higher in Franklinton than in Bogalusa. *Source:* Reprinted from Webber, L.S., and Berenson, G.S., Racial Contrasts of Blood Pressure Levels in Two Southern, Rural Communities, *Preventive Medicine*, Vol. 14, pp. 140–151, with permission of Academic Press, © 1985.

Exhibit 14-2 *Healthy People 2000* Health Status Objectives Targeting High Blood Pressure

2.5   Reduce dietary fat intake to an average of 30% of calories or less and average saturated fat intake to <10% of calories among people aged 2 and older. (Baseline: 36% of calories from total fat and 13% from saturated fat for people aged 20 through 74 in 1976–80; 36% and 13% for women aged 19 through 50 in 1985.)

2.6   Increase complex carbohydrate and fiber-containing foods in the diets of adults to 5+ daily servings for vegetables (including legumes) and fruits, and to 6+ daily servings for grain products. (Baseline: 2½ servings of vegetables and fruits and 3 servings of grain products for women aged 19 through 50 in 1985.)

2.7   Increase to at least 50% the proportion of overweight people aged 12 and older who have adopted sound dietary practices combined with regular physical activity to attain an appropriate body weight. (Baseline: 30% of overweight women and 25% of overweight men for people aged 18 and older in 1985.)

2.9   Decrease salt and sodium intake so at least 65% of home meal preparers prepare foods without adding salt, at least 80% of people avoid using salt at the table, and at least 40% of adults regularly purchase foods modified or lower in sodium. (Baseline: 54% of women aged 19 through 50 who served as the main meal preparer did not use salt in food preparation, and 68% of women aged 19 through 50 did not use salt at the table in 1985; 20% of all people aged 18 and older regularly purchased foods with reduced salt and sodium content in 1988.)

15.4   Increase to at least 50% the proportion of people with high blood pressure whose blood pressure is under control. (Baseline: 11% controlled among people aged 18 through 74 in 1976–80; an estimated 24% for people age 18 and older in 1982–84.)

Special Population Target

High Blood Pressure Control	1976–80 Baseline	1982–84 Baseline	2000 Target
15.4a Men with high blood pressure	6%	16%	40%

15.5   Increase to at least 90% the proportion of people with high blood pressure (>140 mm Hg systolic and/or 90 mm Hg diastolic) who are taking action to help control their blood pressure. (Baseline: 79% of aware hypertensives aged 18 and older were taking action to control their blood pressure in 1985.)

Special Population Targets

Taking Action To Control Blood Pressure	1985 Baseline	2000 Target
15.5a White hypertensive men aged 18–34	51%*	80%
15.5b Black hypertensive men aged 18–34	63%*	80%

*Baseline for aware hypertensive men, 20–74 years.

Source: Reprinted from *Healthy People 2000: National Health Promotion and Disease Prevention Objectives*, U.S. Department of Health and Human Services, Public Health Service, Publication No. 91-50212, 1991.

3. informative food labeling
4. heart-healthy menus in restaurants
5. safe trails for walking and biking
- multiple channels for outreach:
  1. health care settings
  2. schools

3. work sites
4. churches and community centers
5. supermarkets and pharmacies
- media promotion
- second-order prevention efforts directed toward individuals with "normal" risk factor

Exhibit 14-3 Model Nutrition Objective for Reduced Risk Reduction

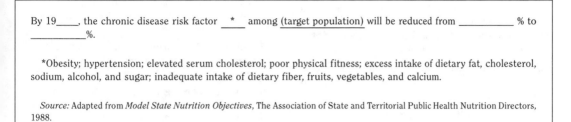

By 19____, the chronic disease risk factor __*__ among (target population) will be reduced from _____ % to _____%.

*Obesity; hypertension; elevated serum cholesterol; poor physical fitness; excess intake of dietary fat, cholesterol, sodium, alcohol, and sugar; inadequate intake of dietary fiber, fruits, vegetables, and calcium.

Source: Adapted from *Model State Nutrition Objectives*, The Association of State and Territorial Public Health Nutrition Directors, 1988.

levels who need education and support to maintain preventive behaviors (i.e., weight control, exercise, and good nutrition)

Modest activities can expand to become comprehensive programs. Coordination with clinicians and other health care providers may increase support of the community program. Advisory boards or community high blood pressure councils facilitate cooperation with professional agencies, local health departments, voluntary health agencies, hospitals, industry, and other interest groups. Community advisory boards or councils can identify community problems and local resources, set priorities, list practical solutions to problems, and formulate methods of evaluating program effectiveness.[92-95] In addition, community involvement fosters a sense of ownership. Ownership strengthens the community's acceptance of responsibility for its health problems and potential solutions.

HEALTHY PEOPLE 2000 ACTIONS

HP2K objectives for lifestyle changes to address high blood pressure prevention and control are presented in Exhibit 14-2. The composition of eating patterns (i.e., fat, complex carbohydrate, fiber, and sodium intake) is the primary focus. Attaining an appropriate body weight and controlling blood pressure are listed as objectives for individuals from adolescence throughout the adult years. An important action is to increase to 90% the proportion of men and women who take direct responsibility for their blood pressure control. Black men and white men are specific high-risk groups targeted by this objective. Community nutrition professionals can direct their program planning toward the lifestyle changes that include eating behavior and support blood pressure prevention and control (see Exhibit 14-3).

REFERENCES

1. Maxwell MH. *Nutritional Medicine in Medical Practice*. Los Angeles, Calif: UCLA Extension; January 22-23, 1993.

2. Stamler J. Epidemiologic findings on body mass and blood pressure in adults. *Ann Epidemiol*. 1991;1:347-362.

3. Chiang BN, Perlman LV, Epstein FH. Overweight and hypertension: A review. *Circulation*. 1969;39:403-421.

4. MacMahon S, Cutler J, Brittain E, et al. Obesity and hypertension: Epidemiological and clinical issues. *Eur Heart J*. 1987;8:57-70.

5. Fortmann SP, Haskell WL, Vranizan K, et al. The association of blood pressure and dietary alcohol: Differences by age, sex, and estrogen use. *Am J Epidemiol*. 1983;118:497-507.

6. Van Itallie TB. Health implications of overweight and obesity in the United States. *Ann Intern Med*. 1985;103: 983-988.

7. Kannel WB, Gordon T. Evaluation of cardiovascular risk in the elderly: The Framingham Study. *Bull NY Acad Med*. 1978;54:573-591.

8. National Institutes of Health Consensus Development Panel on the Health Implications of Obesity. Health implications of obesity: National Institutes of Health Consensus Development. *Ann Intern Med*. 1985;103:981-1077.

9. Shaper AG. Communities without hypertension. In: Shaper AG, Hutt MSR, Fejfar Z, eds. *Cardiovascular Disease in the Tropics*. London, England: British Medical Association; 1974:77-83.

10. Beilin LJ. The fifth George Pickering memorial lecture. Editorial review. Epitaph to essential hypertension—A preventable disorder of known aetiology? *J Hypertension*. 1988;6:85-94.

11. Lian C. L'Alcoolisme cuse d'hypertension arterielle. *Br Acad Med*. 1915;74:525–528.

12. Criqui MH, Meban I, Wallace RB, et al. Multivariate correlates of adult blood pressures in nine North American populations: The Lipid Research Clinics Prevalence Study. *Preventive Med*. 1982;11:391–402.

13. Friedman GD, Klatsky AL, Siegelaub AB. Alcohol, tobacco, and hypertension. *Hypertension*. 1982;4(Suppl III):III-143–III-150.

14. MacMahon SW, Blacket RB, Macdonald GJ, et al. Obesity, alcohol consumption and blood pressure in Australian men and women: The National Heart Foundation of Australia Risk Factor Prevalence Study. *J Hypertension*. 1984;2:85–91.

15. Potter JF, Beevers DG. Pressor effect of alcohol in hypertension. *Lancet*. 1984;1:119–122.

16. Gordon T, Doyle JT. Alcohol consumption and its relationship to smoking, weight, blood pressure and blood lipids: The Albany Study. *Arch Intern Med*. 1986;146:262–265.

17. Puddey IB, Beilin LJ, Vandongen R, et al. Evidence for a direct effect of alcohol consumption on blood pressure in normotensive men: A randomized controlled trial. *Hypertension*. 1985;7:707–713.

18. Dahl LK. Salt and hypertension. *Am J Clin Nutr*. 1972;25:231–244

19. Law MR, Frost CD, Wald NJ. By how much does dietary salt reduction lower blood pressure? I. Analysis of observational data among populations. *Br Med J*. 1991;302:811–815.

20. Fregly MS, Fregly MJ. The estimates of sodium intake by man. In: Fregly MJ, Kare MR, eds. *The Role of Salt in Cardiovascular Hypertension*. New York, NY: Academic Press; 1982;3–15.

21. Watt GCM, Foy CJW. Dietary sodium and arterial pressure: Problems of studies within a single population. *J Epidemiol Community Health*. 1982;36:197–201.

22. Stamler R. Implications of the Intersalt study. *Hypertension*. 1991;17(Suppl I):I-16–I-20.

23. Intersalt Cooperative Research Group. Intersalt: An international study of electrolyte excretion and blood pressure. Results for 24 hour urinary sodium and potassium excretion. *Br Med J*. 1988;297:319–328.

24. Intersalt Cooperative Research Group. Sodium, potassium, body mass, alcohol and blood pressure: The Intersalt Study. *J Hypertension*. 1988;6(Suppl 4):584S–586S.

25. Muntzel M, Drueke T. A comprehensive review of the salt and blood pressure relationship. *Am J Hypertension*. 1992;5:1S–42S.

26. Grobbee DE, Hofman A. Does sodium restriction lower blood pressure? *Br Med J*. 1986;293:27–29.

27. Subcommittee on Nonpharmacological Therapy of the 1984 Joint National Committee on Detection, Evaluation, and Treatment of High Blood Pressure. Nonpharmacological approaches to the control of high blood pressure. *Hypertension*. 1986;8:444–467.

28. Witteman JCM, Willett WC, Stampfer MJ, et al. A prospective study of nutritional factors and hypertension among US women. *Circulation*. 1989;80:1320–1327.

29. Ascherio A, Rimm EB, Giovanucci EL, et al. A prospective study of nutritional factors and hypertension among US men. *Circulation*. 1992;86:1475–1484.

30. The Trials of Hypertension Prevention Collaborative Research Group. The effects of nonpharmacologic interventions on blood pressure of persons with high normal levels. Results of the Trials of Hypertension Prevention, Phase I. *JAMA*. 1992;267:1213–1220.

31. He J, Tell GS, Tang Y-C, et al. Relation of electrolytes to blood pressure in men: The Yi People Study. *Hypertension*. 1991;17:378–385.

32. Treasure J, Ploth D. Role of dietary potassium in the treatment of hypertension. *Hypertension*. 1983;5:864–872.

33. Tannen RL. Effects of potassium on blood pressure control. *Ann Intern Med*. 1983;98:773–780.

34. Whelton PK, Klag MJ. Potassium in the homeostasis and reduction of blood pressure. *Clin Nutr*. 1987;6:76–82.

35. Langford HG. Can black/white differences in blood pressure and hypertensive mortality in the US be explained by differences in potassium intake? In: Whelton PK, Whelton A, Walker WG, eds. *Potassium in Cardiovascular and Renal Medicine—Arrythmias, Myocardial Infarction, and Hypertension*. New York, NY: Marcel Dekker; 1986; 397–400.

36. Medical Research Council Working Party. Medical Research Council trial of treatment of hypertension in older adults: Principal results. *Br Med J*. 1992;304:405–412.

37. Dahlof B, Linholm LH, Hansson L, et al. Morbidity and mortality in the Swedish Trial in Old Patients with Hypertension (STOP-Hypertension). *Lancet*. 1991;338:1281–1285.

38. Kromhout D, Bosschieter EB, Coulander C de L. Potassium, calcium, alcohol intake and blood pressure: The Zutphen Study. *Am J Clin Nutr*. 1985;41:1299–1304.

39. Ackley S, Barrett-Connor E, Suarez L. Dairy products, calcium, and blood pressure. *Am J Clin Nutr*. 1983;38:457–461.

40. Connor SL, Connor WE, Henry H, et al. The effects of familial relationships, age, body weight, and diet on blood pressure and the 24 hour urinary excretion of sodium, potassium, and creatinine in men, women, and children of randomly selected families. *Circulation*. 1984;70:76–85.

41. Gruchow HW, Sobocincki KA, Barboriak JJ. Alcohol, nutrient intake, and hypertension in US Adults. *JAMA*. 1985;253:1567–1570.

42. Harlan WR, Hull AL, Schmouder RL, et al. High blood pressure in older Americans: The First National Health and Nutrition Examination Survey. *Hypertension*. 1984;6:802-809.

43. Harlan WR, Hull AL, Schmouder RL, et al. Blood pressure and nutrition in adults: The National Health and Nutrition Examination Survey. *Am J Epidemiol*. 1984;120:17-28.

44. Iso H, Terao A, Kitamura A, et al. Calcium intake and blood pressure in seven Japanese populations. *Am J Epidemiol*. 1991;133:776-783.

45. Joffres MR, Reed DM, Yano K. Relationship of magnesium intake and other dietary factors to blood pressure: The Honolulu heart study. *Am J Clin Nutr*. 1987;45:469-475.

46. Kesteloot H, Geboers J. Calcium and blood pressure. *Lancet*. 1982;1:813-815.

47. Kok FJ, Vandenbroucke JP, van der Heide-Wessel C, et al. Dietary sodium, calcium, potassium, and blood pressure. *Am J Epidemiol*. 1986;123:1043-1048.

48. Nichaman M, Shekelle R, Paul O. Diet, alcohol, and blood pressure in the Western Electric Study. *Am J Epidemiol*. 1989;130:469-470.

49. Reed D, McGee D, Yano K. Biological and social correlates of blood pressure among Japanese men in Hawaii. *Hypertension*. 1982;4:406-414.

50. Reed D, McGee D, Yano K, et al. Diet, blood pressure, and multicolinearity. *Hypertension*. 1985;7:405-410.

51. Sempos C, Cooper R, Kovar MG, et al. Dietary calcium and blood pressure in National Health and Nutrition Examination Surveys I and II. *Hypertension*. 1986;8:1067-1074.

52. Sowers MR, Wallace RB, Lemke JH. The association of intakes of vitamin D and calcium with blood pressure among women. *Am J Clin Nutr*. 1985;42:135-142.

53. Witteman JCM, Willett WC, Stampfer MJ, et al. A prospective study of nutritional factors and hypertension among US women. *Circulation*. 1989;80:1320-1327.

54. Belizan JM, Villar J, Pineda O, et al. Reduction of blood pressure with calcium supplementation in young adults. *JAMA*. 1983;249:1161-1165.

55. Cappuccio FP, Markandu ND, Beynon GW, et al. Effect of increasing calcium intake on urinary sodium excretion in normotensive subjects. *Clin Sci*. 1986;71:453-456.

56. Elliott P, Fehily AM, Sweetnam PM, et al. Diet, alcohol, body mass, and social factors in relation to blood pressure: The Caerphilly Heart Study. *J Epidemiol Community Health*. 1987;41:37-43.

57. Feinleib M, Lenfant C, Miller SA. Hypertension and calcium. *Science*. 1984;226:384-386.

58. Garcia-Palmieri MR, Costas R Jr, Cruz-Vidal M, et al. Milk consumption, calcium intake, and decreased hypertension in Puerto Rico: Puerto Rico Heart Health Program Study. *Hypertension*. 1984;6:322-328.

59. Hung J-S, Huang T-T, Wu DL, et al. The impact of dietary sodium, potassium, and calcium on blood pressure. *J Formosan Med Assoc*. 1990;89:17-22.

60. McGarvey ST, Zinner SH, Willett WC, et al. Maternal prenatal dietary potassium, calcium, magnesium, and infant blood pressure. *Hypertension*. 1991;17:218-224.

61. Bierenbaum ML, Wolf E, Bisgeier G, et al. Dietary calcium: A method of lowering blood pressure. *Am J Hypertension*. 1988;1:149S-152S.

62. Grobbee DE, Hofman A. Effect of calcium supplementation on diastolic blood pressure in young people with mild hypertension. *Lancet*. 1986;2:703-706.

63. Johnson NE, Smith EL, Freudenheim JL. Effects on blood pressure of calcium supplementation of women. *Am J Clin Nutr*. 1985;42:12-17.

64. Lyle RM, Melby CL, Hyner GC, et al. Blood pressure and metabolic effects of calcium supplementation in normotensive white and black men. *JAMA*. 1987;257:1772-1776.

65. Mascioli S, Grimm R Jr, Launer C, et al. Sodium chloride raises blood pressure in normotensive subjects: The study of sodium and blood pressure. *Hypertension*. 1991;17(Suppl I):I-21-I-26.

66. Whelton PK, Klag MJ. Magnesium and blood pressure: Review of the epidemiologic and clinical trial experience. *Am J Cardiol*. 1989;63:26G-30G.

67. Henderson DG, Schierup J, Schodt T. Effect of magnesium supplementation on blood pressure and electrolyte concentrations in hypertensive patients receiving long term diuretic treatment. *Br Med J*. 1986;293:664-665.

68. Saito K, Hattori K, Omatsu T, et al. Effects of oral magnesium on blood pressure and red cell sodium transport in patients receiving long-term thiazide diuretics for hypertension. *Am J Hypertension*. 1988;1:71S-74S.

69. National Diet-Heart Study Research Group. The National Diet-Heart Study final report. *Circulation*. 1968;37(suppl I):I-1-I-419.

70. Sacks FM, Kass EH. Low blood pressure in vegetarians: Effects of specific foods and nutrients. *Am J Clin Nutr*. 1988;48:795-800.

71. Brussard JH, van Raaij JMA, Stasse-Wolthuis M, et al. Blood pressure and diet in normotensive volunteers: Absence of an effect of dietary fiber, protein, or fat. *Am J Clin Nutr*. 1981;34:2023-2029.

72. Kelsay JL, Behall KM, Prather ES. Effect of fiber from fruits and vegetables on metabolic responses of human subjects: I. Bowel transit time, number of defecations, fecal weight, urinary excretions of energy and nitrogen and apparent digestibilities of energy, nitrogen, and fat. *Am J Clin Nutr*. 1978;31:1149-1153.

73. Margetts BM, Beilin LJ, Vandongen R, et al. A randomized controlled trial of the effect of dietary fibre on blood pressure. *Clin Sci.* 1987;72:343–350.

74. Swain JF, Rouse IL, Curley CB, et al. Comparison of the effects of oat bran and low-fiber wheat on serum lipoprotein levels and blood pressure. *N Engl J Med.* 1990;322:147–152.

75. Stamler J, Caggiula A, Grandits A. Relationships of dietary variables to blood pressure (BP): Findings of the Multiple Risk Factor Intervention Trial (MRFIT). *Circulation.* 1992;85:867. Abstract.

76. Mensink RP, Janssen M-C, Katan MB. Effect on blood pressure of two diets differing in total fat but not in saturated and polyunsaturated fatty acids in healthy volunteers. *Am J Clin Nutr.* 1988;47:976–980.

77. Sacks FM, Rouse IL, Stampfer MJ, et al. Effect of dietary fat and carbohydrate on blood pressure of mildly hypertensive patients. *Hypertension.* 1987;10:452–460.

78. Sacks FM, Stampfer MF, Munoz A, et al. Effect of linoleic and oleic acids on blood pressure, blood viscosity, and erythrocyte cation transport. *J Am Coll Nutr.* 1987;6: 179–185.

79. Kumanyika SK. Feasibility and efficacy of sodium reduction in the trials of hypertension prevention, phase I. *Hypertension.* 1993;22:502–512.

80. Stamler R, Stamler J, Gosch FC, et al. Primary prevention of hypertension by nutritional-hygienic means: Final report of a randomized, controlled trial. *JAMA.* 1989; 262:1801–1807.

81. Hypertension Prevention Trial Research Group. The Hypertension Prevention Trial: Three-year effects of dietary changes on blood pressure. *Arch Intern Med.* 1990;150: 153–162.

82. National Heart, Lung, and Blood Institute. *The Fifth Report of the Joint National Committee on Detection, Evaluation, and Treatment of High Blood Pressure.* Bethesda, Md: National Institutes of Health; January 1993. NIH publication 93-1088.

83. Working Group on Health Education and High Blood Pressure Control, National High Blood Pressure Education Program. *The Physician's Guide: Improving Adherence among Hypertensive Patients.* Bethesda, Md: US Department of Health and Human Services, National Heart, Lung, and Blood Institute; March 1987.

84. National High Blood Pressure Prevention and Control Program. Easy-to-read materials produced by four stroke belt projects. *Info memo.* Bethesda, Md: National Heart, Lung, and Blood Institute; 1993.

85. SHEP Cooperative Research Group. Prevention of stroke by antihypertensive drug treatment in older persons with isolated systolic hypertension. *JAMA.* 1991;265:3255–3264.

86. National High Blood Pressure Education Program Coordinating Committee. *Statement on Hypertension in the Elderly–Final Report.* Bethesda, Md: National Institutes of Health; 1980.

87. Working Group on Hypertension in Diabetes, National High Blood Pressure Education Program. Statement on hypertension in diabetes mellitus: Final report. *Arch Intern Med.* 1987;147:830–842.

88. Epstein M, Sowers JR. Diabetes mellitus and hypertension. *Hypertension.* 1992;19:403–418.

89. National High Blood Pressure Education Program Working Group on High Blood Pressure in Pregnancy. Working group report on high blood pressure in pregnancy. *Am J Obstet Gynecol.* 1990;163:1689–1712.

90. National High Blood Pressure Education Program. *Working Group Report on Primary Prevention of Hypertension.* Bethesda, Md: National Institutes of Health; May 1993. NIH publication 93-2669.

91. Lefebvre RC, Lasater TM, Carleton RA, et al. Theory and delivery of health programming in the community: The Pawtucket Heart Health Program. *Preventive Med.* 1987;16:80–95.

92. Mittelmark MB, Leupker RV, Jacobs DR, et al. Community-wide prevention of cardiovascular disease: Education strategies of the Minnesota Heart Health Program. *Preventive Med.* 1986;15:1–17.

93. Levine DM, Bone L. The impact of a planned health education approach on the control of hypertension in a high risk population. *J Hum Hypertension.* 1990;4:317–321.

94. Farquhar JW, Fortmann SP, Flora JA, et al. Effects of community wide education on cardiovascular disease risk factors: The Stanford Five-City Project *JAMA.* 1990;264:359–365.

95. National High Blood Pressure Education Program. *Measuring Progress in High Blood Pressure Control: An Evaluation Handbook.* Bethesda, Md: US Department of Health and Human Services, National Heart, Lung, and Blood Institute; April 1986. NIH publication 86-2647.

Learning Objectives

- Discuss the epidemiology of obesity in the United States.
- Define the role of eating behavior in the etiology, prevention, and treatment of obesity.
- Discuss voluntary methods practiced by individuals for weight loss and control.
- Identify the *Healthy People 2000* objectives for obesity.
- Describe how community nutritionists can be actively involved in the primary, secondary, and tertiary care of obesity in the United States.

High Definition Nutrition

Qualitative obesity—an abnormally high proportion of body fat.
Quantitative obesity—a body mass index (BMI) >27. BMI classes are:

- class 0: 20–25 kg/m^2 and not obese
- class I: 25–30 kg/m^2 and low risk for illness
- class II: 30–35 kg/m^2 and moderate risk
- class III: 35–40 kg/m^2 and high risk
- class IV: >40 kg/m^2 and very high risk

AN OVERVIEW OF OBESITY

One in six Americans—about 44 million people—are obese,[1] and obesity-related health problems in the United States are complex, serious, and difficult to manage. A National Institutes of Health (NIH) Consensus Development Conference Panel on Obesity reviewed current research and concluded that a body mass index (BMI)—weight in kg/height in meters^2—greater than 26.9 in women and 27.2 in men indicates increased risk for many common diseases, including heart disease, certain cancers, stroke, diabetes mellitus, and atherosclerosis.[1,2] The cost of these diseases is more than $277 billion for health care alone. More than 17% or $39 billion is due to obesity.[3,4]

A BMI of greater than 35 kg/m^2 is associated with a twofold increase in total mortality and a multifold increase in morbidity, yet a 10 to 20% weight loss can forestall or eliminate most obesity-related disease.[5] In addition, a definite reduction in health care costs as a result of improved cardiac function, improved lipid profiles, and improved glucose tolerance and the associated decreased need for medication can be realized with weight loss.[6-8]

Research has contributed to the understanding and management of body weight from three major domains[9]:

1. *descriptive*—identification of characteristics of individuals with obesity
2. *theoretical*—explanation of various theories of human behavior to life situations
3. *experimental*—evaluation of the effectiveness of various nutrition education approaches

In the early 1980s, several researchers proposed a system of classification of levels of obesity, beginning with a standardization manual for data collection,[10] but the attempt has continued to be challenging. Obesity can be defined in terms of amount or distribution of body fat, mortality, or morbidity. Even skills such as the ability to possess eating restraint have been used to characterize or to differentiate individuals with obesity.[11-13]

Due to the multifactorial nature of obesity, there is not a consensus of what is precisely a healthy level of body fatness, but many believe that a healthy or good body weight range is one that is associated with the most favorable mortality experience[14,15] (see Table 15–1). Even with obesity being defined many different ways, the most common definitions are qualitative and quantitative.

Contributions from the theoretical or explanatory domain have evolved over the years. Most contemporary theories about obesity stem from response to the psychodynamic theory, even though the theory is limited to unique situations.[16,17] Other theories that have been tested in obesity research include behavioral theory involving antecedents and consequences or internal and external hunger cues.[18,19] Social learning theory, later termed *social cognitive theory*, explains behavior as the interplay of cognition, personal factors, and environmental factors.[20,21] The theory was expanded to focus on self-efficacy, and a scale with scores explaining a significant portion of the eating behavior of weight control participants has been tested.[22-24]

Self-efficacy has been shown to be associated with adherence, and nutrition education approaches teach individuals to become aware of their defeating thoughts and feelings and substitute negative thoughts with positive ones.[25] Two other theories that have been the basis of intervention programs include (1) the Health Belief Model, which incorporates an individual's perception of the seriousness of obesity with his or her ability to address and to change the problem;[26,27] and (2) the Theory of Reasoned Action, which assumes that humans' behavior can be predicted from their attitude, evaluation, and perception of others toward their behavior.[28]

Data from experimental studies have involved numerous therapeutic approaches that range from increasing the awareness of individuals about the energy content of foods to multifac-

Table 15–1 Descriptive Terminology for Weight

Adjective	Year	Source
Ideal	1942	Metropolitan Life Insurance Company weight and height tables
Acceptable, normal, ideal	1980	Dietary guidelines
Suggested	1980	Dietary guidelines
Desirable	1959	Metropolitan Life Insurance Company weight and height tables
	1985	Dietary guidelines
Acceptable	1975	Fogarty/NIH Conference
Healthy	1990	Dietary guidelines
Suggested	1990	Dietary guidelines

Source: Adapted from Kuczmarski, R.J., Prevalence of Overweight and Weight Gain in the United States, *American Journal of Clinical Nutrition*, Vol. 55, p. 495S, with permission of the American Society for Clinical Nutrition, © 1992.

eted strategies employing exercise, cognition, and skill development. Skill training as an indirect approach to empower individuals before working on changing behaviors has been recommended. Developing social support, buffering the effect of stress, uncovering the factors that bring on disinhibition, and setting up sequential stages of change have been explored.[13,29,30] Factors that appear to predict intention and dropout in weight-loss programs have been identified as demographic, type of program, personal variables, and environmental and attitudinal variables.[31]

The reasons for excess weight are multiple and mirror the characteristics of individuals who are more successful with their weight management. Those who are more successful with maintaining weight loss have achieved higher self-efficacy scores that reflect their taking responsibility for their efforts, defining a fitness or exercise program, developing a lifestyle using multiple resources, and participating in several programs to meet their needs.[32,33] Reality checks about obesity can be administered and reviewed by community health care professionals to plan and to direct programs for individuals with obesity (see Exhibit 15-1).

GENDER AND ETHNIC DIFFERENCES

To standardize comparisons, reference persons in data analysis are adults, 20 to 29 years old. This is because after growth is completed during the 20s there is no further increase in stature. For most national surveys, obesity is defined as individuals whose BMI is above the 85th percentile (often defined as overweight). Excess weight gain is associated with an accumulation of adipose tissue.[34] The 10-year incidence of weight gain for white and black women is presented in Table 15-2.[35]

A greater percentage of minority groups and female minorities are obese.[36,37] Black adult women display the highest prevalence among all groups for both obesity and severe obesity (see Table 15-3). White men and women have the lowest rates.

The prevalence of obesity reaches 50% for Native-American, African-American, and Hispanic women in the United States.[38,39] For Hispanic subgroups in the United States, prevalence of obesity has been reported for the 1982–1984 period using national data. With obesity defined as BMI at or above the 85th percentile and mor-

---

Exhibit 15-1 Reality Checks for Health Care Professionals—Obesity in the United States

- One in six Americans—about 44 million people—are overweight, and obesity-related health problems are complex, serious, and difficult to manage.
- A greater percentage of minority groups and female minorities are obese.
- Weight gain is an important indicator of obesity in the United States.
- Individuals at the extremes of body weight and body mass index (BMI) warrant special concern.
- Body fat placement influences health risk.
- There is a link between obesity and coronary heart disease risk factors.
- The incidence of non-insulin-dependent diabetes mellitus increases with rising BMI, and there is no evidence of a threshold.
- Mortality from all types of cancer increases with increasing weight among women and men.
- Most epidemiological studies report that excess body weight and excess BMI increases mortality.
- Depression appears to be a significant factor causing weight change among adults.
- Obesity can begin early in life; when it begins, it represents a cause for concern.
- One-third of women and one-fourth of men try to lose or control their weight.
- There is no single, effective strategy for weight loss.
- There are definite attitudinal and behavioral barriers to weight loss.
- Eating and exercise changes reinforced by behavior modification is the most common and preferred combined therapy.
- Professionals have a responsibility to assist overweight and obese individuals to lose weight.

Table 15–2   10-Year Incidence of Weight Gain among Women in the NHANES I Epidemiologic Follow-Up Survey by Age and Race

	25–34 Years		35–44 Years	
	White	Black	White	Black
Mean change in BMI	+1.2	+1.8	+0.9	+1.3
Incidence of overweight (%)	12.0	9.5	12.8	23.6
Incidence of major weight gain (%)	8.1	11.2	7.0	8.7

Source: Adapted from Kuczmarski, R.J., Prevalence of Overweight and Weight Gain in the United States, *American Journal of Clinical Nutrition*, Vol. 55, p. 495S, with permission of the American Society for Clinical Nutrition, © 1992.

bid obesity defined as BMI at or above the 95th percentile, the rates for obesity are 39%, 37%, and 34% for Mexican-American, Puerto Rican, and Cuban American women, respectively. For women, morbid obesity was noted for 16%, 14%, and 8% of Mexican Americans, Puerto Ricans, and Cuban Americans, respectively. For men, obesity was noted for 30%, 29%, and 25% of Mexican Americans, Cuban Americans, and Puerto Ricans, and morbid obesity was noted for 10%, 11%, and 8%, respectively.[40]

Data can be analyzed by education and income levels. Education can be stratified into three groups (0–8 years, 9–12 years, and >12 years) and then subclassified by age (20–44 years and 45–74 years). For younger men and women, the majority who were obese had 9 or more years of education. For individuals 45 to 74 years old,

especially Hispanics, a higher percentage of those who were obese were less educated.[34]

For individuals below the poverty level, prevalence of obesity was highest for black, Mexican-American, and Puerto Rican groups. Nearly one-fourth of overweight Mexican-American and Puerto Rican males had incomes below the poverty level; almost one-half of obese Puerto Rican women and one-third of black and Mexican-American obese women were below the poverty level (see Figure 15–1).[34]

A sample of 936 Mexican Americans and 398 Anglo Americans from three culturally and socially distinct San Antonio neighborhoods reported a significantly greater prevalence of non-insulin-dependent diabetes mellitus among Mexican Americans compared with Anglo Americans at all three levels of body fatness.[41]

Table 15–3   Age-Adjusted Percentage of Overweight and Severely Overweight Persons aged 20–74 Years from NHANES II and HHANES by Ethnicity and Sex

	Male		Female	
	Overweight (%)	Severely Overweight (%)	Overweight (%)	Severely Overweight (%)
White	24.4	7.8	24.6	9.6
Black	26.3	10.4	45.1	19.7
Mexican	31.2	10.8	41.5	16.7
Cuban	28.5	10.3	31.9	6.9
Puerto Rican	25.7	7.9	39.8	15.2

Source: Adapted from Kuczmarski, R.J., Prevalence of Overweight and Weight Gain in the United States, *American Journal of Clinical Nutrition*, Vol. 55, p. 495S, with permission of the American Society for Clinical Nutrition, © 1992.

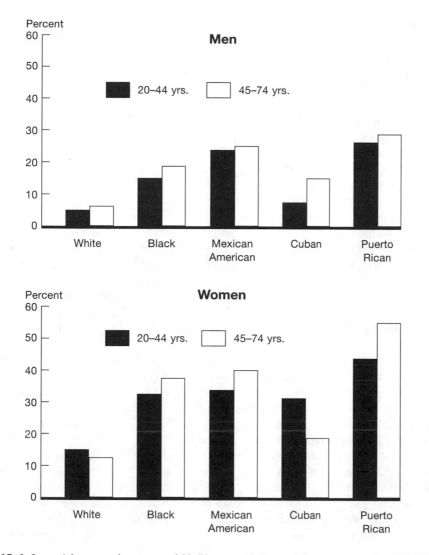

Figure 15-1 Overweight men and women aged 20-74 years with income below poverty levels, NHANES II (1976-80) and HHANES (1982-84). *Source:* Adapted from Kuczmarski, R.J., Prevalence of Overweight and Weight Gain in the United States, *American Journal of Clinical Nutrition*, Vol. 55, p. 495S, with permission of the American Society for Clinical Nutrition, © 1992.

Obesity prevalence remained stable for white men and females and was high but fairly consistent for black females when contrasting the 1960-1962 NHANES with the 1976-1980 surveys. The greatest increase in prevalence of obesity occurred for black males, from 21.7% in 1960-1962 to 27.7% in 1976-1980.[42]

Weight gain in the United States can be described using NHANES I Epidemiologic Follow-Up Survey data.[43] Participants were 25 to 74 years of age at the first measure in 1971-1975 and then remeasured 10 years later (N = 9,862). Weight change was reported in absolute BMI units (kg/m^2). Greatest weight gain occurred in the younger participants.[43]

Based on average gain per decade, men gained about 4.5 kg and woman 7.3 kg between 25 and 54 years of age. Major weight gain of more than 5 BMI units was seen for about 2.3% of men and 5.3% of women. The greatest incidence for women occurred for those 25 to 44 years old who were initially obese 10 years earlier; for men, highest incidence occurred among those who were 45 to 64 years old and underweight at baseline, and those who were 25 to 44 years old and overweight at baseline.[43]

The greatest average increase in BMI over the 10 years occurred for black women compared with white women in both age groups. Ethnicity may not be an independent risk factor for weight gain during adult years; less education, lower income, and marrying during follow-up appeared a more important potential causal factor for women gaining weight.[44] Less education, less income, and marital status (both marrying or staying single) were more strongly linked to weight gain for men.[45]

FAT PLACEMENT AND TIMING

Skinfold thickness on the trunk and extremities, circumference measures of the abdomen and hips and its ratio, and nuclear magnetic resonance imaging arc ways to evaluate fat distribution.[46] Men have more abdominal fat or android fat; women have more gluteal fat and hip circumferences, called gynoid fat. Major complications of obesity (cardiovascular disease, diabetes mellitus, hypertension, and hyperlipidemia) are associated with increased abdominal fat.[47,48] This is true for men with a waist-hip ratio (WHR) greater than 0.95 and for women with WHR greater than 0.80.[49]

The age at which an individual becomes obese is important in relation to health risk. The risk for a comparable degree of obesity seems to be greater among individuals who became obese before age 40 than for those who became obese after age 40.[50] In addition, longitudinal studies show that weight gain accompanies a greater risk of cardiovascular disease than an unchanging level of obesity.[51]

DEVELOPMENT OF OBESITY

At a basic level, excess body fat can only occur when energy ingested exceeds energy require-

ments or when fat intake exceeds fat oxidation. This can occur due to behavioral causes (i.e., high intake of fat or of total energy or low levels of physical activity) or metabolic causes (i.e., low maintenance energy requirement or high energy efficiency).

Obesity Viewed as a Metabolic Problem

Obesity could be considered to be a metabolic problem in someone with an abnormally low rate of essential energy expenditure and an abnormally high food efficiency. However, based on current knowledge, a low rate of essential energy expenditure estimated by resting metabolic rate (RMR) is not a major cause of obesity.

Determinants of RMR are reasonably well understood, with 80% to 90% of the between-subject variation in RMR being explained by fat-free mass, body-fat mass, age, and gender.[52] Some researchers have suggested a familial component to RMR.[52] When these variables are considered, RMR is not substantially different between lean and obese individuals.

Food efficiency can be approximated by the thermic effect of food (TEF), which consists of the costs of digestion, absorption, and metabolism of ingested food. Precise determinants of TEF, and whether a low TEF is a factor in obesity development, are controversial.[53] Any existing between-subject differences in TEF are likely to be small and not of major importance in obesity development.

No general abnormalities in essential energy expenditure or in food efficiency have been identified that would explain development of obesity. Based on current knowledge, the development of obesity cannot be solely blamed on metabolic causes.

Systematic lean-obese metabolic differences are not identified, but small individual differences in essential energy expenditure or in food efficiency could influence the development of obesity under specific nutrition and environmental conditions. For example, individuals whose measured RMR is lower than their predicted RMR have been observed to have a higher incidence of weight gain over time than individuals whose measured

RMR is higher than predicted RMR.[52] During overfeeding, individual differences are seen both in the amount of weight gained and in the composition of weight gain.[54] These differences could result from small individual differences in metabolism.

Obesity Viewed as a Behavioral Problem

Great difficulty occurs when researchers try to avoid classifying obesity as a problem in food intake. Regardless of energy expenditure, weight gain will not occur if energy intake is matched to energy expenditure. Individuals who practice an eating behavior with excess energy or fat intake may be at risk for positive energy and fat balance and ultimate gain in body fat. Similarly, individuals who reduce physical activity may be at risk of positive energy and fat balance if intake is not also adjusted downward.

Dietary composition is a factor in obesity development. High-fat foods promote fat storage by increasing total energy intake without any immediate increase in fat oxidation.[55] Maintenance of a consistent body composition requires that, on average over time, the fuel mixture ingested equals the fuel mixture burned.[56] Acute changes in protein and carbohydrate intake produce rapid changes in their oxidation. Fat oxidation is not acutely affected by changes in fat intake.[55,56]

Excess dietary energy from fat is stored as body fat more efficiently than excess energy from carbohydrate or protein.[56] The notion that high-fat diets promote fat accumulation is consistent with the high prevalence of obesity in Western societies, where high-fat diets are prevalent. Even with the average percentage of calories from fat declining, individuals may be consuming more total energy and exercising less. They are in effect consuming more fat and expending fewer fat calories.

The hypothesis that body fat is related to food composition and not total energy intake has become a popular research topic. Body fat may be closely related to the amount of fat in the foods consumed, as 97% of food energy from fat is available for immediate storage as body fat.[57] Pre and post measures of social characteristics and weight-related attitudes and behaviors and body mass indices were examined for 304 Mexican-American women, 19 to 50 years old living in Starr County, Texas. Path analysis revealed that women with higher socioeconomic characteristic scores had less frequent meals and ate less calorically dense foods. Dietary behaviors (e.g., frequency of meals and snacks, use of high- and low-caloric foods, and eating restraint) explained 17.4% of the variance in weight change.[58]

In another study, three-day dietary records that included a one-day recall were compared for 23 lean men, 17 lean women, 23 obese men, and 15 obese women. No differences were observed in total energy intake or energy intake relative to lean body mass between lean and obese participants. The obese men and women ate significantly more fat and less total carbohydrate than lean men and women; they consumed a similar amount of total sugar, but the obese men and women consumed a significantly greater percentage of added sugar.[59]

Several studies have reported similar results.[60-63] And several studies have reported a preference for highly sugared foods among obese individuals.[64-68] Data suggest that obese individuals prefer a higher fat-to-sugar ratio in their food than normal-weight individuals.[60,69] The high-fat foods may be selected due to taste, and for many high-fat foods, sugar is a complementary ingredient. Lean individuals may consume a substantial amount of sugar in the form of fruits and vegetables but naturally less fat. In other words, the source of the dietary sugar (added versus natural), not the actual amount, and the amount of dietary fat, not the source, appear more important than total energy, fat, and sugar.

An additional consideration is dietary fiber intake. Fiber reduces intestinal transit time and increases postprandial satisfaction and the rate of glucose absorption. Whole grains, fruits, vegetables, and legumes are rich, natural sources of sugar and fiber. The fiber may influence the absorption rate of the natural sugars among lean individuals and retard fat deposition.[70-72] This action is not present in the obese, as their dietary patterns are low in fiber and high in sugar and fat.[60]

Obesity Viewed as a Problem in the Interaction of Behavior and Metabolism

Obesity is not solely a metabolic or a behavioral problem.[73] Whether a person becomes obese under a given set of nutritional circumstances is determined by an interaction between the behavioral response to those circumstances and the metabolic response to the behavior. These processes determine how much and what type of energy enters the system and the disposition of that energy within the body. Whether body weight and body composition remain the same or increase or decrease over time depends on how closely metabolism matches behavior, so that energy intake equals energy expenditure and nutrient intake equals nutrient oxidation.[73]

TREATMENT OF OBESITY TO PRODUCE NEGATIVE ENERGY BALANCE

Reducing body weight requires a negative energy balance. This is usually accomplished by calorie restriction. Since daily energy expenditure declines as body mass is lost, the amount of body energy lost will be less than the amount of negative energy balance produced.

A common problem in obesity treatment is not producing weight loss but maintaining the reduced body weight.[73] Poor success in maintaining weight reduction has led to the hypothesis that after weight reduction, the previously obese person has an abnormally high energy efficiency, virtually ensuring that weight regain will occur even if extremely low intake is maintained.

An examination of the metabolic state after weight reduction may explain the ease of weight gain without the need to hypothesize an altered energy efficiency. Resting metabolic rate declines with weight reduction, since it is related to body mass. The majority of data suggest that the determinants of RMR after weight loss are the same as before.[74] The thermal effect of food (described as a percentage of ingested energy) does not appear to change with weight reduction.

A reduced body mass would lead to a decline in the energy cost of physical activity. Unless the amount of physical activity is increased, energy expenditure during activity may be reduced. Thus, total energy expenditure declines with weight loss, but the decline appears to be appropriate for the loss of body mass.

The composition of fuel burned is also altered by weight loss. The daily rate of fat oxidation seems to be proportional to the body fat mass,[75] and since proportionally more body fat is lost compared to body stores of protein or carbohydrate, fat oxidation may decline to a greater extent than protein or carbohydrate oxidation.[75] Thus, the weight-reduced individual is left with a lower rate of energy expenditure than before weight loss, and with a smaller proportion of this energy expenditure coming from fat than before. This situation favors weight regain, but not because of an abnormally high energy efficiency.[73]

One research report suggests that if weight loss is to be maintained without exercise, sedentary individuals may have to consume 30 to 40% fewer calories than the average daily amount required for their weight.[57] On the other hand, physically active individuals who expend about 200 extra calories per day in physical activity are able to maintain weight loss with a caloric consumption equal to the amount required for their weight.[57]

STRATEGIES TO AVOID WEIGHT REGAIN

Avoiding weight regain involves recognizing that altered body weight and body composition are associated with altered energy requirements, and altering behavior appropriately. Unless permanent changes in behavior are made to ensure that energy and nutrient balance are maintained, weight regain will occur. If the individual who was obese and is now reduced in weight reverts to pre-weight-loss behavior, weight regain will likely occur.

The importance of permanent changes in behavior for weight maintenance is illustrated by data showing that weight maintenance increases with length of behavioral therapy.[76] The problem is that once a target weight is reached, the individual stops behavior therapy and begins to revert to previous behavior.

Important strategies for avoiding a regain in body weight include a reduction in dietary fat (to meet the lower rates of fat oxidation) and an increase in physical activity. Physical activity is particularly important since it increases fat oxidation as well as total energy expenditure.

Obesity cannot be blamed solely on overeating or on a low metabolism. Obesity develops when energy intake exceeds energy expenditure, and this can result from an increased energy intake or a decreased amount of exercise. Individual differences in behavior and metabolism can explain why some people maintain a higher body fat content than others. Obesity treatment involves creating negative energy balance, and differences in metabolism explain differences in weight loss. There is no convincing evidence that the reduced-obese subject has an abnormal metabolic state. Because energy requirements are altered by a loss of body weight, weight regain will occur unless permanent changes are made in behavior to meet the altered energy requirements.

A comprehensive approach to weight loss and weight loss maintenance seems appropriate. Recommended components are as follows[77]:

- behavioral therapy
- cognitive intervention
- social support
- nutrition education

Behavioral therapy involves reducing caloric intake via stimulus control (e.g., reducing environmental food cues and the response to external cues). It involves modification of eating behaviors such as placing utensils on the table between bites, pausing during meals, and planning regularly scheduled meals. Behavior therapy also includes contingency management or providing positive feedback for healthful behavior and self-monitoring with effective problem solving.[78] Behavioral techniques that focus on fat intake reduction and increased energy expenditure should be emphasized.

Cognitive interventions involve restructuring the way an individual thinks and may include self-instructional training and relapse prevention techniques. A six-month behavior, self-monitoring program was tested with 35 obese men and women and showed an average loss of 8 kg of body weight, 6 kg of fat, and 4% of body fat. No change was noted among the control group. The self-administered program included a workbook with simple self-evaluations of fat, carbohydrate, sugar, and water intake. The program emphasized exercise and making changes at home.[59]

Social support can be the common thread that continues after behavioral training if a spouse or significant other supports the weight loss. The significant other can assist with realistic weight goals, provide motivation, and assist with positive self-attitudes.[79]

Nutrition education in the form of teaching individuals how to read labels, plan healthy meals, calculate energy intake and output, and modify recipes for less fat are important ways to assist individuals with how to create a new lifestyle rather than follow a diet at repeated intervals.

THEORIES OF OBESITY DEVELOPMENT

Some researchers believe that obesity develops due to a pathological condition characterized by a defect in the regulation of body weight or body fat content. An alternative view is that an individual's body fat content is not regulated directly but is the consequence or the result of many other regulated metabolic processes.[73] The body fat content can be considered as a "settling point." This represents the body fat content present at the point where the other metabolic processes reach equilibrium so that energy and nutrient balance are achieved.

According to this view, obesity would not be a pathological condition, and no specific metabolic defect would be noted. This still raises important questions, such as why some individuals have such a high body fat content when the systems reach equilibrium and whether the "settling point" can be altered by changing behavior or metabolism.[73]

THE LINK BETWEEN OBESITY AND CHRONIC DISEASE

In epidemiologic studies, the association between obesity and hypertension has been reported for a broad range of socioeconomic, racial, and ethnic groups. The Framingham Study found that relative body weight, body weight change, and skinfold thickness were related to blood pressure levels and to the subsequent development of hypertension. Weight gain and loss were associated with increased and decreased blood pressure, respectively.[80]

The Community Hypertension Evaluation Clinic screened about 1 million Americans. Individuals classifying themselves as overweight had rates of hypertension twice as high as individuals classifying themselves as normal weight. From the Intersalt study, BMI was positively associated with systolic blood pressure and diastolic blood pressure. A 10 kg difference in body weight was associated with a 3 mm Hg diastolic and a 2.2 mm Hg systolic blood pressure difference.[81] In NHANES I, BMI had the strongest relationship to blood pressure of all the nutritional variables.[82] Upper-body obesity (android) correlated best with blood pressure.

Several intervention trials observe that moderate weight reduction lowers blood pressure in normotensive and hypertensive individuals and that blood pressure reduction may not relate to salt intake. Blood pressure reduction does correlate with weight loss and, if weight is regained, blood pressure increases. Sodium restriction and weight loss are additive. Weight reduction reduces other cardiovascular risk factors of hyperlipidemia and glucose intolerance.[80]

Obesity increases the risk of developing non-insulin-dependent diabetes, cardiovascular disease, and several other chronic diseases. (see Chapters 11, 13, 14, and 16). Despite its prevalence and known association with other diseases, its treatment remains largely unsuccessful, in part because of an incomplete understanding of its etiology.

THE LINK BETWEEN OBESITY AND LIPOPROTEIN PROFILE

Obesity, whether indicated by relative weight or by body mass index, has been positively associated with a more atherogenic lipoprotein profile. This is true for total cholesterol, low-density lipoprotein (LDL) cholesterol, and triglycerides. A negative correlation is noted with high-density lipoprotein (HDL) cholesterol.[83-85] These associations have been reported for both adults and children[83,86,87] Framingham Study data predict that for each percentage increase in relative weight, a 1.1 mg/dL increase in serum cholesterol is expected.[84]

The cardiovascular disease cost attributed to obesity can be estimated. About 27% of cardiovascular disease, excluding hypertension, is diagnosed among men and women with BMI ≥29 kg/m². Among the obese, 70% of cardiovascular disease is attributed to obesity. This projects 19% of the total cardiovascular disease due to obesity or health care costs of $22.2 billion.[4]

Android obesity or excess fat deposits located predominantly in the upper body as opposed to gynoid or lower-body obesity is observed in individuals with carbohydrate and lipid abnormalities.[88] Upper-body fat is more frequently associated with hypertriglyceridemia; this association was reported as early as 1965.[89] More recently, the relative contribution of body fatness to serum triglyceride, LDL cholesterol, and HDL cholesterol levels was insignificant compared to the effects of a central- or upper-fat pattern.[90]

Using the Gothenburg study sample, the ratio of waist-to-hip circumference was associated most strongly with the incidence of ischemic heart disease, and waist-to-hip circumference was independently associated with the incidence of myocardial infarction.[91] In the Honolulu Heart Study cohort of 7,692 men, risk of coronary events had a positive association with subscapular skinfold thickness. This was independent of BMI.[92] Men in the highest tertile for subscapular skinfold thickness had more than twice the incidence of coronary heart disease during the 12-year follow up compared with men in the lowest tertile. Abdominal skinfold was significantly and negatively correlated with the serum HDL cholesterol concentration ($r = -0.16$) in a different cohort of 421 healthy men over 18 years old.[93]

A 5% to 10% drop in plasma total-cholesterol and LDL cholesterol levels has been reported for calorie-restricted weight-loss diets.[94-96] Some studies report unchanged posttreatment plasma total cholesterol and LDL-cholesterol levels, with weight loss[95-97]; a few researchers have observed changes after six months of follow up.[94] Reductions in body weight due to exercise training have led to reductions in plasma total cholesterol and LDL cholesterol levels to the extent of 13 and 11 mg/dL, respectively.[98]

HDL level response has varied (e.g., in some studies it has increased,[99-102] in some it has decreased,[103-105] and in some it has remained unchanged[106] after weight loss). In one study, HDL levels increased approximately 21% in obese patients (123% to 209% of ideal body weight) who lost a significant amount of weight.[96] Another study reported a 15.6% increase in HDL levels in six previously sedentary obese men who lost about 5.7 pounds following a moderate exercise and calorie-restricted regimen.[107] A 5% increase in HDL levels was reported for participants who lost weight by exercise training.[98]

OBESITY AND DIABETES

The incidence of non-insulin-dependent diabetes mellitus (NIDDM) increases with rising BMI, and there is no evidence of a threshold. Costs of NIDDM include the following[4]:

- routine care for uncomplicated NIDDM
- morbidity and mortality from complications (e.g., diabetic ketoacidosis, diabetic coma, diabetic retinopathy, and diabetic neuropathy)
- excess prevalence of other disease conditions including visual, renal, and skin disorders

Data from the Nurses' Health Study show that 61% of NIDDM cases were diagnosed among women 30 to 64 years old with BMI 29 kg/m² or greater, and 94% of NIDDM cases were attributed to obesity. Using 1986 population expenditures of $11.6 billion as the direct costs of health care expenditures and $8.2 billion as foregone productivity or indirect costs, and then applying the Nurses' Health Study data, 57% ($0.61 \times 0.94 = .57$) of the costs of NIDDM are attributed to obesity. This equates to $11.3 billion.[4] Additional costs would be added for managing 40% of the costs attributed to morbid obesity.

OBESITY AND CANCER

Mortality from all types of cancer increases with increasing weight among women and for men above desirable weight. Mortality ratios are higher for colon and prostate cancer among obese men, and for breast, endometrial, cervical, ovarian, and gall bladder cancer among obese women.[108] Using a 1986 total estimated cost of cancer in the United States of $75.1 billion and the cost due to cancers attributed in part to obesity, it is estimated that the combined contribution of obesity-promoted colon and breast cancer alone is 2.5% or $1.9 billion.[4]

Cancer epidemiology and clinical experiments have provided data that show an indirect link of obesity to reduced immunocompetence. Overall cancer death rate and the risk of certain types of cancer (i.e., cancer of the endometrium, colon, prostate, and breast) are elevated in obesity.[108,109] Data from Chandra and Kutty show depressed immune function in obese children and adolescents ($N = 28$) attending a weight loss clinic.[110] The impairment in immune function was associated with clinical and subclinical deficiencies of zinc and/or iron, which were more common in the obese versus the control group and reversed following appropriate supplementation therapy.[110]

Other researchers have observed at least a 50% reduction in the number of monocytes that matured into macrophages among obese individuals. Impaired monocyte maturation has been reported in association with certain kinds of cancers.[111] An additional finding has been the lower amount of a macrophage factor or cytokine that concentrates macrophages at an area of infection among obese, nonhyperglycemic individuals compared to normal weight controls.[112]

BODY WEIGHT AND MORTALITY

New weight standards reflect results of several population-based studies that compared body weight to mortality.[73] Body mass index (BMI) is the criterion recommended for defining a desirable weight index. It indicates relative fatness and has a minimal correlation to height. Using BMI, most epidemiological studies report that excess body weight increases mortality and that BMI is influenced by fat patterning, gender, and age.[73]

Similar increases in mortality are seen for individuals with a low BMI. For these individuals, lifestyle factors appear most important. Carefully measured weight and height are the easiest and most useful determinants of nutritional status and important predictors of mortality for the general population.[73]

Ideal, desirable, or healthy body weights are defined as those associated with the lowest mortality. For over 50 years, reference weights developed by the Metropolitan Life Insurance Company have been popular. Their use is limited, however, because they underrepresent the lower socioeconomic class, minorities, and the elderly. They use arbitrary definitions of body frame size and refer to populations rather than individuals. They fail to remove early mortality from the overall analysis.[73,113-115] New standards are available (see Table 15–4).

Gender-specific height-weight tables are not being used. Instead, new standards use the Quetelet or BMI (kilograms/meters²) to define a desirable weight index (see Table 15–5). BMI is not independent of stature (i.e., it declines as height increases).[73] The 1983 Metropolitan Height-Weight Table listed a BMI range of 21.4 to 27.4 kg/m^2 for the shortest women and a range of 18.8 to 24.4 kg/m^2 for the tallest women. BMI is an acceptable surrogate for assessing percentage of body fat in most epidemiological studies. BMI below or above the recommended range is associated with worsened health and increased mortality. This weight and mortality association influences predicting hospitalization and health care expenditures, setting premiums for health insurance, strengthening preventive medicine, and establishing health care policy goals for the nation.

Potential Errors in Data Collection

Potential errors in how weight data are collected reduce the importance of identifying optimal weights for longevity.[73] For example, survival analyses often reflect either a single body weight or a reported weight at one point in time. Individuals at various ages may comprise the sample. Reporting may be inaccurate, the weight scale may not be calibrated, garment weight may vary for different individuals, and individuals may have just eaten or not eaten prior to measurement. Change in body weight due to aging may not be considered during follow up.

Body weight is determined by a complex interaction of behavioral, cultural, socioeconomic, psychological, physiological, and genetic factors. Each factor may independently influence longevity. Body weight may be a surrogate for another variable, which may have a positive or negative impact on mortality (e.g., leisure time activity, functional capacity, or the quantity and composition of the eating pattern).

Body weight and BMI provide only a snapshot view of an individual's fitness and are not sensitive to moderate changes in illness or aging. Men and women with the same BMI may look vastly different and have different body fatness and leanness. Likewise, body fat may accompany aging, but individuals may not see a change in BMI as they age.

Most clinical studies use the Quetelet index (kg/m^2) but a weight-to-height ratio for which the exponent value is population-specific (kg/m^p) is important. In the 1971–1974 National Health and Nutrition Examination Survey (NHANES I), two was the exponent used for men and 1.5 was used for women.[116] An exponent of two was used for both men and women in NHANES II, 1976 to 1980.[36]

Morbidity is rarely reported as an outcome variable. If it were reported as an outcome variable, there might be a shift of optional weight ranges.

The Build and Blood Pressure Studies

The Build and Blood Pressure Studies in 1959 and 1979[117,118] reported that mortality increased

Table 15–4 Recommended Range of Body Mass Index by Source, Age, and Sex

Reference	Sex	Age Group (Years)	Recommended BMI (kg/m²)
US Department of Agriculture/ US Department of Health and Human Services	Male and Female	19–34 ≥35	19–25 21–27
National Academy of Sciences	Male and Female	19–24 25–34 35–44 45–54 55–64 ≥65	19–24 20–25 21–26 22–27 23–28 24–29
National Center for Health Statistics	Male Female	20–74 20–74	20.7–27.8 19.1–27.3
World Health Organization	Male and Female	Adults	20–25
Ministry of National Health and Welfare of Canada	Male and Female	20–65	20–27

Source: Adapted from Sichieri, R., Everhart, J.E., and Hubbard, V.S., Relative Weight Classifications in the Assessment of Underweight and Overweight in the United States, *International Journal of Obesity*, Vol. 16, pp. 303–312, with permission of Macmillan Press, Ltd., © 1992.

as excess body weight increased; the data were confirmed by other prospective studies.[114] A curvilinear relationship between BMI and mortality was reported after review of 40 studies.[119,120] BMI greater than 35 kg/m² was associated with both a twofold increase in total mortality and a multifold increase in morbidity. This is due to diabetes, cerebrovascular and cardiovascular disease, and certain cancers that are more prevalent among men. Limitations of these studies however are as follows:

- fewer than 7,000 participants or less than 5 years follow up
- lack of control for smoking, thereby producing an artifact or high mortality among lean individuals
- no elimination of early mortality during the analysis
- inability to control for hypertension, hyperlipidemia, and diabetes—the adverse consequences of obesity
- false exclusion of some groups
- oversample of low-risk individuals

Other Studies

A prospective eight-year study of obesity and coronary heart disease (CHD), the Nurses' Health Study, was conducted with 115,886 women, 30 to 55 years of age and 98% white.[121] In data analysis, adjustment was made for age and smoking. One important result was that relative weight had a strong positive association with the occurrence of fatal and nonfatal CHD. Obese women with a BMI greater than 29 kg/m² had a relative risk of 3.5 for fatal CHD compared to women with a BMI greater than 21 but less than 29 kg/m². When intermediate risk factors were controlled, the relative risk was under 2.0.

A 15-year follow-up study of 2,731 black females, 40 to 79 years old who were members of the Kaiser Foundation Health Plan between 1966 and 1973, presents a different picture.[122] Smoking, antecedent illness, education, and alcohol use were considered intermediate risk factors and controlled in the analysis. Measures for the first five years of follow up were deleted. The resulting relative risk of death for women with a BMI greater than 25.8 was 1.00, compared to the

Table 15–5 Body Weights in Pounds According to Height and Body Mass Index

Height (in.)	Body Mass Index (kg/m²)													
	19	20	21	22	23	24	25	26	27	28	29	30	35	40
	Body Weight (pounds)													
58	91	96	100	105	110	115	119	124	129	134	138	143	167	191
59	94	99	104	109	114	119	124	128	133	138	143	148	173	198
60	97	102	107	112	118	123	128	133	138	143	148	153	179	204
61	100	106	111	116	122	127	132	137	143	148	153	158	185	211
62	104	109	115	120	126	131	136	142	147	153	158	164	191	218
63	107	113	118	124	130	135	141	146	152	158	163	169	197	225
64	110	116	122	128	134	140	145	151	157	163	169	174	204	232
65	114	120	126	132	138	144	150	156	162	168	174	180	210	240
66	118	124	130	136	142	148	155	161	167	173	179	186	216	247
67	121	127	134	140	146	153	159	166	172	178	185	191	223	255
68	125	131	138	144	151	158	164	171	177	184	190	197	230	262
69	128	135	142	149	155	162	169	176	182	189	196	203	236	270
70	132	139	146	153	160	167	174	181	188	195	202	207	243	278
71	136	143	150	157	165	172	179	186	193	200	208	215	250	286
72	140	147	154	162	169	177	184	191	199	206	213	221	258	294
73	144	151	159	166	174	182	189	197	204	212	219	227	265	302
74	148	155	163	171	179	186	194	202	210	218	225	233	272	311
75	152	160	168	176	184	192	200	208	216	224	232	240	279	319
76	156	164	172	180	189	197	205	213	221	230	238	246	287	328

Note: Each entry gives the body weight in pounds (lb) for a person of a given height and body mass index. Pounds have been rounded off. To use the table, find the appropriate height in the left-hand column. Move across the row to a given weight. The number at the top of the column is the body mass index for the height and weight.

Source: Reprinted from Bray, G.A., and Gray, D.S., Obesity. Part I: Pathogenesis, *Western Journal of Medicine*, Vol. 148, pp. 429–441, with permission of the California Medical Association, © 1988.

lowest-mortality group with a BMI range of 23.5–25.8. A lack of association between BMI and mortality among black women has been reported in two smaller studies.[123,124]

BMI does not account for differences in body composition (e.g., fat distribution at various body sites). Increased central or visceral fat is a predictor of non-insulin-dependent diabetes mellitus, breast cancer, cardiovascular disease, and overall mortality.[48] BMI is an independent predictor of relative weight. The ratio of waist-to-hip circumference indicates body fat distribution. Beginning in the mid-1980s, several longitudinal studies of middle-aged adults reported an association between body fat distribution, increased risk for cardiovascular disease, and all-cause mortality.[91,125–126]

After a 12-year follow up, the unadjusted odds ratio for the incidence of CHD for Swedish adults 54 years old was 3.2 for men compared to women. The ratio decreased to 3.1 after BMI and other cardiovascular risk factors were controlled. When waist-to-hip ratio was controlled, the odds ratio declined to 1.1 and eliminated the sex differences. This suggests that waist-to-hip ratio may be a marker of genetic, hormonal, or lifestyle factors closely related to CHD risk. Thereby, failing to control for body-fat pattern confounds any analysis of the association between excess body weight and mortality.[127]

NHANES II data reported that for overweight adults under 45 years of age, the risk of comorbidity with hypertension, diabetes, and hypercholesterolemia was substantially higher than for overweight persons aged 45 to 75.[128] Minimal mortality was noted with progressively increasing body weight as individuals aged from 20 through 69 years.[129]

A 15-year follow up of 18,403 men, aged 40 to 60 years, who were initially examined between 1968 and 1970, revealed that 1,236 deaths were caused by CHD.[130] No significant association between BMI and cardiovascular disease was noted in men aged 60 to 64 years compared to men under 60 years of age. A second study included nine-year mortality data from NHANES I for 4,710 white men and women, 55 to 74 years old at the time of examination.[131] Mortality risk was approximately 2.5 times greater for the 65-to-74-year-old group compared to the 55-to-64-year-old group. Mortality for all women combined did not vary according to BMI. A positive effect was seen only for men when BMI was greater than 31.8 kg/m^2.

In a 12-year follow up of 22,995 Finnish men, over age 25, minimum mortality was observed for overweight men over age 75 and within a BMI range of 28 to 31 kg/m^2. Life expectancy was highest for healthy Finnish women, over age 65 and in a BMI range of 27 to 31 kg/m^2, compared to younger women with a BMI of 21.0 to 26.0 kg/m^2.[132]

Harris et al[133] analyzed Framingham Study data (N = 1,723 nonsmoking men and women, 65 years old between 1957 and 1981). Individuals in the upper 30% body weight range (BMI >28.5 kg/m^2) had a relative risk of mortality of 1.6 and 1.9 respectively, in contrast to those in the reference BMI range of 23.0 to 25.2 kg/m^2 for men and 24.1 to 26.1 kg/m^2 for women. The Framingham Study strengthened the observation that health risks of excess weight occur for individuals over the age of 65. However, BMI may become less associated with mortality as aging progresses.[134]

MORTALITY AND BEING UNDERWEIGHT

The association of mortality and relative weight is *J*- or *U*-shaped[108,135,136] (see Figure 15-2). Excess mortality occurs at the very low and very high BMI. The nadir of the curve generally occurs at a BMI between 19.0 and 27.0 kg/m^2. It appears that healthy individuals below a desir-

able relative weight are at risk. A systematic overestimation of the influence of being underweight on mortality occurs if there is a failure to control for cigarette smoking or failure to account for subclinical disease precipitating an early mortality.[137,138]

The 14-year American Cancer Society prospective study of mortality (N = 750,000 individuals) confirmed that mortality among smokers in the lowest weight category was almost twice that of nonsmokers in the same category.[139] Mortality ratios of lean but heavy smokers (more than 20 cigarettes per day) were similar to ratios for individuals in the highest weight index. Cigarette smoking confounds mortality data among the underweight group, since the excess mortality of lean smokers is mainly caused by lung cancer and other diseases of the respiratory system. Failure to eliminate early mortality from the analysis due to clinical or subclinical illness can erroneously increase estimates of mortality due to lower weights.[108,118,140,141]

Smoking duration and intensity affect body leanness. Self-reported smoking data were collected from 12,000 adult men and women in NHANES II. As duration increased, BMI decreased for both men and women.[142] BMI of frequent male smokers was significantly greater than that of average smokers, whereas the data on women showed that there was no difference in weights among women having either average or high smoking rates. The Cancer Prevention Study I reported that cigarette smokers may have a higher waist-to-hip ratio than nonsmokers. This is independent of BMI and may increase mortality risk.[143]

Between 1977 and 1988, 11,703 men in good health were followed for all-cause, cardiovascular disease, and cancer mortality. Weight was reported but not measured. Five weight-change categories were defined. During the 11 years, 1,441 men died—345 from heart disease and 459 from cancer. Lowest all-cause mortality occurred for men who kept their weight within 1 kg. In comparison, relative risk (RR) for death was the highest for men who lost more than 5 kg (RR = 1.57) or gained 5 kg (RR = 1.36); for CHD, the RRs were 1.75 and 2.01 for these weight-change categories. The higher RR for total mortality remained when cigarette smoking, physical activ-

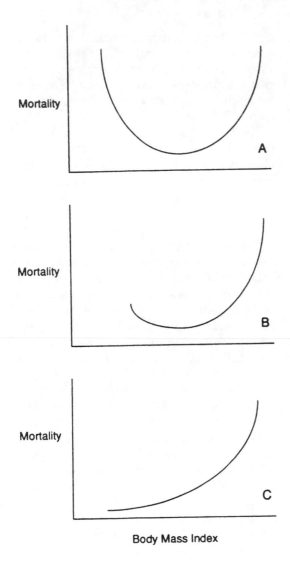

Body Mass Index

Figure 15-2 Schematic representation of the BMI-mortality relationship. Epidemiological studies suggest a *U*-shaped (A), *J*-shaped (B), or direct (C) association. *Source:* Adapted from Kushner, R.F., *Nutrition Reviews*, Vol. 51, No. 5, 1993, page 129.

through 1987. All-cause, cardiovascular disease, and noncardiovascular disease mortality rates were evaluated, considering percent maximum weight loss and BMI. Percent maximum weight loss was calculated by subtracting measured weight from reported highest weight and expressed as a percentage. After adjusting for age, race, smoking, parity, and preexisting illness, the lowest death rate occurred for individuals with BMI less than 26 kg/m^2 and a loss of less than 5% of their maximum weight. A weight loss of more than 15% of maximum weight was associated with higher relative mortality for both men and women, irrespective of maximum BMI. The highest all-cause (RR = 2.8), cardiovascular disease (RR = 3.3), and noncardiovascular disease mortality (RR = 2.3) occurred for women with BMI greater than 29 and with weight loss greater than 15%.[145]

A four-year follow up of 10,529 Multiple Risk Factor Intervention Trial (MRFIT) men was conducted. The men were 35 to 57 years of age and free of cancer.[146] Weight change mirrored a six-to-seven-year time period and was expressed as both the intraindividual standard deviation (ISD) of weight and the type of weight change (e.g., no change, loss, gain, or weight cycling). Results were as follows:

- Men with a stable weight had the lowest adjusted risk of mortality.
- The highest relative risk for all-cause and cardiovascular disease mortality occurred in the highest ISD quartile.
- The average weight change was 1.4 kg.
- Adjusted relative risk of mortality was higher for individuals with sustained weight loss, not sustained weight gain.
- Relative risk for all-cause and cardiovascular mortality was dependent on baseline BMI.
- Men with a baseline BMI less than 28.8 kg/m^2 had a positive association between ISD of weight and mortality.

The trend emerging from various studies is that a sizeable weight loss or gain is associated with higher relative rates of mortality. The causes of the changes in weight are not known. Data from 1794 NHANES I participants identified depres-

ity, and initial BMI (<25 versus >25 kg/m^2) were controlled. Curiously, weight change did not predict cancer mortality, but this may be due to the overall low rate of cigarette smoking of 17.5%.[144]

NHANES I mortality data for 2,140 men and 2,550 women, age 45 to 71 years, was reviewed. Baseline data were collected in NHANES I (1971–1975), and the cohort was followed

sion as a significant factor causing weight change for about 27% of younger adults and 24% of older adults.[147] Voluntary weight loss was reported in 21,673 telephone interviews for approximately 25% of men and 40% of women attempting weight loss.[148]

PSYCHOLOGICAL ASPECTS OF OBESITY

Contempt for obesity appears widespread. Obese individuals are often subjected to intense prejudice that crosses age, sex, race, and socio-economic strata.[149-151] The prejudice appears to begin in childhood.[152] Six-year-old children describe silhouettes of an obese child as ugly, dirty, lazy, and stupid, among other adjectives.[153] When children are shown pictures of handicapped individuals missing limbs along with obese children, the obese children are chosen as the least likeable.[154-156] Interestingly, obese individuals also demonstrate a similar prejudice.[153-155] Several systematic studies have reported that severely obese individuals do not demonstrate unusual levels of psychopathology using standard measures.[157-159]

Disparities are noted in acceptance rates for obese and nonobese individuals into universities and private colleges; employment rates by the armed forces, police, fire departments, and airlines; and salary levels.[27,160-162,163,164] Estimates are that each pound of fat incurs about $1,000 per year for executives.[165]

As many as 78% of severely obese individuals undergoing surgery reported that they had always or usually been treated disrespectfully by medical professionals due to their weight.[166] A survey of 77 physicians documented their description of obese patients as ugly, awkward, and weak-willed.[167] Negative attitudes of medical professionals towards obese individuals may in part be based on unsuccessful attempts at treatment.[152] These data should alert professionals to the importance of their personal attitudes and expressions during contact with obese individuals.

The first publicized case in which obesity was considered a disability was a 1985 decision regarding the New York handicapped employment law, *McDermott versus Xerox Corporation*. After a medical exam, a tentative employment offer

for McDermott—a 5-foot, 6-inch female who weighed 249 pounds—was terminated. The court upheld the state commission's finding of discrimination.[168] Similar court decisions were seen in *Gimello versus Agency Rent-A-Car Systems*, where obesity was considered a disability under New Jersey law, and in *Cassisata versus Community Foods* (1992), where the California Court of Appeals found that an employer had discriminated against a 305-pound female applicant due to her weight.[168-170]

CHILDHOOD OBESITY

Over the past 20 years, there has been an increase in the percentage of obese children and adolescents. Current estimates are that 27% of US children and 21% of US adolescents are obese. These estimates represent a 54% and a 39% increase, respectively. Approximately 12% of children are severely obese.[171,172] Anthropometric reference data (height, weight, and triceps skinfolds) from the US National Health Survey, 1976–1980, are detailed in Chapters 7 and 8.

Hispanic Health and Nutrition Examination Survey data indicate that Mexican-American boys and girls are shorter and relatively heavier than non-Hispanic white children. The excess weight appears to be related to fat of the upper trunk and not to lean body mass.[177] Anthropometric reference data (height, weight, and tricep skinfold measures) from the Hispanic Health and Nutrition Examination Survey, 1982–1984, are detailed in Chapters 7 and 8.

The heights and weights of 1,670 elementary children in three Central Harlem, New York, schools were measured and compared with the National Center for Health Statistics standards. The median weight and height for age of these children exceeded the standard by 1.4 cm and 2.2 kg for boys and 2.7 cm and 2.8 kg for girls. For boys the height-age was advanced by about 0.24 years, and for girls it was advanced by 0.47 years. For both boys and girls, about 14% were above the 95th percentile in weight for height.[174]

Six major factors that contribute to obesity have been identified[175]:

1. genetic factors
2. lifestyle factors
3. emotional overeating
4. indulgence
5. neglect
6. medical factors

An obese child may embody more than one of these contributory factors.[175]

Obesity initiates a chain reaction for many children. It is generally complicated by the additional daily stress of problems with peers, social isolation, psychological distress including low body- and self-esteem, physical limitations, illness, and lack of body skills to enhance participation in dance and sports.

A case-control study of 100 obese participants and 100 age- and sex-matched, always-slender controls were queried about prior sexual abuse and depression. Sexual and nonsexual abuse in infancy, childhood, or adolescence was reported by 25% and 29% of the obese patients, compared with 6% and 14% of the always-slender group. Obesity was described frequently as a sexually protective device by overweight participants who also reported overeating to cope with emotional disturbances.[176]

Obesity in childhood carries a 70% risk of persistence into adulthood, when chronic disease expression occurs. An obese child often experiences adolescence earlier than his or her peers. This creates a shorter period for bone growth and a potentially shorter statute. Acute illnesses may surface (e.g., hyperinsulinemia, elevated serum lipids, and pulmonary and orthopedic problems).[175]

Judgment of body size, attractiveness, and self-concept were compared for 19 diet-intervention mother-daughter pairs and 18 control pairs. Both mothers and daughters ranked large figures as less attractive than thin ones. Daughters wanted to be thinner than they perceived themselves to be; mothers tended to see their daughters as "just right." Daughters' self-concept was inversely related to their age, and their own and their mother's size.[177] Lower self-esteem was noted for girls with large body sizes and girls whose mothers had large body sizes. Control-group mothers

with high BMI measures had lower levels of self-esteem; their daughters identified body size as an important factor in feelings of self-worth.[177]

Attempts to treat childhood obesity during the 1970s consisted of approaches that emphasized dieting, exercise, and behavioral change. Success was limited. Family-based strategies that emerged in the 1980s have been credited with sustained weight loss and a broader base for successful skill development. When the whole family addresses both the problems and the positive aspects of the child's life, each member can reorient attitudes and behaviors.

A decline in physical activity and an increase in television watching and sedentary activities such as video games may contribute to the increased prevalence of obesity among US youths. A 1992 International Food Information Council survey reported that 53% of six-to-nine year olds play outside after school and on weekends, but 80% report watching television.[178] Data from the National Health Examination Surveys show that the prevalence of obesity increased by 2% for each additional hour of television viewed, after controlling for numerous social and family variables.[179]

A reduction in resting metabolic rates may be the promoting factor. Resting metabolic rate declined by 12% for normal-weight girls, 8 to 12 years old, watching 25 minutes of nonviolent television programs; it declined by 16% for obese girls.[180]

One successful approach to treat childhood obesity has been the SHAPEDOWN program. In the program, interdisciplinary teams of highly skilled health professionals work with various aspects of the problem. A biopsychosocial assessment identifies the medical and psychosocial seriousness of the obesity. Intervention tackles the obese child's symptoms and factors that create the excess weight gain. The intervention may include marital, substance abuse, or individual counseling for family members.[175]

Action and commitment at the national level to address the problem of childhood obesity in the United States has been sought. An improvement in the access to care for families with obese children is one direction. Mellin drafted eight specific recommendations and submitted them to President Clinton, political leaders, and nutritional professionals to improve the overall well-being of children and to improve the availability, accessibility, and effectiveness of child obesity services[175]:

1. Create a cabinet-level position on the child and family. This effort is needed to create a national agenda on childhood obesity and support legislation and policies.
2. Provide more economic and social support for low-income children. Support could be in the form of recreational areas; family-oriented programs; low-fat supplemental foods; and increases in fruits, vegetables, and grains.
3. Implement a national plan for high-quality after-school care and day care. Enhance after-school care so parents and children want to participate.
4. Mandate health-promoting environments in public schools. Endorse comprehensive school health that is reflected in required physical activity, healthy meals, nutrition education, and self- and body-esteem.
5. Create an advisory committee on children and nutrition. With the commitment of a national advisory group, childhood obesity and hunger issues would remain priorities until solutions are found.
6. Extend coverage by health insurers to family-based, child-obesity services. Most obese children are denied a safe and effective medical care setting. Medical coverage for services is almost nonexistent, and costs of medical care when obesity is compounded with other chronic diseases is exceptionally high.
7. Designate increased funding for training. A shortage of health care providers for obese children and families escalates the need for training, ranging from undergraduate courses, to university fellowships, to professional education.
8. Designate increased research funding for the prevention and treatment of childhood obesity. Expand research support to address the handicapped, multiethnic groups, and practical approaches for working with young children and families.

VOLUNTARY WEIGHT LOSS

The NIH Nutrition Coordinating Committee and the Office of Medical Applications of Research held a technology assessment conference in the spring of 1992 to evaluate voluntary weight loss and control methods.[15] The conference convened experts in obesity, nutrition, metabolism, epidemiology, biostatistics, behavior, and exercise physiology. Data on diet, exercise, behavior modification, and drug treatment in adults were presented. Surgery, liposuction, medical devices, the economics and ethics of weight-loss practices, and regulatory issues were not covered. This state-of-the-art information from the panel demonstrates the magnitude of the weight-loss challenge in the United States.[15]

Data from four recent national surveys of health practices indicate that 33 to 40% of adult women and 20 to 24% of men currently attempt weight loss; 28% of each group strive to maintain weight. For those trying weight loss, their efforts averaged 6.4 months for women and 5.8 months for men. Women averaged 2.5 attempts to lose weight in the past two years, compared to 2.0 attempts for men. Weight-loss efforts are not restricted to persons with high BMI.[15]

Fewer younger people try to lose weight compared with older persons. Weight-loss attempts increase with higher education, family income, and BMI. A higher percentage of Hispanic men attempt weight loss compared to all ethnic groups; the lowest percentage occurs for African-American men. A higher proportion of African-American and Hispanic women are overweight than are white women, but a similar percentage of all groups try weight-loss regimens.

Forty-four percent of female high school students and 15% of male students reported that they were trying to lose weight; 26% of female and 15% of male students were tying to keep from gaining weight.[15]

Americans attempt weight loss for several reasons:

- to improve their self-image
- to reduce the risk of weight-related health problems
- to improve their perception of their health
- to increase societal acceptance of their weight

Concerns about future and current health, fitness, and appearance are the most important reasons that individuals try to lose weight. Individuals with higher BMI voice health concerns as an issue. Appearance and fitness are identified more frequently for individuals with a lower BMI. Appearance rather than fitness is more important to women. Weight loss after smoking cessation or pregnancy is also a priority.

STRATEGIES FOR WEIGHT LOSS

Women try to lose weight by eating fewer calories (84%) and increasing physical activity (60 to 63%). Men try to lose weight by eating fewer calories (76 to 78%) and increasing physical activity (60 to 62%). Race, education, income, and age influence which methods are used most often.[15]

Other surveys of adults report that more than 80% of men and women who try to lose weight blend eating and exercise regimens. Popular methods used by adults include vitamins or meal replacements, over-the-counter products, weight-loss programs, and diet supplements. An individual's BMI influences the method she or he chooses.[15]

Students who attempted weight loss reported that for the week immediately prior to the survey, they used exercise (51% of females and 30% of males), skipped meals (49% and 18%, respectively), used diet pills (4% and 2%, respectively), and practiced self-induced vomiting (3% and 1%, respectively). The general methods chosen include exercise (80% of females and 44% of males), diet

pills (21% and 5%, respectively), and vomiting (14% and 4%, respectively).[15]

SUCCESS OF VARIOUS METHODS FOR WEIGHT LOSS AND CONTROL

Few scientific studies evaluate the effectiveness and safety of weight-loss methods. Participants lose weight but, after completing a program, they tend to regain the weight with time.

Some weight-loss strategies may be harmful. Individuals should examine the scientific data on effectiveness and safety of the weight-loss program before adopting it. Over $30 billion is spent each year in the United States on weight-loss efforts. The proportion of persons who complete programs, how much weight they lose, and their success in maintaining the weight loss, are not generally reported in peer-reviewed literature.[15]

Success rates are influenced by initial weight, the length of treatment, the magnitude of weight loss desired, and the motivation for wanting to lose weight. Effectiveness of unsupervised efforts to lose weight is suspect, because limited data exist on the personal strategies, individual compliance, and follow up.[15]

Dietary Change

Most individuals try to lose weight by changing their eating pattern. They may reduce total calories; alter the percentage of calories from fat, protein, and carbohydrate; or use protein or fat substitutes. The effectiveness of these methods is unknown, because data are only available for programs following individuals about five years.

Acute weight loss may be greater than 10% of initial body weight, but individuals may regain two-thirds of the weight within one year. Some individuals maintain their weight loss for a few weeks to a few months; dropout rates may be higher than 80%.[15]

Frequently, individuals employ either a caloric restriction of 1,000–1,500 calories per day, which equals about 12 to 15 kcal/kg body weight, or 800 or fewer calories per day, which is approximately 6 to 10 kcal/kg body weight. Adverse side effects and excessive loss of lean body mass are reported for either level. Very-low-calorie diets produce more weight loss than low-calorie diets, but participants often return to preprogram weight within five years. Modifying the proportion of calories from macronutrients has a much smaller effect on weight loss than caloric restriction.

Very-low-calorie diets are generally provided as one part of a comprehensive program. Weight loss may average 1.5 to 2.5 kg/week, with a total loss of about 20 kg after three to four months on the regimen. To preserve lean body mass, foods with protein of a high biological value are needed at the minimum of 1 g per kg of ideal body weight per day. The diet can cause serious complications, with the most common complication being cholelithiasis.[181]

Adjunct Therapy

Weight loss achieved in conjunction with exercise and energy restriction is preferred. Exercise has an independent effect on weight loss. It increases HDL cholesterol and lean body mass. Exercise can offset postprogram weight gain and provide a four-to-seven-pound weight loss in addition to the loss from caloric restriction.[15]

Behavior modification is a technique used for modifying eating and physical activity habits. It focuses on the following components:

- making small, consistent changes
- identifying adverse eating or lifestyle behaviors
- setting specific behavioral goals
- modifying determinants of the behavior(s) to be changed
- reinforcing desirable behavior
- participating in group or individual sessions with professionals or peer therapists

- participating in 16- to 18-week programs that result in a weight loss of 1 to 1.5 pounds per week

About one-third of the weight that is lost in behavior modification programs is regained within one year. Most is regained within five years; however, a few participants maintain their weight loss.[15]

Investigational drugs have produced weight loss, but their prolonged use may slow weight loss and create a weight plateau. Phenyl-propanolamine, an over-the-counter FDA-approved appetite suppressant, has produced weight loss. However, long-term benefit is not well documented, and potential misuse is possible.[15]

Dietary change and exercise, reinforced by behavior modification, is the most common combined therapy. A greater short-term weight loss occurs when diet and exercise are combined than when either is attempted alone. Behavior modification may extend the period of time before weight is regained if participant contact is continuous.[15]

Weight-Loss Enablers and Barriers

Success appears linked to therapies that promote practical dietary behaviors and to therapies or counselors who assist individuals with high-risk emotional and social situations. Success is also linked to behavioral strategies that employ self-monitoring of progress and encourage stress reduction. Barriers to weight loss include the following[15]:

- reduced self-efficacy
- inability to lose weight early in the program, causing individuals to stop their dietary and exercise changes
- lack of social or professional support
- deeply rooted social or psychological problems (e.g., depression)
- cultural norms and mores

Info Line

Beneficial Effect of Medical Nutrition Therapy by an RD in the Weight-Management Outcome of Dyslipidemic Patients

The research aim was to investigate the beneficial effect of medical nutrition therapy by a registered dietitian (RD) in the weight management of dyslipidemic patients. According to the National Cholesterol Education Program Adult Treatment Panel's second report on hyperlipidemia, dietary modification including weight management is an essential first step and RDs have the key responsibility to facilitate dietary behavior changes. Twenty-three dyslipidemic males 50–70 years old in a lipid research trial requiring frequent dietary intervention with an RD were compared with 23 patients in another trial not requiring dietary intervention with an RD. Weight gain of ≥ 3 lbs occurred in 43% of non-RD group versus no weight increase in the RD-treated group ($p < 0.01$). Weight stabilization, i.e., gaining or losing ≤ 2 lbs, occurred in twice as many men or 61% in the RD-treated group versus 30% in the other group ($p < 0.05$). Overall, compared with the non-RD treated group, the RD-treated group experienced a 57% additional health benefit and strengthened their rapport with an RD through medical nutrition therapy.

Source: Reprinted with permission of G Sikand, NA Downey, ML Kashyap, M.D., Lipid Research Clinic, VA Medical Center, Long Beach and U.C. Irvine College of Medicine, Irvine, CA.

BENEFITS AND RISKS OF WEIGHT LOSS

Observational studies of persons who report weight loss and data from clinical trials document the association of weight loss to health. A reduction in the incidence and severity of non-insulin-dependent diabetes mellitus and hypertension in overweight persons is an immediate benefit. Diet and exercise-evoked weight loss can prevent the onset of hypertension and diabetes mellitus. Improved glycemic control and elimination of oral agents may occur for persons with diabetes. Randomized trial data indicate that weight loss among hypertensive patients accompanies significant declines in blood pressure and a decline in continued drug therapy. A positive effect on lipid and lipoprotein levels is also observed. What is not clear is whether short-term improvements confer permanent health benefits.[15]

For morbidly obese individuals, weight loss improves functional status, reduces work absenteeism, lessens pain, and increases social interaction. The prevalence and severity of sleep apnea can be markedly reduced by weight loss.[15]

Very-low-calorie diets and fasting regimens can produce short-term adverse response (e.g., periodic fatigue, hair loss, and dizziness). Gallstones and acute gallbladder disease, cardiac arrhythmia, and death have been reported. Diets with high-quality protein, minerals, and electrolytes have offset serious, life-threatening complications. The effect of weight-loss programs on binge-eating and bulimia needs further study. Many alternatives for weight loss are available to the public (see Exhibit 15–2). For further information about the adverse effects of weight loss, see F. Berg's *Health Risks of Weight Loss*.[182]

As discussed earlier, epidemiologic studies suggest that weight loss is associated with increased mortality and yet the reason for weight loss may not be known (e.g., weight loss could be intentional by a healthy individual or it could be associated with illness and psychosocial distress). People who stop smoking gain weight and complicate the data.

Weight cycling affects energy metabolism and may result in a faster regain of weight. Data about the long-term, negative effects of weight cycling on psychological and physical health are needed. Weight-reducing drugs appear safe in controlled studies, but these studies are short term. They involve older, more stable individuals who are not likely to abuse the drugs. Studies with adolescents and young adults are needed to evaluate the use of weight-reducing drugs among youths.

Exhibit 15–2 Popular Weight-Loss Programs

DO-IT-YOURSELF PROGRAMS

- *Overeaters Anonymous:* Nonprofit international organization that provides volunteer support groups patterned after the 12-step Alcoholics Anonymous program. Physical, emotional, and spiritual recovery aspects of compulsive overeating are addressed.
- *TOPS (Take Off Pounds Sensibly):* Nonprofit support organization of more than 300,000 members who meet weekly in groups. Does not prescribe or endorse particular eating or exercise regimen. Mandatory weigh-in at weekly meetings.

NONCLINICAL PROGRAMS

- *Diet Center:* Focuses on achieving healthy body composition through diet and personalized exercise recommendations under the name "Exclusively You Weight Management Program." A minimum 1,200-calorie diet is based on regular supermarket food. Diet Center prepackaged cuisine is optional. Clients are encouraged to visit center daily for weigh-in.
- *Jenny Craig:* Personal weight management menu based on Jenny Craig's cuisine with additional store-bought foods. Diet ranges from 1,000 to 2,600 kcal.
- *Nutri/System:* Menu plans based on Nutri/System's prepared meals with additional store-bought foods. Clients receive individual calorie levels ranging from 1,000 to 2,200 kcal/day. Multivitamin-mineral supplement available for clients.
- *Weight Watchers:* Emphasis on portion control and healthy lifestyle habits. Dieters choose from regular supermarket food, Weight Watchers Personal Cuisine (available in select markets to members only), or both. Reducing phase: Women average 1,250 kcal daily; men, 1,600 daily.

CLINICAL PROGRAMS

- *Health Management Resources (HMR):* Medically supervised very-low-calorie diet (VLCD) or fortified, high-protein, liquid meal replacements (520 to 800 kcal daily) or a low-calorie option consisting of liquid supplements and prepackaged HMR entrees (800 to 1,300 kcal daily).
- *Medifast:* Medifast is a physician-supervised, very-low-calorie diet program of fortified meal replacements containing 450–500 kcal/day. LifeStyles, The Medifast Program of Patient Support, prepares patients to maintain their goal weight after completing the VLCD. Medifast also provides a low-calorie diet of approximately 860 kcal/day for those not indicated for the VLCD.
- *New Direction:* This system includes a medically supervised VLCD program of fortified meal replacements with 600–840 kcal/day, or programs with 1,000–1,500 kcal/day using regular foods, fortified bars, and beverages.
- *Optifast:* Medically supervised program of fortified liquid meal replacements and/or fortified food bars, eventually including more regular foods. Dieters assigned an 800-, 950-, or 1,200-kcal plan.
- *Physicians in a Multidisciplinary Program:* Multidisciplinary programs are similar to Health Management Resources, New Direction, and Optifast. The approach is food-based and weight-loss oriented but is a modified form of the two. The multidisciplinary approach seeks coordination of services, the availability of individual and/or group counseling, and comprehensive health care.
- *Private Practice RDs:* Highly personalized approach to weight loss and maintenance. Exercise is encouraged as part of a safe, sensible weight-control plan. Clients identify barriers to their weight loss and maintenance and receive education about healthy lifestyles.

Source: Adapted from Ward, E., Programs for and Approaches to Treating Obesity, *Environmental Nutrition*, pp. 1–4, with permission of Environmental Nutrition, Inc., © 1994.

Exhibit 15-3 *Healthy People 2000* Objectives for Reduction of Obesity

2.3   Reduce overweight to a prevalence of no more than 20% among people aged 20 and older and no more than 15% among adolescents aged 12 through 19. (Baseline: 26% for people aged 20 through 74 in 1976-80, 24% for men and 27% for women; 15% for adolescents 12-19 yrs in 1976-80.)

2.5   Reduce dietary fat intake to an average of 30% of calories or less and average saturated fat intake to <10% of calories among people aged 2 and older. (Baseline: 36% of calories from total fat and 13% from saturated fat for people aged 20 through 74 in 1976-80; 36% and 13% for women aged 19 through 50 in 1985.)

2.6   Increase complex carbohydrate and fiber-containing foods in the diets of adults to 5+ daily servings for vegetables (including legumes) and fruits, and to 6+ daily servings for grain products. (Baseline: 2½ servings of vegetables and fruits and 3 servings of grain products for women aged 19 through 50 in 1985.)

2.7   Increase to at least 50% the proportion of overweight people aged 12 and older who have adopted sound dietary practices combined with regular physical activity to attain an appropriate body weight. (Baseline: 30% of overweight women and 25% of overweight men for people aged 18 and older in 1985.)

17.12 Reduce overweight to a prevalence of no more than 20% among people aged 20 and older and no more than 15% among adolescents aged 12 through 19. (Baseline: 26% for people aged 20 through 74 in 1976-80, 24% for men and 27% for women; 15% for adolescents 12-19 yrs in 1976-80.)

Special Population Targets

Overweight Prevalence	1976–80 Baseline for 20+ Year Olds	2000 Target
17.12a Low-income women aged 20 and older	37%	25%
17.12b Black women aged 20 and older	44%	30%
17.12c Hispanic women aged 20 and older		25%
Mexican-American women	39%[*]	
Cuban women	34%[*]	
Puerto Rican women	37%[*]	
17.12d American Indians/Alaska Natives	29-75%[**]	30%
17.12e People with disabilities	36%[$]	25%
17.12f Women with high blood pressure	50%	41%
17.12g Men with high blood pressure	39%	35%

[*]1982-84 baseline for Hispanics aged 20-74.
[**]1984-88 estimates for different tribes.
[$]1985 baseline for people aged 20-74 who report any limitation in activity due to chronic conditions.

Note: For people aged 20 and older, overweight is defined as body mass index (BMI) equal to or >27.8 for men and 27.3 for women. For adolescents, overweight is defined as BMI equal to or greater than 23.0 for males aged 12 through 14, 24.3 for males aged 15 through 17, 25.8 for males aged 18 through 19, 23.4 for females aged 12 through 14, 24.8 for females aged 15 through 17, and 25.7 for females aged 18 through 19. The values for adolescents are the age- and gender-specific 85th percentile values for the 1976-80 National Health and Nutrition Examination Survey (NHANES II), corrected for sample variation. BMI is calculated by dividing weight in kilograms by the square of height in meters. The cut points used to define overweight approximate the 120% of desirable body weight definition used in the 1990 objectives.

Source: Reprinted from *Healthy People 2000: National Health Promotion and Disease Prevention Objectives*, U.S. Department of Health and Human Services, Public Health Service, Publication No. 91-50212, 1991.

Exhibit 15-4 Model Nutrition Objective for Reduced Risk Reduction

---

By 19____, the chronic disease risk factor _____*_____ among (target population) will be reduced from _____%
to _____%.

*Obesity; hypertension; elevated serum cholesterol; poor physical fitness; excess intake of dietary fat, cholesterol, sodium, alcohol, and sugar; inadequate intake of dietary fiber, fruits and vegetables, and calcium.

Source: Adapted from *Model State Nutrition Objectives*, The Association of State and Territorial Public Health Nutrition Directors, 1988.

HEALTHY PEOPLE 2000 ACTIONS

Obesity is a fertile area for community nutrition professionals to apply group counseling skills for individuals at all ages. HP2K objectives that focus on obesity address prevalence of the disorder, nutritionally balance eating patterns with fat replaced by complex carbohydrate, and high-risk ethnic groups (see Exhibit 15-3). A model nutrition objective to reduce risk reduction for obesity is presented in Exhibit 15-4.[183]

REFERENCES

1. US Department of Health and Human Services. *The Surgeon General's Report on Nutrition and Health*. Washington, DC: US Government Printing Office, 1988.

2. National Institutes of Health Consensus Development Conference Panel. Health implications of obesity. *Ann Intern Med*. 1985;103:1073.

3. Berg F. Obesity costs reach $39.3 billion. *Obesity & Health*. 1991;5:95.

4. Colditz GA. Economic costs of obesity. *Am J Clin Nutr*. 1992;55:503S–507S.

5. Kanders BS, Blackburn GL. Reducing primary risk factors by therapeutic weight loss. In: Wadden TA, Van Itallie TB, eds. *Treatment of the Seriously Obese Patient*. New York, NY: Guilford Press; 1992.

6. Benotti PN, Bistrian B, Benotti JR, et al. Heart disease and hypertension in severe obesity: The benefits of weight reduction. *Am J Clin Nutr*. 1992;55(suppl):586S–590S.

7. Gleysteen JJ. Results of surgery: Long-term effects on hyperlipidemia. *Am J Clin Nutr*. 1992;55(suppl):591S–593S.

8. Pories WJ, MacDonald KG Jr, Morgan EJ, et al. Surgical treatment of obesity and its effect on diabetes: 10-year follow-up. *Am J Clin Nutr*. 1992;55(suppl):582S–585S.

9. Parham ES. Nutrition education research in weight management among adults. *J Nutr Ed*. 1993;25:258–267.

10. Schlundt DG, Taylor D, Hill JO, et al. A behavioral taxonomy of obese female participants in a weight-loss program. *Am J Clin Nutr*. 1991;53:1151–1158.

11. Herman CP, Mack D. Restrained and unrestrained eating. *J Personality*. 1975;43:647–600.

12. Stunkard AJ, Messick S. The three-factor eating questionnaire to measure dietary restraint, disinhibition, and hunger. *J Psychosomatic Res*. 1985;29:71–83.

13. Herman CP, Polivy J. A boundary model for the regulation of eating. In: Stunkard AJ, Stellar E, eds. *Eating and Its Disorders*. New York, NY: Raven Press; 1984;141–156.

14. Bray GA, ed. *Obesity in Perspective*. Bethesda, Md: National Institutes of Health; 1978. DHEW publication 75-708. Fogarty International Series on Preventive Medicine. Vol 2, part 1.

15. National Institutes of Health. Technology Assessment Panel Statement. Methods for voluntary weight loss and control. *Nutr Rev*. 1992;50:340–345.

16. McReynolds WT. Toward a psychology of obesity: Review of research on the role of personality and level of adjustment. *Int J Eating Disorders*. 1982;2:37–57.

17. Stuart RB, Davis B. *Slim Chance in a Fat World: Behavioral Control of Obesity*. Champaign, Ill: Research Press; 1972.

18. Brownell KD, Kramer FM. Behavioral management of obesity. *Med Clin North Am*. 1989;73:185–201.

19. Schachter S. Obesity and eating. *Science*. 1968;161:751–756.

20. Bandura A. *Social Learning Theory*. Englewood Cliffs, NJ: Prentice Hall; 1977.

21. Bandura A. *Social Foundations of Thought and Action: A Social Cognitive Theory*. Englewood Cliffs, NJ: Prentice Hall; 1986.

22. Bandura A. Self-efficacy: Toward a unifying theory of behavior change. *Psychol Rev*. 1977;84:191–215.

23. Glynn SM, Ruderman AJ. The development and validation of an eating self-efficacy scale. *Cognitive Therapy and Research*. 1986;10:403–420.

24. Shannon B, Bagby R, Wang MQ, et al. Self-efficacy: A contributor to the explanation of eating behavior. *Health Ed Res.* 1990;5:395-407.

25. Bennett GA. An evaluation of self-instructional training in the treatment of obesity. *Addictive Behaviors.* 1986;11:125-134.

26. Sobal J, Stunkard AJ. Socioeconomic status and obesity: A review of the literature. *Psych Bull.* 1989;105:260-275.

27. Allon N. The stigma of overweight in everyday life. In: Wolman BJ, ed. *Psychological Aspects of Obesity.* New York, NY: Van Nostrand Reinhold Co; 1981:130-174.

28. Ajzen I, Fishbein M. *Understanding Attitudes and Predicting Social Behavior.* Englewood Cliffs, NJ: Prentice Hall; 1980:1-274.

29. Thoits PA. Social support as coping assistance. *J Consulting and Clinical Psychol.* 1987;54:416-423.

30. LaPorte DJ, Stunkard AJ. Predicting attrition and adherence to a very low calorie diet: A prospective investigation of the eating inventory. *Int J Obesity.* 1990;14:197-206.

31. Pratt CA. A conceptual model for studying attrition in weight-reduction programs. *J Nutr Ed.* 1990;22:177-182.

32. Kayman S, Bruvold W, Stern JS. Maintenance and relapse after weight loss in women: Behavioral aspects. *Am J Clin Nutr.* 1990;52.800-807.

33. Graham LE II, Taylor CB, Hovell MF, et al. Five-year follow-up to a behavioral weight-loss program. *J Consulting and Clinical Psychol.* 1983;51:322-323.

34. Kuczmarski RJ. Prevalence of overweight and weight gain in the United States. *Am J Clin Nutr.* 1992;55:495S.

35. McDowell A, Engel A, Massey JT, et al. National Center for Health Statistics. Plan and operation of the Second National Health and Nutrition Examination Survey, 1976-80. *Vital Health Stat*(1). 1981;(15):1-144.

36. Najjar MF, Rowland M. Anthropometric data and prevalence of overweight, United States: 1976-80. *Vital Health Stat* (11). 1987;238. DHHS Pub. No. (PHS) 87-1688, Washington, DC; 1987.

37. Najjar MF, Kuczmarski RJ. Anthropometric data and prevalence of overweight for Hispanics: 1982-84. *Vital Health Stat* (II). 1989;239. DHHS Pub. No. (PHS) 87-1689, Washington, DC; 1989.

38. Harlan WR, Landis JR, Flegal KM, et al. Secular trends in body mass in the United States, 1960-1980. *Am J Epidemiol.* 1988;128:1065-1074.

39. Revicki DA, Israel RG. Relationship between body mass indices and measures of body adiposity. *Am J Public Health.* 1986;76:992-994.

40. Prevalence of overweight for Hispanics: US, 1982-1984. *MMWR.* 1989;38:838-842.

41. Stern MP, Gaskill SP, Hazuda HP, et al. Does obesity explain prevalence of diabetes among Mexican Americans? *Diabetologia.* 1983;24:272-277.

42. National Center for Health Statistics. *Health, United States, 1989.* Washington, DC: US Government Printing Office; 1990. Public Health Service publication 86-1255.

43. Williamson DF, Kahn HS, Remington PL. The 10-year incidence of overweight and major weight gain in US adults. *Arch Intern Med.* 1990;150:665-672.

44. Kahn HS, Williamson DF, Stevens JA. Race and weight change in US women: The roles of socioeconomic and marital status. *Am J Public Health.* 1991;81:319-323.

45. Kahn HS, Williamson DF. The contributions of income, education and changing marital status to weight change among US men. *Int J Obesity.* 1990;14:1057-1068.

46. Lukaski HD. Methods for the assessment of human body composition: Traditional and new. *Am J Clin Nutr.* 1987;46:537-556.

47. Sjostrom L. Morbidity and mortality of severely obese subjects. *Am J Clin Nutr.* 1992;55(suppl):508S-515S.

48. Bouchard C, Bray GA, Hubbard VS. Basic and clinical aspects of regional fat distribution. *Am J Clin Nutr.* 1990;52:946-950.

49. Bray GA. Pathophysiology of obesity. *Am J Clin Nutr.* 1992;55:488S-494S.

50. Bray GA. *The Obese Patient: Major Problems in Internal Medicine.* Volume 9. Philadelphia, Pa: WB Saunders; 1976.

51. National Research Council. *Diet and Health: Implications for Reducing Chronic Disease Risk.* Washington, DC: National Academy Press; 1989.

52. Ravussin E, Bogardus C. A brief overview of human energy metabolism and its relationship to essential obesity. *Am J Clin Nutr.* 1992;55:242S-245S.

53. D'Alessio DA, Kavle EC, Mozzoli MA, et al. Thermic effect of food in lean and obese men. *J Clin Invest.* 1988;81:1781-1789.

54. Bouchard C, Tremblay A, Despres JP, et al. The response to long-term overfeeding identical twins. *N Engl J Med.* 1990;322:1477-1482.

55. Thomas CD, Peters JC, Reed GW, et al. Nutrient balance and energy expenditure during ad libitum feeding of high-fat and high-carbohydrate diets in humans. *Am J Clin Nutr.* 1992;55:934-942.

56. Flatt J. Importance of nutrient balance in body weight regulation. *Diabetes.* 1988;4:571-581.

57. Katahn M, McMinn MR. Obesity: A biobehavioral point of view. *Ann NY Acad Sci.* 1990;602:189-204.

58. Joos SK. Social, attitudinal and behavioral correlates of weight change among Mexican American women. University of Houston. *Dissertation Abstracts International.* 1984;46:131.

59. Miller WC, Eggert KE, Wallace JP, et al. Successful weight loss in a self-taught, self-administered program. *Int J Sports Med.* 1993;14:401-405.

60. Miller WC, Kindeman AK, Wallace JP, et al. Diet composition, energy intake, and exercise in relation to body fat content in men and women. *Am J Clin Nutr.* 1990;52: 426-430.

61. Miller WC. Diet composition, energy intake, and nutritional status in relation to obesity in men and women. *Med Sci Sports Exerc.* 1991;23:280-284.

62. Dreon DM, Frey-Hewitt B, Ellsworth N, et al. Dietary fat: Carbohydrate ratio and obesity in middle-aged men. *Am J Clin Nutr.* 1988;47:995-1000.

63. Romieu I, Willett WC, Stampfer MJ, et al. Energy intake and other determinants of relative weight. *Am J Clin Nutr.* 1988;47:406-412.

64. Rodin J, Moskowitz HR, Bray GA. Relationship between obesity, weight loss, and taste responsiveness. *Physiol Behav.* 1976;17:591-597.

65. Drewnowski A, Halmi KA, Pierce B, et al. Taste and eating disorders. *Am J Clin Nutr.* 1987;46:442-450.

66. Gates JC, Huenemann RL, Brand RJ. Food choices of obese and non-obese persons. *J Am Diet Assoc.* 1975;67:339-343.

67. Thompson DA, Moskowitz HR, Campbell RG. Effects of body weight and food intake on pleasantness ratings for a sweet stimulus. *J Applied Physiol.* 1976;41:77-83.

68. Drewnowski A, Greenwood MRC. Cream and sugar: Human preferences for high fat foods. *Physiol Behav.* 1983;30:629-633.

69. Drewnowski A, Brunzell JD, Sande K, et al. Sweet tooth reconsidered: Taste responsiveness in human obesity. *Physiol Behav.* 1985;35:617-622.

70. Rossner S, Zweigbergk DV, Ohlin A, et al. Weight reduction with dietary fibre supplements—results of two double-blinded randomized studies. *Acta Med Scand.* 1987;222:83-88.

71. Mickelsen O, Makdani DD, Cotton RH, et al. Effects of a high fiber bread diet on weight loss in college-age males. *Am J Clin Nutr.* 1979;32:1703-1709.

72. Rigaud D, Ryttig KR, Angel AL, et al. Overweight treated with energy restriction and a dietary fibre supplement: A 6-month randomized, double-blind, placebo-controlled trial. *Int J Obesity.* 1990;14:763-769.

73. Kushner RF. Body weight and mortality. *Nutr Rev.* 1993;51(5):127-136.

74. Wadden TA, Foster GD, Letizia KA, et al. Long-term effects of dieting on resting metabolic rate in obese outpatients. *JAMA.* 1990;264:707-711.

75. Schutz T, Tremblay A, Weinsier RL, et al. Role of fat oxidation in the long-term stabilization of body weight in obese women. *Am J Clin Nutr.* 1992;55:670-674.

76. Brownell KD, Jeffery RW. Improving long-term weight loss: Pushing the limits of treatment. *Behav Ther.* 1987;18:353-374.

77. Hawks SR, Richins P. Toward a new paradigm for the management of obesity. *J Health Ed.* 1994;25:147-153.

78. Kalodner CR, DeLucia JL. Components of effective weight loss programs: Theory, research, and practice. *J Counseling and Development.* 1990;68:427-433.

79. DeLucia JL, Kalodner CR. An individualized cognitive intervention: Does it increase the efficacy of behavioral interventions for obesity? *Addictive-Behaviors.* 1990;15: 473-479.

80. Hurbert HB, Feinleib M, McNamara PM, et al. Obesity as an independent risk factor for cardiovascular disease: A 26-year follow-up of participants in the Framingham Heart Study. *Circulation.* 1983;67:968.

81. Intersalt Cooperative Research Group. Intersalt: An international study of electrolyte excretion and blood pressure. Results for 24 hour urinary sodium and potassium excretion. *Br Med J.* 1988;297:319-328.

82. Burton BT, Foster WR, Hirsch J, et al. Health implications of obesity: A NIH consensus development conference. *Int J Obesity.* 1985;9:155.

83. Glueck CJ, Taylor HL, Jacobs D, et al. Plasma high-density lipoprotein cholesterol: Association with measurements of body mass. The Lipid Research Clinics Program Prevalance Study. *Circulation.* 1980;62(Suppl IV):62.

84. Kannel WB, Gordon T, Castelli WP. Obesity, lipids, and glucose tolerance: The Framingham Study. *Am J Clin Nutr.* 1979;32:1238.

85. Brennan PJ, Simpson JM, Blacket RB, et al. Effects of body-weight on serum-cholesterol, serum triglycerides, serum urate, and systolic blood pressure. *Aust NZ J Med.* 1980;10:15.

86. Aristimuno GG, Foster TA, Voors AW, et al. Influence of persistent obesity in children on cardiovascular risk factors: The Bogalusa Heart Study. *Circulation.* 1984;69:895.

87. Freedom DS, Burke GL, Harsha DW, et al. Relationship of changes in obesity to serum-lipid and lipoprotein changes in childhood and adolescence. *JAMA.* 1985;254:515.

88. Vague J. The degree of masculine differentiation of obesities: A factor determining predisposition to diabetes, atherosclerosis, gout, and uric calculous disease. *Am J Clin Nutr.* 1956;4:20.

89. Albrink MJ, Meigs JW. The relationship between serum triglycerides and skinfold thickness in obese subjects. *Ann NY Acad Sci.* 1965;131:673.

90. Foster CJ, Weinsein RL, Birch R, et al. Obesity and serum lipids: An evaluation of the relative contribution of body fat and fat distribution and lipid levels. *Int J Obesity.* 1987;11:151.

91. Lapidus L, Bengstsson C, Larrson B. Distribution of adipose tissue and risk of cardiovascular disease and death:

A 12 year follow up of participants in the population study of women in Gothenburg, Sweden. *Br Med J.* 1984;289:1257.

92. Donahue RP, Abbott RD, Bloom E, et al. Central obesity and coronary heart disease in men. *Lancet.* 1987;1:821.

93. Despres JP, Tremblay A, Perusse L, et al. Abdominal adipose tissue and serum HDL-cholesterol: Association independent from obesity and serum triglyceride concentration. *Int J Obesity.* 1988;12:1.

94. Follick MJ, Abrams DB, Smith TW, et al. Contrasting short- and long-term effects of weight loss on lipoprotein levels. *Arch Int Med.* 1984;144:1571.

95. Vaswani AN. Effect of weight-reduction on circulating lipids: An integration of possible mechanisms. *J Am Coll Nutr.* 1983;2:123.

96. Wolf RN, Grundy SM. Influence of weight reduction on plasma lipoproteins in obese patients. *Arteriosclerosis.* 1983;3:160.

97. Thompson PD, Jeffrey RW, Wing RP, et al. Unexpected decrease in plasma high density lipoprotein cholesterol with weight loss. *Am J Clin Nutr.* 1979;32:2016.

98. Tran ZV, Weltman A. Differential effects of exercise on serum lipid and lipoprotein levels seen with changes in body weight. *JAMA.* 1985;254:919.

99. Friedman CI, Falko JM, Patel ST, et al. Serum lipoprotein responses during active and stable weight reduction in reproductive obese females. *J Clin Endocrinol Metab* 1982;55.258.

100. Contaldo F, Strazzullo P, Postiglione A. Plasma high density lipoprotein in severe obesity after stable weight loss. *Atherosclerosis.* 1980;37:163.

101. Streja DA, Boyko E, Rabkin SW. Changes in plasma high-density lipoprotein cholesterol concentrations after weight reduction in grossly obese subjects. *Br Med J.* 1980;281:770.

102. Wolf RN, Grundy SM. Influence of weight reduction on plasma lipoprotein in obese patients. *Arteriosclerosis.* 1983;3:160.

103. Brownell KD, Stunkard AJ. Differential changes in plasma high-density lipoprotein cholesterol levels in obese men and women during weight reduction. *Arch Intern Med.* 1981;141:1142.

104. Wechsler JG, Hutt V, Wenzel H, et al. Lipids and lipoproteins during a very low calorie diet. *Int J Obesity.* 1981;5:325.

105. Thompson PD, Jeffery RW, Wing RR, et al. Unexpected decrease in plasma high density lipoprotein cholesterol with weight loss. *Am J Clin Nutr.* 19879;32:2016.

106. Rabkin SW, Boyko E, Streja DA. Relationship of weight loss and cigarette smoking to changes in high-density lipoprotein cholesterol. *Am J Clin Nutr.* 1981;34:1764–1768.

107. Leon AS, Conrad J, Hunnihake DB, et al. Effects of a vigorous walking program on body composition, carbohy-

drate, and lipid metabolism of obese young men. *Am J Clin Nutr.* 1979;32:1776.

108. Lew EA, Garfinkel L. Variations in mortality by weight among 750,000 men and women. *J Chron Dis.* 1979;32:563–576.

109. Miller AB. Diet and cancer: A review. *Acta Oncol.* 1990;29:87–95.

110. Chandra RK, Kutty KM. Immunocompetence in obesity. *Acta Paediatr Scand.* 1980;69:25–30.

111. Krishan EC, Trost L, Aarons S, et al. Study of function and maturation of monocytes in morbidly obese individuals. *J Surg Res.* 1982;33:89–97.

112. Kolterman OG, Olefsky JM, Kurahara C, et al. A defect in cell-mediated immune function in insulin-resistant diabetic and obese subjects. *J Lab Clin Med.* 1980;96:535–543.

113. Knapp TR. A methodological critique of the "ideal weight" concept. *JAMA.* 1983;250:506–510.

114. Simopolous AP, Van Itallie TB. Body weight, health, and longevity. *Ann Intern Med.* 1984;100:285–295.

115. Harrison GG. Height-weight tables. *Ann Intern Med.* 1985;103:989–994.

116. *Obese and Overweight Adults in the United States.* Hyattsville, Md: National Center for Health Statistics; 1983. Public Health Service publication 83-1680, series 11, no. 230.

117. Society of Actuaries. *Build and Blood Pressure Study, 1959.* Chicago, Ill: Society of Actuaries; 1959:1.

118. Society of Actuaries and Association of Life Insurance Medical Directors. *Build Study, 1979.* Chicago, Ill: Society of Actuaries and Association of Life Insurance Medical Directors; 1980.

119. Sjostrom LV. Mortality of severely obese subjects. *Am J Clin Nutr.* 1992;55:516S–523S.

120. Sjostrom LV. Morbidity of severely obese subjects. *Am J Clin Nutr.* 1992;55:508S–515S.

121. Manson JE, Colditz GA, Stampfer MJ, et al. A prospective study of obesity and risk of coronary heart disease in women. *N Engl J Med.* 1990;322:882–889.

122. Wienpahl J, Ragland, SS. Body mass index and 15-year mortality in a cohort of black men and women. *J Clin Epidemiol.* 1990;43:949–960.

123. Stevens J, Keil JE, Rust PF, et al. Body mass index and body girths as predictors of mortality in black and white women. *Arch Intern Med.* 1992;152:1257–1262.

124. Johnson H, Heineman EF, Heiss G, et al. Cardiovascular disease risk factors and mortality among black women and white women aged 40–69 years in Evans County, Georgia. *Am J Epidemiol.* 1986;123:209–220.

125. Larsson B, Svardsudd K, Welin L, et al. Abdominal adipose tissue distribution, obesity, and risk of cardiovascu-

lar disease and death: 13 year follow up of participants in the study of men born in 1913. *Br Med J*. 1984;288:1401–1404.

126. Donahue RP, Abbott RD, Bloom E, et al. Central obesity and coronary heart disease in men. *Lancet*. 1987;11:821–824.

127. Rogers AE, Longnecker MP. Biology of disease. Dietary and nutritional influences on cancer: A review of epidemiologic and experimental data. *Lab Invest*. 1988;59:729–759.

128. Van Itallie TB. Health implications of overweight and obesity in the United States. *Ann Intern Med*. 1985;103:983–988.

129. Andres R, Elahi D, Tobin JD, et al. Impact of age on weight goals. *Ann Intern Med*. 1985;103:1030–1033.

130. Fitzgerald AP, Jarrett RJ. Body weight and coronary heart disease mortality: An analysis in relation to age and smoking habit. 15 years follow-up data from the Whitehall Study. *Int J Obesity*. 1992;16:119–123.

131. Tayback M, Kumanyika S, Chee E. Body weight as a risk factor in the elderly. *Arch Intern Med*. 1990;150:1065–1072.

132. Rissanen A, Heliovaara M, Knekt P, et al. Weight and mortality in Finnish women. *J Clin Epidemiol*. 1991;44:787–795.

133. Harris T, Cook EF, Garrison R, et al. Body mass index and mortality among nonsmoking older persons. *JAMA*. 1988;259:1520–1524.

134. Andres R. Mortality and obesity: The rationale for age-specific height-weight tables. In: Hazzard WR, Andres R, Bierman EL, et al. eds. *Geriatric Medicine and Gerontology*. 2nd ed. New York, NY: McGraw-Hill, Inc; 1990:759–765.

135. Waaler HT. Hazard of obesity—The Norwegian experience. *Acta Med Scand*. 1988;723(suppl):17–21.

136. Tsukamoto H, Sano F. Body weight and longevity: Insurance experience in Japan. *Diabetes Res Clin Pract*. 1990;10:S119–S125.

137. Garrison RJ, Feinleib M, Castelli WP, et al. Cigarette smoking as a confounder of the relationship between relative weight and long-term mortality. *JAMA*. 1983;249:2199–2203.

138. Manson JE, Stampfer MJ, Hennekens CH, et al. Body weight and longevity: A reassessment. *JAMA*. 1987;257:353–358.

139. Garfinkel L. Overweight and mortality. *Cancer*. 1986;58:1826–1829.

140. Sidney S, Friedman GD, Siegelaub AB. Thinness and mortality. *Am J Public Health*. 1987;77:317–322.

141. Wannamethee G, Shaper AG. Body weight and mortality in middle aged British men: Impact of smoking. *Br Med J*. 1989;299:1497–1502.

142. Albanes D, Jones YJ, Micozzi MS, et al. Associations between smoking and body weight in the US population: Analysis of NHANES II. *Am J Public Health*. 1987;77:439–444.

143. Istvan JA, Cunningham TW, Garfinkel L. Cigarette smoking and body weight in the cancer prevention study I. *Int J Epidemiol*. 1992;21:849–953.

144. Lee I-M, Paffenbarger RS. Change in body weight and longevity. *JAMA*. 1992;268:2045–2049.

145. Pamuk ER, Williamson DF, Madans J, et al. Weight loss and mortality in a national cohort of adults, 1971–1987. *Am J Epidemiol*. 1992;136:686–697.

146. Blair SN, Shaten J, Brownell K, et al. Body weight change, all-cause and cause-specific mortality in the multiple risk factor intervention trial. *Ann Intern Med*. 1993;119:749–757.

147. DiPietro L, Anda RF, Williamson DF, et al. Depressive symptoms and weight change in national cohort of adults. *Int J Obesity*. 1992;16:745–753.

148. Williamson DF, Serdula MK, Anda RF, et al. Weight loss attempts in adults: Goals, duration, and rate of weight loss. *Am J Public Health*. 1992;82:1251–1257.

149. Wadden TA, Stunkard AJ. Social and psychological consequences of obesity. *Ann Intern Med*. 1987;499:55–65.

150. Weissman M, Myers J. Affective disorders in a US urban community. *Arch Gen Psychiatry*. 1978;35:1304–1311.

151. Allon N. Self-perception of the stigma of overweight in relationship to weight-losing patterns. *Am J Clin Nutr*. 1979;32:470–480.

152. Stunkard AJ, Wadden TA. Psychological aspects of severe obesity. *Am J Clin Nutr*. 1992;55:524S–532S.

153. Staffieri JR. A study of social stereotype of body image in children. *J Pers Soc Psychol*. 1967;7:101–104.

154. Goodman N, Dornbusch SM, Richardson SA, et al. Variant reactions to physical disabilities. *Am Sociol Rev*. 1963;28:429–435.

155. Maddox GL, Back K, Liederman V. Overweight as social deviance and disability. *J Health Soc Behav*. 1968;9:287–298.

156. Richardson SA, Goodman N, Hastorf AH, et al. Cultural uniformity in reaction to physical disabilities. *Am Sociol Rev*. 1961;26:241–247.

157. Holland J, Masling J, Copley D. Mental illness in lower class, normal, obese and hyperobese women. *Psychosom Med*. 1970;32:351–357.

158. Halmi KA, Long M, Stunkard AJ, et al. Psychiatric diagnosis of morbidly obese gastric bypass patients. *Am J Psychiatry*. 1980;137:470–472.

159. Gertler R, Ramsey-Stewart G. Pre-operative psychiatric assessment of patients presenting for gastric bariatric

surgery (surgical control of morbid obesity). *Aust NZ J Surg.* 1986;56:157-161.

160. Allon N. The stigma of overweight in everyday life. In: Bray G, ed. *Obesity in Perspective.* Washington, DC: US Government Printing Office; 1975:83-102.

161. Canning H, Mayer J. Obesity—Its possible effects on college admissions. *New Engl J Med.* 1966;275:1172-1174.

162. Pargaman D. The incidence of obesity among college students. *J Sch Health.* 1969;29:621-625.

163. Larkin JE, Pines HA. No fat persons need apply. *Sociol Work Occup.* 1979;6:312-327.

164. Roe DA, Eickwort KR. Relationships between obesity and associated health factors with unemployment among low income women. *J Am Med Wom Assoc.* 1976;31:193-204.

165. Fat execs get slimmer paychecks. *Industry Week.* 1974;180:221,224.

166. Rand CSW, Macgregor AMC. Successful weight loss following obesity surgery and the perceived liability of morbid obesity. *Int J Obesity.* 1991;15:577-579.

167. Maddox GL, Liederman V. Overweight as a social disability with medical implications. *J Med Educ.* 1969;44:214-220.

168. Davis SH. Students with disabilities: Part II. Disability and discrimination. *Dep-line, Summer Newsletter of the Dietetic Educators and Practitioners.* 1994;12(3).

169. Frierson JG. Obesity as a legal disability under the ADA, Rehabilitation Act, and state handicapped employment laws. *Labor Law Journal.* 1993;44:286-296.

170. McEroy SA. Fat change: Employment discrimination against the overweight. *Labor Law Journal.* 1992;42:3-14.

171. Kuczmarski RJ. Trends in body composition for infants and children in the US. *Crit Rev in Food Sci and Nutr.* 1993;33:375-387.

172. Flegal KM. Defining obesity in children and adolescents: Epidemiologic approaches. *Crit Rev in Food Sci and Nutr.* 1993;33:307-312.

173. Kaplowitz H, Martorell R, Mendoza F. Fathers and fat distribution in Mexican-American children and youth from the Hispanic Health and Nutrition Examination Survey. *Am J Human Biol.* 1989;1:631-648.

174. Okamoto E, Davidson LL, Conner DR. High prevalence of overweight in inner-city school children. *Am J Dis Child.* 1993;147:155-159.

175. Mellin L. To: President Clinton, Re: Combatting childhood obesity. *J Am Diet Assoc.* 1993;93:265-266.

176. Felitti VJ. Childhood sexual abuse, depression, and family dysfunctions in adult obese patients: A case study. *South Med J.* 1993;86:732-736.

177. Hall SK. Judgments of body size and attractiveness by Mexican-American mothers and daughters. University of Houston. *Dissertation Abstracts International.* 1987;48:1168.

178. *Kids Make the Nutritional Grade.* Washington, DC: International Food Information Council; 1992.

179. Dietz WH, Bortmaker SL. Do we fatten our children at the television set? Obesity and television in children and adolescents. *Pediatrics.* 1985;75:807-812.

180 Klesges RC, Shelton ML, Klesges LM. The effects of television on metabolic rate. Potential implications for childhood obesity. *Pediatrics.* 1993;91:281-286.

181. National Task Force on the Prevention and Treatment of Obesity. Very low-calorie diets. *JAMA.* 1993;270:967-974.

182. Berg F.M. Health Risks of Weight Loss. *Healthy Weight Journal;* 1995.

183. Kaufman M. *Nutrition in Public Health—A Handbook for Developing Programs and Services.* Gaithersburg, Md: Aspen Publishers, Inc; 1990:570.

16

Debilitating Diseases—Osteoporosis, Alcoholism, Arthritis, and Renal Disease

Learning Objectives

- Describe the occurrence and etiology of osteoporosis, alcoholism, arthritis, and renal disease.
- Identify secondary and tertiary prevention approaches for these diseases.
- List and enumerate the role of dietary components in the secondary prevention of these diseases.

High Definition Nutrition

Alcohol—a chemical compound having a hydroxyl group linked to carbon. It has both negative and positive effects on the body (i.e., it can impair the functioning of the brain, irritate the gastrointestinal tract, and dilate arteries in the arms, legs, and skin, but it can also relax people, reduce their inhibitions, provide an antiviral, and lower blood cholesterol level).

Alcoholic drink—one "drink" is equivalent to one beer, 100 mL of wine, or one ounce of spirits.

Alcoholism or alcohol addiction—predictable, progressive, and often fatal condition with a 4- to 15-year progression from abuse to addiction. Frequency and pattern of consumption may vary. Condition is not determined by amount consumed or frequency of use, rather it depends on events surrounding use of alcohol. There is usually significant impairment and denial. The individual consumes approximately 25% to 60% of total energy from alcohol and has more than eight drunken episodes per year.

Bioavailability—the extent or degree to which a drug, substance, element, or nutrient is available to the target tissue.

Gout—an inherited disorder of purine metabolism; uric acid accumulates in the blood.

Moderated use of alcohol—the consumption of one or two drinks a day, averaging 8% to 14% of total energy intake without physical, mental, emotional, or legal consequences.

Osteomalacia—also known as adult rickets, is a qualitative not quantitative disorder of bone metabolism. It is characterized by an increased, normal, or decreased mass of inadequately mineralized bone matrix.

Placebo effect—when an inactive pill, diet, or device is given to a person with a disease and the person improves. It demonstrates the power of mind over body. The word is derived from the Latin, *placebo* ("I shall please").

Problem drinking—ritual, periodic, or episodic use of more than two drinks per day and more than eight drunken incidents per year. Situation creates some unpredictability. Consequences may include weight gain, physical discomfort, hangover, and possible social or relationship conflicts.

Social drinking—occasional, predictable, guilt-free consumption of alcoholic beverages. No loss of control is noted. Individual is able to stop after one drink. One or two drunken incidents per year.

Tyrosine–an amino acid used as a supplement during drug and alcohol detoxification that affects craving and withdrawal symptoms.

OSTEOPOROSIS

The National Osteoporosis Foundation and the US Administration on Aging estimate that there are 25 million Americans with a bone-thinning disease called osteoporosis. It is called a "silent thief" because it develops in an asymptomatic manner until it is expressed as a fracture either in the hip, wrist, or spine. Fifty percent of women and 20% of men over 65 years of age have osteoporosis.[1] A progressive spinal deformity is common (see Figure 16–1).

Osteoporosis has also been called "a pediatric disease with a geriatric outcome." This is because bone mass is formed early in life and needs to be maintained into the sixth and seventh decades and beyond. The causes of osteoporosis are not known, but select risk factors place an individual at risk for reduced bone health (see Figure 16–2). The simple checklist below can be used with individuals or in group settings to identify the level of risk of an individual. The greater the number of "yes" responses to these questions, the greater the risk of developing osteoporosis[2,3]:

- Do you have a small, thin frame, or are you Caucasian or Asian?
- Do you have a family history of osteoporosis?
- Are you a postmenopausal woman?
- Have you had an early or surgically induced menopause?
- Do you take excessive thyroid medication or high doses of cortisone-like drugs for asthma, arthritis, or cancer?
- Would you describe your daily consumption of dairy products and other calcium-rich foods as low?
- Are you physically active?
- Do you smoke cigarettes or drink alcohol in excess?

- Are you allergic to milk products or are you lactose intolerant?
- Do you spend less than one hour a week participating in activities like aerobics, walking, or bicycling?
- Have you ever had an eating disorder such as bulimia or anorexia nervosa?

Info Line

The National Osteoporosis Foundation is the nation's leading resource for patients and health care professionals seeking up-to-date, medically sound information and educational materials on the causes, prevention, and treatment of osteoporosis. For information, contact National Osteoporosis Foundation, 1150 17th Street, NW, Suite 500, Washington, DC 20036-4603.

Calcium, Vitamin D, and Fractures

Insufficient dietary calcium is one of the possible risk factors for osteoporosis and thereby for fractures. An inadequate intake of calcium is common in women. National Health and Nutrition Examination Survey (NHANES) data show that calcium intake in women is 40% to 50% below that of men; 75% to 80% of women have daily intakes below 800 mg, while 25% have intakes below 300 mg. According to the 1984 National Institutes of Health (NIH) consensus conference on osteoporosis, dietary calcium intake required to prevent negative calcium balance increases from 1,000 mg/day in perimenopausal women to 1,500 mg/day after menopause.[4-6]

Intestinal absorption of calcium declines with advancing age. However, estrogen is known to enhance intestinal calcium absorption and renal calcium conservation. Both estrogen and calcium supplementation then reduce a negative calcium balance. For health-conscious older adults, low-fat eating patterns often mean a reduced intake of dairy products and calcium, which may increase a negative calcium balance.

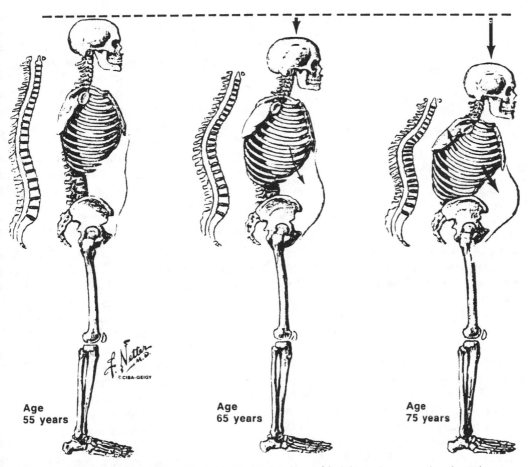

Age 55 years

Age 65 years

Age 75 years

Compression fractures of thoracic vertebrae lead to loss of height and progressive thoracic kyphosis (dowager's hump). Lower ribs eventually rest on iliac crests, and downward pressure on viscera causes abdominal distention

Figure 16-1 Progressive spinal deformity in osteoporosis. *Source:* Reprinted from Kaplan, F.S., Osteoporosis: Pathophysiology and Prevention, *Clinical Symposia*, Vol. 39, No. 1, p. 21, with permission of Ciba-Geigy Corporation, © 1987.

Low dietary calcium intake may be a risk factor for osteoporosis and for fractures. However, data on the effectiveness of calcium supplements vary. This variation may reflect differences in the hormonal status and eating pattern of individuals. For example, in one study of older, postmenopausal women, calcium supplements prevented bone loss for women whose calcium intake was less than 400 mg. Supplementation did not assist women who had higher dietary calcium intakes. Adding vitamin D may increase the effect of supplemental calcium on preventing bone loss.

It is not clear if this is due to an enhanced absorption of calcium or whether vitamin D has an independent effect. The percentage of calcium available in common compounds is shown in Table 16-1. Estrogen therapy reduces bone loss among postmenopausal women. Calcium supplementation for women who receive estrogen may reduce bone loss further.

Research data are not available regarding the efficacy of calcium and vitamin D supplementation. Women are currently taking supplements to reduce fractures. A clinical trial can provide a

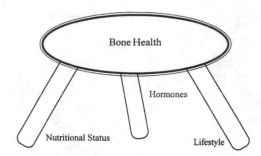

Figure 16–2 Bone health is analogous to a three-legged stool. Three predisposing factors include nutritional status, hormones, and lifestyle.

rational basis for advising women to take such supplementation. The Women's Health Initiative will determine if supplementation can reduce bone loss and fracture rates. The trial will also provide a test for interactions of supplementation alone or in combination with estrogens (see Chapter 9).

Osteoporosis and osteomalacia are both influenced by poor nutrient intake, decreased physical activity, corticosteroid therapy, and lack of sunshine experienced by people who are homebound. Malabsorption of vitamin D in the small bowel is often seen with advanced disease. The deficiency of vitamin D and calcium play a major role in the development of osteomalacia.

The 1994 NIH Consensus Development Conference Statement on Optimal Calcium Intake

In the absence of intervention, women over 45 years experience 5.2 million fractures and in-

Table 16–1 Percent Calcium Available from Common Calcium Supplements

Compounds	Calcium (%)
Calcium carbonate	40
Calcium lactate	13
Calcium gluconate	9

Source: Adapted from *Osteoporosis: Cause, Treatment and Prevention*, p. 21, National Institutes of Health, Publication No. 86-2226, 1986.

cur $45.2 billion in costs to the health care system. There are about 195,000 vertebral fractures in the United States annually. At 50 years of age, a US Caucasian woman has a 32% chance of a vertebral fracture, 16% chance of hip fracture, and 15% chance of wrist fracture.[4] Peak bone mass achieved in the first 30 years of life and the rate at which bone is lost later in life are the major influences on osteoporosis.

In the NIH report of the conference, several questions about osteoporosis were addressed. Six important questions and the response to each are given below.[5]

What Is the Optimal Calcium Intake?

Optimal calcium intake is the level of intake needed to achieve and maintain peak adult bone mass and minimize bone loss later in life (see Table 16–2). Calcium needs are greater during rapid growth in childhood and adolescence, pregnancy, lactation, and later adult life. Ninety-nine percent of total body calcium is located in bones. Body retention of calcium increases as calcium intake increases up to a threshold, above which no further gain in calcium retention is noted.

Peak adult bone mass is usually achieved by 20 years of age, but additional bone mass may form through the third decade. Cross-sectional studies show a positive association between lifelong calcium intake and adult bone mass.[7,8] Data suggest that calcium intake between 1,200 and 1,500 mg/day might result in higher peak adult bone mass.

After adult peak bone mass is achieved, bone turnover stabilizes for both men and women (i.e., bone formation and bone resorption are balanced). For women, resorption rate increases and bone mass decreases as estrogen production declines with menopause. Specifically, the decline in circulating 17 beta-estradiol is the predominant factor in accelerated bone loss. This begins immediately after the onset of menopause and lasts for six to eight years. Hormonal-replacement therapy slows the decline in bone mass, but supplemental calcium at this time does not appear to slow the decline. Later in menopause, calcium intakes of 1,500 mg/day may reduce the rates of bone loss in certain parts of the skeleton (i.e., the femoral neck).[9–11]

Table 16–2 Recommendations of NIH Consensus Development Panel on Optimal Calcium Intake

Age	Gender	NIH Recommendations (mg)	Current RDAs (mg)
Birth–1 yr	M/F	400–600	400–600
1–5 yrs	M/F	800	800
6–10 yrs	M/F	800–1200	1200
11–24 yrs	M/F	1200–1500	1200
25–49 yrs	F	1000	800
Pregnant/nursing	F	1200–1500	1200
Postmenopausal (50–64 yrs)	F		
On estrogen		1000	800
Not on estrogen		1500	800
25–64 yrs	M	1000	800
65 yrs+	M/F	1500	800

Source: Adapted from *Food Insight*, September/October 1994, with permission of the International Food Information Council Foundation, © 1994.

If postmenopausal women receive estrogen-replacement therapy, 1,000 mg/day of calcium is recommended to maintain calcium balance and stabilize bone mass. If women do not take estrogen, 1,500 mg of calcium per day may limit loss of bone mass, but will not replace estrogen.[12]

Low calcium intake has been implicated as a determinant of preeclampsia, colon cancer, and hypertension. A large multicenter trial is currently evaluating the role of increased calcium in preeclampsia, and data should be available in 1996. The Women's Health Initiative will evaluate the effect of vitamin D and calcium supplementation on colorectal cancer and osteoporosis incidence. A number of epidemiologic studies report an inverse association between blood pressure and calcium intake. Few prospective studies have confirmed this association, but beta analyses demonstrate a small reduction in systolic pressure and no effect on diastolic blood pressure with calcium intake.[5]

What Are the Important Cofactors for Achieving Optimal Calcium Intake?

Dietary constituents, hormones, and drugs modify calcium balance and influence bone mass. An individual's age, ethnic and genetic background, gastrointestinal disorders including malabsorption, and liver and renal disease affect bone health. Interactions of these factors may have either a positive or negative effect on efficacy of calcium.

Vitamin D metabolites enhance calcium absorption by stimulating active transport of calcium in the small intestine and colon. Deficiency of 1,25-dihydroxyvitamin D reduces calcium absorption. The deficiency may be due to an inadequate amount or impaired activation of vitamin D or even to an acquired resistance to vitamin D. Vitamin D deficiency is also associated with an increased risk of fractures.

Sex hormone deficiency is linked to excessive bone resorption in women and men. Calcium supplementation can decrease the estrogen dosage required to maintain bone mass in postmenopausal women, but oral calcium will not prevent the postmenopausal bone loss due to estrogen deficiency.[11,12] Endogenous factors (e.g., growth hormone, insulin-like growth factor-I, and parathyroid hormone) enhance overall calcium absorption.

Increased physical activity can enhance the beneficial effect of oral calcium supplementation on bone mass in young adults. Immobilization rapidly decreases bone mass. This is especially true for individuals placed on bed rest or individuals who have paraplegia or quadriplegia. The concern is that increased calcium intake may predispose these individuals to hypercalcemia, ectopic calcification, ectopic ossification, and nephrolithiasis.

Calcium intake, intestinal absorption, urinary excretion, and endogenous fecal loss influence calcium balance. High amounts of sodium and animal protein can significantly increase urinary calcium excretion. For every 2,300 mg of sodium, a 40-mg calcium loss occurs.[13,14]

Primitive hunter-gatherers had calcium and sodium intakes yielding a 1.0 to 0.76 ratio. This equates to four calcium atoms per three sodium atoms. Today, average sodium intakes produce 17 sodium atoms per 1 calcium atom. Protein intake increases calcium requirements due to loss of calcium in the kidneys and the demand for a calcium balance. High oxalate and phytate content of foods can reduce the availability of calcium; wheat bran, fat, phosphate, magnesium, and caffeine have not been found to alter calcium absorption significantly. A 5-ounce cup of coffee creates a loss in calcium balance by about 3 milligrams. Glucocorticoids decrease calcium absorption; excess is associated with negative calcium balance and a dramatic increase in fracture risk. Oral calcium and vitamin D supplements decrease glucocorticoid-associated bone loss.[5]

What Are the Risks Associated with Increased Levels of Calcium Intake?

High levels of calcium intake above 2 grams can have adverse effects (e.g., the efficiency of calcium absorption decreases as intake increases). This occurs as a protective mechanism to reduce calcium intoxication. However, the adaptive mechanism is overcome by a calcium intake greater than 4 grams per day. Calcium toxicity can cause severe renal damage, and ectopic calcium deposition or a milk-alkali syndrome can occur with misuse of calcium carbonate (i.e., antacid abuse). Hypercalcemia or hypercalciuria can occur when individuals consume less than 4 grams if they are susceptible. No adverse renal effects have been noted when moderate supplementation of 1,500 mg/day is used.

Supplementing individuals who have a history of kidney stones can increase both urinary calcium excretion and stone formation. Iron absorption can be lowered by 50% due to calcium supplements. Gastrointestinal side effects including constipation have been reported from calcium supplements. The calcium ion can produce a "rebound hyperacidity" when a calcium carbonate antacid is used extensively. Side effects are not common when a moderate increase is made in calcium intake. Bone meal and dolomite can have significant contamination with lead and other heavy metals, and supplements containing these should be tested for heavy meal contamination.[5,15]

What Are the Best Ways to Attain Optimal Calcium Intake?

The preferred technique to achieve optimal calcium intake is to select foods that are calcium-rich, but calcium-fortified foods or calcium supplements are popular choices. Dairy products are high in calcium content (e.g., 300 mg/8 fluid ounces of milk). Individuals who are lactose intolerant or vegans can achieve adequate calcium by using low and lactose-free dairy products. Broccoli, kale, turnip greens, Chinese cabbage, calcium-set tofu, some legumes, canned fish, seeds, nuts, and certain fortified food products are also good calcium sources and average about 100 to 150 mg/serving. Breads and cereals are fairly low in calcium but are significant contributors because of their high frequency of consumption.

Bioavailability of calcium depends on the total calcium content of the food, the presence of oxalic acid, phytic acid, and wheat bran, which can enhance or inhibit absorption.

Calcium-fortified juices and fruit drinks, breads, and cereals may provide 300 mg/serving. Calcium supplements are most efficient at 500 mg or less. Absorption of calcium carbonate is blocked in fasting individuals due to the absence of gastric acid. Many older adults have a depressed gastric acid production and should take calcium supplements with meals for optimal absorption.

Optimal bone health depends on an adequate calcium intake and a balance of other essential nutrients. Since calcium intakes are generally below recommended levels, intake must be addressed daily. Current Food Guide Pyramid dietary guidelines recommend two to three servings per day of dairy products and three to five servings of vegetables (see Table 16–3).

Table 16–3 The Healthy Eating Pattern: Back to Basics

Food Group	Daily Servings	What Counts as a Serving
Vegetables	3–5 servings	1 cup raw leafy greens ½ cup other vegetables
Fruits	2–4 servings	1 medium apple, banana, orange ½ cup fruit (fresh, cooked, canned) ¾ cup juice
Breads, cereals, rice, and pasta	6–11 servings	1 slice bread ½ bun or bagel 1 ounce dry cereal ½ cup cooked cereal, rice, pasta
Milk, yogurt, and cheese	2–3 servings	1 cup milk (skim or low fat) 8 ounces low-fat yogurt 1½ ounces low-fat natural cheese 2 ounces low-fat processed cheese
Meat, poultry, fish, dry peas and beans, eggs, and nuts	2–3 servings	This totals 6 ounces of cooked lean meat, poultry without skin, or fish per day Count ½ cup cooked beans, 1 egg, or 2 Tbsp. peanut butter as 1 ounce meat Limit the use of egg yolks and organ meats, since they are high in cholesterol.

Source: Adapted from *Dietary Guidelines for Americans*, U.S. Department of Agriculture/U.S. Department of Health and Human Services, 1990.

What Public Health Strategies Are Available and Needed To Implement Optimal Calcium Intake Recommendations?

Data from the National Health and Nutrition Examination Survey (NHANES) III, 1988–1991, reports that 6-to-11-year-old children have lower calcium intakes than children in NHANES II (1976–1980), and a large percentage of US residents do not meet the Recommended Dietary Allowance (RDA) for calcium intakes.[16]

Suboptimal calcium intake increases health care costs, warranting aggressive attention to *Healthy People 2000* objectives to increase calcium intake. Likewise, strategies to promote optimal calcium intake must involve the following:

- Public education to:
    1. Disseminate consensus recommendations.
    2. Convene meetings of leaders and representatives of national groups to disseminate information and develop action plans.
    3. Work with existing national organizations and the mass media to decrease confusion and encourage high-risk groups such as children and adolescent girls to consume calcium-rich foods.
- Health professionals to educate their patients about bone health and calcium intake by:
    1. disseminating consensus recommendations
    2. developing and distributing educational materials
    3. serving as a clearinghouse for calcium-related research and developing curriculum
    4. initiating national sessions focusing solely on calcium-related research
- Private sector to actively promote optimal calcium intake in the following ways:
    1. manufacturers and producers marketing calcium-rich foods for the needs and tastes of a diverse population

2. restaurants, grocery stores, and other food outlets increasing the accessibility and visibility of calcium-rich products

3. biotechnology researchers developing inexpensive technologies to screen the public and identify those at high risk of fracture who would also be candidates for high calcium intakes

- Public sector to solicit the federal government to:

1. Instruct the National Center for Health Statistics and the US Department of Agriculture to disseminate US nutrient intake data and food consumption patterns, giving data specific to age, gender, ethnic group, region, and socioeconomic status.

2. Ensure that existing federal food and food subsidy programs and facilities for infants, children, low-income populations, and the elderly promote optimal calcium intake for program recipients.

3. Address use of calcium supplements for individuals who cannot reach optimal calcium intake with foods.

4. Use government food facilities to promote optimal calcium intake by serving calcium-rich foods, labeling foods, and distributing educational brochures.

5. Ensure that government guidelines reflect the current state of knowledge about calcium needs and requirements.

What Are the Recommendations for Future Research on Calcium Intake?

- prospective longitudinal studies to investigate long-term effects of calcium in postmenopausal women and in men
- prospective longitudinal studies in adolescent girls and boys to observe the long-term effects of different calcium levels on peak bone mass
- studies of long-term effects of calcium on bone remodeling
- studies of interactions between calcium supplementation and nutrient absorption

- evaluation of dose-response association between calcium requirement and estrogen-replacement therapy
- determination of optimal calcium requirements among different ethnic populations
- evaluation of the effect of long-term calcium supplementation on the development or prevention of kidney stones
- development of a cost-effective method to identify calcium-deficient individuals
- initiation of health-promoting programs to effect change in population behavior regarding calcium intakes
- development of methods to achieve and maintain optimal dietary intake of calcium among all ages of individuals.

ALCOHOLISM

Alcohol is the most commonly abused drug in our society. About two-thirds of Americans drink alcohol, and 9% are addicted to alcohol. Over 100,000 deaths per year are alcohol-related. Alcohol abuse costs billions of dollars and is linked to thousands of divorces, about 50% of the incidents of family violence, and millions of hours of school and job absenteeism. Alcohol abuse is also linked to several diseases (e.g., pancreatitis, Wernicke's syndrome, Korsakoff's syndrome, alcoholic cardiomyopathy, and liver cirrhosis).[17]

Alcohol intake may account for 10% of the hypertension in men. Epidemiologic studies show a short-term pressor effect of alcohol consumption. A decline in blood pressure occurs from abstinence or less than one drink per day in heavy drinkers. Individuals who are previous drinkers have the same blood pressure as nondrinkers.

Alcoholic beverages contain ethyl alcohol, which is toxic. The amount of alcohol in beer and wine is given as a percentage. Beer averages 4% alcohol, wine about 12% alcohol. Labels on distilled liquors (i.e., scotch, vodka, bourbon, tequila, and rum) state a *proof*, a number that equals twice the percentage of alcohol in the product. A 100-proof scotch is 50% alcohol. Standard portions of alcoholic beverages have about

½ ounce of ethyl alcohol. A 2-ounce jigger of rum that is 40% alcohol is 0.80 ounces of alcohol. Alcohol has 7 kcal per gram, which are considered "empty-calories."

Alcohol is absorbed into the body through the gastrointestinal tract with 20% absorbed by the stomach and the rest by the small intestine. Alcohol is carried to all body tissues and organs. High-fat foods or proteins slow the absorption of alcohol. Nonalcoholic substances in beverages can slow absorption of alcohol; carbon dioxide in champagne, sparkling wines, beer, and carbonated mixed drinks increase the rate of alcohol absorption. Individuals experience intoxication more quickly when drinking champagne or beer, especially on an empty stomach. A higher alcohol content increases the absorption rate.[17]

About 10% of alcohol is excreted unchanged in sweat, urine, or breath. Alcohol that is not excreted is metabolized at a rate of about ½ ounce per hour, primarily by the liver into carbon dioxide and water. Table 16–4 outlines the characteristics of various alcohols and the time required to metabolize different alcohols.

Alcohol Abuse

Alcohol abuse is the most common type of drug abuse in the United States, affecting 12 million people. More than 3 million US teenagers have a drinking problem. Over one-third of all suicides involve alcohol. Six million adults are "alcoholics." They are unable to control their drinking.[18] Warning signs of alcoholism are listed in Exhibit 16–1.[17] Tyrosine, an amino acid, can be used during drug and alcohol detoxification. A therapeutic dose of tyrosine may effect the nervous system by regulating the heart rate, blood flow, muscle contractions, and sensitivity. Caution should be taken to recognize side effects producing serious adverse conditions.[18]

Table 16–4 Metabolic Characteristics of Various Alcoholic Drinks

Number of Drinks	Ounces of Alcohol	Blood Alcohol Content (g/100 mL)	Metabolism (Hrs)	Effects
1 beer, glass of wine, or mixed drink	0.5	0.02	1.0	Feeling relaxed or "loosened up"
2½ beers, glasses of wine, or mixed drinks	1.25	0.05	2.5	Feeling "high"; decrease in inhibitions; increase in confidence; judgment impaired
5 beers, glasses of wine, or mixed drinks	2.5	0.10	5.0	Memory impaired; muscular coordination reduced; slurred speech; euphoric or sad feelings
10 beers, glasses of wine, or mixed drinks	5.0	0.20	10.0	Slowed reflexes; erratic changes in feelings
15 beers, glasses of wine, or mixed drinks	7.5	0.30	15.5	Stuporous; complete loss of coordination; little sensation
20 beers, glasses of wine, or mixed drinks	10.0	0.40	20.0	Comatose; breathing may cease
25–30 beers, glasses of wine, or mixed drinks	18.0	0.50	26.0	Fatal for most people

Source: Data from *Health and Wellness: A Holistic Approach*, 4th ed., by G. Edlin and E. Golanty, pp. 285–294, Jones and Bartlett Publishers, © 1992.

Exhibit 16-1 12 Warning Signs of Alcoholism

---

1. Gulps drinks.
2. Drinks to modify uncomfortable feelings.
3. Changes behavior after drinking.
4. Drinks frequently.
5. Experiences "blackouts."
6. Has frequent accidents or illness.
7. Prepares self with alcohol before a social event.
8. Refuses to talk about negative consequences of drinking.
9. Is preoccupied with alcohol.
10. Focuses on social situations around alcohol.
11. Sneaks drinks or clandestine drinking.
12. Has redness of face and skin.

Source: Edlin, G., and Golanty, E., *Health and Wellness: A Holistic Approach*, 4th ed., © 1992, Boston: Jones and Bartlett Publishers. Adapted with permission.

Alcoholism develops across three phases[19]:

- *Warning phase:* Person develops an increased tolerance to alcohol and a preoccupation with drinking.
- *Crucial phase:* Person loses control over amount drunk and rationalizes that there are good reasons for heavy drinking.
- *Chronic phase:* Person is totally dependent on alcohol, and drinking consumes all aspects of life.

Alcoholic Liver Disease

This disease is the ninth most common cause of death in the United States, with about 200,000 patients dying annually. Men drink more than women, but women are more susceptible to alcohol. Risk of alcoholic liver disease is greater in women who have three drinks each day, compared to six drinks per day for men. A schema showing alcoholic liver diseases and other disorders common with alcohol abuse is shown in Figure 16-3.[17]

Susceptibility to liver disease is linked to the effects of heredity and gender on the metabolism of alcohol. The effect of alcohol as a toxin and causing a nutrient imbalance both contribute to the development of alcoholic liver disease.

Numerous animal models have demonstrated that substitution of alcohol for carbohydrate in diets fed to baboons, rats, and pigs lead to features of alcoholic liver disease and increase fibrosis in the liver.

Malnutrition is a universal feature of alcoholic cirrhosis. A Veterans Administration cooperative study of more than 300 patients with alcoholic cirrhosis showed 100% incidence of protein-calorie malnutrition. Other surveys showed greater than 50% incidence of low serum folate, thiamine, and pyridoxine in alcoholic liver disease. Liver biopsies indicate universal depletion of hepatic vitamin A in alcoholic liver disease. The manifestations of malnutrition in alcoholism include altered cellular immunity due to protein and zinc deficiency; anemia due to combinations of folate, iron, and pyridoxine deficiencies; night blindness due to vitamin A deficiency; and Wernicke's or Korsakoff's syndrome due to thiamine deficiency.

Energy wasting during excessive binge drinking is well documented, and is probably due to the increased calorie cost of metabolizing alcohol by the microsomal system. Heavy drinkers often substitute alcohol for other essential micronutrients, and alcoholic beverages are nearly all devoid of micronutrients. Intestinal malabsorption, which is common, is due to alteration of the intestinal mucosa from chronic binge drinking. Alcohol has a direct effect on the mucosa, with secondary effects due to folate deficiency. Malabsorption of folic acid, thiamine, glucose, and several amino acids have been documented in binge drinkers.

At least 50% of patients with alcoholic cirrhosis have fat and fat-soluble vitamin malabsorption due to decreased secretion and transfer of bile salts to the intestine. Pancreatic insufficiency is also common in alcoholic liver disease. The metabolism of alcohol is known to lead to destruction of certain vitamins, including folic acid and pyridoxine. Cirrhotic patients have been shown to have increased energy expenditure per unit of lean body mass. Protein turnover is normal in stable cirrhotics but increases in individuals with active alcoholic hepatitis.[20,21] See Appendix 16-A for more information about the effects of alcohol.

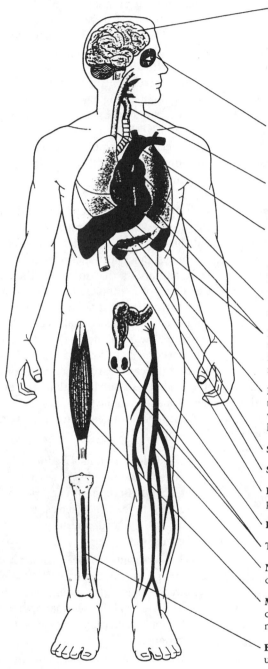

Brain. *Wernicke's syndrome*, an accute condition characterized by ataxia, mental confusion, and ocular abnormalities. *Korsakoff's syndrome*, a psychotic condition characterized by impairment of memory and learning, apathy, and degeneration of the white brain matter.

Eyes. Tobacco-alcohol blindness. Wernicke's ophthalmoplegia, a reversible paralysis of the muscles of the eye.

Pharynx. Cancer of the pharynx is increased tenfold for drinkers who smoke.

Esophagus. Esophageal varices, an irreversible condition in which the person can die by drowning in his own blood when the varices open.

Heart. Alcoholic cardiomyopathy, a heart condition.

Lungs. Lowered resistance is thought to lead to greater incidences of tuberculosis, pneumonia, and emphysema.

Liver. An acute enlargement of the liver, which is reversible, as well as the irreversible alcoholic's liver (cirrhosis).

Spleen. Hypersplenism.

Stomach. Gastritis and ulcers.

Pancreas. Acute and chronic pancreatitis.

Rectum. Hemorrhoids.

Testes. Atropy of the testes.

Nerves. Polyneuritis, a condition characterized by loss of sensation.

Muscles. Alcoholic myopathy, a condition resulting in painful muscle contractions.

Blood and bone marrow. Coagulation defects and anemia.

Figure 16-3 Frequently observed diseases and disorders when alcohol abuse is present. *Source:* Edlin, G., and Golanty, E., *Health and Wellness: A Holistic Approach*, 4th ed., © 1992, Boston: Jones and Bartlett Publishers. Reprinted with permission.

Info Line

Alcoholics Anonymous (AA) is an international, nonprofit self-help organization. AA aims for total sobriety, anonymity, and a step-by-step program for recovery of alcoholics. AA addresses sobriety as a state of mind. It presents recovery as a change in values, attitudes, and lifestyles. The AA program assists problem drinkers by asking them to examine their feelings, recognize their limitations, and accept responsibility for past wrongs. For more information, contact Alcoholics Anonymous General Service Office, 475 Riverside Drive, New York, NY 10015; (212) 870-3400. Or write to PO Box 459, Grand Station, New York, NY 10163.

ARTHRITIS

Arthritis is a pain for people of all ages. Each year, a million people learn they have arthritis. One in every seven people is affected by some form of arthritis. It is the nation's most common chronic disease and its number one crippler. There are more than 100 kinds of arthritis or rheumatoid disease, and the disease affects all age groups, from the very young to the very old. About a quarter of a million children suffer from some form of juvenile arthritis.[22]

Juvenile rheumatoid arthritis attacks infants and children. It can cripple a child for life; but if it is diagnosed early, the effects can be minimized, often leaving little trace. Sometimes the attack is acute, with soaring temperature, a rash, and pain or tenderness in one or more joints. In other cases, the disease begins mildly with a general, "I don't feel well all over." In children, arthritis may last only a few weeks, it may go on for years, or it may disappear only to recur years later.

Arthritis is a discriminatory disease—it prefers women. Regardless of age, race, or occupation, women are the prime target of arthritis. It has been shown that arthritis symptoms often decrease during pregnancy, only to return later. Thus, hormonal change probably has something to do with susceptibility. Women must be more aware of the early warning signs.[23,24]

The arthritic disease process can be defined as any destruction that occurs to joints—which include cartilage, ligaments, tendons, and bones. This destruction may occur at repeated times during inflammation. The pathological changes combined with the mechanical stress of carrying an individual's weight, muscle pull, and other stresses produce the deformities seen with the disease.[25]

Systemic changes occur due to the nature of the disease. These systemic changes affect the individual's ability to function and metabolism. These systemic and functional changes initiate body alterations that influence the nutritional well-being of the individual. These changes can alter the nutrients that become available to the individual. Many individuals may not be able to consume the food they need. Medications can influence the digestion and, if foods are limited, absorption can be reduced. Excretion can be modified due to nutrients that are not available for normal metabolic processes.

Functional changes from arthritis include the following[25]:

- Wrist destruction, a reduced hand-gripping ability, and a decreased functioning mobility all interfere with arthritic individual's ability to feed themselves, to shop for the foods they need, and to prepare their own meals.

- A decreased shoulder rotation or an increased involvement with the elbow decreases the ability to bring food to the mouth with the hand. These situations result in frustration, and eating becomes a negative experience.

- With increased involvement with the mandibular areas, individuals cannot chew well. This reduces the ability to eat fresh, raw foods (such as vegetables and salads) and especially decreases the ability to chew fibrous meats and vegetables that require a tremendous amount of jaw action.

- A restriction in movement of the oral area means individuals may not be able to cleanse and brush the teeth properly or open and move the jaw freely. Dental caries and periodontal disease can increase.

Generally, the causes of nutritional alteration in individuals with arthritis are related to two major factors. One is the spontaneous arthritis attacks and the other is related to the stages of remission. The inability to feed or to eat deprives the individual of nutrients. When the spontaneous attacks occur, the individual does not receive adequate nutrition. The changes in diet can change the immune response of the individual and further affect the manifestations of the disease. During periods of spontaneous remission, individuals may believe that a "quack" or a "magic food" produced the change, and they may lose their commitment to a healthy, balanced eating pattern.[26]

A potential link between diet and rheumatoid arthritis is that the reactions or symptoms experienced by the individual may be an allergic reaction to substances in food. Food then becomes a negative substrate, and the patient may be unaware that the food is initiating the problem. The only known diet link with arthritis is the link between diet and gout. Individuals with gout are not able to eat foods with purines (i.e., sweetbreads, liver, alcohol, kidney, and brain). Individuals with gout cannot rid their body of purines, which worsen the symptoms and pain. Physicians prescribe colchicine for acute attacks to reduce the pain, but gastrointestinal problems such as diarrhea can occur.[27]

Sjögren's syndrome is a chronic, inflammatory disorder that occurs in about 10% to 15% of arthritic patients. This syndrome is characterized by a decreased secretion of salivary juices and the onset of gingivitis; the production of a stiff, white mucosa in the mouth; and altered taste and smell. All of these symptoms are likely to occur.[28]

Secondary and Tertiary Prevention

Nutrition has an important effect on the health of individuals with arthritis. Eating behavior is one element in the base of the treatment pyramid for rheumatoid arthritis (see Figure 16–4). Some people, however, go far beyond a sensible approach to eating. Because the exact causes of arthritis are not yet known, the door is left open for many unproven ideas about how to help or cure it. People often hear that one diet or another can cure arthritis.

Supplements such as vitamins and minerals are advertised and sold as remedies for arthritis. The claims sound reasonable until they are weighed against what is known. Many unusual behavioral remedies and diet plans, such as a diet free of "nightshades" (foods such as peppers and tomatoes) have made people with arthritis feel better. Most of these benefits, however, are due to natural improvement—which can occur by itself in any kind of arthritis—or to a placebo effect. If a person truly believes that something he or she takes, eats, or rubs on the joints is going to work, it can often relieve arthritis symptoms temporarily.[29]

Info Line

The Arthritis Foundation
PO Box 19000
Atlanta, GA 30326
1-800-283-7800

Community nutrition professionals need to become actively involved in secondary and tertiary prevention efforts to help improve the quality of life of patients with arthritis. Generally, one of the first goals is to evaluate patients' ability to feed themselves. This involves considering their functional status, any of the secondary manifestations of the arthritis, and the medical treatment they receive. Multiple feeding modalities may be required. A combination of oral supplements, tube feedings, and even parenteral nutrition may be needed to meet the nutritional needs of individuals with arthritis.

Eating behavior must be considered in the management of arthritic patients. One problem is the nutrient/drug interaction and gastrointes-

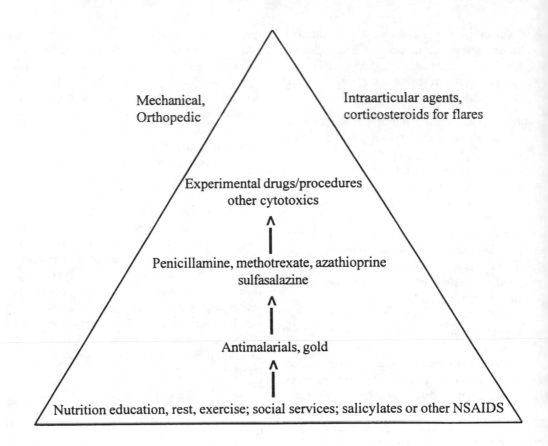

Figure 16-4 Treatment pyramid for rheumatoid arthritis *Source:* From the *Primer on the Rheumatic Diseases*, tenth edition, © 1993. Used by permission of the Arthritis Foundation.

tinal functioning. There are seven major drug therapies for arthritis: salicylates (e.g., aspirin), nonsteroidal anti-inflammatory agents, anti-malarial compounds, gold shots, penicillin, steroids, and immunosuppressive agents.[30-32] Possible nutrient-drug interactions associated with these therapies include the following:

- Aspirin is a mild pain reliever and a major anti-inflammatory drug. When an individual takes a high dose of aspirin, there is a possibility of potential blood loss through the bowels. Aspirin can irritate the stomach and alter platelet function. Aspirin can also act as minor blood-thinning agent. High doses of aspirin can cause nausea and vomiting. This upsets the gastrointestinal tract and causes an altered eating behavior.

- Many of the nonsteroidal anti-inflammatory agents irritate the lining of the gastrointestinal tract (e.g., indocin, Naprosyn, ibuprofen, Nalfon, and Feldene). Some anti-inflammatory agents may cause slight fluid retention. Some individuals self-prescribe a salt-restricted diet if they are retaining fluid. This may not have an adverse effect immediately, but it can place the individual on a roller coaster. Food becomes the target for change in order to appease the actual symptoms.

- Antimalarial agents, penicillin, and gold salts inhibit the disease process, but have minimal anti-inflammatory properties. The body reacts to these medications with a process called chelation, a binding of zinc, copper, and iron in the gastrointestinal tract. This reduces their absorption, and a potential deficiency can occur.

- Corticosteroids are the most potent anti-inflammatory agents. However, they demonstrate a high degree of toxicity. A common reaction is a decrease in the synthesis and breakdown of protein (e.g., muscle, skin, connective, and adipose tissue). Calcium can spill into the urine. If a restriction of vitamin D activity occurs, this reduces the overall intestinal calcium absorption, and increases chances for osteoporosis.

- Prednisone reduces inflammation, suppresses immunological response, increases appetite, and may enhance loss of bone. Long-term side effects of prednisone can be reduced if vitamin D and calcium supplements are given. Prednisone influences fluid retention, suggesting that salt intake should be moderated.

- Immunosuppressive agents are slow-acting drugs. Their action can have a direct effect, which is often dose-related, on calcium absorption. Folate may become deficient.

The overall recommended eating pattern for individuals with arthritis involves weight control and a low-fat and low-saturated-fat eating pattern. Individuals with arthritis who are overweight need to lose weight to avoid putting unnecessary stress on diseased joints.

If weight changes drastically, the quick weight loss may mean a variety of things:

- overactive thyroid, which increases the basal metabolic rate
- difficulty swallowing and eating
- a possible serious infection with tissue disease and destruction
- depression from the arthritis

If weight loss is rapid due to insufficient calories, an impaired antibody production can occur. Increased rejection of skin grafts, increased delayed hypersensitivity, and increased lymphokine production may occur.

If depression leads to a fasting stage, a number of other complications are possible. A zinc deficiency can occur. Low-fat and low-calorie diets taken to the extreme can affect the autoimmune process.[33]

Nontraditional Remedies

There are many approaches to treating arthritis, and some of these are questionable. For example, prayer has been seen as effective in reducing pain for some individuals. One of the more common and unproven nutrition regimens is the vegetarian diet. The rationale is that meats may cause or potentially aggravate arthritis. The vegetarian diet is thought to cleanse the body. Another popular practice is to eliminate foods that are thought to cause an allergic reaction (e.g., corn, wheat, coffee, beef, peanuts, tomatoes, chocolate, eggs, apples, oranges, and cola drinks). An extreme nutrition regimen that is unproven and not safe is fasting for three to five days before adding back a few foods at a time. Another practice is the use of enemas, which are thought to rid the body of toxins.[34,35]

Another unproven practice is a diet that includes apple cider vinegar and honey three times a day and a drop of iodine solution a few times a week, plus a restriction on total amount of foods eaten. The thought is that vinegar will thin the blood fluids and make tissues around the joints more tender, and that honey will relieve pain. Garlic, alfalfa, wheat germ oil, and blackstrap molasses are also thought to give relief from the arthritic symptoms.[34,35]

Megadoses of certain vitamins and minerals and fat modification are also considered to be ways to relieve pain and complications.[36-43] Vitamin A megadoses of 25,000 International Units (IU) have been used, whereas 5,000 is the RDA. Chronic vitamin A toxicity can occur at a 25,000 IU level if taken daily over an extended period. For vitamin D, the RDA is 200 IU or 5 milligrams. The megadoses recommended are between 2,500 and 600,000 IU. For vitamin E, 15 IU is the RDA, and dosages up to 20,000 IU have been recommended. Toxicity can occur at these levels if taken for a long period.

Vitamin C is water soluble. In fairly high dosages, there have been reports of an alleviation of the low platelet level and low plasma vitamin C level, especially if individuals with arthritis are taking aspirin. Dosages over 4,000 milligrams can cause some gastrointestinal symptoms, and large dosages can interfere with copper absorption and uric acid excretion. These dosages greatly exceed the RDA of 60 milligrams.

Thiamine is a B-vitamin that is known to be decreased in rheumatoid arthritis patients. In addition, older adults may not use thiamine efficiently. There is very little evidence for toxicity. However, amounts that have been recommended, 10 milligrams, exceed the 1.2 milligram RDA.

For vitamin B_{12}, the RDA is 3 micrograms. For individuals with arthritis, levels as high as 500 micrograms have been used. Vitamin B_{12} is not toxic, and high levels may give false negative results for pernicious anemia due to the very high circulating blood levels.

Mineral regimens are often listed by the popular press as ways to alter arthritic symptoms.[36-39] Calcium, zinc, and copper head the list. Calcium levels are commonly found to be low in people with arthritis, which is generally the rationale for people taking it. Women, especially after menopause, may need to take more than 800 milligrams per day, which is the RDA. However regimens of 3,000 milligrams per day have been reported.

Iron supplementation (e.g., 25 to 75 milligrams per day) is probably safe. Additional iron may be beneficial for those with some blood loss due to heavy aspirin use.[37] For zinc, the RDA is 15 milligrams per day. Intakes tend to be low in individuals with arthritis. Some studies have shown that taking about 200 milligrams three times a day can be beneficial. However, toxicity has been shown when more than 2,000 milligrams is taken. As a rule, if a supplement is given, its dosage is from 15 to 50 milligrams per day. These levels are clinically unproven as beneficial in remediating arthritic conditions.

Excess zinc intake can lower blood copper levels. The RDA for copper is 2 to 3 milligrams per day, and 5 to 10 milligrams seems fairly safe. Toxicity has been shown with ingestion of 20 milligrams of copper sulfate on a routine basis.

Two other minerals reported as aiding arthritis are selenium and choline. The RDA for selenium is 50 to 100 micrograms; levels of 2.5 or 3 milligrams per day are considered harmful. It is estimated that some individuals take 50 to 100 micrograms per day. The average choline intake is around 500 to 800 milligrams a day, and intake often depends on egg consumption. Toxicity has not been documented at levels as high as 16 grams per day when taken for four months. It appears that 0.5 to 1 gram, or 500 to 1,000 milligrams is safe.

Assessing Eating Behavior

The following steps are needed to conduct a careful review of the nutritional well-being of individuals with arthritis:

- A diet history that includes the names, amounts, and types of foods and supplements that an individual takes is needed.
- The amount of raw food consumed should be assessed. Raw foods are often ingested in the "therapeutic concoctions" that individuals prepare, because people believe they are a magic cure. These preparations may actually be detrimental to the individual. For example, bone meal, which is often recommended by health food establishments to supplement calcium intake, may contain toxic amounts of lead.
- Major pain or physical complaints (e.g., stomach irritation or diarrhea) should be assessed. Individuals often follow their own self-prescribed practices, such as enemas to rid themselves of what they believe are harmful substances in their system.
- Food elimination practices or patterns should be assessed. Individuals may abstain from eating a type of food such as milk, milk products, or fruits because they believe they are harmful.
- Compliance with drug therapy should be assessed, because adherence to medications may be weak. Food may be substituted as the sole therapy, and this may be harmful if physicians are not aware that medication is not being taken.

- A comparison of costs for the multiple therapies that a patient self-prescribes is informative. A placebo effect may occur with some therapies. Individuals, especially older adults, are being hooked on potential cures that are costly and not beneficial. Some of these "cures" may be harmful. It is important to inform patients that the times they feel exceptionally good might be the result of a temporary remission, which is common, rather than the result of a magic potion. Treatment that coincides with a spontaneous remission may be viewed as a miracle cure.
- It is important to identify the positive aspects of an individual's efforts so he or she remains active in the treatment.

Community nutritional professionals should remain sympathetic to individuals with arthritis, encouraging them to follow the most medically sound regimens. Their immobility, which restricts their activities and adds additional pain, should be documented. Often the restriction of independent living is the major impetus for individuals to search for a cure or remedy.

Manipulation problems common to individuals with arthritis include opening jars, tearing plastics, reaching shelves, and holding dishes and utensils. Several ways to help arthritic individuals to take part in their food procurement and preparation are as follows:

- Mount a wedge-shaped gripper on the kitchen wall.
- Break suction on vacuum lids with a lid-lifter.
- Use a fork handle as a lever to pull up ring-top openers.
- Lay boxes on sides and cut tops with a knife.
- Use scissors for sealed plastic or cellophane.
- Use an electric can opener with a "power stroke."
- Use the palm and not the fingers to open jars.
- Use large-handled utensils.
- Put damp sponges or thin rubber disks under plates.

- Use sharp utensils, "T" handle cups, and cover cups with terry cloth or foam coasters.
- Use straws to avoid lifting.
- Take careful bites and chew gently; eat and swallow slowly.
- Eat small, frequent meals with soft foods.
- Drink liquids with meals to aid swallowing.

Exercise for overall body tone and conditioning, as well as for expending calories, is important. Protection of muscles and joints from temperature and contact insults can lessen pain and damage. Weight control with careful dieting and response to the manipulation problems of patients is important.

RENAL DISEASE

Chronic renal failure is a gradual progression in the loss of kidney function. Slowly there is a loss of excretory, endocrine, and metabolic activity of the kidney.[44] The extent of renal disease is defined by serum creatinine level:

- advanced renal insufficiency: 8–10 mg/dL
- moderate insufficiency: 4–8 mg/dL
- mild insufficiency: 2–4 mg/dL

If 70 to 80% of renal function is lost, water, electrolyte, and acid-base balance are not possible. The incidence of end-stage renal disease (ESRD) is estimated at about 83 people per million. A 6.5% annual increase has occurred from 1978 to 1983, with individuals under 25 and over 65 years of age showing the largest increase.[45] ESRD is a common manifestation of diabetes mellitus, especially Type I, but it can develop from polycystic renal disease, from a streptococcal infection, or as an outcome of renal damage.[45-47] Other high-risk groups include African-American hypertensives, Native American Indians with non-insulin-dependent diabetes mellitus, and individuals with overt proteinuria.[44,48,49]

Individuals with ESRD must receive tertiary prevention or they will not survive. Hemodialysis, continuous ambulatory peritoneal dialysis, or a renal transplant are required if the individual is to live. Individuals without intervention develop vitamin D deficiency, hyperparathyroidism, and osteodystrophy, which result from the accumulation of toxic substances and associated endocrine and metabolic disturbances. Manifestations of ESRD include dyslipidemia, anemia, muscle weakness and atrophy, peripheral and central nervous system impairment, and depression. Coronary heart disease is a major cause of death in dialysis patients, possibly due to hyperlipidemia causing glomerular injury.[45,46] Malnutrition is common, because the metabolism of nutrients is impaired and dialysis leaches nutrients out of the body fluids.[50] Thiamine, riboflavin, vitamin B_6, and vitamin C deficiencies are common and contrast with high-plasma vitamin A.[46,51-54]

Current medical nutritional therapy reflects the National Renal Diet, which includes recommendations for protein, phosphorus, sodium, and potassium intakes (see Table 16–5). Because the disease is chronic, modification of protein and

phosphorus is essential when managing mild renal failure. If individuals are pre-ESRD, a low-protein diet of 0.6 g/kg per 24 hours with greater than 35 kcal/kg per 24 hours protects against uremia.[46,47,55] Since individuals with renal disease retain phosphorus, a limit of less than 900 mg/24 hours and use of phosphate-binding compounds is required.

The National Institute of Diabetes, Digestive and Kidney Diseases of NIH sponsored a consensus symposium entitled Prevention of Progression in Chronic Renal Disease Management Recommendations. The meeting was held in April 1994, with the objective to establish timely, basic recommendations to manage individuals with progressive renal disease. Because these individuals are generally not institutionalized but live independently, community nutrition professionals have a role in the management and monitoring of these individuals.

Recommendations for dietetic practice for secondary and tertiary prevention include the following[44,56]:

Table 16–5 General Dietary Recommendations for Renal Patients

Dietary Component	Renal Insufficiency	Hemodialysis	Peritoneal Dialysis
Protein (g/kg IBW)[a]	0.6–0.8[b]	1.1–1.4	1.2–1.5
Energy (kcal/kg IBW)	35–40	30–35	25–35
Phosphorus (mg/kg IBW)	8–12[c]	≤17[d]	≤17
Sodium (mg/day)	1,000–3,000	2,000–3,000	2,000–4,000
Potassium (mg/kg IBW)	Typically not restricted	40	Typically not restricted
Fluid (mL/day)	Typically not restricted	500–750 plus Daily urine output or 1,000 if anuric	≥2,000
Calcium (mg/day)	1,200–1,600	Depends on serum level	Depends on serum level

[a]IBW = ideal body weight.

[b]The upper end of this range is preferred for patients with diabetes or malnutrition. Suggested protein intake for persons with nephrotic syndrome is 0.8 to 1.0 g/kg IBW.

[c]Intake of 5 to 10 mg phosphorus per kg IBW is frequently quoted in the scientific literature, but 5 mg/kg IBW is practical only when used in conjunction with a very-low-protein diet supplemented with amino acids or ketoacid analogs.

[d]It may not be possible to meet the optimum phosphorus prescription on a higher-protein diet.

Source: Reprinted from Meeting the Challenge of the Renal Diet, Journal of the American Dietetic Association, Vol. 93, No. 6, p. 637, with permission of the American Dietetic Association, © 1993.

Exhibit 16-2   *Healthy People 2000* Objectives for Individuals with Renal Disease, Osteoporosis, Alcoholism, and Arthritis

---

2.5   Reduce dietary fat intake to an average of 30% of calories or less and average saturated fat intake to <10% of calories among people aged 2 and older. (Baseline: 36% of calories from total fat and 13% from saturated fat for people aged 20 through 74 in 1976–80; 36% and 13% for women aged 19 through 50 in 1985.)

2.6   Increase complex carbohydrate and fiber-containing foods in the diets of adults to 5+ daily servings for vegetables (including legumes) and fruits, and to 6+ daily servings for grain products. (Baseline: 2½ servings of vegetables and fruits and 3 servings of grain products for women aged 19 through 50 in 1985.)

2.7   Increase to at least 50% the proportion of overweight people aged 12+ who have adopted sound dietary practices combined with regular physical activity to attain an appropriate body weight. (Baseline: 30% of overweight women and 25% of overweight men for people aged 18 and older in 1985.)

2.8   Increase calcium intake so at least 50% of youth aged 12 through 24 and 50% of pregnant and lactating women consume 3 or more servings daily for foods rich in calcium, and at least 50% of people aged 25 and older consume 2+ servings daily. (Baseline: 7% of women and 14% of men aged 19 through 24, and 24% of pregnant and lactating women consumed 3 or more servings, and 15% of women and 23% of men aged 25 through 50 consumed 2 or more servings in 1985–86.)

 Note: The number of servings of foods rich in calcium is based on milk and milk products. A serving is considered to be 1 cup of skim milk or its equivalent in calcium (302 mg). The number of servings in this objective will generally provide approximately three-fourths of the 1989 Recommended Dietary Allowance (RDA) of calcium. The RDA is 1200 mg for people age 12 through 24, 800 mg for people age 25 and older, and 1200 mg for pregnant and lactating women.

4.2   Reduce cirrhosis deaths to no more than 6 per 100,000 people. (Age-adjusted baseline: 9.1 per 100,000 in 1987.)

Special Population Targets

Cirrhosis Deaths (per 100,000)		*1987 Baseline*	*2000 Target*
4.2a	Black men	22	12
4.2b	American Indians/Alaska Natives	25.9	13

Baseline data sources: National Vital Statistics System, CDC; Indian Health Service Administrative Statistics, IHS.

4.5   Increase by at least 1 year the average age of first use of cigarettes, alcohol, and marijuana by adolescents aged 12 through 17. (Baseline: Age 11.6 for cigarettes, age 13.1 for alcohol, and age 13.4 for marijuana in 1988.)

 Baseline data source: National Household Survey of Drug Abuse, American Drug, Alcohol and Mental Health Association.

4.6   Reduce the proportion of young people who have used alcohol, marijuana, and cocaine in the past month, as follows:

Substance/Age	*1988 Baseline*	*2000 Target*
Alcohol/aged 12–17	25.2%	12.6%
Alcohol/aged 18–20	57.9%	29%

---

continues

Exhibit 16–2 continued

4.7   Reduce the proportion of high school seniors and college students engaging in recent occasions of heavy drinking of alcoholic beverages to no more than 28% of high school seniors and 32% of college students. (Baseline: 33% of high school seniors and 41.7% of college students in 1989.)

  Note: Recent heavy drinking is defined as having 5 or more drinks on 1 occasion in the previous 2-week period as monitored by self-reports.

  Baseline data source: Monitoring the Future (High School Senior Survey), ADAMHA.

4.8   Reduce alcohol consumption by people aged 14 and older to an annual average of no more than 2 gallons of ethanol per person. (Baseline: 2.54 gallons of ethanol in 1987.)

  Baseline data source: National Institute on Alcohol Abuse and Alcoholism, ADAMHA.

4.9   Increase the proportion of high school seniors who perceive social disapproval associated with the heavy use of alcohol, occasional use of marijuana, and experimentation with cocaine, as follows:

Behavior	1989 Baseline	2000 Target
Heavy use of alcohol	56.4%	70%
Occasional use of marijuana	71.1%	85%
Trying cocaine once or twice	88.9%	95%

  Note: Heavy drinking is defined as having 5 or more drinks once or twice each weekend.

  Baseline data source: Monitoring the Future (High School Senior Survey), ADAMHA.

4.10   Increase the proportion of high school seniors who associate risk of physical or psychological harm with the heavy use of alcohol, regular use of marijuana, and experimentation with cocaine, as follows:

Behavior	1989 Baseline	2000 Target
Heavy use of alcohol	44%	70%
Regular use of marijuana	77.5%	90%
Trying cocaine once or twice	54.9%	80%

  Note: Heavy drinking is defined as having 5 or more drinks once or twice each weekend.

  Baseline data source: Monitoring the Future (High School Senior Survey), ADAMHA.

4.13   Provide to children in all school districts and private schools primary and secondary school educational programs on alcohol and other drugs, preferably as part of quality school health education. (Baseline: 63% provided some instruction, 39% counseling, and 23% referred students for clinical assessments in 1987.)

  Baseline data source: Report to Congress and the White House on the Nature and Effectiveness of Federal, State, and Local Drug Prevention/Education Programs, U.S. Department of Education, 1987.

4.14   Extend adoption of alcohol and drug policies for the work environment to at least 60% of worksites with 50 or more employees. (Baseline data available in 1991.)

4.16   Increase to 50 the number of States that have enacted and enforce policies, beyond those in existence in 1989, to reduce access to alcoholic beverages by minors.

  Note: Policies to reduce access to alcoholic beverages by minors may include those that address restriction of the sale of alcoholic beverages at recreational and entertainment events at which youth make up a majority of participants/consumers, product pricing, penalties and license-revocation for sale of alcoholic beverages to minors, and other approaches designed to discourage and restrict purchase of alcoholic beverages by minors.

4.17   Increase to at least 20 the number of States that have enacted statutes to restrict promotion of alcoholic beverages that is focused principally on young audiences. (Baseline data available in 1992.)

15.3   Reverse the increase of end-stage renal disease (requiring maintenance dialysis or transplantation) to attain an incidence of no more than 13 per 100,000. (Baseline: 13.9 per 100,000 in 1987.)

continues

Exhibit 16-2 continued

	Special Population Target	
ESRD Incidence (per 100,000)	*1987 Baseline*	*2000 Target*
15.3a Blacks	32.4	30

Source: Reprinted from *Healthy People 2000: National Health Promotion and Disease Prevention Objectives*, U.S. Department of Health and Human Services, Public Health Service, Publication No. 91-50212, 1991.

- A sufficient number of calories is required to spare dietary protein, which is needed for tissue repair.
- Protein restriction can slow progression of the disease.
- Strict glycemic control among diabetics can blunt the occurrence of nephropathy, neuropathy, and retinopathy.[56,57]
- Active and aggressive medical nutrition therapy preserves nutritional status.[58]
- Moderate dietary sodium restriction (2-4 grams per 24 hours) should be considered.[59]

HEALTHY PEOPLE 2000 ACTIONS

Specific HP2K objectives target the general population at risk for cardiovascular disease and obesity, as well as individuals who abuse alcohol or are at risk for osteoporosis or end-stage renal disease (see Exhibit 16-2). Community nutrition professionals can support efforts to meet these HP2K objectives and extend their scope to general public education and school-based education about alcohol abstinence and basic healthy eating.

REFERENCES

1. National Osteoporosis Foundation. *Osteoporosis—Can It Happen to You?* Washington, DC: National Osteoporosis Foundation; 1991.

2. American Osteoporosis Association. General information. 1990.

3. *Osteoporosis—What You Don't Know May Hurt You.* Evanston, Ill: Wyeth—Ayerst Laboratories; May 1991:3-4.

4. Heaney RP. *Research Update: Nutritional Medicine in Medical Practice—Putting Nutrition to Work in the Prevention and Treatment of Common Disease and Chronic Diseases.* Santa Monica, Calif: University of California Nutrition Research Unit, UCLA School of Medicine; January 22-23, 1993.

5. National Institutes of Health. Consensus statement. Optimal calcium intake. June 6-8, 1994. *JAMA.* NIH Consensus Statement, 1994;12(4):1-31.

6. Turner LW, Whitney EN. Nature versus nurture: The calcium controversy. *Nutr Clin.* 1989;4:1.

7. Kaplan FS. Osteoporosis—Pathophysiology and prevention. *Clinical Symposia.* 1987;39(1):2-32.

8. Pollitzer WS, Anderson JJB. Ethnic and genetic differences in bone mass: A review with an hereditary versus environmental perspective. *Am J Clin Nutr.* 1989;50:1244.

9. Riggs BL, Wahner HW, Melton LJ III, et al. Dietary calcium intake and rates of bone loss in women. *J Clin Invest.* 1987;80:979-982.

10. Ettinger B, Genant HK, Cann CE. Postmenopausal bone loss is prevented by treatment with low-dosage estrogen with calcium. *Ann Intern Med.* 1987;106:40-45.

11. Riis B, Thomsen K, Christiansen C. Does calcium supplementation prevent postmenopausal bone loss? *N Engl J Med.* 1987;316:173.

12. Rodysill KJ. Postmenopausal osteoporosis—Intervention and prophylaxis: A review. *J Chron Dis.* 1987;40;743-760.

13. Raisz LG. Local and systematic factors in the pathogenesis of osteoporosis. *N Engl J Med.* 1988;318:818.

14. Schuette SA, Linkswiler HM. Calcium. In: Olson RE, ed. *Nutrition Review's Present Knowledge in Nutrition.* Washington, DC: The Nutrition Foundation, Inc; 1984.

15. Peck WA, Riggs BL, Bell NH. *Physician's Resource Manual on Osteoporosis.* Washington, DC: National Osteoporosis Foundation; 1987.

16. Wotecki CE. Nutrition in childhood and adolescence—Parts 1 and 2. *Contemporary Nutr.* 1992;17(2):1-2.

17. Edlin G, Golanty E. *Health and Wellness: A Holistic Approach*. 4th ed. Boston, Mass: Jones and Bartlett Publishers; 1992:285–294.

18. Beckley L. *Taking Control: Diet, Drug Abuse and Addiction*. Nutrition Dimension. San Marcos, Calif: Author; 1987.

19. Jellinek EM. *The Disease Concept of Alcoholism*. New Haven, Conn: College and University Press; 1960.

20. Mendelson JH, Mello NK. *Alcohol: Use and Abuse in America*. Boston, Mass: Little, Brown & Co; 1985.

21. Olson S. *Alcohol in America: Taking Action to Prevent Abuse*. Washington, DC: National Academy Press; 1985.

22. Utsinger PD, Zvaifler NJ, Ehrlich GE, eds. *Rheumatoid Arthritis: Etiology, Diagnosis and Treatment*. Philadelphia, Pa: JB Lippincott Co; 1985.

23. Dugowson CE, Keopsell TD, Voigt LF, et al. Rheumatoid arthitis in women: Incidence rate in group health cooperative. Seattle, Washington, 1987–1989. *Arthritis Rheum*. 1991;34:1502–1507.

24. Goemaere S, Ackerman C, Goethals K, et al. Onset of symptoms of rheumatoid arthritis in relation to age, sex, and menopausal transition. *J Rheumatol*. 1990;17:1620–1622.

25. Ragan C, Farrington E. The clinical features of rheumatoid arthritis. Prognosis indices. *JAMA*. 1959;2:16.

26. Bollet AJ. Nutrition and diet in rheumatic disease. In: Shils ME, Young VR, eds. *Modern Nutrition in Health and Disease*. 7th ed. Philadelphia, Pa: Lea & Febiger; 1988.

27. Levinson D, Becker MA. Clinical gout and pathogenesis of hyperuricemia. McCarty DJ, Koopman WJ, eds. In: *Arthritis and Allied Conditions*. 12th ed. Philadelphia, Pa: Lea & Febiger; 1993:1773–1805.

28. Bloch KJ, Buchanan WW, Wohl MJ, et al. Sjögren's syndrome: A clinical, pathological, and serological study of 62 cases. *Medicine*. 1965;44:187–231.

29. Lasagna L. The placebo effect. *J Allergy Clin Immunol*. 1986;78:161–165.

30. Weiss MM. Corticosteriods in rheumatoid arthritis. *Semin Arthritis Rheum*. 1989;19:9–21.

31. Situnayake RD, Grindulis KA, McConkey B. Longterm treatment of rheumatoid arthritis with sulfasalazine, gold, or penicillamine: A comparison using life table methods. *Ann Rheum Dis*. 1987;46:177–183.

32. Paulus HE. The use of combinations of disease-modifying antirheumatic agents in rheumatoid arthritis. *Arthritis Rheum*. 1990;33:113–120.

33. Touger-Decker R. Nutritional considerations in rheumatoid arthritis. *J Am Diet Assoc*. 1988;88:327.

34. Panush RS. Controversial arthritis remedies. *Bull Rheum Dis*. 1984;34:1–10.

35. Dlesk A, Ettinger MP, Longley S, et al. Unconventional arthritis therapies. *Arthritis Rheum*. 1982;25:1145–1147.

36. Borglund M, Akesson A, Akesson B. Distribution of selenium and glutathione peroxidase in plasma compared in healthy subjects and rheumatoid arthritis patients. *Scand J Clin Lab Invest*. 1988;48:27.

37. Blake D, Bacon PA. Iron and rheumatoid disease. *Lancet*. 1982;1:623.

38. Darlington LG, Ramsey NW, Mansfield JR. Placebo-controlled, blind study of dietary manipulation therapy in rheumatoid arthritis. *Lancet*. 1986;1:236.

39. Hicklin JA, McEwen LM, Morgan JE. The effect of diet in rheumatoid arthritis. *Clin Allergy*. 1980;10:463.

40. Kremer JM, Michalek AV, Lininger L, et al. Effects of manipulation of dietary fatty acids on clinical manifestations of rheumatoid arthritis. *Lancet*. 1985;1:184–187.

41. Kremer JM, Jubiz W, Michalek A, et al. Fish-oil fatty acid supplementation in active rheumatoid arthritis. *Ann Intern Med*. 1987;106:497–503.

42. Pearson DJ. Food allergy, hypersensitivity and food intolerance. *J Roy Coll Phys Lond*. 1985;19:154–162.

43. Tarp U, Hansen JC, Overvad K, et al. Glutathione peroxidase activity in patients with rheumatoid arthritis and in normal subjects: Effects of long-term selenium supplementation. *Arthritis Rheum*. 1987;30:1162–1166.

44. Beto JA. Highlights of the consensus conference on prevention of progression in chronic renal disease: Implications for practice. *J Renal Nutr*. 1994;4(3):122–126.

45. Ahmed FE. Effect of diet on progression of chronic renal disease. *J Am Diet Assoc*. 1991;91:1266–1270.

46. Coulston AM, Rock CL. A summary of the current state of knowledge in clinical nutrition and dietetic practice: Suggestions for future research in dietetic practice and implications for health care. *The Research Agenda for Dietetics: Conference Proceedings ADA*. Chicago, Ill: ADA; 1993.

47. Kopple JD. Nutrition, diet, and the kidney. In: Shils ME, Young VR, eds. *Modern Nutrition in Health and Disease*. 7th ed. Philadelphia, Pa: Lea & Febiger; 1988:1230–1268.

48. Rostand SG. US minority groups and end-stage renal disease: A disproportionate share. *Am J Kidney Dis*. 1992;19:411–413.

49. McClellan WM. The epidemic of end-stage renal disease in the United States: A public health perspective on ESRD prevention. *AKF Nephrol Letter*. 1993;10:29–40.

50. Makoff R. Water-soluble vitamin status in patients with renal disease treated with hemodialysis or peritoneal dialysis. *J Renal Nutr*. 1991;1:56–73.

51. Stein G, Sperschneider H, Koppe S. Vitamin levels in chronic renal failure and need for supplementation. *Blood Purif*. 1985;3:52–62.

52. Muth I. Implications of hypervitaminosis A in chronic renal failure. *J Renal Nutr*. 1991;1:2–8.

53. Gleghort E, Eisenberg L, Hack S, et al. Observations of vitamin A toxicity in three patients with renal failure receiving parenteral alimentation. *Am J Clin Nutr.* 1986;44: 107–112.

54. Wolfson M, Cohen AH, Kopple JD. Vitamin B-6 deficiency and renal function and structure in chronically uremic rats. *Am J Clin Nutr.* 1991;53:942–953.

55. Renal Dietitians Practice Group. *Suggested Guidelines for Nutrition Care of Renal Patients.* Chicago, Ill: The American Dietetic Association; 1986.

56. Diabetes Control and Trial Research Group. The effect on intensive treatment of diabetes on the development and progression of long-term complications in insulin-dependent diabetes mellitus. *N Engl J Med.* 1993;329: 977–986.

57. Gilbert RE, Tsalamandris C, Bach LA, et al. Long-term glycemic control and the rate of progression of early diabetic kidney disease. *Kidney Int.* 1993;44:855–859.

58. Morbidity and mortality of renal dialysis: NIH consensus statement. *Ann Intern Med.* 1994;121:62–70.

59. Bigazzi R, Bianchi S, Baldari D, et al. Microalbuminuria in salt-sensitive patients. *Hypertension.* 1994;23: 195–199.

Appendix 16–A

Effects of Alcohol

Physiological/Metabolic Consequence	Nutritional Implications	Recommendations
Oral cavity		
Deficient care and neglect Trauma	Reduction of variety, quantity of food	Nutrient-calorie-dense diet
Manifestations of malnutrition • loss of taste buds • irritation, lesions of lips, gums, and tongue	Loss of appetite	Limit food poorly tolerated (spicy, acidic, salty, hot/cold)
Periodontal Disease • gum infection • bone degeneration • impaired healing • hypersensitivity	Poorly fitting dentures Increased nutrient need for repletion from infection	Limit cariogenic foods Vitamin B, vitamin C, Ca
Esophagus		
Pyloric valve relaxation/reflux Erosion	Heartburn Impaired food intake resulting in malnutrition	Six small meals Fluid between meals
Esophageal varices		Soft texture Sodium restriction
Stomach		
20% of alcohol absorbed directly via gastric cavity resulting in gastritis and ulceration	Impaired nutrient intake and absorption Malnutrition	Nutrient-dense diet, six small meals, avoid poorly tolerated foods
Intestines		
80% alcohol absorbed	Malabsorption of dairy and fatty foods	Low-fat diet
Duodenal-gastric reflux/ulcer		Minimize poorly tolerated foods
Enzyme inhibition	Impaired transport of B_1, C, folic acid	Therapeutic vitamin
Diminished integrity/repletion causing diarrhea Hyper/hypo motility	Potential vitamin K, B_{12} deficiency	Nutrient-dense diet

continues

Source: Adapted from Beckley, L. *Taking Control: Diet, Drug Abuse and Addiction.* Nutrition Dimension. 1990.

Physiological/Metabolic Consequence	Nutritional Implications	Recommendations
Liver		
Impaired detoxification resulting in fatty acid and uric acid synthesis and impaired gluconeogenesis and protein synthesis	Hyperlipidemia Gout Periodic hypoglycemia	Low-fat diet Low-purine diet Complex CHO
Inefficient use of calories	Compromised immunity Maldigestion	Supplementation
Fatty liver	Malabsorption	High-calorie plan
Hepatitis	Impaired storage and metabolism, causing malnutrition	
Cirrhosis	Weight loss Anemia	
Central nervous system		
Cerebrum cortex		
Impaired cognitive, perceptive systems	Impulsive food selection, poor nutritional quality	Nutrient-dense diet
Hypothalamus irritant		
Alcohol-withdrawal syndrome	Stimulate or impair hunger	Supplement
Atrophy (memory loss)	Fatigue, high sugar intake	Simple written guidelines
Cerebellum		
Visual disturbances	Multiple deficiencies	Neurotransmitter nutrients
Polyneuropathy	Questionable history	
Wernicke-Korsakoff Syndrome	Increased calorie expenditure	
Autonomic nervous system		
Elevated temperature		
Hypertension		
Heart		
Increased risk of heart disease	Hyperlipidemia Hypertension	Low-fat diet; exercise Gradual repletion of calories
Beriberi heart disease	Wasting of tissue	
Cardiomyopathy	Vitamin B_1, Mg	Supplementation deficiency Sodium restriction
Kidneys		
Suppressed antidiuretic hormone, diuresis of fluids and nutrients	Hyperexcretion of Mg, Zn, Ca, B, K	Nutrient-dense diet
Inflammation of nephrons, frequent infections	Dehydration, rebound fluid retention Impaired active vitamin D	Potassium foods Minimize caffeine Supplement vitamin D_3

continues

Physiological/Metabolic Consequence	Nutritional Implications	Recommendations
Hormones		
Exaggerated estrogen retention resulting in gynecocomastia, premenstrual syndrome (PMS)	Adipose tissue Craving and appetite Fluid retention	Low-fat diet and weight loss PMS precautions
Sexual reproduction		
Testicular atrophy, impotence	Abuse of vitamin E and Zn	Education
Skeletal system		
Osteoporosis, osteomalacia	Inactive D_3	Exercise
Calcium mobilization from bone	Dairy foods as tolerated	Supplement Ca, D_3, Mg Vitamin C foods
Somatic tissues		
High percentage body fat	Chronic caloric deficit	Long-term fat loss High CHO, low-fat diet
Muscle wasting		Exercise

17

Single and Cluster Diseases

- Identify common diseases that cluster, causing morbidity and mortality.
- Differentiate between primary, secondary, and tertiary prevention.
- Describe the content, purpose, and benefits of health-risk appraisals.
- Discuss the self-management approach in health care reform.
- Outline the traditional components of health education.

High Definition Nutrition

Self-management—taking responsibility for one's own treatment activities. This often occurs in collaboration with health care professionals.

Deadly quartet—The clustering in a single individual of hyperinsulinemia, hypertension, hypertriglyceridemia, and obesity.

Health-risk appraisal—Method to evaluate an individual's probability or risk for morbidity or mortality of chronic diseases.

Andragogy—The teaching of adults.

Pedagogy—The art or profession of teaching.

WHAT DO WE KNOW?

Coronary Heart Disease

We know the three major risk factors for coronary heart disease (CHD): elevated serum total cholesterol, hypertension, and smoking. The primary risk factor is serum total cholesterol. Studies of infants and children provide insight to the changes in serum total cholesterol early in life. Cholesterol in cord blood at birth averages 71 mg%; between 6 months and 2 years of age, it increases to about 140 mg%. Average serum total cholesterol of school-age children is about 170 mg%. High-density lipoprotein (HDL) cholesterol decreases in adolescence, bringing total cholesterol down briefly, but low-density lipoprotein (LDL) dips and then increases to offset the decline. This is especially true for boys.[1]

Dietary intake is a very important regulating factor in both the etiology and prevention of CHD. Studies show the following[2]:

- Dietary cholesterol and saturated fat in food lower the LDL receptor activity on the liver cell. This decreases the amount of LDL cholesterol that leaves the blood.
- Antioxidants in fruits, vegetables, grains, and beans reduce the oxidation of LDL.

- Excess energy intake is generally precipitated by an excess amount of dietary fat. Men and women consume about one pound of fat every four days and six days, respectively. The fat constituents that influence the health of the individual may not be measured in the fasting blood cholesterol or cholesterol fractions. Rather, chylomicron remnants may enter and remain in the artery wall, forming a building block for the atherosclerotic plaque. More highly saturated fats encourage blood clot formation within hours of food ingestion.
- Fat in fish reduces clot formation via a clearing mechanism.
- LDL cholesterol reductions are greater for men who have elevated blood levels prior to medical nutrition therapy (i.e., Step 1 and Step 2 diets).[3] The blood lipid response may be enhanced greatly by weight reduction (e.g., a 25% reduction of total cholesterol can be expected for men consuming high saturated fat if they reduce body weight to a healthy level and practice the Step 2 diet).[4,5]

Assessment of an individual's knowledge of CHD risk factors may be important. Several true-false, one-page instruments have been developed by the National Institutes of Health (NIH) to administer to individuals and groups for awareness and focused education for CHD prevention (see Exhibit 17–1).

Cancer

Many factors motivate the ultimate effect of eating behavior on cancer prevention. A high-fat eating pattern may be an intermediate marker for a distinct eating pattern and lifestyle. Studies show the following[6]:

- Some studies of breast cancer report a correlation with fat intake, yet other studies have found no correlation. Obesity is associated with an increased recurrence of breast cancer and with a lower survival rate. An increasing body weight in adulthood is recognized as a predictor of breast cancer risk;

excess energy intake and reduced physical activity have been shown to increase cancer risk. The abdominal or "apple" shape is more highly associated with breast cancer. Weight loss of 14.5 kg may lessen breast cancer risk by 45%.[7-24]

- Several case-control studies report a significant association between fat intake and colon cancer. Eating patterns high in fat, which increase bile acid secretion, promote tumor development and cell proliferation. Bacterial flora common among omnivores form mutagenic secondary bile acids, placing individuals at high risk for colon cancer. The opposite occurs for individuals who have a high fruit and vegetable intake. Dietary fiber and calcium supplementation can decrease, whereas dietary fat can increase the proliferation rates of cells in the rectal mucosa.[25-39]
- Multicountry studies have helped to unravel various dietary associations with prostate cancer. Among postmenopausal women, obesity and an eating pattern high in fat have been associated with uterine cancer.[40,41]
- High energy intake fueled by fat, especially polyunsaturated fat, accelerates cell proliferation. Polyunsaturated fat also promotes prostaglandin synthesis. Conversely, energy restriction stops tumor growth in some animal models. Aromatization of adrenal androgens produces estrogens in postmenopausal women; estradiol increases and promotes tumor growth[42-49] (see Chapter 12).

Diabetes Mellitus

Patients with non-insulin-dependent diabetes mellitus (NIDDM) often exhibit a clustering of risk factors. Research shows the following.[50]

The clustering in a single individual of hyperinsulinemia, hypertension, hypertriglyceridemia, and obesity (in particular, upper-body obesity) is termed "the deadly quartet."[51] A lifestyle modification program with a very-low-fat, high-carbohydrate, high-fiber diet and daily aerobic exercise was set up for 13 NIDDM patients. The diet comprised 10% of its calories from fat, 75% from unrefined carbohydrates, with 35 to 40 grams of dietary fiber per 1,000 kcal. After 21 days, fasting serum insulin, glucose, and triglycerides declined significantly by 33%, 28%, and 44%, respectively. Systolic and diastolic blood pressures, body weight, and body mass index (BMI) were all significantly reduced by the intervention. Total cholesterol and LDL cholesterol levels were significantly reduced by 22% and 26%, respectively, and HDL cholesterol levels fell significantly by 13.5%.[52]

Diabetic retinopathy or other visual abnormalities require care by an ophthalmologist experienced in the management of people with diabetes. The individual with abnormal renal function may develop proteinuria or elevated serum creatinine, which require heightened attention and control of other risk factors (e.g., hypertension and smoking). Such a situation requires consultation with a specialist in diabetic renal disease.

Individuals with cardiovascular risk factors should be carefully monitored. If symptoms of cardiovascular disease occur (i.e., angina, decreased pulses, and ECG abnormalities), then efforts should be aimed at correction of contributing risk factors (e.g., obesity, smoking, hypertension, sedentary lifestyle, hyperlipidemia, and poorly regulated diabetes). Treatment of the specific cardiovascular problem should be monitored. A questionnaire to evaluate an individual's weight and heart IQ can be used to assist treatment (see Exhibit 17–2).

Diabetic neuropathy may result in painful paresthesia, muscle weakness, and loss of sensation. Autonomic involvement can affect the function of the gastrointestinal, cardiovascular, and genitourinary systems and may require consultation with an appropriate medical specialist.

Upper-body obesity accompanies an increased prevalence of hypertension, diabetes, and dyslipidemia. A similar clustering of metabolic disturbances in nonobese, hypertensive patients has been called syndrome X.[50] Syndrome X contributes to a marked increase in the risk of CHD for individuals with or without clinically defined diabetes. A syndrome that includes both syndrome X and "the deadly quartet" is "insulin-resistance syndrome," because both conditions are associated with and likely caused by resistance to the peripheral actions of insulin with subsequent hyperinsulinemia.[51] All obese hypertensives and about one-half of nonobese hypertensives are insulin resistant.

Multiple mechanisms appear responsible for insulin resistance,[50,53–57] but the specific etiologic factor observed in obese and nonobese patients with hypertension is uncertain.[51] Excess body weight distributed in the upper body may be the responsible factor for obese individuals. The degree of hyperinsulinemia may be even greater if weight gain is induced by high carbohydrate intake. Continual stress-induced, sympathetic nervous system activation may also lead to insulin resistance. An increased proportion of Type IIB muscle fibers, reflecting either genetic or acquired processes, may be responsible. These fibers are more resistant to the effects of insulin than are Type I and Type IIA fibers.[57]

Irrespective of the process by which insulin resistance is initiated, the outcome of hyperinsulinemia may be responsible for increased systemic blood pressure, dyslipidemia, and CHD. Drug and medical nutrition therapy to reduce insulin resistance seem appropriate and potentially of great benefit. Targeted nutritional programs are an essential part of the approach. Suggested lifestyle changes to overcome insulin resistance are as follows[58]:

- weight reduction if obesity is present
- regular aerobic exercise
- moderate consumption of alcohol
- use of antihypertensive agents, such as captopril and doxazosin, which improve insulin sensitivity
- avoidance of diuretics and beta-blockers, which complicate insulin sensitivity
- use of metformin, which increases insulin sensitivity and decreases hyperinsulinemia.

Hypertension

Hypertension is a major risk factor for CHD, which enhances the progression of several other debilitating diseases. Research shows the following:

Exhibit 17-1 Check Your Healthy Heart IQ

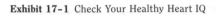

CHECK YOUR

Healthy Heart I.Q.

Answer "true" or "false" to the following questions to test your knowledge of heart disease and its risk factors.
Be sure to check the answers and explanations on the back of this sheet to see how well you do.

1. The risk factors for heart disease that you *can do something about* are: T   F
   high blood pressure, high blood cholesterol, smoking, obesity, and physical inactivity.

2. A stroke is often the first symptom of high blood pressure, and a heart attack is   T   F
   often the first symptom of high blood cholesterol.

3. A blood pressure greater than or equal to 140/90 mm Hg is generally   T   F
   considered to be high.

4. High blood pressure affects the same number of blacks as it does whites.   T   F

5. The best ways to treat and control high blood pressure are to control your weight,   T   F
   exercise, eat less salt (sodium), restrict your intake of alcohol, and take your high
   blood pressure medicine, if prescribed by your doctor.

6. A blood cholesterol level of 240 mg/dL is desirable for adults.   T   F

7. The most effective dietary way to lower the level of your blood cholesterol is   T   F
   to eat foods low in cholesterol.

8. Lowering blood cholesterol levels can help people who have already   T   F
   had a heart attack.

9. Only children from families at high risk of heart disease need to have their blood   T   F
   cholesterol levels checked.

10. Smoking is a major risk factor for four of the five leading causes of death including   T   F
    heart attack, stroke, cancer, and lung diseases such as emphysema and bronchitis.

11. If you have had a heart attack, quitting smoking can help reduce your chances of   T   F
    having a second attack.

12. Someone who has smoked for 30 to 40 years probably will not be able to   T   F
    quit smoking.

13. The best way to lose weight is to increase physical activity and eat fewer calories.   T   F

14. Heart disease is the leading killer of men **and** women in the United States.   T   F

Prepared by the National Heart, Lung, and Blood Institute   NATIONAL INSTITUTES OF HEALTH

continues

Exhibit 17-1 continued

Healthy Heart I.Q.

1. TRUE High blood pressure, smoking, and high blood cholesterol are the three most important risk factors for heart disease. On the average, each one doubles your chance of developing heart disease. So, a person who has all three of these risk factors is 8 times more likely to develop heart disease than someone who has none. Obesity increases the likelihood of developing high blood cholesterol and high blood pressure, which increase your risk for heart disease. Physical inactivity increases your risk of heart attack. Regular exercise and good nutrition are essential to reducing high blood pressure, high blood cholesterol, and overweight. People who exercise are also more likely to cut down or stop smoking.

2. TRUE A person with high blood pressure or high blood cholesterol may feel fine and look great; there are often no signs that anything is wrong until a stroke or heart attack occurs. To find out if you have high blood pressure or high blood cholesterol, you should be tested by a doctor, nurse, or other health professional.

3. TRUE A blood pressure of 140/90 mm Hg or greater is generally classified as high blood pressure. However, blood pressures that fall below 140/90 mm Hg can sometimes be a problem. If the diastolic pressure, the second or lower number, is between 85-89, a person is at increased risk for heart disease or stroke and should have his/her blood pressure checked at least once a year by a health professional. The higher your blood pressure, the greater your risk of developing heart disease or stroke. Controlling high blood pressure reduces your risk

4. FALSE High blood pressure is more common in blacks than in whites. It affects 29 out of every 100 black adults compared to 26 out of every 100 white adults. Also, with aging, high blood pressure is generally more severe among blacks than among whites, and therefore causes more strokes, heart disease, and kidney failure.

5. TRUE Recent studies show that lifestyle changes can help keep blood pressure levels normal even into advanced age and are important in treating and preventing high blood pressure. Limit high-salt foods which make many snack foods, such as potato chips, salted pretzels, and salted crackers; processed foods, such as canned soups; and condiments, such as ketchup and soy sauce. Also, it is **extremely important** to take blood pressure medication, if prescribed by your doctor, to make sure your blood pressure stays under control.

6. FALSE A total blood cholesterol level of under 200 mg/dL is **desirable** and usually puts you at a lower risk for heart disease. A blood cholesterol level of 240 mg/dL or above is **high** and increases your risk of heart disease. If your cholesterol level is high, your doctor will want to check your levels of LDL-cholesterol ("bad" cholesterol) and HDL-cholesterol ("good" cholesterol). A HIGH level of LDL-cholesterol increases your risk of heart disease, as does a LOW level of HDL-cholesterol. A cholesterol level of 200-239 mg/dL is considered **borderline-high** and usually increases your risk for heart disease. If your cholesterol is borderline-high, you should speak to your doctor to see if additional cholesterol tests are needed. All adults 20 years of age or older should have their blood cholesterol level checked at least once every 5 years.

7. FALSE Reducing the amount of cholesterol in your diet is important; however, eating foods **low in saturated fat** is the most effective dietary way to lower blood cholesterol levels, along with eating less total fat and cholesterol. Choose low-saturated fat foods, such as grains, fruits, and vegetables; low-fat or skim milk and milk products; lean cuts of meat; fish; and chicken. Trim fat from meat before cooking; bake or broil meat rather than fry; use less fat and oil; and take the skin off chicken and turkey. Reducing overweight will also help lower your level of LDL-cholesterol as well as increase your level of HDL-cholesterol.

8. TRUE People who have had one heart attack are at much higher risk for a second attack. Reducing blood cholesterol levels can greatly slow down (and, in some people, even reverse) the buildup of cholesterol and fat in the walls of the coronary arteries and significantly reduce the chances of a second heart attack.

9. TRUE Children from "high risk" families, in which a parent has high blood cholesterol (240 mg/dL or above) or in which a parent or grandparent has had heart disease at an early age (at 55 years of age or younger), should have their cholesterol levels tested. If a child from such a family has a cholesterol level that is high, it should be lowered under medical supervision, primarily with diet, to reduce the risk of developing heart disease as an adult. For most children, who are not from high-risk families, the best way to reduce the risk of adult heart disease is to follow a low-saturated fat, low cholesterol eating pattern. All children over the age of 2 years and all adults should adopt a heart-healthy eating pattern as a principal way of reducing coronary heart disease.

10. TRUE Heavy smokers are 2 to 4 times more likely to have a heart attack than nonsmokers, and the heart attack death rate among all smokers is 70 percent greater than that of nonsmokers. Older male smokers are also nearly twice as likely to die from stroke than older men who do not smoke, and these odds are nearly as high for older female smokers. Further, the risk of dying of lung cancer is 22 times higher for male smokers than male nonsmokers and 12 times higher for female smokers than female nonsmokers. Finally, 80 percent of all deaths from emphysema and bronchitis are directly due to smoking.

11. TRUE One year after quitting, ex-smokers cut their extra risk for heart attack by about half or more, and eventually the risk will return to normal in healthy ex-smokers. Even if you have already had a heart attack, you can reduce your chances of having a second attack if you quit smoking. Ex-smokers can also reduce their risk of stroke and cancer, improve blood flow and lung function, and help stop diseases like emphysema and bronchitis from getting worse.

12. FALSE Older smokers are more likely to succeed at quitting smoking than younger smokers. Quitting helps relieve smoking-related symptoms like shortness of breath, coughing, and chest pain. Many quit to avoid further health problems and take control of their lives.

13. TRUE Weight control is a question of balance. You get calories from the food you eat. You burn off calories by exercising. Cutting down on calories, especially calories from fat, is key to losing weight. Combining this with a regular physical activity, like walking, cycling, jogging, or swimming, not only can help in losing weight but also in maintaining weight loss. A steady weight loss of 1/2 to 1 pounds a week is safe for most adults, and the weight is more likely to stay off over the long run. Losing weight, if you are overweight, may also help reduce your blood pressure, lower your LDL-cholesterol, and raise your HDL-cholesterol. Being physically active and eating fewer calories will also help you control your weight if you quit smoking.

14. TRUE Coronary heart disease is the #1 killer in the United States. Approximately 489,000 Americans died of coronary heart disease in 1990, and approximately half of these deaths were women.

Source: Reprinted from *Check Your Healthy Heart IQ*, National Heart, Lung, and Blood Institute, National Institutes of Health, Publication No. 92-2724, October 1992.

Exhibit 17-2 Check Your Weight and Heart Disease IQ

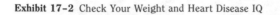

CHECK YOUR WEIGHT AND HEART DISEASE

I.Q.

Prepared by the National Heart. Lung, and Blood Institute • NATIONAL INSTITUTES OF HEALTH

The following statements are either true or false.
The statements test your knowledge of overweight and heart disease.
The correct answers can be found on the back of this sheet.

[T] [F]   **1** Being overweight puts you at risk for heart disease.

[T] [F]   **2** If you are overweight, losing weight helps lower your high blood cholesterol and high blood pressure.

[T] [F]   **3** Quitting smoking is healthy, but it commonly leads to excessive weight gain which increases your risk for heart disease.

[T] [F]   **4** An overweight person with high blood pressure should pay more attention to a low-sodium diet than to weight reduction.

[T] [F]   **5** A reduced intake of sodium or salt does not always lower high blood pressure to normal.

[T] [F]   **6** The best way to lose weight is to eat fewer calories and exercise.

[T] [F]   **7** Skipping meals is a good way to cut down on calories.

[T] [F]   **8** Foods high in complex carbohydrates (starch and fiber) are good choices when you are trying to lose weight.

[T] [F]   **9** The single most important change most people can make to lose weight is to avoid sugar.

[T] [F]   **10** Polyunsaturated fat has the same number of calories as saturated fat.

[T] [F]   **11** Overweight children are very likely to become overweight adults.

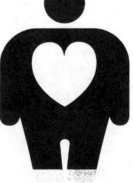

YOUR SCORE: How many correct answers did you make?

10–11 correct = Congratulations! You know a lot about weight and heart disease. Share this information with your family and friends. **8–9 correct** = Very good. **Fewer than 8** = Go over the answers and try to learn more about weight and heart disease.

NHLBI OBESITY EDUCATION INITIATIVE

continues

Exhibit 17-2 continued

A N S W E R S   T O   Y O U R   W E I G H T   A N D   H E A R T   D I S E A S E   I Q   T E S T

1 True. Being overweight increases your risk for high blood cholesterol and high blood pressure, two of the major risk factors for coronary heart disease. Even if you do not have high blood cholesterol or high blood pressure, being overweight may increase your risk for heart disease. Where you carry your extra weight may affect your risk too. Weight carried at your waist or above seems to be associated with an increased risk for heart disease in many people. In addition, being overweight increases your risk for diabetes, gallbladder disease, and some types of cancer.

2 True. If you are overweight, even moderate reductions in weight, such as 5 to 10 percent, can produce substantial reductions in blood pressure. You may also be able to reduce your LDL-cholesterol ("bad" cholesterol) and triglycerides and increase your HDL-cholesterol ("good" cholesterol).

3 False. The average weight gain after quitting smoking is 5 pounds. The proportion of ex-smokers who gain large amounts of weight (greater than 20 pounds) is relatively small. Even if you gain weight when you stop smoking, change your eating and exercise habits to lose weight rather than starting to smoke again. Smokers who quit smoking decrease their risk for heart disease by about 50 percent compared to those people who do not quit.

4 False. Weight loss, if you are overweight, may reduce your blood pressure even if you don't reduce the amount of sodium you eat. Weight loss is recommended for all overweight people who have high blood pressure. Even if weight loss does not reduce your blood pressure to normal, it may help you cut back on your blood pressure medications. Also, losing weight if you are overweight may help you reduce your risk for or control other health problems.

5 True. Even though a high sodium or salt intake plays a key role in maintaining high blood pressure in some people, there is no easy way to determine who will benefit from eating less sodium and salt. Also, a high intake may limit how well certain high blood pressure medications work. Eating a diet with less sodium may help some people reduce their risk of developing high blood pressure. Most Americans eat more salt and other sources of sodium than they need. Therefore, it is prudent for most people to reduce their sodium intake.

6 True. Eating fewer calories and exercising more is the best way to lose weight and keep it off. Weight control is a question of balance. You get calories from the food you eat. You burn off calories by exercising. Cutting down on calories, especially calories from fat, is key to losing weight. Combining this with a regular exercise program, like walking, bicycling, jogging, or swimming, not only can help in losing weight but also in maintaining the weight loss. A steady weight loss of 1 to 2 pounds a week is safe for most adults, and the weight is more likely to stay off over the long run. Losing weight, if you are overweight, may also help reduce your blood pressure and raise your HDL-cholesterol, the "good" cholesterol.

7 False. To cut calories, some people regularly skip meals and have no snacks or caloric drinks in between. If you do this, your body thinks that it is starving even if your intake of calories is not reduced to a very low amount. Your body will try to save energy by slowing its metabolism, that is decreasing the rate at which it burns calories. This makes losing weight even harder and may even add body fat. Try to avoid long periods without eating. Five or six small meals are often preferred to the usual three meals a day for some individuals trying to lose weight.

8 True. Contrary to popular belief, foods high in complex carbohydrates (like pasta, rice, potatoes, breads, cereals, grains, dried beans and peas) are lower in calories than foods high in fat. In addition, they are good sources of vitamins, minerals, and fiber. What adds calories to these foods is the addition of butter, rich sauces, whole milk, cheese, or cream, which are high in fat.

9 False. Sugar has not been found to cause obesity; however, many foods high in sugar are also high in fat. Fat has more than twice the calories as the same amount of protein or carbohydrates (sugar and starch). Thus, foods that are high in fat are high in calories. High-sugar foods, like cakes, cookies, candies, and ice cream, are high in fat and calories and low in vitamins, minerals, and protein.

10 True. All fats—polyunsaturated, monounsaturated, and saturated—have the same number of calories. All calories count whether they come from saturated or unsaturated fats. Because fats are the richest sources of calories, eating less total fat will help reduce the number of calories you eat every day. It will also help you reduce your intake of saturated fat. Particular attention to reducing saturated fat is important in lowering your blood cholesterol level.

11 False. Obesity in childhood does increase the likelihood of adult obesity, but most overweight children will not become obese. Several factors influence whether or not an overweight child becomes an overweight adult: (1) the age the child becomes overweight; (2) how overweight the child is; (3) the family history of overweight; and (4) dietary and activity habits. Getting to the right weight is desirable, but children's needs for calories and other nutrients are different from the needs of adults. Dietary plans for weight control must allow for this. Eating habits, like so many other habits, are often formed during childhood, so it is important to develop good ones.

For more information, write:
NHLBI Obesity Education Initiative
P.O. Box 30105
Bethesda, MD 20824-0105

Source: Reprinted from *Check Your Weight and Heart Disease IQ*, National Heart, Lung, and Blood Institute, National Institutes of Health, Publication No. 93-3034, May 1993.

- Hypertension contributes to the development and progression of chronic complications of diabetes.
- Hypertension should be treated aggressively to achieve and maintain blood pressure in the normal range.
- Eating and exercise behavior change can moderate blood pressure levels. Community nutrition professionals can begin by assessing individuals' knowledge about high blood pressure (see Exhibit 17–3).
- If medication is needed, selection of an antihypertensive drug should be individualized to minimize the number and severity of side effects. For example, beta-blockers should be used with caution in insulin-treated individuals, because these drugs may mask early symptoms of hypoglycemia and prolong recovery from hypoglycemia.[54]
- Attention has been given to both the negative and positive effects of different types of antihypertensive agents on the multiple risk factors for premature CHD[59–61] (see Table 17–1). Various lifestyle therapies can reduce the major adverse effects of hypertension and the risk factors that frequently accompany high blood pressure (see Exhibit 17–4).

Smoking

One of the major risk factors for CHD is cigarette smoking. Smoking cessation is a major lifestyle change recommended for men and women with a smoking habit. Medical nutrition therapy to support smoking cessation can involve replacing lost nutrient intake, increasing soluble fiber, weight management, and substituting alkaline foods during withdrawal symptoms (see Exhibit 17–5).

WHAT ARE THE NATIONAL DIRECTIVES?

The Surgeon General's Report on Nutrition and Health[62] and *Nutrition and Your Health: Dietary Guidelines for Americans*[63] clearly docu-ment the relationship between what people eat and their health. Based on decades of research and the resulting consensus of numerous scientific groups, these documents direct primary and secondary prevention activities via planning healthy eating patterns for individuals or groups or providing nutrition education programs. The direction is risk reduction, and the target is chronic disease (e.g., CHD, cancer, hypertension, and diabetes).

Healthy People 2000: National Health Promotion and Disease Prevention Objectives offers a vision for the next century, which sees the United States as a nation that could experience significantly less death and disability from preventable diseases, an improved quality of life, and a great reduction in the disparities of health status among select groups of people.[64] Certain ethnic groups such as African Americans experience a greater proportion of CHD deaths and cancer deaths; Native Americans and Latinos have a higher incidence of obesity, diabetes, and hypertension.

The *Healthy People 2000* vision has set the current nutrition agenda for US educational institutions, health care facilities, state and local health agencies, nonprofit organizations, and the food industry. The National Cholesterol Education Program (NCEP) underscores those *Healthy People 2000* objectives specific to CHD, with a national campaign emphasizing the importance of low-fat eating for all individuals two years and older.[65]

Throughout the United States, the "5-A-Day" campaign links food industry activities with the National Cancer Institute initiative to increase fruit and vegetable intake to reduce cancer risk. Specific programs at the state and local levels complement these national initiatives. In many cases, individual states have formalized their own programs to address the nutritional needs of their residents. For example:

- In 1988, the California Department of Health Services established the "California 5-a-Day-for-Better Health!" campaign to promote fruit and vegetable consumption as part of a low-fat, high-fiber eating pattern. This was possible due to a five-year grant awarded by

Exhibit 17-3 Check Your High Blood Pressure Prevention IQ

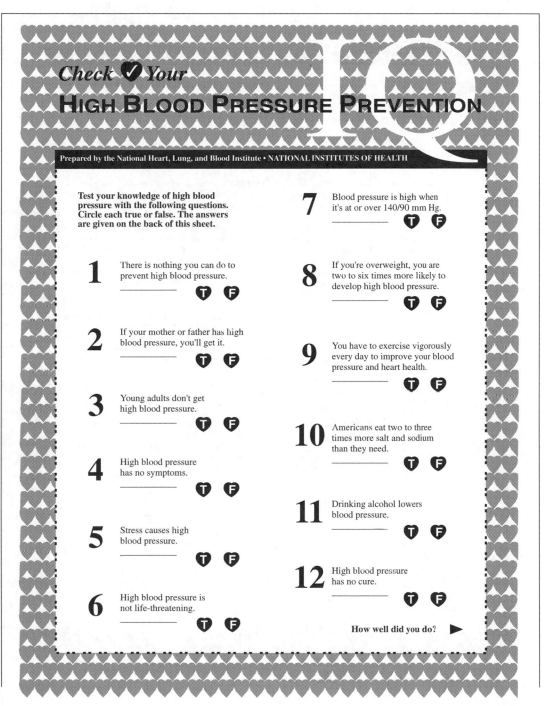

Check ✓ Your
HIGH BLOOD PRESSURE PREVENTION

Prepared by the National Heart, Lung, and Blood Institute • NATIONAL INSTITUTES OF HEALTH

Test your knowledge of high blood pressure with the following questions. Circle each true or false. The answers are given on the back of this sheet.

1 There is nothing you can do to prevent high blood pressure. ——— T F

2 If your mother or father has high blood pressure, you'll get it. ——— T F

3 Young adults don't get high blood pressure. ——— T F

4 High blood pressure has no symptoms. ——— T F

5 Stress causes high blood pressure. ——— T F

6 High blood pressure is not life-threatening. ——— T F

7 Blood pressure is high when it's at or over 140/90 mm Hg. ——— T F

8 If you're overweight, you are two to six times more likely to develop high blood pressure. ——— T F

9 You have to exercise vigorously every day to improve your blood pressure and heart health. ——— T F

10 Americans eat two to three times more salt and sodium than they need. ——— T F

11 Drinking alcohol lowers blood pressure. ——— T F

12 High blood pressure has no cure. ——— T F

How well did you do? ►

continues

Exhibit 17–3 continued

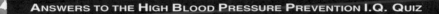

ANSWERS TO THE HIGH BLOOD PRESSURE PREVENTION I.Q. QUIZ

1. FALSE. High blood pressure can be prevented with four steps: keep a healthy weight; become physically active; limit your salt and sodium use; and, if you drink alcoholic beverages, do so in moderation.

2. FALSE. You are more likely to get high blood pressure if it runs in your family, but that doesn't mean you must get it. Your chance of getting high blood pressure is also greater if you're older or an African American. But high blood pressure is NOT an inevitable part of aging and everyone can take steps to prevent the disease—the steps are given in answer 1.

3. FALSE. About 15 percent of those ages 18–39 are among the 50 million Americans with high blood pressure. Once you have high blood pressure, you have it for the rest of your life. So start now to prevent it.

4. TRUE. High blood pressure, or "hypertension," usually has no symptoms. In fact, it is often called the "silent killer." You can have high blood pressure and feel fine. That's why it's important to have your blood pressure checked—it's a simple test.

5. FALSE. Stress does make blood pressure go up, but only temporarily. Ups and downs in blood pressure are normal. Run for a bus and your pressure rises; sleep and it drops. Blood pressure is the force of blood against the walls of arteries. Blood pressure becomes dangerous when it's always high. That harms your heart and blood vessels. So what does cause high blood pressure? In the vast majority of cases, a single cause is never found.

6. FALSE. High blood pressure is the main cause of stroke and a factor in the development of heart disease and kidney failure.

7. TRUE. But even blood pressures slightly under 140/90 mm Hg can increase your risk of heart disease or stroke.

8. TRUE. As weight increases, so does blood pressure. It's important to stay at a healthy weight. If you need to reduce, try to lose 1/2 to 1 pound a week. Choose foods low in fat (especially saturated fat), since fat is high in calories. Even if you're at a good weight, the healthiest way to eat is low fat, low cholesterol.

9. FALSE. Studies show that even a little physical activity helps prevent high blood pressure and strengthens your heart. Even among the overweight, those who are active have lower blood pressures than those who aren't. It's best to do some activity for 30 minutes, most days. Walk, garden, or bowl. If you don't have a 30-minute period, do something for 15 minutes, twice a day. Every bit helps—so make activity part of your daily routine.

10. TRUE. Americans eat way too much salt and sodium. And some people, such as many African Americans, are especially sensitive to salt. Salt is made of sodium and chloride, and it's mostly the sodium that affects blood pressure. Salt is only one form of sodium—there are others. So you need to watch your use of both salt and sodium. That includes what's added to foods at the table and in cooking, and what's already in processed foods and snacks. Americans, especially people with high blood pressure, should eat no more than about 6 grams of salt a day, which equals about 2,400 milligrams of sodium.

11. FALSE. Drinking too much alcohol can raise blood pressure. If you drink, have no more than two drinks a day. The "Dietary Guidelines" recommend that for overall health, women should limit their alcohol to no more than one drink a day. A drink would be 1.5 ounces of 80 proof whiskey, or 5 ounces of wine, or 12 ounces of beer.

12. TRUE. But high blood pressure can be treated and controlled. Treatment usually includes lifestyle changes—losing weight, if overweight; becoming physically active; limiting salt and sodium; and avoiding drinking excess alcohol—and, if needed, medication. But the best way to avoid the dangers of high blood pressure is to prevent the condition.

For more information on high
blood pressure,
call 1-800-575-WELL,
or write to the
National Heart, Lung, and Blood
Institute Information Center,
P.O. Box 30105,
Bethesda, MD
20824-0105.

National High Blood Pressure   U.S. DEPARTMENT OF HEALTH
   Education Program   AND HUMAN SERVICES
National Heart, Lung, and   Public Health Service
   Blood Institute   National Institutes of Health
                                   NIH Publication No. 94-3671
                                   September 1994

Source: Reprinted from *Check Your High Blood Pressure Prevention IQ*, National Heart, Lung, and Blood Institute, National Institutes of Health, Publication No. 94-3671, September 1994.

Table 17–1 Effects of Antihypertensive Drugs on Cardiovascular Risk Factors

Risk Factor	Diuretic	Beta-Blocker	Alpha-Blocker	Calcium Blocker	ACE Inhibitor
Blood pressure	+	+	+	+	+
Cholesterol	–	NC	+	NC	NC
HDL cholesterol	NC	–	NC	NC	NC
Glucose intolerance	–	–	+	NC	+
Hyperinsulinemia	–	–	+	NC	+
Physical activity	NC	–	+	NC	NC
Left ventricular hypertrophy	–	+/–	+	+	+

Note: + = positive; – = negative; NC = no change.

Source: Adapted from Kaplan, N.M., The Deadly Quartet: Upper Body Obesity, Glucose Intolerance, Hypertriglyceridemia, and Hypertension, *Archives of Internal Medicine*, Vol. 149, pp. 1514–1520, with permission of the American Medical Association, © 1989.

Exhibit 17–4 Lifestyle Approaches for Hypertension

PROVEN FAVORABLE EFFECT

- Weight reduction (especially for upper-body obesity)
- Moderate sodium restriction to 2 grams sodium (88 mmol)/day
- Moderation of alcohol to no more than 2 drinks/day
- Regular isotonic exercise
- Potassium supplements

UNPROVEN FAVORABLE EFFECT

- Calcium supplements
- Magnesium supplements
- Fish oil supplements
- Relaxation
- Moderation of caffeine

Source: Adapted from Kaplan, N.M., The Deadly Quartet: Upper Body Obesity, Glucose Intolerance, Hypertriglyceridemia, and Hypertension, *Archives of Internal Medicine*, Vol. 149, pp. 1514–1520, with permission of the American Medical Association, © 1989.

---

the National Cancer Institute. Currently, California's program reaches millions of adults and children with media and point-of-purchase information. California's "Project LEAN–Low-fat Eating for Americans Now!"

campaign has reached major population segments and various ethnic groups throughout California.

- The *Food Guide Pyramid*[66] is the visual presentation of the *Dietary Guidelines for Americans* (see Chapter 2). The pyramid was preceded in 1989 by California's Assembly Bill 2109. AB 2109 mandated development of "the California Daily Food Guide," which is currently used for all nutrition programs in California. The guide provides quantitative, life-cycle dietary recommendations with ethnic-, age-, and gender-specific food guides. It provides continuity for programs and for the public. If the eating pattern begins in childhood, transition to adolescence and adulthood is easier and probable.

- The California Department of Education developed nutrition guidelines for all food and beverages sold on school campuses in California. The resulting *Nutrition Guidelines for California School Foods*[67] presents a three-tiered approach to dietary modification of lunch and breakfast menus. This model has been used to establish the "new shape menu planning," which is frequently adopted nationally for school menu planning to reduce fat, salt, and sugar and to increase whole grains, vegetables, and fruits, which

Exhibit 17-5 Nutrition Guidelines To Assist Smoking Cessation

---

EAT A NUTRIENT-DENSE DIET

Recover lost nutrients emphasizing vitamin A, beta-carotene, vitamin B$_{12}$, folic acid, vitamin C, and zinc. Consume more yellow/orange fruits and vegetables, citrus and fresh fruits, dark green leafy vegetables, lean red meat, and low-fat milk and yogurt.

INCREASE FIBER

Include more roughage in the diet, adequate water, and exercise to reduce constipation. Eat fresh fruits and vegetables with skins such as potatoes, squash, apples, pears, and peaches.

CONTROL WEIGHT

Start to lose weight before quitting. A 500-calorie daily deficit equals one pound of weight loss per week. Plan a 250 kcal deficit a day and burn 250 additional kcal each day by increasing exercise (such as 45 minutes of aerobic walking or bicycling or 30 minutes of swimming or jogging).

REDUCE WITHDRAWAL SYMPTOMS AND CRAVINGS WITH ALKALINE FOODS

Alkaloid foods enhance reabsorption of nicotine. Alkaline-forming foods are high in potassium, calcium, magnesium, and sodium. Acid-forming foods, which are high in phosphorous, sulfur, and chloride, should be limited.

Limit intake of the following:

- protein foods
- poultry
- fish
- eggs
- seafood
- cranberry
- plums
- prunes

Increase intake of the following:

- milk
- yogurt
- shrimp
- coffee
- tea
- soda
- water
- mineral water
- fruits and vegetables
- dried fruit
- olives
- almonds
- brazil nuts

Eat moderate amounts of the following:

- grains
- starches
- corn
- asparagus

RESTRUCTURE EATING

Alter your snack and meal environment. Reduce contact with smoking. Practice behavior modification techniques. Experiment with altering your tastes by choosing among these alternatives, which also enhance oral gratification:

- special coffee blends, strong blends
- lemon drops, Lifesavers, diet candy, and gum
- raw vegetables when feeling anger or aggressive
- yogurt to comfort or sooth
- diet soda, diet lemonade, fruit juice, and mineral water
- melba toast, Rye Crisp, Rusk crackers
- use a straw, a toothpick

Source: Adapted from Beckley, L. *Taking Control: Diet, Drug Abuse and Addiction.* Nutrition Dimension. 1990.

---

increase fiber, vitamins, and minerals (see Chapter 8).

The Recommended Dietary Allowances (RDAs) are the quantitative standards used throughout the United States for planning and evaluating the nutritional adequacy of a population's food intake. These standards are used for meal planning in schools, hospitals, extended-care facilities, penal institutions, congregate feeding sites, and military installations. The RDAs do not currently address the modifications of nutrient intakes to reduce chronic disease risk. Healthy menu planning must blend the nutrient needs to avoid deficiencies, represented by RDAs, with health-promoting meal composition to forestall chronic disease, represented by *Dietary Guidelines for Americans* and *The Food Guide Pyramid.*

Because today's food and health consumers or buyers range from preadolescents to older adults who live alone, nutrition education for all age groups is essential. What US residents see on food labels in grocery stores has changed dramatically during the past few years. The Nutrition Labeling Education Act of 1990 has revamped food labels, defined common terms describing the health-promoting attributes of foods, and set criteria for making nutrition and health claims about foods. The food label has become a major teaching tool to educate children and adults about healthy food choices, and it has enlarged the responsibility of nutrition education to include industry.

The National Action Plan to Improve the American Diet[68] recognizes that no individual organization or initiative can create the massive dietary changes needed to reduce chronic disease in the majority of the US population. This plan recommends a coordinated approach to complement current interventions to reach the *Healthy People 2000* goals.

WHAT CAN WE DO?

Health-Risk Appraisals

Between 5 and 15 million Americans have completed a health-risk appraisal (HRA).[69] The HRA, which has gained popularity as a means of assessing a person's health status, provides an estimate of the likelihood of mortality or morbidity from disease using risk factors such as blood pressure, weight, smoking habits, and medical history.

In addition, appraisal questionnaires are a form of health education, because they make people aware of the outcome or result of their lifestyles and health habits.[70] Many organizations administer HRAs to employees as a part of their health insurance and health benefits package and as a method to evaluate the effectiveness of health promotion programs.

HRAs vary in the way risk is defined and estimated. Computations to predict risk levels generally create a score or a more easily interpreted number. Four different scoring methods are as follows[71]:

1. The probability of dying from leading causes of death over a period of time (e.g., 10 years). Estimates for CHD and stroke are independently estimated. Mortality risk estimates are based on an actuarial approach called the Geller-Gesner method.
2. A focus on heart attacks and heart disease using scales divided into low-, average-, and high-risk ranges. Pencil-and-paper tests are summed for each item.
3. Life expectancy as a surrogate for risk. These HRAs contain the major CHD factors and are scored by hand.
4. Broad measures of overall health (e.g., lifestyle, wellness, stress, or health risk). This format is simple to score by hand, but it may provide only a crude measure of risk.

Many HRAs do not address dietary habits. Some include only one or two items, none of which are used to compute risk. The responses may only serve to trigger changes for improving dietary habits.

The reasons nutrition may not be central to a health-risk appraisal are as follows:

- Dietary status is difficult to measure. Twenty-four-hour dietary recalls may underestimate, whereas frequencies may overlook detail or specific foods. Detailed dietary inventories are not practical for most HRAs.[72]
- The strength of a direct correlation between dietary components and mortality is not established. For example, CHD risk computations are often based on prospective surveys, and those studies may not collect a sufficient volume of detailed dietary data.
- HRAs are driven by physiological precursors of morbidity and mortality. Eating and exercise behavior are intermediate mediators to these precursors. The immediate precursors include blood pressure, plasma cholesterol, lipid fractions, and body mass.

Guidelines for Selecting an HRA

With more than 200 HRAs in the United States, selection guidelines and questions are needed. The following may be useful[71]:

- What is the validity or accuracy of the risk estimates? With diversity of scoring methods and databases, discrepant estimates of risk for an individual are expected. Forty-one popular appraisal instruments were evaluated for similarity of CHD risk estimates. They were compared with projections from the Framingham Heart Study and the UCLA Risk Factor Update Project.[73] HRAs based on logistic regression equations or the Geller-Gesner method with additive scales were the most accurate. Comprehensiveness of the assessment items was a major indicator of accuracy. The least accurate instruments were those that do not include major risk factors, that ignore sex and age, or that employ two or three broad categories to measure a factor.
- What does the report form contain? How easy is it to read and to understand? What and how much feedback is most appropriate for clients? Generally, simple identification of below average, average, and above average risk may be sufficient, but in some instances a detailed estimate of life expectancy or probability of dying is needed. An individual's actual age can be contrasted with the "appraised" age (the average age at which members of the general population have the same risk). Risks associated with select factors (e.g., smoking or physical activity) are informative and directive. If HRA data are to be used to evaluate a health promotion or dietary intervention, a matrix defining risk and future action may be appropriate.
- Are the appraisal questionnaires expensive if self-administered? Usually self-administered questionnaires are available in bulk at a nominal charge. However, versions for personal computers are available. The cost varies from $50 to more than $300. Complete HRA assessments are often available, and for a fee they include personalized charts, detailed explanations, and summary reports. This is the most expensive option, but it can be cost-effective when an entire work site or large population is evaluated.

Limitations of HRAs

The major limitations of HRAs are as follows[71]:

- Clients may not comprehend or interpret the results accurately, because probability estimates are difficult to grasp. This uncertainty can reduce the educational and motivational potential.
- Clients may not know how to assess the accuracy of the appraisal. If blood pressure and cholesterol levels are missing, and an average value is used, then an artificially low risk estimate can be given.
- Self-scored HRAs may contain simple math errors and mislead individuals about their actual status.
- If HRAs are administered in an unsupervised environment, then the results may cause unnecessary fear and anxiety.

Info Line

For more information on HRAs, contact Carter Center Health Risk Appraisal Project, 1989 North Williamsburg Drive, Suite E, Decatur, GA 30033.

Food-Scoring Systems

These systems vary from a comprehensive approach to a rapid or quick assessment of a food record. Nutrient-based analysis is more revealing if based on reliable and accurate records.[71]

Two useful food-scoring systems that provide a quick estimation of the effect of eating pattern on serum cholesterol are the Food Record Rating and the Dietary Achievement Score. They are practical for groups or individuals.[74,75]

The Food Record Rating (FRR) was used in the Multiple Risk Factor Intervention Trial

(MRFIT); the Dietary Achievement Score was used in the Heart Saver Program of the Chicago Heart Association. Both methods estimate adherence and indirectly predict changes in serum cholesterol. Both instruments can be used for self-monitoring and teaching clients about food selection. The food score averages three days of food records. The use of food-scoring systems in nutrition counseling has been described in detail and should be considered as a way to monitor behavior after establishing a baseline.[74,75]

An exchange system has been used to assess intake and evaluate compliance. Foods appearing on a record can be converted into exchanges. The quality of the eating pattern is then based on the number of exchanges consumed compared with the number recommended.[76,77]

The Cholesterol-Saturated-Fat Index (CSI) has become a useful indicator of the hypercholesterolemic potential of foods. The atherogenic effect of a given food varies with the cholesterol and saturated fatty acid content. Foods high in saturated fatty acids and cholesterol increase an individual's plasma total cholesterol level (see Chapter 11).[78]

Because foods vary in cholesterol and saturated fatty acid content, it is difficult to calculate the exact hypercholesterolemic effect of a single food. An index or single score can account for the various amounts of cholesterol and saturated fatty acids in a given food (see Table 17–2). The value identifies the food as hypercholesterolemic or atherogenic. The CSI demonstrates why some foods (e.g., cheeses or frozen desserts) that have vegetable oil instead of butterfat are better choices.[78] Vegetable oils have no cholesterol and a small amount of saturated fat and, thus, a low CSI value.

Assessment of Sodium Intake

Multiple days of records are needed to quantify an individual's sodium intake.[79] For populations, a one-day food record can give a reasonable estimate of intake. However, assessing sodium intake with a combination of methods is being used.[80] Another approach is to use a regression equation that reflects the independent contribution of the following:

- the daily quantity of table salt used over seven days
- the contribution of sodium from sodium-rich foods assessed in a seven-day food frequency checklist
- an estimate of sodium in the overall foods and beverages consumed

Table 17–2 The Cholesterol-Saturated-Fat Index (CSI) of Selected Fish, Poultry, and Red Meat

Food	Description	Portion	CSI
Whitefish	Snapper, perch, sole, cod, halibut, shellfish (clams, oysters, scallops), water-packed tuna	3.5 oz or 100 g	4
Salmon		3.5 oz or 100 g	5
Shellfish	Shrimp, crab, lobster	3.5 oz or 100 g	6
Poultry	No skin	3.5 oz or 100 g	6
Beef, pork, and lamb	10% fat (ground sirloin, flank steak)	3.5 oz or 100 g	9
	15% fat (ground round)		10
	20% fat (ground chuck, pot roasts)		13
	30% fat (ground beef, pork, steaks, lamb steaks, ribs, pork chops, lamb chops, roasts)		18

Source: Adapted from Conner, S.L., Gustafson, J.R., Artaud-Wild, S.M., et al., The Cholesterol/Saturated-Fat Index: An Indication of the Hypercholesterolemic and Atherogenic Potential of Food, *Lancet*, Vol. 1, p. 1229, with permission of The Lancet Ltd., © 1986.

WHAT COMMUNITY APPROACHES ARE AVAILABLE?

The decade of the 1990s began with a health care system structured for acute care and crisis intervention. It depended almost exclusively on end-stage intervention (e.g., dialysis for renal failure, amputation for diabetes mellitus, or percutaneous transluminal coronary angioplasty for arteriosclerosis). This approach cannot respond efficiently to chronic disease.[81,82] Medical crises often reflect an individual's behavior and lifestyle. Traditional medicine does not produce positive change, and only 5% of adults with chronic disease are institutionalized.[83] The "hidden health care system" at work sites and at home must be fueled to provide the intervention needed to alter the onset and progression of disease.[81,84]

Radical change in the delivery of health care services shifts certain health care activities to the individual or the consumer rather than continuing and strengthening existing services. The goal should be to empower individuals in the management of their own health. "In the health care policy debate, the time has come for a major conceptual shift from viewing people as consumers of health care to seeing them as they really are: its primary providers."[81(p1)] This shift in responsibility can help to control health care expenditures and address the largest challenge to our health care system—the prevention and management of chronic disease.

In the 1940s health education gained identity as a profession, with health education professionals following standardized training and education programs.[85] Currently, professionals can take a national exam and become a Certified Health Education Specialist. The practice of health education is founded on the following traditions[86]:

- *Pedagogy:* This emphasizes the importance of a needs assessment, instruction tailored to the progress of the learner, and instruction seeking the "teachable moment." *Andragogy* or adult education fosters self-diagnosis of educational needs and problem-oriented instruction.[87]
- *Mass media:* This includes radio, television, newspapers, magazines, billboards, posters, and direct mail. The media in the 1930s and 1940s were used to promote public acceptance of immunizations and family planning or to promote awareness of lifestyle and health.[88]
- *The community organization:* This approach began in England in 1844 to educate the public about the sanitary problems in the growing industrial society. Three approaches to organizing a community include[89]:
  1. community development using a model that involves skills and understanding of the whole community
  2. social action, which is a response to the needs of a disadvantaged subgroup in a population by redistribution of resources (This may involve petitions, demonstrations, or boycotts.)
  3. social planning and organizational development, in which experts address social or organizational problems by discussion, debate, and planned change
- *Social psychology:* This approach applies psychological research to solving societal problems. It was the foundation for the Health Belief Model (HBM) in the late 1950s, and it directed the research agenda and attention to attitude change, persuasive communications, fear arousal, and the information-processing system. The HBM is now a model that combines psychological readiness and environmental influences.[90]
- *Group dynamics:* This approach actively involves individuals in making decisions about their own health behaviors and lifestyles. Group dynamics have been and are currently used for smoking cessation, weight management, and a variety of self-help programs.

In health education today these diverse approaches are usually combined. The effective aspects of each add to and create an overall and potentially more powerful outcome.[91-93] Using mass media is one innovative primary prevention approach to teach nutrition education or general health education on a large scale. Social-marketing techniques that use mass media have become common components of nutrition education efforts. The marketing task is to sell nutrition. The immediate goal is to persuade health consumers to act. The long-range goal is for individuals or groups to learn and to integrate certain behaviors into their lifestyle.

A marketing mix comprising four decision areas (product, promotion, price, and distribution) is the basis of the technique. The marketing mix has been used to foster healthy eating and to encourage the food industry, health agencies, and the media to work together for a coordinated approach to nutrition education of the public.[94]

A secondary or tertiary prevention approach can be initiated in the community setting amid the private practice of a physician, registered dietitian (RD), or other health care professional. Although a physician may be responsible for secondary and tertiary prevention of a specific disease (e.g., hyperlipidemia and obesity), the community nutrition specialist, often an RD, can serve an important role in the health care process. For example, the community nutrition professional defines eating behavior goals for patients who are at increased risk of heart disease, imparts skills and knowledge to patients for improved quality of life and risk reduction, and monitors and reports success or failure of patients' efforts to the primary physician. Developing an integrated approach to medical nutrition therapy benefits not only the physician and the community nutrition professional but also the patient.[95]

The Adult Treatment Panel II of the National Cholesterol Education Program outlined practical dietary recommendations to reduce blood cholesterol levels of clients 2 years of age and above. It is the recommendation of the panel that medical nutrition therapy "should not be prematurely disregarded" and, for most patients, "should be continued at least 6 months before deciding whether to add drug treatment."[96] The treatment involves a two-step plan. Step 1 recommends an intake of saturated fat of less than 10% of calories, total fat of less than 30% of calories, and dietary cholesterol of no more than 300 mg/day. Step 2 emphasizes further reduction of saturated fat intake to less than 7% of calories, and dietary cholesterol to less than 200 mg/day. Movement from Step 1 to Step 2 involves lowering saturated and total fat and increasing carbohydrate, while stabilizing protein. Both steps promote weight loss in the overweight patient by eliminating excess fat calories.

Creating effective implementation guidelines is part of the challenge. Dietary modifications must become a reality in the daily lives of individuals. An operational timeline is presented in Table 17–3 for a slightly different approach with a three not two-phase program. The timeline is recommended to simplify the progression and complexity. Alteration of specific dietary components can be targeted to alter the lipid or lipoprotein aberration.[97]

No less than three months should be allowed for achievement of each phase. Not all individuals can make the dietary changes and retain them as a new, preferred eating behavior, even within three months. But after a total of nine months, the result of a serious effort can be noted. A timeline can also blend instruction with measurement for evaluating both dietary and biochemical objectives, a combination that helps the physician and community nutrition professional to monitor each patient's goals and progress.

INTERVENTIONS TO ENHANCE EATING BEHAVIORS

Behavioral approaches should be carefully planned to fit into primary, secondary, and tertiary prevention programs and to appeal to health-conscious consumers in light of their personal characteristics, geographic area, ethnic foods, festivals, and opportunities for physical activity. Communication techniques are essential (see Exhibit 17–6). Initial components of a medical nutrition therapy program include a one-year timeline, a computerized food intake analysis, a weight and cholesterol grid, and sound educational materials.

The health care professional should make a diligent effort to make no changes until 6 to 10 patients have completed the program. The three main reasons physicians give for not initiating medical nutritional services are perceived lack of patient interest, lack of a patient goal, and

Table 17–3 Timeline for Introducing Selected Dietary Components for Secondary Intervention of Hyperlipidemia

	Monthly Consultation Visit								
	Phase I (Months)			Phase II (Months)			Phase III (Months)		
Activity/Instruction	1	2	3	4	5	6	7	8	9
Assessment*									
Anthropometric	X	X	X	X	X	X	X	X	X
Record of food intake	X	X			X		X		
Computerized analysis of food intake			X		X			X	
Lipid/lipoprotein determination				X			X		X
Instructions									
Energy reduction	X		X		X			X	X
Fat modification									
• Total fat	X	X		X			X		
• Fat ratios		X		X			X		X
Cholesterol		X					X		X
Alcohol			X	X		X			
Complex CHO			X	X			X		
Fiber			X					X	

*Initial visit after evaluation of serum lipids/lipoproteins.

Source: Frank, G.C., Nutritional Therapy for Hyperlipidemia and Obesity: Office Treatment Integrating the Roles of the Physician and the Registered Dietitian, *Journal of the American College of Cardiology*, Vol. 12, No. 4, pp. 1098–1100. Reprinted with permission of the Helen Dwight Reid Educational Foundation. Published by Heldref Publications, 1319 18th Street, NW, Washington, D.C. 20036-1802. Copyright © 1988.

nonadherence to the service.[98] A structured program provides direction for the patient and permits evaluation by the clinician and community nutrition professional.

Computerized Analysis of Food Intake

Assessment has two purposes. It indicates adherence to dietary change, and it is an educational tool to direct further change. Computerized analysis of usual food intake is a practical way to evaluate dietary adherence. Using a computerized analysis system, one can ask and answer specific questions, such as the following:

• Is total fat approaching 30% of the total energy intake?

• Is there an increase in complex versus simple carbohydrates?

The DINE System, a computerized database that clinicians and patients have used fairly extensively, produces a record for the medical chart and a handout for the patient. The handout is tangible and helps the patient to refine and alter specific food choices before the next office visit[99] (see Chapter 9).

Individuals tend to consume set meals once they find foods and recipes they like within the allowed food list. The first follow-up food record should be incorporated on the timeline about two weeks after the initial consultation. The record may illustrate a common practice noted among clients (e.g., consumption of modular 300 to 500 kcal entrees, which clients buy, freeze, and cook

Exhibit 17-6 Counseling Techniques To Improve Communication and Adherence for Behavioral Change

- Listening
- Identifying behaviors
- Values clarification
- Feelings assessment
- Self-directed treatment
- Confrontation
- Step 1, 2, 3
- Relapse prevention
- Cognitive/reality therapy
- Mirroring
- Positive affirmation
- Behavior modification
- Written assignments
- Visualization
- Laughter therapy

Source: Adapted from Beckley, L. *Taking Control: Diet, Drug Abuse and Addiction.* Nutrition Dimension. 1990.

in the microwave oven within a few minutes in the evening or at work).

Although the sodium content may be prohibitive (in excess of 750 to 1,000 mg per entree) and the fat type more saturated than desired, the frozen meals are practical. Fish and fowl entrees can be selected to reduce saturated fat and, if the entree is high in sodium, high-sodium foods can be avoided during the remainder of the day. When possible, individuals should be allowed to make gradual changes and to make food choices they can live with daily, rather than forbidden from trying new alternatives and food products. Aiding individuals to make cumulative changes increases the likelihood of dietary success (see Exhibit 17-7). It also increases the likelihood that clients will continue to come in for follow-up visits because they know a receptive rather than a restrictive environment exists.

Weight and Cholesterol Grids

Although charting body weights has been common for decades, clients do not seem to be motivated by a chart on file. It is important to emphasize eating behavior changes to produce permanent weight loss, rather than mere "pounds off."

A weight chart can be an effective teaching tool. For example, on initial eating behavior instruction, the community nutrition professional can chart the patient's current weight and project the weight at six or nine months. Using a 2 lb (0.9 kg), as an example, weight loss per week, one can place an asterisk on the graph six months in the future, showing a projected 24 lb (11 kg) weight loss. One copy can be retained for the chart and another given to the client. Recommend that the client tape the chart near the scale at home and graph his or her weight once a week. This technique shifts the responsibility for weight loss to the patient rather than the community nutrition professional. Further, it defines a manageable goal, rather than merely saying, "You have to lose weight." The same instructional technique can be used with a cholesterol grid.

Educational Materials

There are many diet books on the market. Recommend the nutritionally sound ones, so interested and skilled clients can make sizable, long-term changes in their eating patterns. The American Diabetes Association/American Dietetic Association *Exchange Lists for Meal Planning* is an excellent, user-friendly guide for energy, fat, and carbohydrate modifications.[100] The American Heart Association's *Dietary Treatment of Hypercholesterolemia* is a detailed manual for patients.[101] By using *The New American Diet*[102] as a blueprint for formulating specific staging of fat changes, the community nutrition professional can help the client achieve an eating behavior with no more than 20% of the total energy obtained from fat. Consumption of fish, not fish oil supplements, is espoused, and the program recommends a three-step progression to a permanent dietary pattern low in fat and high in complex carbohydrates.

When concentrating on interventions to enhance eating behavior objectives, primary, secondary, and tertiary prevention are needed in an integrative, comprehensive manner (see Figure 17-1). A worksheet to identify primary, secondary, and tertiary prevention approaches to reduce risk specific to a disease is pre-

Exhibit 17-7 A Self-Contract as a Contingency Plan To Commit to Small Behavioral Changes

HEART HEALTHY EATING

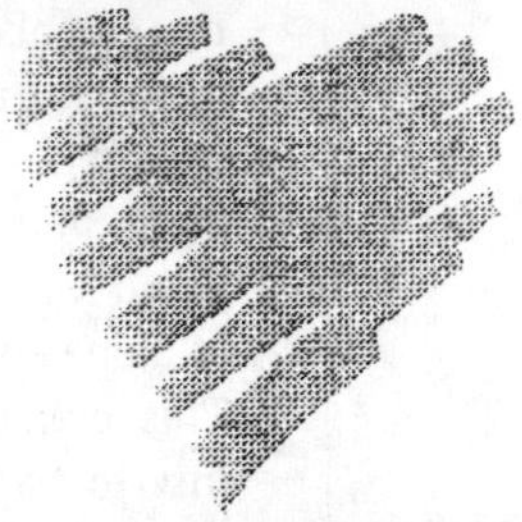

SELF-CONTRACT

I, _____, agree with the following
small steps to reduce my fat intake.

❑ I pledge to use the Food Guide Pyramid **twice a week** to
choose foods to make a healthy meal.

❑ I pledge to eat a fruit or vegetable for a snack **everyday**.

❑ I pledge to select low fat foods **more often** & my favorite
high fat food, _____, only **once a week**.

Within the next 4 weeks, by _____ , I'll be following
these pledges **regularly**.

If I do, I will reward myself with/by _____
_____.

If I do not, I will <u>revise the contract and start over</u>.

_____   _____
Signature   Date

_____   _____
Witness   Date

UNDERSTANDING LEVEL

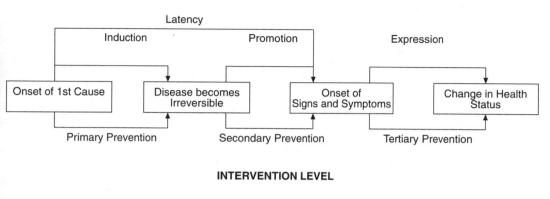

Figure 17-1 A model to blend understanding of disease progression with levels of intervention. *Source:* Adapted from *Epidemiologic Research: Principles and Quantitative Methods Solution Manual* by D.G. Kleinbaum and L.L. Kupper, p. 22, with permission of Lifetime Learning Publications, © 1982.

sented in Exhibit 17-8. One axis lists the approach, and the other axis lists different age-specific groups.

Examples of approaches for heart health of adults who need either primary, secondary, or tertiary intervention are as follows:

- *Primary*—weight loss, increased physical activity or leisure-time activity, daily warm-up and stretching of the body, increased fruit/vegetable intake, Step 1 eating pattern, healthy snacking, preparing healthy appetizers, eating out wisely, increased soluble fiber intake, following the Food Guide Pyramid, and increasing intake of foods that are low in sodium

- *Secondary*—Step 2 eating pattern, healthy eating with attention to sucrose-to-starch ratio if diabetic, decreased sodium eating pattern, increased calcium intake if at risk for osteoporosis, vitamin or mineral supplementation if iron-deficiency anemia exists, wellness/fitness plan and/or counseling if sedentary, and weight-loss program if obese

- *Tertiary*—Step 2 eating pattern for heart health with routine follow up and contingency plans, consistent aerobic activities, and drug therapy if required

BROAD STROKES

Broad strokes with a population approach are needed to shift US eating patterns to a healthier track and to insult the chronic disease process. The major health education framework currently used to orchestrate change is the PRECEDE model. This stands for predisposing, enabling, and reinforcing constructs that can be used to diagnose and evaluate any education and behavior-oriented intervention. PRECEDE is considered a diagnostic framework. Four disciplines are innate to the framework: epidemiology, social and behavioral sciences, management, and education. Application of the PRECEDE model involves working through seven steps[92]:

1. Assess the social problems in the target group.
2. Identify specific health problems that contribute.
3. Identify the specific health-related behaviors (e.g., cigarette smoking, nonadherence) that are causally linked to the health problems.
4. Identify the factors that influence performance of specified health-related behaviors: *predisposing factors* (i.e., attitudes, beliefs, values, perceptions); *enabling factors* (i.e.,

Exhibit 17–8 Disease Exploration and Prevention–A Worksheet To Identify and Define the Community Nutrition Approach for Different Age Groups

Target Disease: _____

| | Age Group | | | |
Prevention/Treatment Approach	Infant/ Preschooler	Youth	Adult	Older Adult
Primary				
Secondary				
Tertiary				

supportive forces within the system); and *reinforcing factors* (i.e., social support from family, peers, and health professionals).

5. Set priorities, choosing among the various factors as the nucleus of the intervention.
6. Develop and implement the intervention.
7. Evaluate the intervention for achievement of program objectives.

The PRECEDE framework can be applied to any health problem, but often the process for change is limited to clinical trials or demonstrating studies and not total community approaches. For example, several clinical trials demonstrate that a basic low-fat eating pattern is feasible and that individuals can follow the pattern and create a new way of eating.[103-105] If dietary cholesterol is limited to 100 mg/day, saturated fat is kept to 5 to 6% of total calories, and fish is eaten a minimum of twice a week, then a maximum lowering of LDL cholesterol can occur.

Dietary studies in free-living individuals show that an eating pattern reflecting a Step 1 diet reduces serum cholesterol by 3% to 14%.[4] Dietary equations such as those developed by Keys[3] and Hegsted and colleagues[3,106] predict that the Step 1 diet will reduce total cholesterol levels by 5% to 7% in men who consume an average of 13 to 14% of their calories as saturated fat. An additional 3% to 7% reduction in serum total cholesterol is anticipated by following a Step 2 diet.

A heart-healthy pattern can be phased into an individual's or family's lifestyle. A strategy of slow but steady changes in the type and amount of foods has been found successful by proponents of The New American Diet and The New American Diet System.[107,108] Plasma cholesterol levels of men have responded to their three stages with an average decline of serum total cholesterol of 5% to 7% per phase (see Figure 17–2).

Although data are limited for women, projections are that women would respond in a similar manner. Focused research in clinical trials such as the Women's Health Initiative (see Chapter 9) is necessary to answer the question of how postmenopausal women respond to heart-healthy eating when their CHD risk normally escalates with age.

Success in reducing the fat content of one's eating pattern may also be linked to one's stage of change.[109] Behavioral change is considered dynamic and reflects five stages[109]:

1. Precontemplation–Individual has no intention of changing.
2. Contemplation–Individual seriously considers change.
3. Preparation–Individual makes decisions and commitments to change.
4. Action–Individual makes distinguishable efforts toward change.
5. Maintenance–Person enters a period of behavior stabilization.

Understanding whether individuals are changing or resistant to change appears to be a new

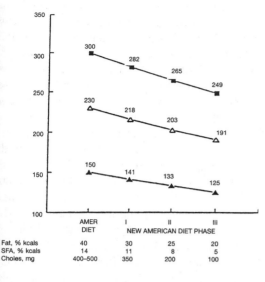

	AMER DIET	I	II	III
		NEW AMERICAN DIET PHASE		
Fat, % kcals	40	30	25	20
SFA, % kcals	14	11	8	5
Choles, mg	400–500	350	200	100

Figure 17-2 Response of individuals at different baseline plasma cholesterol levels to three phases of the New American Diet. *Source:* Reprinted from *The New American Diet System* by S.L. Connor and W.E. Connor with permission of Simon & Schuster, © 1991.

and enlightening variable for successful medical nutrition therapy.

Structural variables for change may be as visible as informative food labels. For example, the Nutrition Labeling and Education Act of 1990 requires a listing of the fat, saturated fat, and cholesterol composition of foods. Any food manufacturer who makes a claim about specific food and its association with heart disease is required to print the claim in a certain format (see Chapter 2). Educating the public about food labels and how to apply the nutrient content to food choices and health promotion must be continuous and consistent.

Blending daily food choices for each age-specific group within the age spectrum with quantity and quality guides such as those in the Food Guide Pyramid is an elemental and instructive action toward healthy eating for individuals and their families. The Public Health Nutrition dietetic practice group of The American Dietetic Association has formalized a call to action for its members to strategically shape food choices for the United States.[110]

SPECTRUM OF PREVENTION: A MODEL FOR PUBLIC HEALTH PLANNING

Individual education aimed at changing behavior is not enough to effectively prevent illness or injury. Programs must address environmental factors, which are some of the largest determinants of health status, and actively involve the community in planning and implementing activities. "Spectrum of Prevention" is a framework for development of multilevel public health programs that integrate client, professional, organizational, and communitywide efforts.

The spectrum ranges from some of the more familiar interventions such as individual and community education to long-term solutions such as legislative and policy changes. Aspects of the spectrum are dependent upon and interrelated to one another. Legislation cannot be enacted and implemented without well-informed, vocal, involved, and committed individuals working together. By combining these approaches, a preventive health program builds on the strengths of each and promotes permanent, effective change. The whole becomes greater than the sum of its parts.[111]

A working model for service providers exists to demonstrate primary prevention in the community. Community-directed models usually aim to promote planning and implementation of scientifically acceptable, preventive interventions. The models are strengthened by real-life settings and attention to research requirements and practical issues facing community members and health care providers.[112,113] Community models serve as the basis for intervention programs amid challenges of the scientific community. A common question is, "Is the intervention supported by valid baseline data, and will the outcome withstand an evaluation?" Challenges from the recipient community include those from individuals who need to know if their important needs are met, if their rights are protected, what they must pay, and what they receive.

The community-directed model provides an umbrella for thought (e.g., the scope, the players, the program, and the potential outcome). The model requires evaluating why certain actions are proposed and who should be involved in each component. In the model, multilevel program-matic and evaluation decisions are enumerated. The process saddles the various activities and yields a comprehensible program. The model pro-motes an open forum for discussion of skills and approaches. As the magnitude of the program is understood, alternate strategies can be compared to identify their various levels of success.[111] The spectrum of prevention, a community model that has been adopted by the Prevention Program of Contra Costa County Health Services Depart-ment, in California, is described below.

Level 1 involves strengthening individual knowledge and skills. Health education programs are designed to reach out to individuals at risk of disease and encourage them to change their be-havior. Such educational efforts provide informa-tion and opportunities to learn new skills and/ or change attitudes. As a common example, ado-lescents are taught the basics of good nutrition and how to plan healthy menus.

Level 2 involves educating the community. A well-coordinated, multidimensional campaign raises community awareness about a particular health issue. Assessing the perceptions of health care professionals and community members about the nutritional needs of the community may tar-get education (see Chapter 1). Events, posters, and use of mass media deliver a specific, inte-grated message. For example, the prevention pro-gram sponsors an annual Healthy Holiday Open House in November. The event provides the com-munity with free samples of healthy holiday foods and recipes, gives community members an op-portunity to learn about nutrition programs in the county, and generates extensive media cov-erage that reaches a broad audience of citizens and community leaders.

Level 3 trains providers. Any preventive ap-proach needs the cooperation and aid of existing health care providers and other service provid-ers. Providers have regular contact with people at risk and can encourage adoption of healthy behavior and screen for additional risks. They can help improve community education, change poli-cies within their institutions, and advocate for legislation. Many providers who work with chil-dren and adolescents do not know the importance of good nutrition or sound nutrition behaviors.

Level 4 builds coalitions. Coalitions combine individual and organizational strengths in new ways. Coalitions and other networking activities also lend themselves to maximizing community resources. Through the work of local coalitions, the national Project LEAN program has been ef-fective in spreading a low-fat eating message through the local media.

Level 5 changes organizational practices and environments. Established organizations can di-rectly change their policies that affect the health of their members/clients. The local Department of Social Services office in Contra Costa allowed the prevention program to insert flyers in the June Aid to Families with Dependent Children (AFDC) checks. These flyers promoted free sum-mer lunches for eligible children. As a result, there was a 25% increase in participation in the free meals program. Another agency in the county established a healthy-snacks policy for its employ-ees; the daily doughnut break became a bagel and fruit break.

Level 6 is directed toward influencing policy and legislation. Legislation and policy represent perhaps the strongest and broadest means for bringing about environmental changes to de-crease the incidence of illness in a community. For example, local communities can institute policies and legislation mandating the availabil-ity of federal food programs for low-income chil-dren.

Formulating nutrition policy to instill positive changes at the national and state levels can complement grassroots efforts and make the *Healthy People 2000* objectives a reality in the United States.

REFERENCES

1. Berenson GS, McMahan CA, Voors AW, et al. *Cardiovas-cular Risk Factors in Children*. New York, NY: Oxford Uni-versity Press; 1980.

2. Connor S. *Facing Fats: The Dietary Challenge of the 90's. Nutritional Medicine in Medical Practice*. Los Ange-les, Calif: UCLA Clinical Research Center; January 1993.

3. Keys A, Anderson JT, Grande F. Prediction of serum cho-lesterol responses of man to changes in fats in the diet. *Lancet*. 1957;ii:959–966.

4. Caggiula AW, Christakis G, Farrand M, et al. The Multiple Risk Factor Intervention Trial (MRFIT), IV: Intervention on blood lipids. *Preventive Med.* 1981;10:443.

5. Gordon T, Kagan A, Garcia-Palmicri M, et al. Diet and its relation to coronary heart disease and death in three populations. *Circulation.* 1981;63:500.

6. Herber D. *The Role of Diet in Cancer Prevention and Control. Nutritional Medicine in Medical Practice.* Los Angeles, Calif: UCLA Clinical Research Center; January 1993.

7. Miller AB, Kelly A, Choi NW. A study of diet and breast cancer. *Am J Epidemiol.* 198;107:499–509.

8. Howe GR, Hirohata T, Hislop G, et al. Dietary factors and risk of breast cancer: Combined analysis of 12 case-control studies. *J Natl Cancer Inst.* 1990;82:561–569.

9. Willett WC, Stampfer MJ, Colditz GA, et al. Dietary fat and the risk of breast cancer. *N Engl J Med.* 1987;316: 22–28.

10. Jones DY, Schatzkin A, Green SB, et al. Dietary fat and breast cancer in the National Health and Nutrition Survey I: Epidemiologic follow-up study. *J Natl Cancer Inst.* 1987;79:465–471.

11. Camoriano JK, Loprinzi CL, Ingle JN, et al. Weight change in women with adjuvant therapy or observed following mastectomy for node-positive breast cancer. *J Clin Oncol.* 1990;8:1327–1334.

12. Tretli S. Height and weight in relation to breast cancer morbidity and mortality. A prospective study of 570,000 women in Norway. *Int J Cancer.* 1989;44:23.

13. Newman SC, Miller AB, Howe GR. A study of the effect of weight and dietary fat on breast cancer survival time. *Am J Epidemiol.* 1986;123:767.

14. deWaard F, Poortman J, Collette BJ. Relationship of weight and obesity on breast cancer incidence and recurrence in Auckland, New Zealand. *Breast Cancer Res Treat.* 1987;9:145.

15. McNee RK, Mason BH, Neave LM, et al. Influence of height, weight, and obesity on breast cancer incidence and recurrence in Auckland, New Zealand. *Breast Cancer Res Treat.* 1987;9:145.

16. Eberlein I, Simon R, Fisher S, et al. Height, weight, and risk of breast cancer relapse. *Breast Cancer Res Treat.* 1985;5:81.

17. Hebert JR, Augustine A, Barone J, et al. Weight, height, and body mass index in the prognosis of breast cancer: Early results of a prospective analysis. *Int J Cancer.* 1988;42: 315–318.

18. Lubin F, Ruder AM, Wax Y, et al. Overweight and changes in weight throughout life in breast cancer etiology: A case-control study. *Am J Epidemiol.* 1985;122:579.

19. Le Marchand L, Kolonel LN, Earle ME, et al. Body size at different periods of life and breast cancer risk. *Am J Epidemiol.* 1988;128:137.

20. London SJ, Colditz GA, Stampfer MJ, et al. Prospective study of relative weight, height and risk of breast cancer. *JAMA.* 1989;262:2853.

21. Schapira DV, Kumar NB, Lyman GH, Estimate of breast cancer risk reduction with weight loss. *Cancer.* 1991;67:2622.

22. deWaard F. Body size and breast cancer risk. In: Pike M, Siiteri P, Welsch C, eds. *Hormones and Breast Cancer.* New York, NY: Cold Springs Harbor Laboratory; 1981;21–261. Report 8.

23. Adami MO, Rimstein A, Stenquist B, et al. Influence of height, weight and obesity on risk of breast cancer in unselected Swedish population. *Br J Cancer.* 1977;36: 787–792.

24. Staszewshi J. Breast cancer and body build. *Preventive Med.* 1977;6:410–415.

25. Jain M, Cook GM, Davis FG, et al. A case-control study of diet and colo-rectal cancer. *Int J Cancer.* 1980;26: 757–768.

26. Potter JD, McMichael AJ. Diet and cancer of the colon and rectum: A case-control study. *J Natl Cancer Inst.* 1986;76:557–569.

27. Lyon JL, Mahoney AW, West DW, et al. Energy intake: Its relationship to colon cancer risk. *J Natl Cancer Inst.* 1987;78:853–861.

28. Graham S, Marshall J, Haughey B, et al. Dietary epidemiology of cancer of the colon in western New York. *Am J Epidemiol.* 1988;128:490–503.

29. Bristol JB, Emmett PM, Heaton KW, et al. Sugar, fat and the risk of colorectal cancer. *Br Med J.* 1985;291: 1467–1470.

30. Chomchai C, Bhadrachari N, Nigro ND. The effect of bile on the induction of experimental intestinal tumors in rats. *Dis Colon Rectum.* 1974;17:310.

31. Narisawa T, Magadia NE, Weisberger JH, et al. Promoting effect of bile acid on carcinogenesis after intrarectal installation of N-methyl-N'-nitro-nitrosoguanidine in rats. *J Natl Cancer Inst.* 1974;53:1093.

32. Ranken R, Wilson R, Bealmer PM. Increased turnover of intestinal mucosal cells of germ free mice induced by cholic acid. *Proc Soc Exp Biol Med.* 1971;138:270.

33. Goldin BR, Swenson L, Dwyer J, et al. Effect of diet and lactobacillus acidophilus supplements on human fecal bacterial enzymes. *J Natl Cancer Inst.* 1980;64:255.

34. Reddy BS, Hanson D, Mangat B, et al. Effect of high fat, high beef diet and of mode of cooking of beef in the diet on fecal bacterial enzymes and fecal bile acids and neutral sterols. *J Nutr.* 1980;110:1880.

35. Willett WC, Stampfer MJ, Colditz GA, et al. Relation of meat, fat and fiber intake to the risk of colon cancer in a prospective study among women. *N Engl J Med.* 1990; 232:1664.

36. Lipkin M, Uehara K, Winawer S, et al. Seventh-Day Adventist vegetarians have a quiescent proliferative activity in colonic mucosa. *Cancer Lett*. 1985;26:139.

37. Lipkin M, Newmark H. Effect of added dietary calcium on colonic epithelial cell proliferation in subjects at high-risk for familial colon cancer. *N Engl J Med*. 1985;313:1381.

38. Alberts DS, Einspahr J, Rees-McGee S, et al. Effects of dietary wheat bran fiber on rectal epithelial cell proliferation in patients with resection for colorectal cancers. *J Natl Cancer Inst*. 1990;82:1280.

39. Stadler J, Stern HS, Sing Yeung KA, et al. Effect of high fat consumption on cell proliferation activity of colorectal mucosa and on soluble faecal bile acids. *Gut*. 1988;20:1326.

40. Graham S, Haughey G, Marshall J, et al. Diet in the epidemiology of cancer of the prostate gland. *J Natl Cancer Inst*. 1983;70:687–692.

41. La Vecchia C, DeCarli A, Fasoli M, et al. Nutrition and diet in the etiology of endometrial cancer. *Cancer*. 1986;57:1248–1253.

42. Lissner L, Levitsky DA, Strupp BJ, et al. Dietary fat and the regulation of energy intake in human subjects. *Am J Clin Nutr*. 1987;46:886.

43. Oscai L, Brown MM, Miller WC. Effect of dietary fat on food intake, growth and body composition in rats. *Growth*. 1984;48:415.

44. Kritchevsky D, Webber, MM, Klurfeld DM. Dietary fat versus caloric content in the initiation and promotion of 7,12 dimethylbenzanthracene-induced mammary tumorigenesis in rats. *Cancer Res*. 1984;44:3174.

45. Zhang L, Bird RP, Bruce WR. Proliferative activity of murine mammary epithelium as affected by dietary fat and calcium. *Cancer Res*. 1987;47:4905.

46. Welsch CW, Dehoog JV, O'Connor DH, et al. Influence of dietary fat levels on development and hormone responsiveness of the mouse mammary gland. *Cancer Res*. 1985;45:6147.

47. Kort WJ, Weijma, IM, Westbrook DL. Is the 7,12 DMBA-induced fat mammary tumor model suitable as a preclinical model to study mammary tumor malignancy? *Cancer Invest*. 1987;5:443.

48. Carroll KK, Khor HT. Effect of level and type of dietary fat on incidence of mammary tumors induced in female Sprague-Dawley rats by 7,12 dimethylbenzanthracene. *Lipids*. 1971;6:415.

49. Karmali RA, Marsh J, Fuchs C. Effects of omega-3 fatty acids on growth of a rat mammary tumor. *J Natl Cancer Inst*. 1984;73:457.

50. Reaven GM. role of insulin resistance in human disease. *Diabetes*. 1988;37:1595–1607.

51. Kaplan NM. The deadly quartet: Upper-body obesity, glucose intolerance, hypertriglyceridemia, and hypertension. *Arch Intern Med*. 1989;149:1514–1520.

52. Barnard RJ. Role of diet and exercise in the management of hyperinsulinemia and associated atherosclerotic risk factors. *Am J Cardiol*. 1992;69:440–444.

53. Ferrannini E, Buzzigoli G, Bonadonna R, et al. Insulin resistance in essential hypertension. *N Engl J Med*. 1987;317:350–357.

54. Kannel WB. Risk factors in hypertension. *Cardiovascular Pharmacol*. 1989;13(Suppl 1):S4–S10.

55. Kaplan NM. Hyperinsulinemia in diabetes and hypertension. *Clin Diabetes*. 1991;9:1–9.

56. Pollare T, Lithell H, Berne C. Insulin resistance is a characteristic feature of primary hypertension independent of obesity. *Metabolism*. 1990;39:167–174.

57. Rodnick KJ, Haskell WL, Swislocki ALM, et al. Improved insulin action in muscle, liver, and adipose tissue in physically trained human subjects. *AM J Physiol*. 1987;253:E489–E495.

58. Kaplan NM. Primary hypertension: Pathogenesis. In: *Clinical Hypertension*. 5th ed. Baltimore, Md: Williams & Wilkins; 1990:54–112.

59. Kaplan NM. Long-term effectiveness of nonpharmacological treatment of hypertension. *Hypertension*. 1991;18(Suppl I):I-153–I-160.

60. Landin D, Tengborn L, Smith U. Treating insulin resistance in hypertension with metformin reduces both blood pressure and metabolic risk factors. *J Intern Med*. 1991;229:181–187.

61. Lithell HOL. Effect of antihypertensive drugs on insulin, glucose, and lipid metabolism. *Diabetes Care*. 1991;14:203–209.

62. *The Surgeon General's Report on Nutrition and Health*. Washington, DC: US Department of Health and Human Services; 1988. Public Health Service publication 88-50210.

63. US Department of Agriculture/US Department of Health and Human Services. *Nutrition and Your Health: Dietary Guidelines for Americans*. 2nd ed. Washington, DC: US Government Printing Office; 1985. HG-232.

64. *Healthy People 2000: National Health Promotion and Disease Prevention Objectives*. Washington, DC: US Department of Health and Human Services; 1991. Public Health Service publication 91-50212.

65. National Cholesterol Education Program Expert Panel. Report on detection, evaluation, and treatment of high blood cholesterol in adults. *Arch Intern Med*. 1988;148:36.

66. *The Food Guide Pyramid*. Washington, DC: US Department of Agriculture; 1992.

67. California Department of Education. Child Nutrition and Food Distribution Division. *Nutrition Guidelines for California School Foods*. Sacramento, Calif: California Department of Education; 1991.

68. Trumpfheller W, Foerster SB, Palombo R, eds. *The National Action Plan to Improve the American Diet: A*

Public/Private Partnership. Washington, DC: Association of State and Territorial Health Officials; 1993.

69. Kannel WB, Schatzkin A. Risk factor analysis. *Prog Cardiovasc Dis.* 1983;26:309.

70. Schoenbach VJ. Appraising health risk appraisal. *Am J Public Health.* 1987;77:409.

71. Kris-Etherton P, ed. *Cardiovascular Disease: Nutrition for Prevention and Treatment.* Chicago Ill: The American Dietetic Association; 1990:64–107.

72. Willett W. Nutritional epidemiology: Issues and challenges. *Int J Epidemiol.* 1987;16:312.

73. Smith KV, McKinlay SM, Thorington BD. The validity of health risk appraisal instruments for assessing coronary heart disease risk. *Am J Public Health.* 1987;77:419.

74. Anderson JT, Jacobs DR, Foster N, et al. Scoring systems for evaluating dietary pattern effect on serum cholesterol. *Preventive Med.* 1979;8:525.

75. *Heart to Heart.* Washington, DC: Public Health Service, National Institutes of Health; 1983. US Dept of Health and Human Services NIH publication 83-1528.

76. Boyar AP, Loughridge JR. The fat portion exchange list: A tool for teaching and evaluating low fat diets. *J Am Diet Assoc.* 1985;85:589.

77. Ney D, Fischer C. A tool for assessing compliance with a diet for diabetes. *J Am Diet Assoc.* 1983;82:287.

78. Connor GL, Gustafson JR, Artaud-Wild SM, et al. The cholesterol/saturated-fat index: An indication of the hypercholesterolemic and atherogenic potential of food. *Lancet.* 1986;1:1229.

79. Caggiula AW, Wing RR, Norwalk MP, et al. The measurement of sodium and potassium intake. *Am J Clin Nutr.* 1985;42:391.

80. Sowers M, Stumbo PA. A method to assess sodium intake in populations. *J Am Diet Assoc.* 1986;86:1196.

81. Levin LS, Idler EL. *The Hidden Health Care System: Mediating Structures and Medicine.* Cambridge, Mass: Ballinger; 1981.

82. Anderson SV, Bauwens EE. The challenge of chronic illness. In: Anderson SV, Bauwens EE, eds. *Chronic Health Problems: Concepts and Applications.* St. Louis, Mo: CV Mosby; 1981.

83. American Hospital Association. *Report of a Conference on Care of Chronically Ill Adults.* Chicago, Ill: American Hospital Association; 1971.

84. Holroyd KA, Cheer TL. *Self-Management of Chronic Disease—Handbook of Clinical Interventions and Research.* New York, NY: Academic Press; 1986.

85. Creswell WH. Professional preparation: A historical perspective. In: *National Conference for Institutions Preparing Health Educators.* Washington, DC: US Government Printing Office; 1981. DHHS publication 81-50171.

86. Parcel GS, Bartlett EE, Bruhn JG. The role of health education in self-management. In: Holroyd KA, Cheer TL, eds. *Self-Management of Chronic Disease—Handbook of Clinical Interventions and Research.* New York, NY: Academic Press; 1986:3–27.

87. Knowles M. *The Modern Practice of Adult Education: Andragogy versus Pedagogy.* New York, NY: Associated Press; 1970.

88. Office of Disease Prevention and Health Promotion. *Evaluation of the National Health Promotion Media Campaign: Executive Summary.* Washington, DC: US Government Printing Office; 1982.

89. Rothman J. Three models of community organization practice. In: Cox FM, Erlich JL, Rothman J, et al, eds. *Strategies of Community Organization: A Book of Readings.* Itasca, Ill: FE Peacock Publishers; 1970.

90. Rosenstock IM. The health belief model and preventive health behavior. *Health Education Monographs.* 1974;2:354–386.

91. Bartlett EE. Behavioral diagnosis: A practical approach to patient education. *Patient Counseling and Health Ed.* 1982;4:29–35.

92. Green LW, Kreuter MS, Deeds SG, et al. *Health Education Planning: A Diagnostic Approach.* Palo Alto, Calif: Mayfield Press; 1980.

93. Kanfer FH, Saslow G. Behavioral diagnosis. In: Franks CM, ed. *Behavior Therapy: Appraisal and Status.* New York, NY: McGraw-Hill; 1969.

94. Campbell-Lindzey LS. Teaching nutrition to fast food freaks: The application of marketing principles to teaching nutrition at the elementary school level. *J Am Diet Assoc.* 1988;88(Suppl):S69–S72.

95. Frank GC. Nutritional therapy for hyperlipidemia and obesity: Office treatment integrating the roles of the physician and the registered dietitian. *J Am Coll Cardiol.* 1988;12:1098–1101.

96. Highlights of the Report of the Expert Panel on Detection. *Evaluation and Treatment of High Blood Cholesterol in Adults. National Cholesterol Education Program.* Bethesda, Md: National Heart, Lung, and Blood Institute; November 1987. NIH publication 88-2926.

97. Hoeg JM, Brewer HB Jr. Definition and management of hyperlipoproteinemia. *J Am Coll Nutr.* 1987;6:157–163.

98. Kottke TE, Foels JK, Hill C, et al. Nutrition counseling in private practice: Attitudes and activities of family physicians. *Preventive Med.* 1984;13:219–225.

99. Dennison D, Dennison KF, Frank GC. The DINE System: Improving food choices of the public. *J Nutr Ed.* 1994;26(2):87–92.

100. American Diabetes Association/American Dietetic Association. *Exchange Lists for Meal Planning.* Alexandria, Va: American Diabetes Association/American Dietetic Association; 1986:32.

101. American Heart Association. *Dietary Treatment of Hypercholesterolemia*. Dallas, Tex: American Heart Association;1988.

102. Connor SL, Connor WE. *The New American Diet*. New York, NY: Simon & Schuster; 1986:410.

103. Rose DP, Boyar A, Haley N, et al. Low fat diet in fibrocystic disease of the breast with cyclical mastalgia: A feasibility study. *Am J Clin Nutr*. 1985;42:856.

104. Lee-Han H, Cousins M, Beaton M, et al. Compliance in a randomized clinical trial of dietary fat reduction in patients with breast dysplasia. *Amer J Clin Nutr*. 1988;48: 575–586.

105. Insull W, Henderson MM, Prentice RL, et al. Results of a randomized feasibility study of a low fat diet. *Arch Intern Med*. 1990;150:421–427.

106. Hegsted DM, McGandy RB, Myers ML, et al. Quantitative effects of dietary fat on serum cholesterol in man. *Am J Clin Nutr*. 1965;17:281.

107. Connor WE, Hodges RE, Bleiler RE. The serum lipids in men receiving high cholesterol and cholesterol-free diets. *J Clin Invest*. 1961;40:894.

108. Connor WE, Connor SL. *The New American Diet System*. New York, NY: Simon & Schuster; 1991.

109. Greene GW, Rossi SR, Reed GR, et al. Stages of change for reducing dietary fat to 30% of energy or less. *J Am Diet Assoc*. 1994;94:1105–1112.

110. The Public Health Nutrition Dietetic Practice Group. *A Call to Action—Shaping Food Choices for the Nation*. Chicago, Ill: American Dietetic Association; 1994.

111. Swift M, Healey KN. Translating research into practice. In: Kessler M, Goldston SE, eds. *A Decade of Progress in Primary Prevention*. Hanover, NH: University Press of New England; 1986.

112. Goldstein SE. An overview of primary prevention programming. In: Klein DC, Goldston SE, eds. *Primary Prevention: An Idea Whose Time Has Come*. Washington, DC: US Government Printing Office; 1977. DHEW publication (ADM) 77-447.

113. Litwak E. An approach to linkage in "grass roots" community organization. In: Cott F, Rothman J, Tropman J, eds. *Strategies of Community Organization*. Itasca, Ill: FE Peacock Publishers, Inc; 1971:126–138.

Index